STEP-UP

TO

USMLE Step 1

2014

STEP-UP

TO

USMLE Step 1

2014

Brian Jenkins, MD

Family Medicine
President, and Chief Educator
Doctors in Training.com, LLC
Fort Worth, Texas

Samir Mehta, MD

Assistant Professor
Department of Orthopaedic Surgery
Chief, Orthopaedic Trauma Service
The Hospital of the University of
Pennsylvania
Philadelphia, Pennsylvania

Michael McInnis, MD

Internal Medicine
Chief Educator
Doctors in Training.com, LLC
Fort Worth, Texas

Chris Lewis, MD

Family Medicine
Chief Educator
Doctors in Training.com, LLC
Austin, Texas

Sonia Mehta, MD

Fellow
Emory Eye Center
Emory University
Atlanta, Georgia

LCDR Edmund A. Milder, MC USNR

Department of Pediatrics
Naval Medical Center
San Diego, California

Sonul Mehta, MD

Assistant Professor
Department of Ophthalmology
Hospital of the University of Pennsylvania
Philadelphia, Pennsylvania

Adam J. Mirarchi, MD

Assistant Professor
Department of Orthopaedic Surgery
Oregon Health & Science University
Portland, Oregon

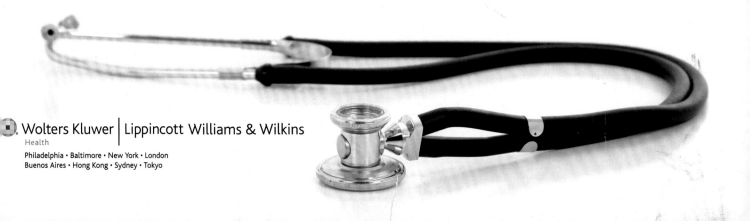

. Wolters Kluwer | Lippincott Williams & Wilkins
Health

Philadelphia · Baltimore · New York · London
Buenos Aires · Hong Kong · Sydney · Tokyo

Publisher: Michael Tully
Acquisitions Editor: Tari Broderick
Product Development Editor: Jennifer Verbiar
Marketing Manager: Joy Fisher-Williams
Designer: Doug Smock
Compositor: Absolute Service, Inc.

351 West Camden Street   Two Commerce Square
Baltimore, MD 21201   2001 Market Street
                                          Philadelphia, PA 19103

Printed in China

9 8 7 6 5 4 3 2 1

Library of Congress Cataloging-in-Publication Data

Jenkins, Brian, 1977- author.
  Step-up to USMLE step 1 : 2014 / Brian Jenkins, Michael McInnis, Samir Mehta,
Chris Lewis, Sonia Mehta, Sonul Mehta, Adam J. Mirarchi.
      p. ; cm.
  Includes index.
  Preceded by: Step-up to USMLE step 1 : 2013 / Samir Mehta ... [et al.]. c2013.
  ISBN 978-1-4511-9277-3
  I. Title.
  [DNLM: 1. Clinical Medicine--United States--Outlines. WB 18.2]
  R834.5
  616.0076--dc23
                    2013035527

DISCLAIMER

Care has been taken to confirm the accuracy of the information present and to describe generally accepted practices. However, the authors, editors, and publisher are not responsible for errors or omissions or for any consequences from application of the information in this book and make no warranty, expressed or implied, with respect to the currency, completeness, or accuracy of the contents of the publication. Application of this information in a particular situation remains the professional responsibility of the practitioner; the clinical treatments described and recommended may not be considered absolute and universal recommendations.

The authors, editors, and publisher have exerted every effort to ensure that drug selection and dosage set forth in this text are in accordance with the current recommendations and practice at the time of publication. However, in view of ongoing research, changes in government regulations, and the constant flow of information relating to drug therapy and drug reactions, the reader is urged to check the package insert for each drug for any change in indications and dosage and for added warnings and precautions. This is particularly important when the recommended agent is a new or infrequently employed drug.

Some drugs and medical devices presented in this publication have Food and Drug Administration (FDA) clearance for limited use in restricted research settings. It is the responsibility of the health care provider to ascertain the FDA status of each drug or device planned for use in their clinical practice.

To purchase additional copies of this book, call our customer service department at **(800) 638-3030** or fax orders to **(301) 223-2320**. International customers should call **(301) 223-2300**.

Visit Lippincott Williams & Wilkins on the Internet: http://www.lww.com. Lippincott Williams & Wilkins customer service representatives are available from 8:30 am to 6:00 pm, EST.

Contributors

We would like to extend our thanks to all the reviewers and contributors to previous editions and extend special thanks to the contributors to this edition who have helped review and update this text to reflect the most current knowledge in their respective fields.

JENNIFER SHUFORD, MD
Infectious Disease
Austin, Texas

HAMPTON RICHARDS, MD
Obstetrics and Gynecology
Dallas, Texas

ADAM ODEH, PhD
Microbiology and Immunology
Fort Worth, Texas

How to Contribute

Interested in medical publishing? Contribute to Step-Up!

Student suggestions and feedback are always welcomed and appreciated by the Step-Up team. Please send feedback and suggestions for new study material and test-taking strategies by writing to the authors at the website provided. Students can also directly submit new mnemonics, quick hits, tables, and figures. For each original entry incorporated into the text, students' names will be listed and personally acknowledged in the next edition. If duplicate entries are received, the first to submit will be acknowledged.

To make an entry or provide feedback and suggestions, simply visit http://www.lww.com and click Contact LWW.

Disclaimer:
Please note: submissions become the property of LWW.

Contents

Chapter 3. The Cardiovascular System

Chapter 4. The Respiratory System

Chapter 5. The Gastrointestinal System

Chapter 6. The Renal System

Chapter 7. The Endocrine System

Chapter 8. The Reproductive System

Chapter 9. The Musculoskeletal System

Chapter 10. The Hematopoietic and Lymphoreticular System

Chapter 11. Biochemistry and Genetics

Chapter 12. Microbiology

Crunch Time Review 380

Where do I find...?

Strategies for Success: A Guide to Effective Preparation for the USMLE Step 1

As the first national licensure exam encountered during a medical career, the USMLE Step 1 is often a source of anxiety for the medical student.

As with most things in life, having a systematic plan can be helpful in approaching what at first seems like an enormous task—preparing for the boards. The authors of *Step-Up to the USMLE Step 1* have created this guide below to direct you in effectively preparing for and excelling on the boards.

The first section of the guide will introduce you to the exam and the test makers. It will also familiarize you with the exam structure, content, testing environment, and interface. Finally, it will review how the test is scored and how to register for the exam.

The second section of the guide details successful preparation strategies. In this section, you will learn tips for creating study schedules and gathering study materials as well as strategies for effective studying. At the end of this section, you will find a blank study schedule you can use as a basis for creating your personalized study schedule.

THE EXAM: THE USMLE STEP 1

The National Board of Medical Examiners

The USMLE is a joint endeavor by the National Board of Medical Examiners (NBME) and Federation of State Medical Boards (FSMB). Step 1 is the first of three exams medical students and graduates need to pass in order to become licensed physicians in the United States. The NBME was founded in 1915 in Philadelphia, Pennsylvania, and administered its first exam in 1916. The first exams were largely essay based and were organized around testing the basic science subjects of anatomy, physiology, biochemistry, pathology, pharmacology, microbiology, and behavioral science. The exam has evolved over the years. In the early 1990s, after years of culminated efforts, the USMLE was introduced. This test embraced the systems-based practice of medicine and adopted a clinically oriented question format. In 1992, Step 1 replaced the Federation Licensing Examination (FLEX) and now serves as the single exam for international medical graduates seeking U.S. medical licensure. In 1999, the test became computer based and in 2005, the FRED software was adopted.

Test Structure

The exam consists of 322 questions administered in seven blocks of 46 questions each with 60 minutes per block (Table 1). The eighth block is a survey consisting of 11 questions. Students are allotted 45 minutes of authorized break time that can be taken anytime between blocks. At the beginning of the exam, you will be presented with a 15-minute tutorial. This tutorial is also available on the NBME website: http://www.usmle.org/practice-materials/index.html. If the tutorial is taken prior to the exam date, it can be skipped on exam day—allowing you an extra 15 minutes for break time. You can also gain extra break time by finishing blocks earlier.

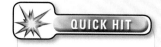

The USMLE Step 1 is designed to test basic science points in clinical vignettes. Know the test and you will prepare for it better!

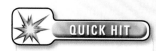

After the seventh block, a screen appears to move on to the eighth block. The eighth block is not a question block. It is a survey of your testing experience consisting of 11 questions. Don't be fooled!

TABLE 1 Time Breakdown of the USMLE Step 1 Exam	
Tutorial	15 min (added to break time if skipped)
Question blocks	7 h (60 min per block)
Break time	45 min (includes time for lunch)

Breaks can be taken between blocks when you wish. Figure 1 shows two suggested test day schedules. The first schedule is the traditional one-break schedule made for the student who likes one large midday break (Figure 1). The second schedule is for those students who prefer multiple breaks in order to stay fresh and to prevent testing fatigue. Both schedules may be modified to individual preferences.

Test Content

The exam consists of multiple-choice questions; each question contains a question stem followed by five or more answer choices. Nearly 75% of questions begin with a clinical vignette or patient scenario. Students may also be asked direct questions. What kinds of

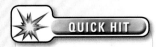

Prior to test day, take the exam tutorial offered on the NBME website. On exam day, skip the tutorial and gain an extra 15 minutes of break time.

FIGURE
1 Structure of the USMLE Step 1 Exam

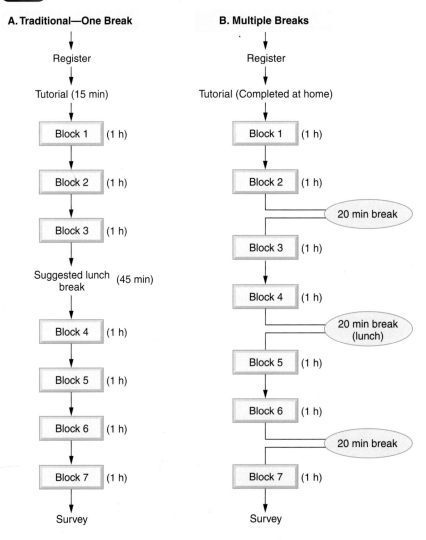

questions are not seen on the test? Question stems including "all of the following except," "not," and matching-style questions are never included in Step 1 exams.

Often, examinees will be presented with answer choices that are partially correct. In these instances, it is important to pick the option that best answers the statement in the question stem and move on.

Questions may range in difficulty from medium to hard. Although the questions vary from test to test and year to year, the proportion of question difficulty does not.

Something important for you to remember: Anywhere from 10% to 20% of questions seen on exam day are experimental questions that are not scored. Therefore, when presented with a difficult question with options that seem partially correct, it is important to select an answer that best fits and move on.

Test Environment

In general, Prometric centers share a generic design. There is the reception area where you will register on the morning of the exam, place your belongings in a locker, and return to take breaks. Beyond this is the examination area where only certain items are allowed: a government-issued identification card (typically a driver's license or passport) and a locker key. Everything else, including cell phones, pagers, digital watches, PDAs, books, notes, wallets, food, and beverages, goes into the locker. The examination area consists of a series of cubicles with computers. Test-takers are given noise reducer muffs, a dry-erase board, markers, and a dry eraser to use as needed during the exam. Proctors walk through the rooms periodically to make sure test rules are obeyed. When taking an authorized break after a block is completed, you will need to leave the examination area, present an identification card, and sign a book. The process is repeated when you return to the testing area after the break. When you return to the cubicle, the computer will ask for your candidate identification number, which is written at the top of the dry erase board. As soon as you enter the candidate identification number into the computer, the next testing block begins.

Test Interface

The NBME offers an online tutorial that reviews exam procedures and the testing interface. Briefly, the testing interface for each block consists mainly of a single question and answer choices below it (Figure 2). Above this is a panel with several icons. Clicking on the appropriate icons allows you to perform that specific function. Clicking on the "mark" button will mark the question for that block, allowing you to return to the question at the end of the set. Next to the mark button are navigation buttons including a "previous" button and "next" button. These move you back one question or forward one question. Clicking on the "labs" button displays the normal lab values screen. Four options are offered: blood, hematologic, cerebrospinal, and sweat/urine/BMI. You can also write a note next to the text by clicking on the "notes" button. Finally, clicking the "calculator" button brings up a calculator to use for basic math functions.

On the left part of the screen is a panel with a running list of 46 questions. The question that is currently being viewed is highlighted in blue. Incomplete questions have a dot next to the item number and completed questions have no dot. When you mark questions with the mark function, a red flag appears next to that question. You can directly click on that question to return to it at any time before the block ends.

Test Scoring

Examinees receive their score via an electronic score report 3 to 6 weeks after taking the exam. The score report consists of three key pieces of information. First, it states whether the examinee has passed or failed. Second, it displays a score in a three-digit scale and two-digit scale that reflects how well the examinee performed on the content of the exam. The mean score on the exam is 225 with a standard deviation of 21. Passing on the three-digit scale is 188, which corresponds to 75 on the two-digit scale. The minimum passing score is subject to change by the NBME, although it is not expected to change for a few years. Finally, there is a table depicting the examinee's performance profile by basic science subject and organ system. The examinee's medical school also receives a report containing

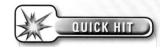

Not everyone will be taking the Step 1. All types of testing take place at the Prometric center and tests are started at different times of the day. Don't be surprised when other test-takers come and go at different times than you do.

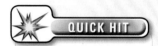

The testing interface allows you to annotate text in the question stem. These can be helpful tools, but be wary of the clock; they can also cause you to waste valuable testing time.

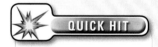

There is no penalty for guessing or benefit in leaving a question blank on the USMLE Step 1. Select answer choices as you move through and complete the block. If you are unsure of your answer, mark the question. If you have time at the end of the block, you can easily return to it and reconsider your initial response.

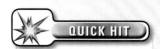

If you have concerns about or fear of taking computer-based tests, consider visiting a Prometric center ahead of time to take a practice exam with the testing interface.

FIGURE
FIGURE 2 Testing interface

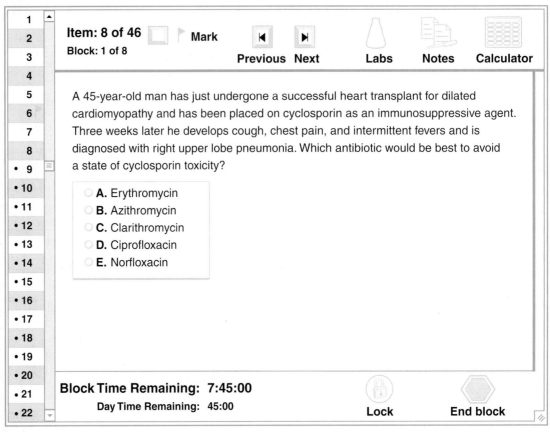

Item: 8 of 46 ☐ ▷ Mark ◀ ▶ Previous Next   Labs   Notes   Calculator
Block: 1 of 8

A 45-year-old man has just undergone a successful heart transplant for dilated cardiomyopathy and has been placed on cyclosporin as an immunosuppressive agent. Three weeks later he develops cough, chest pain, and intermittent fevers and is diagnosed with right upper lobe pneumonia. Which antibiotic would be best to avoid a state of cyclosporin toxicity?

○ **A.** Erythromycin
○ **B.** Azithromycin
○ **C.** Clarithromycin
○ **D.** Ciprofloxacin
○ **E.** Norfloxacin

Block Time Remaining: 7:45:00
Day Time Remaining: 45:00

Lock   End block

(Adapted from http://www.usmle.org/Orientation/2009/menu.html.)

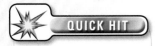

QUICK HIT

The minimum passing score on the USMLE Step 1 is 188. This number generally corresponds to getting 60% to 70% of exam questions right.

pass/fail status, digit score, and group performance profile. During the residency application process, residency programs receive a transcript containing pass/fail status and the digit score without the performance profile (Figure 3).

When preparing for the exam, the goal is two-tiered. Your first objective should be to pass the exam so that you can be on your way to becoming a licensed physician in the United States. Also, passing the exam is often linked to proceeding to the third year of medical school and getting your medical degree. The second objective is doing the best

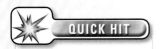

QUICK HIT

88% to 93% of the United States and Canadian medical students pass the exam on their first attempt. Compare this to the U.S. bar exam, which has a passing rate of 67%.

FIGURE 3 **Mean scores for matched U.S. seniors by specialty.** The numbers displayed are mean values for USMLE Step 1 Score for matched U.S. seniors by specialty.

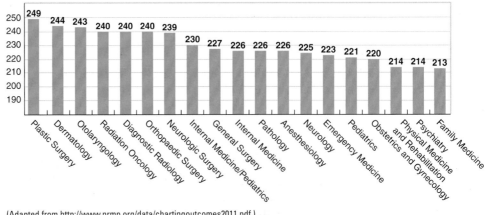

(Adapted from http://www.nrmp.org/data/chartingoutcomes2011.pdf.)

you can so that you can make yourself a competitive applicant for the residency of your choice. Certain highly competitive residency programs such as orthopaedic surgery and ophthalmology use Step 1 scores in the selection process.

It is important to note that the Step 1 score is only one of many factors that weigh in on the residency selection process. Programs make use of other applicant characteristics such as clinical rotation grades, research, publications, and reference letters. Having insight into your academic portfolio and defining your personal goals may be helpful in guiding your studies for Step 1.

Registering to Take the Exam

Six to 8 months prior to the anticipated exam date, you will likely be prompted by your school to begin the registration process for taking the exam. The Step 1 application packet can be downloaded from the USMLE website: http://www.usmle.org. Applicants must select a 3-month time period to take the exam (e.g., April–May–June, June–July–August). The application includes a form requiring a passport-sized photo that must be certified by the school registrar. The NBME processes the submitted application and sends out a scheduling permit.

The scheduling permit contains a unique candidate identification number, which is necessary in order to schedule the exam and take the exam. After receiving the scheduling permit, you should attempt to schedule your exam as soon as possible in order to receive the location and time of your choice. Scheduling occurs on a first-come, first-served basis, and testing centers fill up quickly during popular testing times of the year. Specific instructions on scheduling the test are delineated on the scheduling permit and require calling Prometric 1-800-633-3926 or logging into the Prometric site at http://www.prometric.com. A list of Prometric testing centers nearest you can be found on the Prometric website. Of note, testing centers are closed for the first 2 weeks of January, during major holidays, and generally on Sundays. Also, the exam can be started at different times of the day for those preferring the early or late hours of the day. Generally, Step 1 is taken by second-year medical students finishing their second year of medical school. Some relevant information to consider when scheduling your exam is your second year end date and third year start date. Because most curricula end in May, and students allow themselves a study time of 1 month, most students take the exam in June.

If for some reason you need to reschedule your exam, you will need to call or visit the Prometric website. The rescheduled date must fall within the 3-month eligibility period selected earlier during the registration process (also found on your scheduling permit). Also, to avoid a rescheduling fee, Prometric should be contacted before noon EST 5 business days prior to the testing date.

PREPARING FOR THE EXAM: STUDY STRATEGIES

Study Materials

The first step to preparing for the exam is collecting and familiarizing yourself with study materials. You can start this step years before you actually take the exam. When starting medical school, consider purchasing a comprehensive review text such as *Step-Up to the USMLE Step 1*. The purpose of this is to begin reading, annotating, and familiarizing yourself with the test and content of the book. You might also consider investing early in subject-based reviews as you study those subjects in medical school. Finally, consider purchasing one or a series of question banks. Question banks allow you the opportunity to practice and apply learned concepts, solidifying the exam preparation process.

You should also take advantage of USMLE resources officially provided by the NBME. The NBME offers a free sample test consisting of 143 questions: http://www.usmle.org /practice-materials/index.html. For those examinees who would like to practice taking the exam with the testing interface, a mock testing situation can be set up at a Prometric center. This additional service costs $42. Students are provided with a score report at the end, although no explanations are offered online or at the testing center. The Comprehensive Basic Science Self-Assessment (CBSSA) is a 200-question test offered by the NBME, presented in four blocks of 50 questions each. Students must register to take the exam online and are charged $50 for this service. The website to create an account is https://nsasnbme .org/nsasweb/servlet/mesa_main. After taking the test, students are provided with a performance profile outlining the student's strengths and weaknesses.

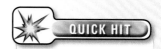

QUICK HIT

You should register for the exam 6 to 8 months prior to your anticipated exam date.

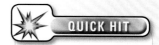

QUICK HIT

Schedule your test as soon as possible after receiving the scheduling permit in order to receive the location and time of your choice.

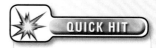

QUICK HIT

The scheduling permit needs to be presented on the day of the exam. Put it in a safe place. Copies will not be accepted.

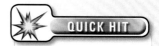

QUICK HIT

To avoid a rescheduling fee, contact Prometric before noon EST 5 business days before the scheduled testing date.

FIGURE
4 Suggested study schedule: organ systems based

Sunday	Monday	Tuesday	Wednesday	Thursday	Friday	Saturday
1	2	3	4	5	6	7
	NERVOUS			CARDIO		
8	9	10	11	12	13	14
RESPIR		GASTRO		RENAL		
15	16	17	18	19	20	21
ENDO		REPRO		MUSCULO		HEME
22	23	24	25	26	27	28
LYMPH	BASIC CONCEPTS		WRAP UP DAYS			
29	30					

Study Schedule

After collecting study materials, the next step is creating a study schedule. Preparation for the USMLE Step 1 can start years before actually taking the exam. As mentioned earlier, as you prepare for your medical school classes, read and annotate review texts along with studying syllabi and textbooks for classes. The purpose of this is to familiarize yourself with the text.

In the months prior to the exam, you should register for the exam, schedule the exam, and collect study materials including a question bank. Familiarize yourself with your study materials and attend campus review sessions.

The month before the exam, create and follow a study schedule. The purpose of the study schedule is to cover each of the disciplines tested on the exam. Typically, most medical students are provided 1 month to study for the exam. When students are creating a study schedule, oftentimes, the most challenging feat is determining how many days to allocate toward one discipline. Figures 4 and 5 are suggested study schedules that have been successful for students in the past. The first study schedule is organized by organ

FIGURE
5 Suggested study schedule: basic science based

Sunday	Monday	Tuesday	Wednesday	Thursday	Friday	Saturday
1	2	3	4	5	6	7
	PATHOLOGY			PHYSIOLOGY		
8	9	10	11	12	13	14
	PHARMACOLOGY				MICRO/	
15	16	17	18	19	20	21
IMMUNO		BIOCHEM		BEHAV SCI		
22	23	24	25	26	27	28
ANATOMY (including embryology, histology)	NEURO		WRAP UP DAYS			
29	30					

TABLE 2 Order for Organ System and Basic Science Schedule	
Order for Organ System Schedule	**Order for Basic Science Schedule**
Basic concepts/general	Physiology
Endocrine	Pathology
Nervous	Behavioral science
Cardiovascular	Microbiology/immunology
Respiratory	Pharmacology
Renal	Biochemistry
Gastrointestinal	Neuroanatomy
Musculoskeletal	Gross anatomy/embryology/histology
Reproductive	
Heme/lymph	

system and the second by basic science discipline. These schedules are only suggested schedules. Individual schedules should be tailored to your needs, keeping in mind your individual strengths and weaknesses, high-yield topics for the exam, and available time to study.

The suggested study schedules in Figures 4 and 5 assume 28 days available for study, including the day before the USMLE. If you have more or fewer days, adjust the schedule accordingly. For example, if you have 31 days, add ½ day to Behavioral Science, ½ day to Gross Anatomy/Embryology, 1 day off, and 1 day to wrap up. In these suggested schedules, 2 to 3 days are allocated for wrap-up before the exam, 1 to 2 days are scheduled as days off as rewards for doing your work, and 24 days are full study days. In general, when determining the order of subjects to study, the general strategy should be longer term memory subjects early and shorter term memory subjects late (Table 2). Also, when determining how many days to allocate certain subjects or organ systems, provide more days for heavily tested subjects like pathology and physiology (Table 3).

TABLE 3 Allocation of Days			
Allocation of Days by Organ System		**Allocation of Days by Basic Science**	
Organ System	**Days**	**Basic Science**	**Days**
Nervous	3.5	Pathology	4
Cardiovascular	3	Physiology	4
Respiratory	2.5	Pharmacology	4
Gastrointestinal	2	Microbiology/immunology	4
Renal	2.5	Biochemistry	3
Endocrine	2.5	Behavioral science	1.5
Reproductive	2	Gross anatomy/embryology/histology	1.5
Musculoskeletal	2	Neuroanatomy	2
Heme/lymph	2		
Basic concepts/general	2		

TABLE 4 Suggested Daily Study Schedule	
Time	**Activity**
8:00 a.m.–12:00 p.m.	Study
12:00 p.m.–1:00 p.m.	Lunch
1:00 p.m.–5:00 p.m.	Study
5:00 p.m.–8:00 p.m.	Exercise, dinner, errands, phone calls
8:00 p.m.–10:00 p.m. (or 11:00 p.m.)	Questions

In the month prior to the exam, you should also create and follow a daily schedule. Table 4 contains a sample daily study schedule. The daily schedule should allot time for studying review texts, reading cases/clinical vignettes, and doing questions. While studying texts, you should not only read but also spend time understanding concepts and memorizing key facts. Tools that help with understanding and memorizing information include organizing information into tables, charts, and figures; using mnemonics; and applying information in daily practice, such as in clinics and caring for patients. Books with clinical cases and vignettes are based on this premise and provide an opportunity to integrate studied information. Doing questions is another excellent method of reinforcing and remembering learned information. An online question bank of more than 450 USMLE format questions based on commonly tested facts has been included with this text and can be accessed via this website: www.thePoint.lww.com/StepUp4e. Moreover, clinical vignettes and questions simulate the test day experience. Make sure you also include in your schedule time to relax and do other things that are important to you (work out, spend time with friends and family, etc.).

The night before the exam, relax and gather your required materials (orange permit slip, government-issued photo ID). Make sure you know how to get to the testing center and have confirmed with the testing center your test time and date. Get a good night's rest!

Study Strategies

Studying is a two-stage process. First, learn the basic definitions and concepts. The best method of accomplishing this is reading. Second, recognize and remember key facts. This is the hardest stage and one that most students neglect. Helpful strategies include:

1. Memorization—Use study aids like mnemonics, flashcards, tables, and figures.
2. Active learning—Engage in active learning by applying the concepts to scenarios, clinical settings, and mini-case presentations.
3. Questions—Apply learned concepts by doing questions.
4. Study groups—Discuss studied material and quiz each other; these activities are helpful in retaining information.

ONLINE RESOURCES

Table 5 summarizes important NBME websites and online resources available to you as you prepare for the USMLE.

PERSONALIZED STUDY SCHEDULE

Use the blank study schedule (Figure 6) on the following page to build your own based on the tips included in this chapter and your own areas of strength and weakness.

TABLE 5 Important Websites for Preparing for the USMLE Step 1

	Website	Description	Cost
NBME	http://www.nbme.org	Find general information and updates on the USMLE Step 1	N/A
Application materials	http://www.usmle.org	Apply to take the USMLE Step 1	$560
Scheduling the exam	http://www.prometric.com	Schedule your exam	N/A
FRED software tutorial and practice questions	http://www.usmle.org/practice-materials/index.html	Select option "Tutorial and Practice Test Items For Multiple Choice Questions." This contains a tutorial on the FRED software, familiarizes you with the testing interface, and contains over 140 sample questions. After taking this tutorial, you may skip the tutorial on test day, providing yourself with an extra 15 min in break time	Free
CBSSA	http://www.nbme.org/Students/sas/overview.html	The CBSSA contains USMLE Step 1 format questions designed by the NBME. There are 200 questions in four blocks of 50 questions each. Register to create an account and then follow instructions for CBSSA	$50
Step-Up to the USMLE Step 1 Question Bank	www.thePoint.lww.com/StepUp4e	Includes more than 350 questions in USMLE format with explanations preparing you for the most commonly tested facts on the USMLE	Free
Step-Up to the USMLE Step 1 website	http://www.lww.com/Step-Up	Ask the authors questions, become a student contributor for the next edition, provide feedback on this text	N/A

FIGURE 6 Blank study schedule

PERSONALIZED STEP 1 STUDY SCHEDULE

Use this blank calendar to create your own personalized Step 1 study schedule. Determine your preference for systems-based review or subject-based review, identify your strong areas and weak areas, and create your study schedule.

_____ SYSTEMS BASED   _____ SUBJECT BASED

Strong areas: _____

Weak areas: _____

Sunday	Monday	Tuesday	Wednesday	Thursday	Friday	Saturday
1	2	3	4	5	6	7
8	9	10	11	12	13	14
15	16	17	18	19	20	21
22	23	24	25	26	27	28
29	30					

TEST DAY TIPS

- Bring a cooler with ice, water, juice, or a sports drink. Pack a lunch. Bring some fruits and snacks. (You may not be able to predict what you're going to want to eat, so it's better to bring too much than too little.) Eat light, not heavy.
- Consider getting out in the sun and/or stretching during your breaks.
- Bring a light sweater or sweatshirt in case the testing center is cold.
- Don't forget your ID and USMLE pass.
- Take your breaks when you need them. (Example: 2 sections → break → 2 sections → break → 1 section → break → 2 sections) Some breaks may need to be longer than others. Don't be afraid to take a small 5-minute bathroom break.
- Expect 5 to 10 questions in each section that you have never seen before. If you expect this, then you won't become anxious when it happens (and it *will* happen).
- Bring your own watch to keep track of your break time!
- Consider answering 10 practice questions prior to going into the test center for "warm-up" (but don't look at the answers, in case you are incorrect).

What should I put on my markerboard prior to the start of the test?

- Don't write on your markerboard for more than 5 minutes before you start your test.
- Put whatever you want, but you may want to consider the following:
  - Developmental milestones
  - Important pharmacokinetic equations
  - Error square
  - Sensitivity, specificity, PPV, NPV, OR, RR, equations, and square
  - Lung volume diagram

Basic Concepts

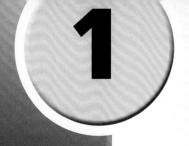

 ENZYME KINETICS

I. Enzymes

A. An enzyme is a protein or nucleic acid molecule that decreases the **energy of activation for a reaction** (*Figure 1-1*).

B. Enzymes interact specifically with substrates at an enzyme active site.

C. By lowering the energy of activation, enzymes increase the rate of reaction.

D. Enzymes **do not alter the equilibrium** of substrates and products, which is concentration dependent, or the free energy released from the reaction.

E. Enzymatic reactions generally require cofactors, such as metals, derivatives of vitamins, or small organic molecules. The vitamins and small organic molecules are often referred to as coenzymes.

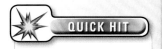

FIGURE 1-1 Enzyme effect on a chemical reaction

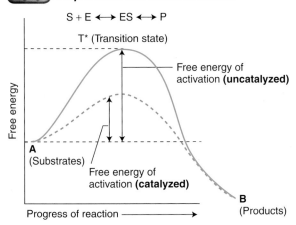

S + E ⟷ ES ⟷ P

An enzyme (E) acts as a catalyst to decrease the amount of free energy required to convert a substrate (S) to a product (P). An uncatalyzed reaction (represented by the solid blue line) requires a much higher amount of free energy than an enzyme-catalyzed reaction (dashed green line).

II. Kinetics

A. **Velocity** (*V*) is the rate of reaction and is dependent on enzyme concentration, substrate concentration, temperature, and pH.

  1. Enzyme concentration: increased enzyme concentration leads to faster rate of reaction.

  2. Substrate concentration: increased concentration leads to increased rate of reaction until a maximum is reached when all enzyme receptor sites are saturated.

  3. Temperature: increased temperature leads to increased rate of reaction up to a maximum, after which enzymes denature.

  4. pH: velocity of a reaction is maximum at its optimal pH. A pH that is either too high or too low leads to a slower reaction or may denature the enzyme.

B. Michaelis–Menten equation

1. Enzymatically catalyzed reactions can be characterized by the Michaelis–Menten equation:

$$V = V_{max} \times [S]/(K_m + [S])$$

where V is the velocity of the reaction.

V_{max} is the maximum velocity of the reaction.
$[S]$ is the substrate concentration.
K_m is the Michaelis constant (the substrate concentration at which velocity is one-half of the maximum velocity of a given reaction; $V = \frac{1}{2} V_{max}$).

2. Effect of substrate concentration on reaction velocity (*Figure 1-2*)

FIGURE
1-2 **Effect of substrate concentration on reaction velocity**

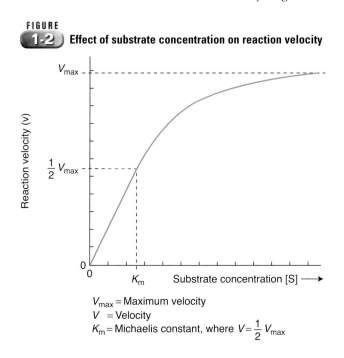

V_{max} = Maximum velocity
V = Velocity
K_m = Michaelis constant, where $V = \frac{1}{2} V_{max}$

C. Lineweaver–Burk plots (*Figure 1-3*)

1. A Lineweaver–Burk plot is a linear representation of the Michaelis–Menten equation, which allows for easier interpretation of the maximum velocity of an equation.

   a. Competitive inhibitors increase the K_m by competing with substrate binding to enzyme at the active site.

   b. Noncompetitive inhibitors decrease the V_{max} by bonding to the enzyme (E or ES) outside of the active site.

   c. Irreversible inhibitors inactivate the enzyme with kinetics similar to noncompetitive inhibition. Example: Aspirin inhibition of cyclooxygenases.

2. Regulatory enzymes in metabolic pathways are influenced by allosteric interactions and will have nonlinear Lineweaver–Burk plots for their kinetics.

FIGURE
1-3 Lineweaver–Burk plot

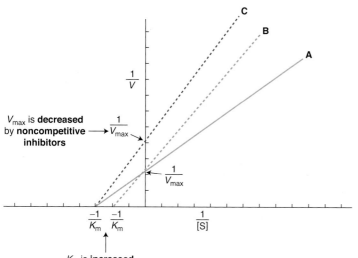

V_{max} is **decreased** by **noncompetitive inhibitors**

$\frac{1}{V}$

$\frac{1}{V_{max}}$

$\frac{1}{V_{max}}$

$\frac{-1}{K_m}$ $\frac{-1}{K_m}$

$\frac{1}{[S]}$

K_m is **increased** by **competitive inhibitors**

A = No inhibitor
B = Competitive inhibitor
C = Noncompetitive inhibitor

[S] = Substrate concentration
V = Reaction velocity
V_{max} = Maximum velocity
K_m = Michaelis constant

$\frac{1}{V_{max}}$ is where the plot crosses the y-axis

$\frac{-1}{K_m}$ is where the plot crosses the x-axis

CONCEPTS IN PHARMACOLOGY

I. Absorption

A. There are many routes of administration (*Figure 1-4*).

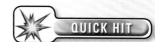
QUICK HIT

When infusing a drug, it takes 4.3 half-lives to achieve 95% of the steady-state concentration.

FIGURE
1-4 Routes of drug administration

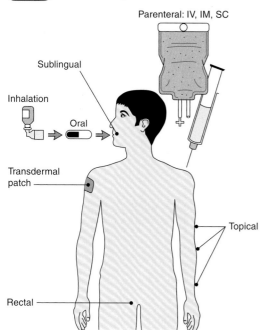

Parenteral: IV, IM, SC

Sublingual

Inhalation

Oral

Transdermal patch

Topical

Rectal

IM, intramuscular; IV, intravenous; SC, subcutaneous. (Adapted from Mycek M, Harvey RA, Champe PC. *Lippincott's Illustrated Reviews: Pharmacology.* 2nd ed. Philadelphia, PA: Lippincott-Raven Publishers; 1996:2. Used with permission of Lippincott Williams & Wilkins.)

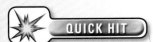

QUICK HIT

If a drug is rapidly metabolized by the liver, the amount reaching the target tissues is significantly reduced. Such drugs include propranolol, lidocaine, verapamil, and meperidine.

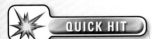

QUICK HIT

Charged species do not cross the gastrointestinal membrane as readily as uncharged species. Therefore, the percentage of drug in the uncharged state determines the rate of absorption.

$$pH = pK_a + log \frac{protonated}{unprotonated} \ species$$

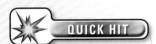

QUICK HIT

Acidophilic drugs bind to albumin, whereas basophilic drugs bind to globulins. The administration of a drug that binds to sites already occupied by a drug can displace the first drug. This leads to a surge in free drug, which, in turn, leads to increased activity and elimination.

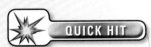

QUICK HIT

Efficacy is equivalent to maximum velocity (V_{max}) in enzyme kinetics.

B. Oral administration is the most common route.
C. Most drugs are absorbed in the **duodenum**.
  1. Drugs enter the portal circulation.
  2. They are subject to **first-pass metabolism** by the liver.
D. Other factors that affect absorption include:
  1. Intestinal pH
  2. Whether taken with food (slows transit, allowing for further acid digestion)
  3. Whether the drug is a sustained-release preparation
  4. Whether gastrointestinal diseases or malabsorption syndromes are present

II. Distribution

$$V_d = D/C$$

A. V_d, volume of distribution; D, amount of drug in body; C, plasma concentration.
B. Distribution occurs more rapidly with high blood flow, high vessel permeability, and a **hydrophobic drug**.
C. Binding to **plasma proteins** (albumin and globulins) accelerates absorption into plasma but slows diffusion into tissues.
D. Many disease states alter distribution:
  1. Edematous states (e.g., cirrhosis, heart failure, nephrotic syndrome) prolong distribution and delay clearance.
  2. Obesity allows for greater accumulation of lipophilic agents within fat cells, increasing distribution and prolonging half-life.
  3. Pregnancy increases intravascular volume, thus increasing V_d.
  4. Hypoalbuminemia allows drugs that are protein bound to have increased availability because of lack of albumin for binding.

III. Pharmacokinetics

A. The effect an agonist has on its receptors depends on concentration.
B. **Efficacy** is a measure of the maximum effect a drug can produce.
C. **Potency** is a measure of the amount of drug needed to produce a given effect (*Figure 1-5*).

FIGURE
1-5 Dose–response curve

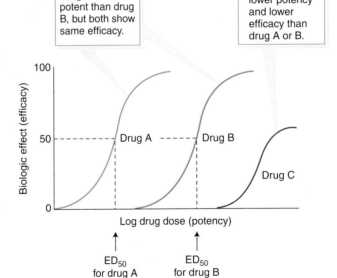

ED_{50}, dose effective in 50% of population.

D. Effective dose (ED) and lethal dose (LD)
  1. ED is the dose of the drug that produces the desired effect.
  2. ED_{50} is the dose of the drug that produces the desired effect in 50% of the population.
  3. LD is the dose of the drug that produces death.

FIGURE
1-6 **Therapeutic range**

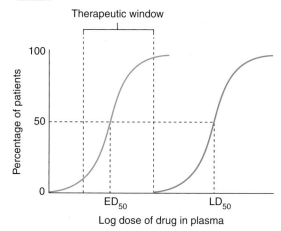

Therapeutic window

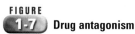

ED_{50}, dose effective in 50% of population; LD_{50}, dose that is lethal in 50% of population.

4. LD_{50} is the dose of the drug that produces death in 50% of the population.
5. Separation of ED and LD determines therapeutic range (*Figure 1-6*).
6. A drug's **therapeutic index** (TI) is a measure of how safe it is to use. TI = LD_{50}/ED_{50}
E. Antagonists (*Figure 1-7*)
 1. **Competitive antagonist**: competes for the same binding site as the agonist or drug
  a. Increases K_m
  b. Does not affect V_{max}
 2. **Noncompetitive antagonist**: prevents binding of the agonist or drug to the receptor or prevents activation of the receptor by the agonist
  a. Decreases the efficacy of the agonist
  b. Decreases V_{max} but does not affect K_m
 3. **Complete antagonist**: prevents all pharmacologic action(s) of the agonist or drug
 4. **Partial agonist**: binds to the same receptor site as the agonist or drug but has a lower efficacy

FIGURE
1-7 **Drug antagonism**

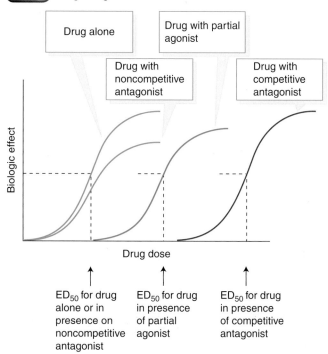

ED_{50}, dose effective in 50% of population.

F. Pharmacokinetics are affected by disease states:
1. Hyperthyroidism increases the heart's sensitivity to catecholamines.
2. Patients with cirrhosis are more sensitive to sedative-hypnotics.
3. Patients with cirrhosis and congestive heart failure (CHF) will retain fluids if taking nonsteroidal anti-inflammatory drugs (NSAIDs) because of the role of prostaglandins in maintaining renal function.

IV. Metabolism
A. Drugs may be chemically altered, varying activity or aiding excretion.
B. The enzymatic transformation of drugs usually follows one of two kinetics:
1. **First-order kinetics**: a constant **fraction** of drug is metabolized in a certain unit of time—by far the most common. This arises because drugs have higher affinities for their receptors (K_d) than their metabolizing enzymes (K_m).
2. **Zero-order kinetics**: a constant **amount** of drug is metabolized in a certain unit of time (e.g., ethanol)—rare.
C. The liver is the primary site of metabolism and uses two sets of reactions:
1. **Phase 1**: drugs are modified or portions are removed (cytochrome P450 oxidation, enzymatic reduction, hydrolysis).
2. **Phase 2**: conjugation reactions add chemical groupings to the drug (e.g., glucuronidation, sulfate or glutathione conjugation, acetylation, methylation).
D. **Prodrugs** are drugs that are administered in an inactive form and are metabolically activated by the body.
E. Some drugs are metabolized to toxic products (e.g., acetaminophen).

V. Elimination
A. Most drugs are eliminated in the urine or bile.
B. Volatile drugs can be eliminated through the lungs.
C. **Renal excretion**
1. Substances with a molecular weight (MW) <5,000 that are free in the plasma are filtered in the glomerulus.
2. Higher concentrations of a substance within the tubules may favor some reabsorption.
3. The proximal convoluted tubule (PCT) may actively secrete a drug.
4. The urine pH, molecular size, lipid solubility, and negative logarithm of the acid ionization constant (pK_a) of the drug affect renal excretion.
D. Biliary excretion
1. Hepatocytes actively take up the drug from plasma, store it or metabolize it, and release it into the bile duct.
2. Some drugs are excreted in feces.
3. Some drugs are reabsorbed in the terminal ileum (enterohepatic cycling).

VI. Special circumstances
A. Geriatric patients
1. These patients often use multiple prescriptions and over-the-counter medications.
2. Decreased body size, body water, and serum albumin, along with increased body fat, alter drug distribution.
3. **Decreased phase 1 reactions**, liver mass, and liver blood flow all slow metabolism.
4. Decreased kidney mass, renal blood flow, glomerular filtration rate, and tubular function hamper drug excretion.
B. Pediatric patients
1. **Most drugs cross the placenta** to some extent, and their possible effects on the fetus are ranked as category A, B, C, D, and X (A = no evidence of first trimester risk in well-controlled human studies, X = positive evidence of fetal risk, and the risks outweigh the potential benefits).
2. Absorption
   a. High gastric pH and delayed emptying affect enteral absorption.
   b. High surface area-to-volume ratio affects transdermal administration.
   c. Low muscle mass limits intramuscular (IM) administration to the **vastus lateralis** in infancy.
3. Albumin does not reach adult levels until 1 year of age.

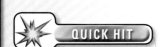

QUICK HIT

Ethanol, barbiturates, and phenytoin **induce** cytochrome P450 enzymes, whereas cimetidine, ketoconazole, and macrolide antibiotics **inhibit** cytochrome P450 enzymes, increasing and decreasing the metabolism of other drugs, respectively (e.g., warfarin).

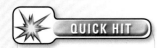

QUICK HIT

Filtration is dependent on the amount of free drug in the blood, whereas active secretion is dependent on the total plasma concentration (free and bound drug).

4. Both phases of metabolism are deficient to varying degrees until 12 years of age.
5. Specific antibiotics avoided in childhood include **quinolones** (articular cartilage erosion and tendon damage) and **tetracycline** (depression of bone and teeth formation).

C. **Pharmacogenetics**
   1. Acetylation of isoniazid
      a. In patients who are **slow acetylators**, there is increased incidence of neuropathy, bladder cancer, and familial Parkinson disease.
      b. Patients who are **rapid acetylators** are the majority of the population.
      c. Rate of acetylation also affects metabolism of hydralazine, dapsone, and phenytoin.
   2. Succinylcholine sensitivity
      a. Atypical **pseudocholinesterase** does not hydrolyze succinylcholine effectively.
      b. It leads to prolonged paralysis (succinylcholine apnea).
      c. It is **autosomal recessive**.
   3. Ethanol metabolism
      a. Ethanol is metabolized by two enzymes:
         i. **Alcohol dehydrogenase** (converts ethanol to acetaldehyde)
         ii. **Aldehyde dehydrogenase** (converts acetaldehyde to acetate)
      b. Aldehyde dehydrogenase shows diminished activity in certain patients (e.g., approximately 30%–40% of Chinese and Japanese individuals have diminished activity).
      c. Acetaldehyde accumulation leads to facial flushing, headache, nausea, and vomiting.

D. Toxicology (Table 1-1)

TABLE 1-1 Toxicology

Poison	Therapy
Acetaminophen	*N*-acetylcysteine
Amphetamine	Ammonium chloride (acidify urine)
Arsenic	Dimercaprol, succimer, penicillamine
Aspirin	Activated charcoal, sodium bicarbonate (alkalinize urine), dialysis
Atropine	Physostigmine
Benzodiazepines	Flumazenil
β-Blockers	Atropine, activated charcoal, glucagon, calcium chloride
Carbon monoxide	100% oxygen, hyperbaric oxygen
Cocaine	Supportive care, benzodiazepines, calcium channel blockers
Copper	Penicillamine
Cyanide	Sodium thiosulfate; amyl nitrite plus sodium nitrite
Digitalis	Activated charcoal, digoxin immune Fab, potassium (if serum potassium level is low), possibly atropine
Ethylene glycol (antifreeze)	Fomepizole, ethanol, dialysis
Heparin	Protamine sulfate
Iron	Deferoxamine
Isoniazid	Vitamin B_6
Isopropyl alcohol	Supportive care
Lead	Succimer, EDTA, dimercaprol
Mercury	Dimercaprol
Methanol	Fomepizole, ethanol, dialysis

(continued)

TABLE 1-1 Toxicology (Continued)

Poison	Therapy
Methemoglobin	Methylene blue
Opioids	Naloxone, naltrexone
Organophosphates	Atropine, pralidoxime
Sulfonylureas	Dextrose, octreotide
tPA, streptokinase	Aminocaproic acid
Tricyclic antidepressants	Gastric lavage, sodium bicarbonate (serum alkalinization), diazepam for seizures
Warfarin	Vitamin K, fresh frozen plasma

EDTA, ethylenediaminetetraacetic acid; tPA, tissue plasminogen activator.

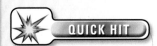

QUICK HIT

High-sensitivity tests are better suited for screening purposes, whereas high-specificity tests are used as confirmatory tests.

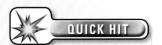

QUICK HIT

For chronic conditions (e.g., diabetes or cirrhosis), the prevalence is higher than the incidence because the long length of the disease process increases prevalence. For conditions that resolve quickly (e.g., strep throat) or are rapidly fatal (e.g., pancreatic cancer), the incidence and prevalence are approximately equal.

● BIOSTATISTICS AND EPIDEMIOLOGY

I. Sensitivity and specificity (*Table 1-2*)

II. Incidence and prevalence (*Table 1-2*)
  A. Incidence is the number of new individuals who develop an illness in a given time period divided by the total number of individuals at risk for the illness.
  B. Prevalence is the number of individuals in the population who have an illness divided by the total population.
  C. Example: **Incidence** is the number of intravenous (IV) drug abusers newly diagnosed with HIV in 2013 divided by the number of HIV-negative IV drug abusers in the population in 2013. **Prevalence** is the number of IV drug users in the United States who are currently HIV positive divided by the total population of IV drug users.

TABLE 1-2 Sensitivity and Specificity

			Disease	
			Yes	**No**
Test Results:		**Positive**	True Positive (A)	False Positive (B)
		Negative	False Negative (C)	True Negative (D)

Terminology	Equation	Definition
Sensitivity (positive in disease)	$\dfrac{A}{(A+C)}$	Probability that a person having a disease will be correctly identified
Specificity (negative in healthy)	$\dfrac{D}{(D+B)}$	Probability that a person who does not have a disease will be correctly identified
Positive predictive value (PPV)	$\dfrac{A}{(A+B)}$	Probability that an individual who tests positive has the disease
Negative predictive value (NPV)	$\dfrac{D}{(C+D)}$	Probability that an individual who tests negative does not have the disease
Prevalence	$\dfrac{A+C}{(A+B+C+D)}$ Generally calculated by incidence $\times$ duration of disease	Total number of cases in a population at a given time
Incidence	Generally calculated by number of new cases/susceptible population	Number of new cases of disease in the population over a given time

III. Key relationships among statistical variables

A. **Sensitivity (Sn), false-negative ratio (FNR), negative predictive value (NPV)**
1. Sn and FNR are inversely related: $Sn = 1 - FNR$.
2. Therefore, increasing the Sn of a test decreases the FNR (the number of false negatives) and increases the NPV.
3. Example: A fasting blood sugar (FBS) >126 mg/dL is used to diagnose diabetes. If we lower the threshold to 110 mg/dL, then we will catch more individuals with diabetes. Statistically, this means decreasing the number of false negatives (those individuals who test negative but actually have the disease) and increasing sensitivity.

B. **Specificity (Sp), false-positive ratio (FPR), positive predictive value (PPV)**
1. Sp and FPR are inversely related: $Sp = 1 - FPR$
2. Therefore, increasing the Sp of a test decreases the FPR (the number of false positives) and increases the PPV.
3. Example: Western blot testing is used as a confirmatory test for HIV because of its high specificity. The initial screening test is highly sensitive (catches all true positives, plus some false positives). Western blot is specific, therefore the false positives on the first test are shown to be true negatives on the Western blot test.

C. **Specificity and sensitivity** are inversely related: as Sp increases, Sn decreases and vice versa.

D. **Treatment**
1. Treatment decreases prevalence by shortening duration (remember that prevalence = incidence × duration of disease) (Table 1-2).
2. Treatment has no effect on incidence.
3. Adherence, therapy, physician access, early detection → decreases duration → decreases prevalence.

IV. Research study designs *(Table 1-3)*

A. Cohort studies
1. Observational and can be prospective or retrospective

> **QUICK HIT**
>
> A screening test is more useful in a population where the disease is highly prevalent. As prevalence increases, PPV increases, and clinical usefulness is reflected in PPV.

TABLE 1-3 Research Study Designs

Study	Purpose	Notes
Case series	A study reporting on a consecutive collection of patients treated in a similar manner; no control group	
Case-control	Retrospective study designed to determine the association between an exposure and outcome: Patients are sampled by outcome (e.g., patients with the disease are compared to patients without the disease); the investigator then examines the proportion of patients with the exposure in the two groups.	Information reported as odds ratio. Example: Individuals with and without lung cancer are identified (outcome = lung cancer). The number of individuals who smoke within each group are counted (exposure = smoking).
Cohort	Prospective study of the factors that might cause a disorder; begins with identification of a specific population (cohort) free of outcome; one cohort is exposed to the putative cause and compared with a concurrent cohort not exposed to the putative cause; both cohorts are then followed to compare the incidence of the outcome of interest.	Information reported as relative risk. Example: Two groups are made: one is exposed to UV radiation, the other is not (exposure = UV radiation). The number of individuals developing skin cancer is then counted within each group (outcome = skin cancer).
Crossover	A study design in which all patients receive both experimental and control treatments in sequence	Subjects act as own control
Cross-sectional	Provide information on possible risk factors and health status of a group of individuals at one specific point in time	Assess prevalence
Meta-analysis	Pooling data from several studies to achieve greater statistical power: often done via literature searches	
Controlled trial	Type of cohort study in which a cohort receiving one treatment/intervention is compared with a cohort receiving a different treatment or placebo	Example: Two groups are made: one is applied sunscreen, the other is applied a placebo cream (intervention = sunscreen). The number of individuals developing skin cancer is then counted within each group (outcome = skin cancer).

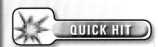

QUICK HIT

The most rigorous form of a clinical trial is the double-blind study, in which neither the subject nor the examiner knows which drug the subject is receiving. Single-blind, double-blind, randomized, crossover, and placebo studies are done to reduce bias.

2. After assessment of exposure to a risk factor, subjects are compared with each other for a period of time.
3. Clinical treatment trial
   a. Highest quality cohort study
   b. Compares the therapeutic benefits of two or more treatments
4. Relative risk
   a. Calculated only for cohort studies
   b. Compares incidence rate in exposed group with incidence rate in unexposed individuals

B. Case-control studies
   1. Retrospective and observational
   2. Subjects with and without disorder are identified, and information on exposure to risk factors is assessed

C. **Odds ratio**
   1. Calculated in case-control studies; approximates the relative risk
   2. Based on disease occurring with or without exposure
   3. Odds ratio = (A × D)/(B × C) = (A/C)/(B/D) = (A/B)/(C/D)
      Where

		Disease	
		Yes	**No**
Exposure: Yes		A	B
No		C	D

V. Biases—A systematic tendency to produce an outcome that differs from the underlying truth
   A. **Sampling bias**—Volunteer subjects in a study may not be representative of the population being studied; as a consequence, the results of the study may not be generalizable to the entire population.
   B. **Selection bias**—Occurs when there is a systematic difference in the way study groups are chosen. One method of decreasing this bias is randomization.
   C. **Expectancy bias**—Occurs when a physician knows which patients are in treatment versus placebo group, causing the physician to draw conclusions supporting the expected outcome. One method of decreasing this bias is a double-blind design.
   D. **Late-look bias**—Results from information being gathered too late to draw conclusions about the disease or exposure of interest from the entire study population. For instance, the more severe cases may have already died.
   E. **Measurement bias**—Describes how information gathered affects information collected. For example, the Hawthorne effect describes how people act differently when being watched.
   F. **Proficiency bias**—This is an issue when comparing the effects of different treatments administered at multiple sites. Physicians at one site may have more skill, thereby providing better treatment.
   G. **Recall bias**—Patients who experience an adverse outcome have a different likelihood of recalling an exposure than do patients who do not have an adverse outcome, independent of the true extent of the exposure.

VI. Disease prevention
   A. **Primary prevention** stops disease occurrence; for example, encouraging use of sun protection to prevent skin cancer.
   B. **Secondary prevention** detects disease early; for example, physician checking for suspicious growths.
   C. **Tertiary prevention** decreases devastating complications of the disease; for example, administering insulin to a diabetic.

VII. Testing and statistical methods
    A. Reliability vs. validity
        1. **Reliability** refers to the reproducibility of test results, which reflects the absence of random variation. Also known as precision.
        2. **Validity** refers to the appropriateness of a test's measurements; that is, how closely the test results reflect the truth. Also known as accuracy.
        3. **Sensitivity** and **specificity** are measures of validity.
    B. Bell curve (*Figure 1-8*)
        1. In a normal distribution, the mean, median, and mode are equal.
           a. Mean: average
           b. Median: middle value in a sequentially ordered group of numbers
           c. Mode: number that appears most often in a group
        2. Skew refers to the way a peak may be offset.
           a. **Positive skew**: peak is to the left (most scores at low end; mean > median > mode)
           b. **Negative skew**: peak is to the right (most scores at high end; mean < median < mode)
        3. A bimodal distribution has two peaks.

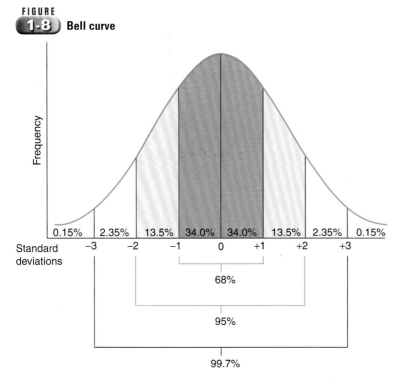

FIGURE 1-8 Bell curve

    C. The **null hypothesis** (H$_0$)
        1. Postulates that there is no significant difference between groups
        2. A **type I error** occurs when the null hypothesis is rejected when it is true. The α is the probability of making a type I error.
           a. The α value is set by the investigator, usually at 0.05.
           b. The *p* value is the probability that the study results occurred due to chance alone, given the null hypothesis is true.
           c. If *p* is less than α (usually 0.05), the results are considered "significant," and the null hypothesis is rejected.
        3. A **type II error** occurs when the null hypothesis is accepted when it is not true. The β is the probability of making a type II error.
        4. **Power** is the probability of rejecting the null hypothesis when the null hypothesis is false. Power $= 1 - \beta$. Increasing the sample size increases power. If $p < 0.05$, then the null hypothesis can be rejected.

5. Example
   a. A study is conducted on the influence of medical school on dating frequency.
   b. The null hypothesis would be that medical school students, when compared with 22- to 26-year-olds in the working population, have no difference in dating frequency.
   c. If the p value of the study is less than 0.05 (meaning that there is a statistical difference), then the null hypothesis can be rejected. Thus, it can be stated that medical school decreases dating frequency.

EXTREME ENVIRONMENTS

I. High altitude
   A. Barometric pressure at sea level is 760 mm Hg. At 20,000 feet above sea level, barometric pressure is 349 mm Hg. Partial pressure of O_2 is 21% of the barometric pressure, regardless of altitude.
   B. To compensate for this lower PO_2 at high altitude, the body makes several physiologic adjustments:

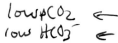
low pCO_2 ←
low HCO_3^- ←

   1. Ventilatory rate increases both acutely and chronically.
   2. Renal excretion of bicarbonate increases to compensate for the respiratory alkalosis caused by increased ventilation.
   3. Erythropoietin production increases to increase red blood cell (RBC) mass.
   4. Numbers of mitochondria and oxidative enzymes increase slightly.
   C. Rapid ascent to high altitude without sufficiency acclimatization can result in **acute mountain sickness.**
   1. Usually occurs 2 hours to 2 days after ascent
   2. Common symptoms include headache and fatigue
   3. Severe illness can result in **acute cerebral edema** or **acute pulmonary edema.**
   4. Can be treated with acetazolamide → excrete HCO_3^-
   D. Individuals who remain at high altitude too long can also develop **chronic mountain sickness.** The clinical features include:
   1. Increased RBC mass and hematocrit
   2. Increased blood viscosity and decreased tissue blood flow
   3. Elevated pulmonary artery pressure (pulmonary arteries constrict in response to hypoxia)
   4. Right-sided heart enlargement
   5. Systemic arterial pressure begins to fall
   6. CHF

II. Aviation and space flight
   A. Gravitational force
   1. 1 G is a force equal to the pull of gravity, and −1 G is an equal force in the opposite direction.
   2. Positive G forces will move blood away from the head (toward the feet), and negative G forces move blood toward the head (away from the feet)
   B. High G environments
   1. Individuals experience a visual "blackout" at 4–6 G, due to pooling of blood in the abdomen and legs, insufficient return of blood to the heart, and insufficient pumping of blood to the brain.
   2. Specialized "G suits" apply pressure to the lower abdomen and legs, to prevent blackouts during high G situations.
   3. During liftoff of a spacecraft liftoff, G forces may reach 8–9 G. To prevent blackout, astronauts liftoff in a semireclining position, transverse to the axis of acceleration.
   C. Individuals who live at **zero gravity** for extended period undergo several physiological changes:
   1. Decreased blood volume and RBC mass
   2. Decreased muscle strength and work capacity

3. Decreased maximum cardiac output

4. Decreased bone mass due to loss of calcium and phosphate

III. Deep sea medicine

A. **Nitrogen narcosis**

1. Atmospheric gas is roughly 78% nitrogen. During prolonged exposure to hyperbaric conditions (such as ocean depths), nitrogen dissolves into the neural membranes, causing reduced neuronal excitability.

2. Symptoms of nitrogen narcosis resemble alcohol intoxication. The diver will first become jovial and careless, then drowsy, then he or she experiences loss of strength and coordination.

B. **Decompression sickness**

1. At the high pressures associated with a deep sea dive, additional nitrogen gas dissolves in the blood.

2. When the diver returns to sea level too rapidly, those gases begin to escape the dissolved state, forming actual bubbles that can occlude blood vessels.

3. Symptoms of decompression sickness (caisson disease, "the bends") include:

   a. Pain in the joints and muscles of the extremities

   b. Neurologic problems (dizziness, paralysis, or syncope) in 5%–10% of patients

   c. Dyspnea and pulmonary edema, due to occlusion of pulmonary capillaries in approximately 2% of patients

4. Treatment is to put the patient in a hyperbaric chamber and redissolve the gas bubbles, then gradually return the patient to sea-level pressure.

 ETHICS AND THE ROLE OF THE PHYSICIAN

I. Ethical principles

A. **Beneficence**—The physician must act in the patient's best interest.

B. **Autonomy** ("self-rule")

1. **Patient autonomy**—The patient has the right to make decisions regarding his or her own body. This includes the right to refuse treatment, or to choose treatments for himself or herself (within reason).

2. **Physician autonomy**—The physician has the right to choose which treatments he or she will or will not provide.

C. **Nonmaleficence**—The physician must not intentionally harm the patient.

D. **Justice**—The physician must strive to treat patients fairly/equitably.

II. Patient consent

A. **Informed consent**—The principle of patient autonomy dictates that before a physician performs any procedure or administers treatment, the patient must give consent. The patient must have some understanding of the procedure/treatment, including the risks involved, the expected benefits, and the alternatives to the procedure.

B. **Decision-making capacity**—In order to give consent, the patient must be determined to have the capacity to make healthcare decisions for himself or herself.

1. The patient must be able to make a treatment decision and communicate that choice to the healthcare team.

2. The patient must also be informed of the risks, benefits, and alternatives.

3. The decision must be consistent with patient's values.

4. The patient's decision has to be stable over time. (However, the patient retains the right to change his or her mind and revoke consent.)

5. The decision is not based on delusions or hallucinations.

C. **Directives**—There are several mechanisms that allow a patient to exercise his or her right to patient autonomy in the event that he or she becomes incapacitated.

1. **Power of attorney for healthcare**—The patient formally designates an individual to consent in the event of incapacitation.

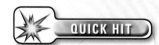

QUICK HIT

Patients also have the right for their medical histories to be kept private and confidential.

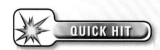

QUICK HIT

In most states, if the patient hasn't assigned power of attorney, the law establishes the succession of surrogates (e.g., the patient's spouse, adult children, parents, etc.) responsible for making healthcare decisions and giving consent.

   2. **Advance directive**—The patient gives instructions in advance about the kinds of procedures and treatments he or she would or would not consent to. This can be in oral or written form.
   3. A **living will** is a legal document that gives treatment instructions to the healthcare team. It is the responsibility of the designated agent to follow the patient's wishes as outlined.
D. **Surrogate decision maker**
   1. If a patient lacks the capacity to give informed consent, the decision-making responsibilities fall to a surrogate decision maker.
   2. **Substituted judgment**—The surrogate's decision should be consistent with the patient's stated values, as if the patient were making the decision for himself or herself. Surrogate decisions carry the same legal weight as the patient's decisions.
E. **Consent for minors**—Treatment of minors requires consent of the parent (or other responsible adult), with certain exceptions:
   1. Emancipated minors ($\geq$16 years old, living on his or her own, and managing his or her own finances)
   2. Treatment of sexually transmitted infections
   3. Treatment related to pregnancy (other than abortion)
   4. Treatment of drug addiction/dependency
   5. Treatment of the child *of* a minor
   6. Treatment of minor serving a sentence of confinement
   7. Emergency situations where parental consent cannot be obtained

III. Medical malpractice—The four basic elements of a malpractice claim are:
A. **Duty:** The physician had an obligation to provide medical care to the plaintiff.
B. **Breach of duty:** The physician failed to meet that obligation.
C. **Harm:** The breach of duty caused some harm or injury to the plaintiff.
D. **Damage:** The patient has suffered some physical, financial, or emotional loss as a result of the injury.

The Nervous System

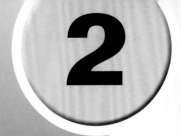

DEVELOPMENT

I. Central nervous system (CNS)

A. The CNS includes the **brain** and **spinal cord**.

B. The CNS forms from the neural tube.
  1. The **basal plate** of the neural tube forms **motor neurons**.
  2. The **alar plate** of the neural tube forms **sensory neurons**.
  3. The basal and alar plates are **separated** by the sulcus **limitans**.

C. **Oligodendrocytes** are responsible for **myelination**, which begins 4 months after conception and is completed by the second year of life.

D. The distal end of the spinal cord, the conus medullaris, is at the level of the third lumbar vertebra (**L3**) at **birth**. As the body grows, the cord "ascends" to its final resting position at the first lumbar vertebra (**L1**) (Figure 2-1).

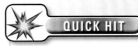

FIGURE 2-1 Adult derivatives of embryonic structures in the nervous system

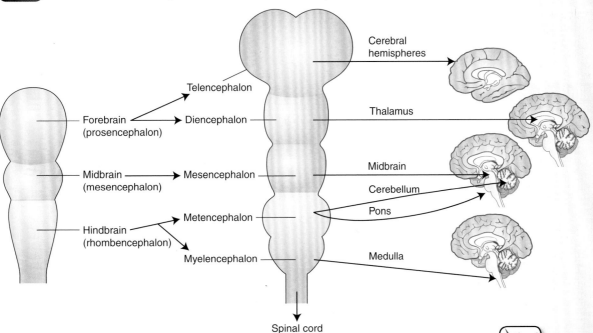

II. Peripheral nervous system (PNS)

A. The PNS includes the **peripheral nerves** and the **autonomic** and **sensory ganglia**.

B. It is **derived from neural crest cells**, which give rise to:
  1. Schwann cells
  2. Pseudounipolar cells of the spinal and cranial nerve (CN) ganglia

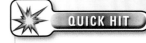

3. Multipolar cells of the autonomic ganglia
4. Pia and arachnoid mater (not part of PNS)
5. Melanocytes (not part of PNS)
6. Epinephrine-producing chromaffin cells of the adrenal gland (not part of PNS)

C. **Schwann cells** are responsible for **myelination**, which begins 4 months after conception and is completed by the second year of life.

CONGENITAL MALFORMATIONS OF THE NERVOUS SYSTEM

Abnormal development of the embryonal components of the nervous system can result in some of the malformations described in Table 2-1.

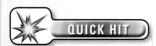

The risk of spina bifida can be decreased by taking folate supplements prior to conception and during pregnancy.

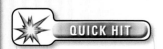

Noncommunicating (obstructive) hydrocephalus refers to increased intracranial pressure caused by a block in cerebrospinal fluid (CSF) flow. In communicating (nonobstructive) hydrocephalus, there is a normal flow of CSF but with abnormal absorption.

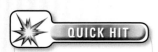

Syringomyelia is associated with formation of Arnold–Chiari malformation.

TABLE 2-1 Congenital Malformations of the Nervous System

Condition	Clinical Features
Fetal alcohol syndrome	• **Most common cause of mental retardation** • **Cardiac septal defects** (VSD) • Facial malformations including widely spaced eyes and long philtrum • Growth retardation

Spina bifida	• Improper closure of posterior neuropore
	• Several forms
	  • **Spina bifida occulta** (mildest form)—failure of vertebrae to close around spinal cord (tufts of hair often evident)
	  • Spinal meningocele (spina bifida cystica)—meninges extend out of defective spinal canal
	  • Meningomyelocele—meninges and spinal cord extend out of spinal canal
	  • Rachischisis (most severe form)—neural tissue is visible externally

Hydrocephaly	• Accumulation of CSF in ventricles and subarachnoid space • Caused by congenital blockage of cerebral aqueducts • May be caused by **cytomegalovirus** or **toxoplasma infection** • Increased head circumference in neonates
Dandy–Walker malformation	• Dilation of fourth ventricle, leading to hypoplasia of cerebellum • Failure of foramina of Luschka and Magendie to open • May result from riboflavin inhibition, posterior fossa trauma, or viral infection
Anencephaly	• Failure of brain to develop • Caused by lack of closure of anterior neuropore • Associated with increased maternal α-fetoprotein (AFP) • Decreased head circumference in neonates
Arnold–Chiari malformation	• Herniation of the **cerebellar vermis** through the foramen magnum • Hydrocephaly • Myelomeningocele

CSF, cerebrospinal fluid.

MAJOR RECEPTORS OF THE NERVOUS SYSTEM

I. **Receptors of the sympathetic and parasympathetic nervous systems**
   A. The sympathetic and parasympathetic nervous systems exert their effects via various receptors scattered throughout the body (Table 2-2).
   B. These effects are mediated by the substances shown in Figure 2-2.

II. **Neurotoxins and their effects** (Figure 2-3)

TABLE 2-2 Receptors of the Sympathetic and Parasympathetic Nervous Systems

Site of Action	Sympathetic Nervous System Receptor	Sympathetic Nervous System Effect on Site	Parasympathetic Nervous System Receptor	Parasympathetic Nervous System Effect on Site
Smooth muscle, skin and viscera	α_1	Contract	Muscarinic	Relax
Smooth and skeletal muscle	α_1 β_2	Contract Relax	Muscarinic	Relax
Smooth muscle of the lung	β_2	Relax	Muscarinic	Contract
Smooth muscle of the gastrointestinal tract	β_2 α_1	Relax intestinal wall Contract sphincters	Muscarinic	Contract intestinal wall, relax sphincter
Heart, SA node	β_1	Increase heart rate	Muscarinic	Decrease heart rate
Heart, ventricles	β_1	Increase contractility and conduction velocity	Muscarinic	Small decrease in contractility
Eye, radial muscle	α_1	**Mydriasis** (dilation of pupil)	N/A	N/A
Eye, sphincter muscle	N/A	N/A	Muscarinic	**Miosis** (constriction of pupil)
Eye, ciliary muscle	β_2	**Relax**	Muscarinic	**Contract** (near vision)
Bladder	β_2 α_1	Relax wall Contract sphincter	Muscarinic	Contract wall, relax sphincter
Uterus	α_1 β_2	Contract Relax	Muscarinic	Contract
Penis	α_2	Emission, ejaculation	Muscarinic	Erection
Sweat glands	Muscarinic	Secrete	N/A	N/A
Pancreas	α_2	**Decrease insulin secretion**	N/A	N/A
	β_2	**Increase insulin secretion**	N/A	N/A
Liver	α_1, β_2	Glycolysis, gluconeogenesis	N/A	N/A
Adipose tissue ' *	β_1, β_3	Lipolysis	N/A	N/A

N/A, not applicable; SA, sinoatrial.

α₁ contracts smooth muscle, radial eye, bladder sphincter, uterus
stimulates liver glycolysis, gluconeogenesis

α₂ ejaculation, decrease insulin

β₁ HR, contractility ↑lung, GI

β₂ Relax smooth muscles, ciliary eye, bladder, uterus
increase insulin, liver glycolysis, gluconeogenesis

FIGURE
2-2 Major receptors of the nervous system

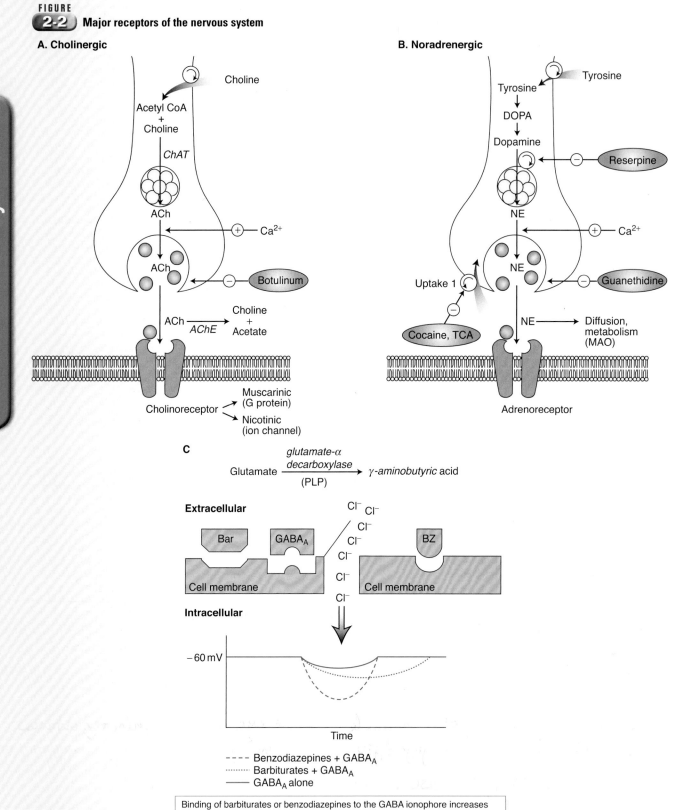

A. Cholinergic

B. Noradrenergic

C

$$\text{Glutamate} \xrightarrow[\text{(PLP)}]{\begin{array}{c}\textit{glutamate-}\alpha\\\textit{decarboxylase}\end{array}} \gamma\textit{-aminobutyric acid}$$

---- Benzodiazepines + GABA$_A$
·········· Barbiturates + GABA$_A$
—— GABA$_A$ alone

Binding of barbiturates or benzodiazepines to the GABA ionophore increases chloride ion conductance. Barbiturates increase the duration of chloride channel opening while benzodiazepines increase the amplitude of depolarization.

Ach, acetylcholine; AChE, acetylcholinesterase; Bar, barbiturates; BZ, benzodiazepine; ChAT, choline acetyltransferase; CoA, coenzyme A; DOPA, dihydroxyphenylalanine; GABA, γ-aminobutyric acid; MAO, monoamine oxidase; NE, norepinephrine; PLP, pyridoxal phosphate; TCA, tricyclic antidepressant.

FIGURE 2-3 Neurotoxins and their effects

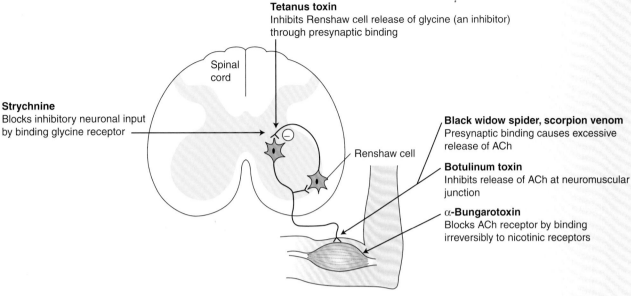

Tetanus toxin
Inhibits Renshaw cell release of glycine (an inhibitor) through presynaptic binding

Spinal cord

Strychnine
Blocks inhibitory neuronal input by binding glycine receptor

Renshaw cell

Black widow spider, scorpion venom
Presynaptic binding causes excessive release of ACh

Botulinum toxin
Inhibits release of ACh at neuromuscular junction

α-Bungarotoxin
Blocks ACh receptor by binding irreversibly to nicotinic receptors

ACh, acetylcholine.

MENINGES, FLOW OF CEREBROSPINAL FLUID, AND PATHOLOGIC TRAUMA (Figure 2-4)

FIGURE 2-4 Meninges, flow of cerebrospinal fluid, and pathologic trauma

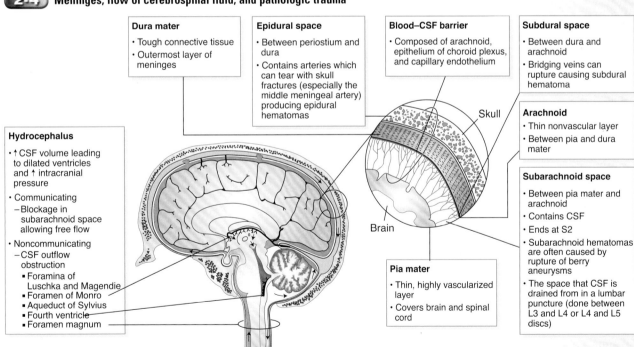

Dura mater
• Tough connective tissue
• Outermost layer of meninges

Epidural space
• Between periostium and dura
• Contains arteries which can tear with skull fractures (especially the middle meningeal artery) producing epidural hematomas

Blood–CSF barrier
• Composed of arachnoid, epithelium of choroid plexus, and capillary endothelium

Subdural space
• Between dura and arachnoid
• Bridging veins can rupture causing subdural hematoma

Skull

Arachnoid
• Thin nonvascular layer
• Between pia and dura mater

Hydrocephalus
• ↑ CSF volume leading to dilated ventricles and ↑ intracranial pressure
• Communicating
  – Blockage in subarachnoid space allowing free flow
• Noncommunicating
  – CSF outflow obstruction
    ▪ Foramina of Luschka and Magendie
    ▪ Foramen of Monro
    ▪ Aqueduct of Sylvius
    ▪ Fourth ventricle
    ▪ Foramen magnum

Brain

Subarachnoid space
• Between pia mater and arachnoid
• Contains CSF
• Ends at S2
• Subarachnoid hematomas are often caused by rupture of berry aneurysms
• The space that CSF is drained from in a lumbar puncture (done between L3 and L4 or L4 and L5 discs)

Pia mater
• Thin, highly vascularized layer
• Covers brain and spinal cord

CSF, cerebrospinal fluid.

BLOOD SUPPLY TO THE BRAIN (*Figure 2-5*)

Cerebrovascular disease is the most common cause of CNS pathology and the third major cause of death in the United States (Table 2-3).

FIGURE 2-5 Blood supply to the brain

A. Arteries of the base of the brain and brain stem

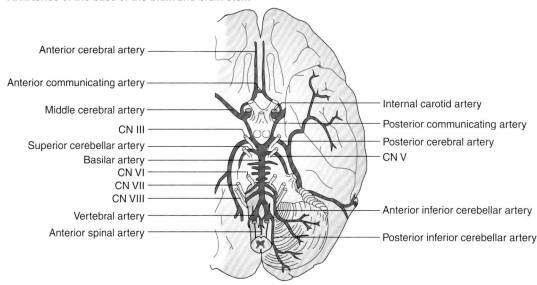

B. Arterial blood supply to the cortex

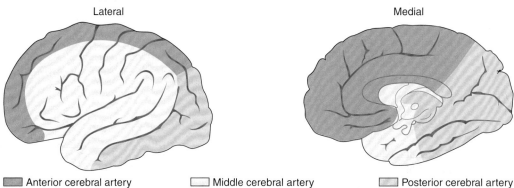

Lateral   Medial

■ Anterior cerebral artery   □ Middle cerebral artery   ▨ Posterior cerebral artery

C. Venous drainage of the brain

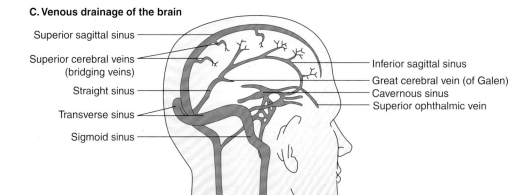

CN, cranial nerve.

TABLE 2-3 Cerebrovascular Disease

Disease	Predisposing Factor	Common Sites
Infarction (more frequent than hemorrhage)		
Thrombosis	Atherosclerosis	Arterial obstruction of internal and external carotid arteries in neck, vertebral and basilar arteries, and vessels branching from circle of Willis to middle cerebral artery
Embolus	Cardiac mural thrombi Valvular vegetation Fat emboli	Middle cerebral artery: leads to contralateral paralysis, motor and sensory deficits, aphasias Smaller vessels: leads to **lacunar strokes**
Hemorrhage		
Intracerebral (bleeding into brain substance)	Hypertension, coagulation disorders, hemorrhage within tumor	Rupture of **Charcot–Bouchard** aneurysms (long-standing hypertension), basal ganglia, pons, frontal lobe, cerebellum
Subarachnoid (bleeding into subarachnoid space)	Associated with **berry aneurysm** in circle of Willis	Circle of Willis, bifurcation of middle cerebral artery

Clinical Vignette 2-1

CLINICAL PRESENTATION: A 26-year-old man was pushed down a flight of stairs in a fight. He **briefly lost consciousness,** then regained consciousness and went to dinner. **After 1 hour** at the restaurant, the man lost consciousness again. He was rushed to the emergency room, and after airway, breathing, and circulation were assessed and secured, a computerized tomography (CT) scan of the head was performed. The scan (Figure 2-6A) showed a convex mass over the right parietal lobe. An eye exam showed a fixed and dilated **right pupil**.

DIFFERENTIALS: Epidural hematoma, subdural hematoma, concussion, brain stem herniation

DIAGNOSTIC TESTS: A **CT scan of the head** is essential for diagnosis in patients with a history of head trauma with loss of consciousness. **An epidural hematoma** is seen on CT as a **convex mass,** which overlays the brain with high attenuation (Figure 2-6A). **(Mnemonic: Epidural = convEx).** An epidural hematoma is a blood clot between the skull and the dura, caused by laceration of the **middle meningeal artery** when the temporal bone is fractured. The "classic" presentation is a patient who has a brief loss of consciousness followed by a lucid interval, after which the patient goes into a coma as the hematoma enlarges and compresses the midbrain.

In contrast, a **subdural** hematoma forms between the dura and the brain (under the dura). It results from **venous bleeding** (as opposed to arterial in epidural hematomas) after blunt head trauma. The movement of brain relative to the skull causes rupture of **bridging veins.** Patients at higher risk for incurring a subdural hematoma after trauma are alcoholics and elderly patients. This is because of brain atrophy, which results in more "space" for the superficial bridging veins to move in response to rapid movement, thus increasing the risk of vessel rupture. Another risk factor for a subdural hematoma is anticoagulation therapy. A subdural hematoma on a CT scan appears as a crescent-shaped (**concave**) hematoma, which is usually less dense than an epidural hematoma because the blood is diluted with cerebrospinal fluid (Figure 2-6B).

CONCUSSION: Brain injury following blunt trauma that usually results in a brief loss of consciousness. Some refer to concussion as a "brain bruise." Those at increased risk include patients with a history of previous concussions. Concussion is caused by dysfunction of the electrophysiology of the midbrain secondary to impact. Patients experience confusion, dizziness, problems with concentration, and inability to answer questions (or a delay in answering) after awakening.

MANAGEMENT: Treatment for an epidural hematoma includes rapid surgical decompression. Conversely, an acute subdural hematoma can be managed by observation or craniotomy with evacuation, depending on size and severity of symptoms. There is no treatment for a concussion.

FIGURE
2-6 A. Epidural hematoma

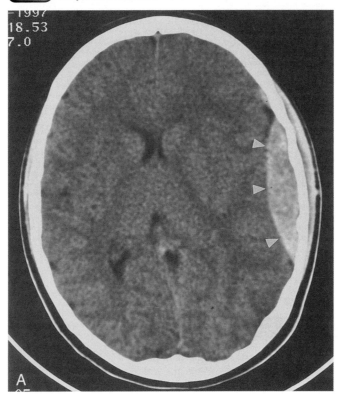

(Reproduced from Daffner RH, Ed. *Clinical Radiology: The Essentials.* 2nd ed. Philadelphia, PA: Lippincott Williams & Wilkins; 1999:513, with permission.)

B. Subdural hematoma

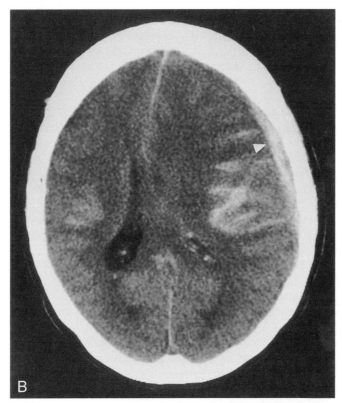

(Reproduced from Daffner RH, Ed. *Clinical Radiology: The Essentials.* 2nd ed. Philadelphia, PA: Lippincott Williams & Wilkins; 1999: 513.9, with permission.)

LESIONS OF THE CEREBRAL CORTEX (Figure 2-7)

2-7 Lesions of the cerebral cortex

A. Lateral view

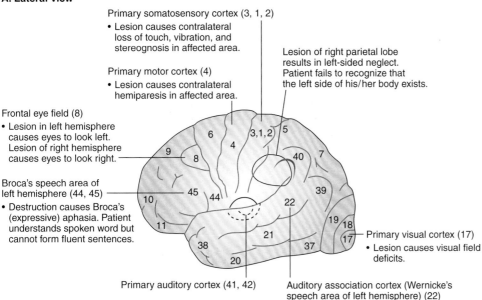

Primary somatosensory cortex (3, 1, 2)
• Lesion causes contralateral loss of touch, vibration, and stereognosis in affected area.

Primary motor cortex (4)
• Lesion causes contralateral hemiparesis in affected area.

Lesion of right parietal lobe results in left-sided neglect. Patient fails to recognize that the left side of his/her body exists.

Frontal eye field (8)
• Lesion in left hemisphere causes eyes to look left. Lesion of right hemisphere causes eyes to look right.

Broca's speech area of left hemisphere (44, 45)
• Destruction causes Broca's (expressive) aphasia. Patient understands spoken word but cannot form fluent sentences.

Primary visual cortex (17)
• Lesion causes visual field deficits.

Primary auditory cortex (41, 42)

Auditory association cortex (Wernicke's speech area of left hemisphere) (22)
• Destruction causes Wernicke's aphasia. Patient cannot understand spoken word, and speech is fluid but does not make sense.

B. Medial view

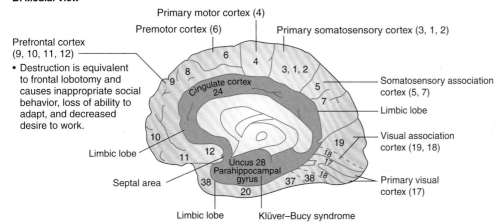

Primary motor cortex (4)
Premotor cortex (6)
Primary somatosensory cortex (3, 1, 2)

Prefrontal cortex (9, 10, 11, 12)
• Destruction is equivalent to frontal lobotomy and causes inappropriate social behavior, loss of ability to adapt, and decreased desire to work.

Somatosensory association cortex (5, 7)

Limbic lobe

Visual association cortex (19, 18)

Primary visual cortex (17)

Limbic lobe
Septal area
Uncus 28
Parahippocampal gyrus
Limbic lobe
Klüver–Bucy syndrome

(Adapted from Fix JD. *High-Yield Neuroanatomy*. Baltimore, MD: Lippincott Williams & Wilkins; 1995:102, with permission.)

IMPORTANT PATHWAYS OF THE SPINAL CORD (Figure 2-8)

I. Posterior white column (dorsal column medial lemniscus pathway)

A. The posterior white column is the ascending pathway that conveys **discriminatory touch (two-point touch), vibration, proprioception,** and **stereognosis.**

B. The posterior white column receives information at all spinal cord levels from pseudounipolar cells of dorsal root ganglia. This information is conveyed from a variety of receptors:
1. Meissner corpuscles (rate of applied stimulus)
2. **Pacinian corpuscles (vibration stimulus)**
3. Joint receptors (joint position; proprioception)

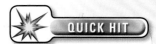
QUICK HIT
Klüver–Bucy syndrome is a bilateral lesion of the amygdala nuclei. It results in hypersexuality, docility, and hyperorality.

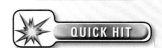
QUICK HIT
Muscle spindles function as the afferent limb of the myotactic (stretch) reflex (e.g., tapping knee with reflex hammer). Ventral horn motor neurons function as the efferent limb.

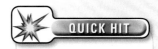
QUICK HIT
Muscle spindles are arranged **in parallel** with the extrafusal muscle fibers; **Golgi tendon organs** are arranged in **series**.

The Nervous System

FIGURE 2-8 Important pathways of the spinal cord

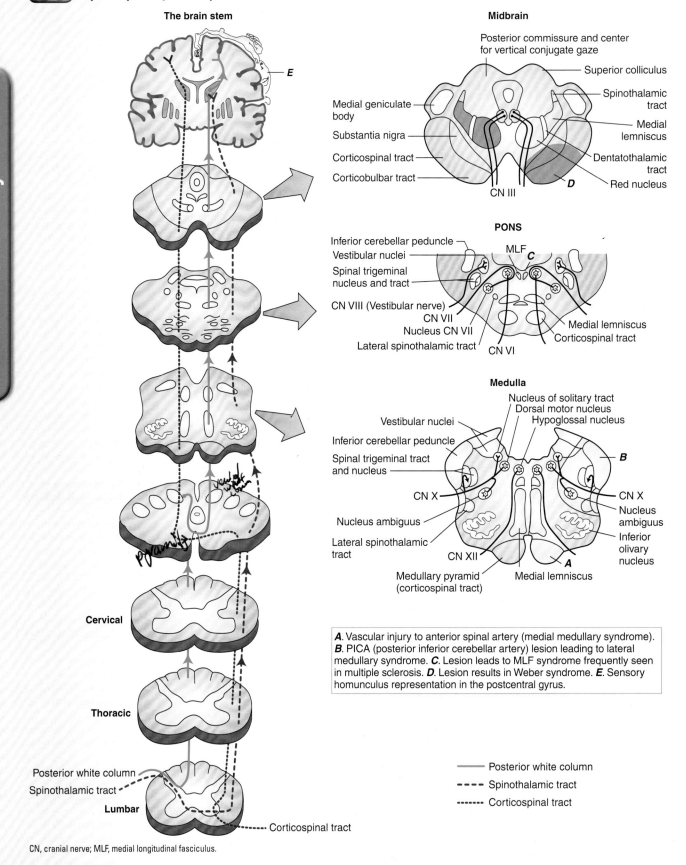

The brain stem

E

Midbrain

Posterior commissure and center for vertical conjugate gaze
Superior colliculus
Spinothalamic tract
Medial geniculate body
Medial lemniscus
Substantia nigra
Dentatothalamic tract
Corticospinal tract
Red nucleus
Corticobulbar tract
CN III
D

PONS

Inferior cerebellar peduncle
MLF
C
Vestibular nuclei
Spinal trigeminal nucleus and tract
CN VIII (Vestibular nerve)
CN VII
Medial lemniscus
Nucleus CN VII
Corticospinal tract
Lateral spinothalamic tract
CN VI

Medulla

Nucleus of solitary tract
Dorsal motor nucleus
Hypoglossal nucleus
Vestibular nuclei
Inferior cerebellar peduncle
B
Spinal trigeminal tract and nucleus
CN X
CN X
Nucleus ambiguus
Nucleus ambiguus
Inferior olivary nucleus
Lateral spinothalamic tract
CN XII
A
Medullary pyramid (corticospinal tract)
Medial lemniscus

Cervical

Thoracic

Posterior white column
Spinothalamic tract
Lumbar
Corticospinal tract

A. Vascular injury to anterior spinal artery (medial medullary syndrome). *B*. PICA (posterior inferior cerebellar artery) lesion leading to lateral medullary syndrome. *C*. Lesion leads to MLF syndrome frequently seen in multiple sclerosis. *D*. Lesion results in Weber syndrome. *E*. Sensory homunculus representation in the postcentral gyrus.

——— Posterior white column
- - - - Spinothalamic tract
······ Corticospinal tract

CN, cranial nerve; MLF, medial longitudinal fasciculus.

4. Muscle spindles (length of a muscle) *parallel*
5. **Golgi tendon organs** (**tension** on a muscle) *series*
C. First-order neurons of the dorsal root ganglia enter at the dorsal horn, ascend in the **fasciculus gracilis (lower limb)** and **fasciculus cuneatus (upper limb)**, and synapse in the nucleus gracilis and cuneatus.
D. Second-order neurons arise from these two nuclei, decussate at the level of the inferior medulla, and ascend as the **medial lemniscus**.
E. Medial lemniscus fibers synapse in the **ventral posterolateral (VPL) nucleus** of the thalamus, and third-order neurons project to the **primary somatosensory cortex**.
F. Lesions below the decussation produce ipsilateral loss of discriminatory touch, proprioception, and vibration, whereas lesions above the decussation produce contralateral loss of these sensations.

II. Spinothalamic tract
A. The spinothalamic tract is the ascending pathway that conveys **pain** and **temperature** from the body.
B. It receives input from free nerve endings of fast (A-type) and slow (C-type) pain fibers.
C. First-order neurons originate in the dorsal root ganglion, enter the spinal cord, and synapse on second-order neurons in the dorsolateral tract of Lissauer (thoracic vertebra level 2 [T2] to lumbar vertebra level 3 [L3]).
D. Second-order neurons ascend while decussating through the **ventral white commissure** and continue to ascend in the lateral spinothalamic tract, terminating in the VPL nucleus of the thalamus.
E. Third-order neurons originate in the VPL and project to the primary somatosensory **cortex**.
F. Lesions of the spinothalamic tract produce contralateral loss of pain and temperature sensation beginning **one level below that of the lesion**.

III. Corticospinal tract
A. The corticospinal tract is the descending pathway that originates in the **primary motor cortex**.
B. It mediates **voluntary movement** of striated muscle.
C. First-order neurons project to the posterior limb of the internal capsule, descend through the middle three-fifths of the midbrain's **crus cerebri** and base of the pons, **decussate in the pyramids of the medulla**, and continue down the spinal cord as the corticospinal tract.
D. Corticospinal fibers synapse on second-order neurons of the ventral horn via interneurons.
E. Lesions above the pyramids (upper motor neurons [**UMNs**]) produce **contralateral spastic paresis** and a positive Babinski sign (upgoing toes).
F. Lesions below the pyramids (**UMNs**) produce **ipsilateral spastic paresis** and a positive Babinski sign.
G. Lesions of the second-order neurons (lower motor neurons [**LMNs**]) produce **flaccid paralysis** and fasciculations.

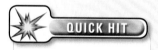

QUICK HIT

In amyotrophic lateral sclerosis (ALS), there is damage to both upper and lower motor neurons, producing symptoms of both spastic and flaccid paresis.

IMPORTANT PATHWAYS OF THE BRAIN STEM AND CEREBRUM

I. Trigeminothalamic pathway
A. The trigeminothalamic pathway is the ascending pathway that conveys **pain** and **temperature from the face** (analogous to the spinothalamic tract).
B. It receives input from free nerve endings of fast (A-type) and slow (C-type) pain fibers.
C. First-order neurons originate in the **trigeminal** ganglion and synapse on second-order neurons in the spinal trigeminal nucleus (ventral trigeminothalamic tract) or principal sensory nucleus of the trigeminal nerve (dorsal trigeminothalamic tract).

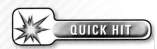

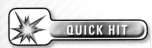

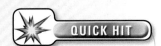

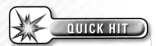

D. Second-order neurons of the ventral tract decussate while ascending; however, the dorsal tract neurons remain uncrossed, with termination in the ventral posteromedial (VPM) nucleus of the thalamus.

E. Third-order neurons originate in the VPM nucleus and project to the **primary somatosensory cortex**.

II. Corticobulbar tract

A. The corticobulbar tract is the descending pathway that originates in the **primary motor cortex**.

B. It mediates voluntary movement of the muscles of facial expression (analogous to the corticospinal tract).

C. First-order neurons project to the genu of the **internal capsule**, descend through the anterior one-third of the midbrain's crus cerebri, and synapse in the nucleus of CN VII (facial nucleus).

D. Second-order neurons innervate the muscles of facial expression (orbicularis oculi, orbicularis oris, buccinator, frontalis, and platysma) via the **facial** nerve.

E. The upper face (orbicularis oculi and frontalis muscles) receives bilateral input from the UMN and therefore is unaffected by unilateral cortical lesions.

F. The lower face (buccinator, orbicularis oris, and platysma) receives only contralateral input.

III. Cerebellar pathway

A. The cerebellar pathway controls posture and balance, maintains muscle tone, and coordinates motor activity.

B. The **dentatothalamic** tract is the major cerebellar tract.
   1. It originates in the dentate nucleus of the cerebellum.
   2. It projects to the **ventrolateral** nucleus of the thalamus (not the VPL nucleus) via the superior cerebellar peduncle.
   3. Thalamic fibers within the tract project to area 4 (primary motor cortex; see Figure 2-7A).
   4. Cerebral fibers within the tract project to corticospinal neurons.
   5. The pons receives cerebral fibers and sends fibers to the cerebellum, where they terminate on mossy fibers.

C. Damage to one side of the vestibulocerebellum results in ipsilateral findings. Patient will fall toward the affected side (**positive Romberg sign**).

IV. Vestibulocochlear pathways

A. **Auditory pathway**
   1. The auditory pathway originates from hair cells in the organ of Corti in the cochlea.
   2. Signals are sent down bipolar cell axons and are then relayed to the cochlear nuclei of the pons via the spiral ganglion.
   3. Signals are sent to higher CNS areas and relayed to the cerebral hemisphere via the **medial geniculate body of the thalamus**.
   4. Fibers terminate in the transverse temporal gyri.
   5. Because of the bilateral projection of information in the auditory pathway, one-sided lesions of this pathway at any point beyond the cochlear nuclei do not produce hearing loss.
   6. Lesions of the cochlear nerve itself will produce ipsilateral hearing loss.

B. **Vestibular pathway**
   1. Hair cells of the three **semicircular canals** encode **angular acceleration** and **deceleration**.
   2. Hair cells of the **utricle** encode **linear acceleration**.
   3. Information is passed via the vestibular nerve to the vestibular nuclei of the low pons.
   4. Fibers then project to:
      a. The spinal cord
      b. The cerebellum

Form of Nystagmus	Direction of Movement during Fast Phase	Direction of Movement during Slow Phase
Rotary nystagmus (i.e., while spinning in a circle)	Same as direction of rotation	Opposite direction of rotation
Postrotary nystagmus (i.e., after spinning in a circle)	Opposite direction of rotation	Same as direction of rotation
Caloric nystagmus		
• Warm water placed in one ear	**Toward the ear with warm water placed in it**	**Away from the ear with warm water placed in it**
• Cold water placed in one ear	**Away from the ear with cold water placed in it**	**Toward the ear with cold water placed in it**

TABLE **2-4** **Direction of Movement in Types of Nystagmus**

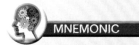

MNEMONIC

Remember **COWS: c**old **o**pposite, **w**arm **s**ame side for the direction of movement during fast phase of caloric nystagmus.

    c. The thalamus
    d. CNs III, IV, and VI via the medial longitudinal fasciculus (MLF)
  5. **Nystagmus** is mediated by the vestibular and oculomotor nuclei, the MLF, and the muscles of ocular movement controlled by CNs III, IV, and VI (Table 2-4).

V. Visual pathways and vision abnormalities (*Figure 2-9*)
  A. Muscles of the eye (Figure 2-10)
  B. **Horner syndrome**
    1. It is caused by a lesion of the sympathetic trunk in the neck.
    2. Clinical features of the syndrome include ipsilateral **ptosis, anhydrosis, flushing of skin**, and **miosis**.
  C. **Argyll Robertson pupil**   *♂ constricts*
    1. A pupil that **accommodates** to near objects but **does not react to light**
    2. Seen in syphilis, systemic lupus erythematosus (SLE), and diabetes mellitus
  D. **Marcus Gunn pupil** (aka afferent defect)   *Pretectal area issue*
    1. It is caused by a relative deficit in the afferent portion of the light reflex pathway.
    2. Shining a light in the affected pupil causes minimal bilateral constriction, but shining light in the unaffected pupil causes normal constriction of both pupils.
  E. **MLF syndrome**
    1. Caused by a lesion of the MLF and can be unilateral or bilateral.
    2. **Clinical features**
      a. The ipsilateral eye (the eye on the side of the MLF lesion) is unable to adduct, and the contralateral eye (the opposite eye) has nystagmus. For example, in the cases of right MLF lesions, the right eye is unable to adduct and the left eye has nystagmus when looking left.
      b. Convergence is unaffected.
    3. Often seen in **multiple sclerosis (MS)** and may be seen in stroke.
  F. **Uncal herniation**
    1. The uncus of the temporal lobe is forced through the opening of the tentorium.
    2. Clinical features include (Figure 2-9):
      a. Compression of CN III occurs, leading to fixed and dilated ("blown") pupil on ipsilateral side
      b. Ophthalmoplegia (paralysis of one or more of the ocular muscles)
      c. Compression of the corticospinal tract leading to ipsilateral hemiparesis
      d. Compression of the posterior cerebral artery leading to contralateral homonymous hemianopsia

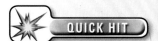

QUICK HIT

Injury to CN III (oculomotor) results in **ptosis** because of loss of the levator palpebrae superioris muscle, **exotropia** because of the unopposed pull of the lateral rectus, **dilation** of the pupil because of unopposed pull of the dilator pupillae muscle, and **impairment of near vision** as a result of loss of accommodation of the ciliary muscle.

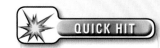

QUICK HIT

Horner syndrome is often caused by **Pancoast tumor**, a lung neoplasm that invades the cervical sympathetic chain.

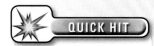

QUICK HIT

The Marcus Gunn pupil can be diagnosed using the **swinging flashlight test**. Shining a flashlight in the normal pupil causes constriction of both pupils. Swinging the flashlight quickly to the affected eye causes paradoxical dilation of the pupils.

The Nervous System

The Nervous System

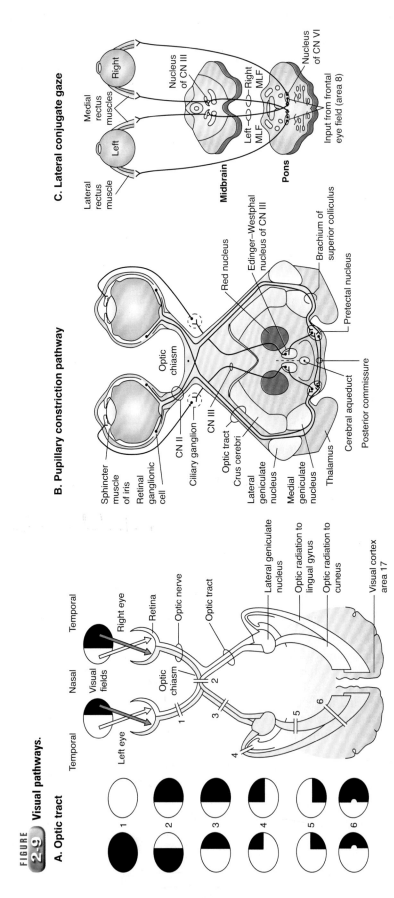

FIGURE 2-9 Visual pathways.

A. Legend for lesions: (1) total blindness; (2) bitemporal hemianopsia—common lesion caused by superiorly growing pituitary tumor; (3) right hemianopsia; (4) right upper quadrantanopia; (5) right lower quadrantanopia; (6) right hemianopsia with macular sparing. **B.** Light shined in one eye causes constriction of both pupils. **C.** Abduction of one eye results in adduction of the other eye in individuals with an intact medial longitudinal fasciculus and normal lateral conjugate gaze. CN, cranial nerve; MLF, medial longitudinal fasciculus. (Adapted from Chung, Kyung Won. *BRS Gross Anatomy*. 2nd ed. Baltimore, MD: Lippincott Williams & Wilkins; 1991:302, with permission.)

FIGURE 2-10 Muscles of the eye

Superior rectus muscle
- Innervated by CN III (oculomotor)
- Causes eye to look upward
- Loss of function causes deviation downward

Superior oblique muscle
- Innervated by CN IV (trochlear)
- Causes eye to look downward and laterally, also intorts the eye
- Loss of function causes deviation medially and superiorly

Medial rectus muscle
- Innervated by CN III (oculomotor)
- Causes adduction of the eye
- Loss of function causes abduction

Trochlea

Cornea

Common tendinous ring

Optic nerve

Inferior oblique muscle
- Innervated by CN III (oculomotor)
- Causes eye to look upward and laterally, also extorts the eye
- Loss of function causes deviation medially and inferiorly

Lateral rectus muscle
- Innervated by CN VI (abducens)
- Causes abduction of the eye
- Loss of function causes adduction

Inferior rectus muscle
- Innervated by CN III (oculomotor)
- Causes eye to look downward
- Loss of function causes deviation upward

CN, cranial nerve. (Adapted from Chung, Kyung Won. *BRS Gross Anatomy.* 2nd ed. Baltimore, MD: Lippincott Williams & Wilkins; 1991:302, with permission.)

TABLE 2-5 Common Ocular Pathology

Disorder	Etiology	Pathology	Clinical Features
Diabetic retinopathy	Proposed mechanism: accumulation of sorbitol in capillary pericytes results in loss of function, leading to retinal ischemia	Nonproliferative type observes microaneurysms, flame hemorrhages, dot and blot hemorrhages, soft exudates (cotton-wool spots), hard exudates (deposits of protein that have leaked from damaged capillaries), venous beading; proliferative type also observes neovascularization and fibrosis	Loss of visual acuity; advanced disease is the major cause of blindness
Age-related macular degeneration	Proposed mechanism: genetic	Pigmentary changes (drusen), macular hemorrhage or edema	Loss of central vision
Cataract	Aging, diabetes, galactosemia, Hurler disease, congenital causes (trisomy, myotonic dystrophy, hypoglycemia, TORCH infections)	Opacity of lens as a result of precipitation of sorbitol (diabetes), galactitol (galactosemia), mucopolysaccharide (Hurler disease), lens proteins (senile)	Decreased visual acuity, glare
Hypertensive retinopathy	High blood pressure → damages capillary walls	Copper wiring, flame hemorrhages, arteriovenous nicking, optic disc swelling (acute rise in blood pressure)	
Atherosclerosis	Atherosclerotic plaque from carotid artery embolizes into ipsilateral retinal artery	Hollenhorst plaque, copper wiring, flame hemorrhages, arteriovenous nicking	Amaurosis fugax (transient loss in vision, classically described as "shade falling over eye")
Papilledema	Increased intracranial pressure	Optic disc swelling (bilateral)	Headache; no changes in visual acuity until advanced disease
Angle-closure glaucoma	Acutely increased intraocular pressure	The lens abuts the posterior surface of the iris, pushing the iris forward and blocking the flow of aqueous humor	Acutely red, painful, rock-hard eye; decreased vision; halos around lights
Open-angle glaucoma	Chronically increased intraocular pressure	Less well understood; may be due to degeneration of the trabecular meshwork and canal of Schlemm	Gradual onset of loss of peripheral vision

TORCH, toxoplasmosis, other infections, rubella, cytomegalovirus, and herpes simplex virus.

FIGURE
2-11 Age-related macular degeneration

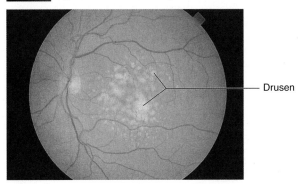

— Drusen

(Reproduced from Tasman W, Jaeger E. *The Wills Eye Hospital Atlas of Clinical Ophthalmology.* 2nd ed. Baltimore, MD: Lippincott Williams & Wilkins; 2001, with permission.)

FIGURE
2-12 Diabetic retinopathy

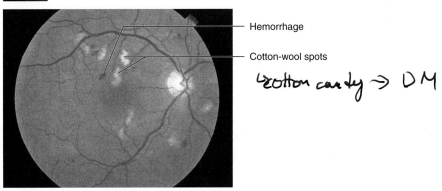

— Hemorrhage

— Cotton-wool spots

cotton canty → DM

(Reproduced from Tasman W, Jaeger E. *The Wills Eye Hospital Atlas of Clinical Ophthalmology.* 2nd ed. Baltimore, MD: Lippincott Williams & Wilkins; 2001, with permission.)

VI. Taste

A. The **solitary** nucleus of the medulla receives taste sensation via the solitary tract from three sources:
  1. The anterior two-thirds of the tongue via the **chorda tympani** nerve of the facial nerve (CN VII)
  2. The posterior third of the tongue via the **glossopharyngeal** nerve (CN IX)
  3. The epiglottic region of the pharynx via the **vagus** nerve (CN X)

B. Neurons carrying taste sensations ascend in the ventral tegmental tract to the VPM nucleus of the thalamus.

C. The VPM nucleus of the thalamus sends fibers to the parietal lobe.

VII. Limbic system

A. Mediates behavior and emotion, specifically:
  1. Feeding
  2. Feeling (emotions)
  3. Fighting
  4. Fleeing
  5. Sexual activity

B. Primarily controlled by the hypothalamus and autonomic nervous system

C. Primary components
  1. Anterior nucleus of thalamus
  2. Cingulate gyrus
  3. Mammillary bodies
  4. Septal area
  5. Hippocampus
  6. Amygdala (Table 2-5 and Figs. 2-11 and 2-12)

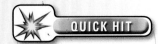

QUICK HIT

Lesions of the mammillary bodies occur in thiamine deficiency, commonly seen in chronic alcoholism due to malnutrition. Damage results in **Korsakoff syndrome,** characterized by confusion, severe memory impairment, and confabulation, which is **irreversible.**

CLASSIC LESIONS OF THE SPINAL CORD (Figure 2-13)

FIGURE 2-13 Classic lesions of the spinal cord

Tabes dorsalis
- Seen in tertiary syphilis
- Bilateral loss of touch, vibration, and tactile sense from lower limbs due to lesion of fasciculus gracilis

A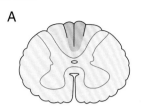

B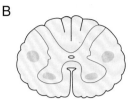

Amyotrophic lateral sclerosis
- Combined UMN and LMN lesion of corticospinal tract
- Spastic paresis (UMN sign)
- Flaccid paralysis with fasciculations (LMN)

Brown–Séquard syndrome
- Ipsilateral loss of touch and vibration and tactile sense below lesion due to posterior white column lesion
- Contralateral loss of pain and touch due to loss of spinothalamic tract
- Ipsilateral spastic paresis below lesion due to lesion of corticospinal tract
- Ipsilateral flaccid paralysis at level of lesion due to loss of LMN
- If lesion occurs above T1, Horner syndrome on side of lesion will result

C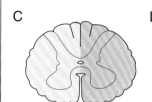

D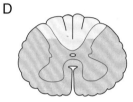

Spinal artery infarct
- Bilateral loss of pain and temperature one level below lesion due to loss of spinothalamic tract
- Bilateral spastic paresis below lesion due to lesion of corticospinal tract
- Bilateral flaccid paralysis at level of lesion due to loss of LMN
- Loss of bladder control due to lesion of corticospinal tract innervation of S2–S4 parasympathetics
- Bilateral Horner syndrome if above T2

Subacute combined degeneration (Vitamin B₁₂ deficiency)
- Bilateral loss of touch, vibration, and tactile sense due to posterior white column lesion
- Bilateral spastic paresis below lesion due to lesion of corticospinal tracts

E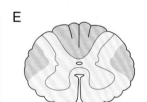

F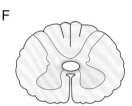

Syringomyelia
- Bilateral loss of pain and temperature one level below due to lesion of ventral white commissure (spinothalamic tract)
- Bilateral flaccid paralysis of level of lesion due to loss of LMN

LMN, lower motor neuron; UMN, upper motor neuron.

HYPOTHALAMUS (Figure 2-14)

FIGURE 2-14 Hypothalamus

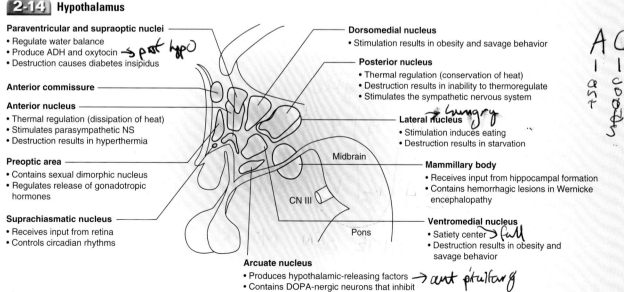

Paraventricular and supraoptic nuclei
- Regulate water balance
- Produce ADH and oxytocin → post hypo
- Destruction causes diabetes insipidus

Anterior commissure

Anterior nucleus
- Thermal regulation (dissipation of heat)
- Stimulates parasympathetic NS
- Destruction results in hyperthermia

Preoptic area
- Contains sexual dimorphic nucleus
- Regulates release of gonadotropic hormones

Suprachiasmatic nucleus
- Receives input from retina
- Controls circadian rhythms

Dorsomedial nucleus
- Stimulation results in obesity and savage behavior

Posterior nucleus
- Thermal regulation (conservation of heat)
- Destruction results in inability to thermoregulate
- Stimulates the sympathetic nervous system

Lateral nucleus hungry
- Stimulation induces eating
- Destruction results in starvation

Midbrain

Mammillary body
- Receives input from hippocampal formation
- Contains hemorrhagic lesions in Wernicke encephalopathy

CN III

Pons

Ventromedial nucleus
- Satiety center → full
- Destruction results in obesity and savage behavior

Arcuate nucleus
- Produces hypothalamic-releasing factors → ant pituitary
- Contains DOPA-nergic neurons that inhibit prolactin release

ADH, antidiuretic hormone; CN, cranial nerve; NS, nervous system. (Redrawn from Fix JD. *High-Yield Neuroanatomy.* Baltimore, MD: Lippincott Williams & Wilkins; 1995:84, with permission.)

THALAMUS *(Figure 2-15)*

FIGURE 2-15 Thalamus

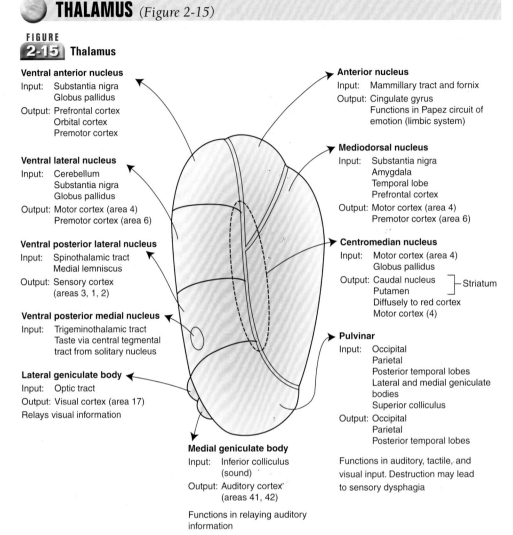

Ventral anterior nucleus

Input: Substantia nigra
Globus pallidus

Output: Prefrontal cortex
Orbital cortex
Premotor cortex

Ventral lateral nucleus

Input: Cerebellum
Substantia nigra
Globus pallidus

Output: Motor cortex (area 4)
Premotor cortex (area 6)

Ventral posterior lateral nucleus

Input: Spinothalamic tract
Medial lemniscus

Output: Sensory cortex
(areas 3, 1, 2)

Ventral posterior medial nucleus

Input: Trigeminothalamic tract
Taste via central tegmental
tract from solitary nucleus

Lateral geniculate body

Input: Optic tract

Output: Visual cortex (area 17)

Relays visual information

Medial geniculate body

Input: Inferior colliculus
(sound)

Output: Auditory cortex
(areas 41, 42)

Functions in relaying auditory
information

Anterior nucleus

Input: Mammillary tract and fornix

Output: Cingulate gyrus
Functions in Papez circuit of
emotion (limbic system)

Mediodorsal nucleus

Input: Substantia nigra
Amygdala
Temporal lobe
Prefrontal cortex

Output: Motor cortex (area 4)
Premotor cortex (area 6)

Centromedian nucleus

Input: Motor cortex (area 4)
Globus pallidus

Output: Caudal nucleus ⎤
Putamen ⎦ Striatum
Diffusely to red cortex
Motor cortex (4)

Pulvinar

Input: Occipital
Parietal
Posterior temporal lobes
Lateral and medial geniculate
bodies
Superior colliculus

Output: Occipital
Parietal
Posterior temporal lobes

Functions in auditory, tactile, and
visual input. Destruction may lead
to sensory dysphagia

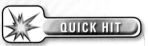

> **QUICK HIT**
>
> Tic douloureux (trigeminal neuralgia) is marked by severe stabbing bursts of pain in the distribution of CN V.

CRANIAL NERVES

The 12 CNs arise from various nuclei within the brain stem and cortex and serve multiple functions in the body. Their extracranial course is important for locating lesions, which can be tested by asking the patient to perform simple tasks. Table 2-6 outlines important information about CNs I to XII.

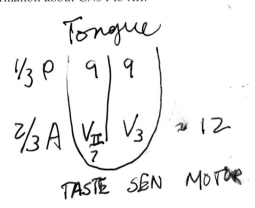

TABLE 2-6 Cranial Nerves

Nerve	Site of Exit from Skull	Function	Common Lesions	Test
I—Olfactory	Cribriform	Smell	Cribriform plate fracture, Kallmann syndrome	Smell
II—Optic	Optic canal	Sight	Figure 2-9	Snellen chart, peripheral vision
III—Oculomotor	Superior orbital fissure	**Parasympathetic** to **ciliary and sphincter muscles,** medial rectus, superior rectus, inferior rectus, inferior oblique	Transtentorial (uncal) herniation, **diabetes,** Weber syndrome	"H" in space, pupillary light reflexes, convergence
IV—Trochlear	Superior orbital fissure	Superior oblique muscle	Head trauma	"H" in space
V—Trigeminal V1—Ophthalmic	Superior orbital fissure	Sensory from medial nose, forehead	Tic douloureux (trigeminal neuralgia)	Facial sensation, open jaw (**deviates toward lesion**)
V2—Maxillary	Foramen rotundum	Sensory from lateral nose, upper lip, superior buccal area		
V3—Mandibular	Foramen ovale	**Muscles of mastication,** tensor tympani, tensor veli palatini; sensory from lower lip, lateral face to lower border of mandible		
VI—Abducens	Superior orbital fissure	Lateral rectus muscle	**Medial inferior pontine syndrome**	"H" in space
VII—Facial	Internal acoustic meatus	Parasympathetic to lacrimal, submandibular, and sublingual glands; **muscles of facial expression and stapedius, stylohyoid muscle; posterior belly of digastric muscle,** sensory from anterior two-thirds of tongue (including taste **via chorda tympani**)	**Bell palsy**	Wrinkle forehead, show teeth, puff out cheeks, close eyes tightly
VIII—Vestibulocochlear	Internal acoustic meatus	Equilibrium, hearing	**Acoustic schwannoma**	Hearing, nystagmus (slow phase toward lesion)
IX—Glossopharyngeal	Jugular foramen	Parasympathetic to parotid gland; stylopharyngeus muscle; sensory from pharynx, middle ear, auditory tube, carotid body and sinus, external ear, posterior third of tongue (including taste)	Posterior inferior cerebellar artery **(PICA)** infarct	Gag reflex (no response ipsilateral to lesion)
X—Vagus	Jugular foramen	Parasympathetic to body viscera; laryngeal and pharyngeal muscles; sensory from trachea, esophagus, viscera, external ear, epiglottis (including taste)	Thyroidectomy, **PICA** infarct	Gag reflex (**uvula deviates away from lesion**)
XI—Accessory	Jugular foramen	Sternocleidomastoid and trapezius muscles	**PICA** infarct	Turning head (weakness turning away from lesion), raising shoulder against resistance (ipsilateral)
XII—Hypoglossal	Hypoglossal canal	Intrinsic tongue muscles	Anterior spinal artery infarct	Tongue protrusion (**deviates toward lesion**)

Handwritten mnemonic annotations (Nerve column): COME, ON, SOFIA, SOFIA, SOFIA, RIGHT, ON, SOFIA, I'M, INTO, JUGS, JOE, SUE, MORE

Handwritten mnemonic annotations (Function column): SOME, SAY, MARRY, MONEY, BUT, MY, BROTHER, SAYS, BIG, BOOBS, MATTER, MORE

CONTENTS OF THE CAVERNOUS SINUS (Figure 2-16)

FIGURE
2-16 Contents of the cavernous sinus

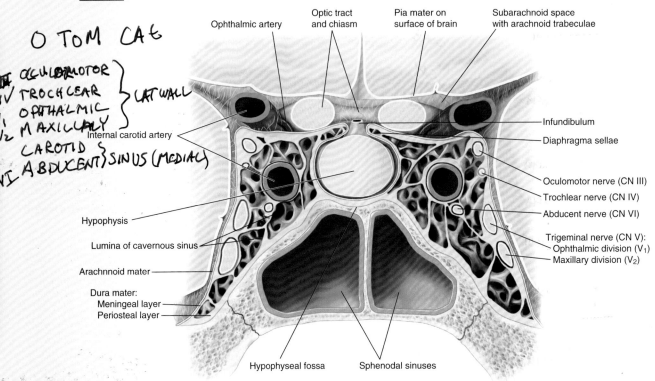

O TOM CAt

III OCULOMOTOR
IV TROCHLEAR } *LAT WALL*
V₁ OPTHALMIC
V₂ MAXILLARY
CAROTID } *SINUS (MEDIAL)*
VI ABDUCENT

CN, cranial nerve. (From Tank PW, Gest TR. Lippincott *Williams & Wilkins Atlas of Anatomy.* Baltimore: Wolters Kluwer Health, 2009. Used with permission)

SLEEP (Figure 2-17)

FIGURE
2-17 The sleep cycle

Stages of rapid eye movement (REM) sleep in the young adult. As sleep progresses, slow-wave sleep decreases and REM sleep episodes increase in duration and frequency. In the elderly, there is decreased slow-wave sleep, increased awakenings, early sleep onset, and early morning awakenings. Solid bars indicate REM sleep.

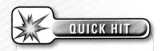

QUICK HIT

The time spent in stage N3 sleep decreases with age and with the use of some drugs (e.g., benzodiazepines).

I. Sleep–wake cycles

A. Based on circadian rhythms controlled by the suprachiasmatic nucleus of the hypothalamus

B. **Serotonin** (5-HT) released from the raphe nuclei of the brain stem is important in initiating sleep, whereas the **reticular activating system** maintains alertness.

C. Sleep is divided in the three non–rapid eye movement (REM) stages (N1, N2, and N3), and REM sleep.
1. An awake, alert individual shows low amplitude, high-frequency (12 to 30 Hz) **beta** waves on electroencephalogram (EEG).
2. A relaxed individual (still awake but with eyes closed, in preparation for sleep) shows lower frequency (8 to 12 Hz) **alpha** waves.
3. **Stage N1** of sleep (light sleep) shows alpha waves giving way to low-frequency (4 to 7 Hz) **theta** waves.
4. Stage N2 sleep shows **sleep spindles** and **K-complexes** on EEG.
5. Stage N3 sleep ("slow-wave sleep," deep sleep) shows very low-frequency (0 to 4 Hz) **delta** waves. Dreaming is possible (though less common than in REM sleep).
6. REM sleep normally occurs at 90-minute intervals and is characterized by high-frequency **beta** waves, which mirror those seen in the alert individual in the waking state. Most dreaming occurs during REM sleep along with increased brain oxygen consumption, nocturnal erections, and loss of skeletal muscle tone. REM sleep is thought to be important for memory processing and consolidation.

II. Common sleep disorders

A. Insomnia affects 30% of the U.S. population. It is associated with anxiety and leads to daytime sleepiness.
B. Restless leg syndrome is the sensation of unpleasant paresthesias that compels the patient to have voluntary, spontaneous, continuous leg movements. It is usually a primary idiopathic disorder, but it can occur secondary to iron deficiency, end-stage renal disease, diabetic neuropathy, Parkinson disease, pregnancy, rheumatic diseases, varicose veins, and excessive caffeine intake.
C. Nightmares versus night terrors
1. Nightmares are frightening dreams that occur during REM sleep, and patients actually awake from sleep.
2. Night terrors occur during non-REM sleep, and patients may appear to be awake (frightened/screaming, tachycardic, and diaphoretic) but are not actually fully awake. They are often difficult to arouse and usually fall right back to sleep after the episode.
D. Central sleep apnea, affecting less than 0.5% of the population, involves an absence of respiratory effort (for a discussion of obstructive sleep apnea, see Chapter 4).
E. Narcolepsy is seen in 0.04% of the population and is characterized by sudden onset of sleep with rapid onset of REM sleep. It may be associated with hallucinations and cataplexy (sudden loss of muscle tone).
F. Nocturnal enuresis is overnight bed-wetting after 5 years of age (developmental age), when daytime bladder control has been achieved. It is often familial.
1. Treatment is usually delayed until the child is at least 7 years of age.
2. Behavioral interventions are usually first line, including motivational therapy (e.g., star charts), nighttime fluid restriction, scheduled wakening, and enuresis alarms (most effective long-term therapy).
3. Pharmacologic interventions are usually second line and may include short-term imipramine, oral desmopressin, or indomethacin. There is a high likelihood of recurrence upon discontinuation.

SEIZURE TYPES

Seizures are paroxysmal events caused by abnormal and excessive discharges from CNS neurons triggered by a variety of causes (Table 2-7).

The antiepileptic agents, which include several different medications, affect **ion channels** (Table 2-8). The side effects of these agents are often significant. Because it is frequently necessary to take these agents for long periods, it is important to understand these side effects.

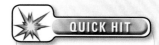

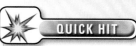

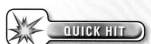

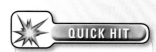

The Nervous System

TABLE 2-7 Seizure Types

Type	Patient	Presentation	Pathology	Treatment
Simple partial seizures	All ages	Malfunction of one muscle or muscle group No loss of consciousness Sensory distortions	Single focus in brain No spread, localized muscular manifestations With chronicity, may progress to generalized muscular manifestations	Phenytoin, carbamazepine
Jacksonian seizures	All ages (subtype of simple partial)	Expanding area of motor malfunction	Original focus spreads to adjacent areas of cortex	Carbamazepine
Complex partial seizures	First seizure during first two decades of life may be caused by fever in children 6 months to 5 years of age (febrile seizure)	Incontinence Jaw movements (or other automatisms) Loss of consciousness Elaborate sensory distortions	Single focus	Phenytoin, carbamazepine (febrile seizures do not require antiseizure medication)
Absence (petit mal) seizures	Begin at 2–3 years of age Often end with puberty	1–5 second loss of consciousness Several episodes per day Blank stare with rapid blinking	Original focus rapidly spreads across both hemispheres	Ethosuximide, valproic acid
Tonic–clonic (grand mal) seizures	Most common type Encountered in different clinical settings, often in patients with metabolic disorders	Sudden loss of consciousness Loss of postural control and continence Tonic phase (static extension) Clonic phase (jerking movements) Recovery period with exhaustion and disorientation	Original focus rapidly spreads across both hemispheres	Phenytoin, carbamazepine *Valproic acid*

TABLE 2-8 Antiepileptic Agents

Drug	Mechanism of Action	Type(s) of Seizure(s) Controlled	Side Effects	Notes
Carbamazepine	Blocks voltage-gated **sodium channels** by increasing the refractory period	Tonic–clonic (grand mal), partial, Jacksonian	Liver enzyme induction, ataxia, diplopia, blood dyscrasias (agranulocytosis, aplastic anemia), teratogenesis, **induction of cytochrome P450** *, SJS*	Can be used to treat trigeminal neuralgia
Ethosuximide	Inhibits certain ~~sodium~~ channels, *T-type Ca²⁺* particularly in certain parts of thalamus that produce cyclic cortical discharges	Absence	Headache, lethargy, diarrhea, urticaria, Stevens–Johnson syndrome	
Phenytoin	Blocks voltage-gated **sodium channels** by increasing refractory period *Zero-order kinetics*	Tonic–clonic (grand mal), partial	Liver enzyme induction, ataxia, diplopia, megaloblastic anemia, lupus-like syndrome, nystagmus, sedation, teratogenesis (fetal hydantoin syndrome), peripheral neuropathy, **hirsutism, gingival hyperplasia, induction of cytochrome P450,** malignant hyperthermia (rare)	
Valproic acid	May affect **po~~ta~~ssium channels** to cause hyperpolarization of neuronal membranes *Na, GABA*	Absence, tonic–clonic (grand mal), partial	Liver enzyme induction, diarrhea, rarely hepatotoxic, tremor, weight gain, neural tube defects in fetus (spina bifida)	Contraindicated in pregnancy
Phenobarbital (barbiturate)	Increase inhibitory effects of γ-aminobutyric acid (GABA) by increasing **duration of chloride channel** opening	Tonic–clonic (grand mal), partial	Liver enzyme induction, sedation, tolerance, dependence, induction of cytochrome P450	First line in pregnant women, children

First Line

(continued)

TABLE 2-8 Antiepileptic Agents (Continued)

Drug	Mechanism of Action	Type(s) of Seizure(s) Controlled	Side Effects	Notes
Benzodiazepines (diazepam, lorazepam)	Increase inhibitory effects of GABA by increasing **frequency of chloride channel** opening	First line for acute <u>status epilepticus</u>	Sedation, tolerance, dependence	Used for seizures of eclampsia
Lamotrigine	Blocks voltage-gated sodium channels *+ glutamate*	Tonic–clonic (grand mal), partial	<u>Stevens–Johnson syndrome</u>	
Gabapentin	Increases GABA release	Tonic–clonic (grand mal), partial	Sedation, ataxia	Used for peripheral neuropathy
Topiramate	Blocks sodium channels, increases GABA action	Tonic–clonic (grand mal), partial	Sedation, weight loss, nephrolithiasis	Also used for migraine prophylaxis

DEGENERATIVE DISEASES

Degeneration in specific parts of the CNS can lead to focal or systemic loss of function. Many of the degenerative diseases affecting the CNS are irreversible and are listed in Table 2-9.

Parkinson disease, a movement disorder, results from deterioration of the **basal ganglia**. **Dopamine** production decreases, which in turn increases the relative effects of **acetylcholine**. Treatment is symptomatic and is aimed at trying to restore the balance between the two hormones (Table 2-10).

TABLE 2-9 Degenerative Diseases

Disease	Etiology	Clinical Manifestation	Notes
Vitamin B$_{12}$ deficiency	Strict vegetarian diet, **pernicious anemia,** fundal gastritis type A, *Diphyllobothrium latum*	**Megaloblastic anemia, peripheral neuropathy, myelin degeneration of posterior white columns** and lateral corticospinal tracts	Megaloblastic anemia component of vitamin B$_{12}$ deficiency can be treated with folate; however, this will not resolve the peripheral neuropathy component of the deficiency
Parkinson disease	**Decrease in dopamine** caused by depletion of cells of substantia nigra and locus coeruleus; similar symptoms may be caused by depression, hydrocephaly, MPTP intoxication	**Resting tremors, masked facies, muscular rigidity,** shuffling gait, **Lewy bodies**	Usually appears after 55 years of age; therapy with dopamine precursors or ACh inhibitors
Poliomyelitis	Poliovirus (RNA); *enterovirus* fecal–oral; replicates in pharynx; spreads to CNS	Aseptic meningitis, **death of anterior horn cells** in spinal cord, paralysis	Killed (Salk) and live-attenuated (Sabin) vaccine available; Sabin vaccine given to children because of IgA response, longer action, and availability of oral form
Rabies	**Rhabdovirus** (RNA); spread via saliva *+ ss RNA - icosahedral non-enveloped CD155 epithelial cells*	Laryngeal spasm resulting in fear of water, CNS excitability, **Negri body** inclusions, hippocampal degeneration	Treatment via passive and active immunization at distant sites *IG vaccine*
Spongiform encephalopathies (a) Animals – Scrapie (sheep) – Bovine spongiform encephalopathy (BSE; cows; aka mad cow disease)	Prions: an abnormally folded variant of a normal cell protein; only infectious agent with no nucleic acid	Vacuolization of brain tissue, dementia, ataxia, depositions of the abnormal protein, long incubation (years), rapid death after onset (months)	Diagnosed at autopsy; no treatment; new-variant CJD acquired by eating BSE-contaminated meat; Kuru spread by nonalignment of neurologic tissue; CJD has been spread by corneal transplant and on contaminated neurosurgical equipment

(continued)

The Nervous System

The Nervous System

TABLE **2-9** **Degenerative Diseases** (*Continued*)

Disease	Etiology	Clinical Manifestation	Notes

(b) Humans
  – Creutzfeldt–Jakob disease (CJD)
  – New-variant CJD
  – Kuru			

Tay–Sachs disease	Autosomal recessive; **deficiency of hexosaminidase A** with increase in G_{M2}, ganglioside seizures	Mental retardation, **cherry-red spot on macula,** muscular weakness	Fatal, prenatal diagnosis possible, usually affects cells of CNS
Thiamine deficiency	Severe malnutrition (may be secondary to alcoholism)	**Degeneration of mammillary bodies**, Wernicke–Korsakoff syndrome—psychosis manifested with confusion, ataxia, and confabulation Dry beriberi—polyneuropathy with peripheral sensorimotor loss Wet beriberi—dry beriberi with cardiovascular symptoms	**Wernicke** encephalopathy **(reversible)** and **Korsakoff** syndrome **(irreversible)** are both secondary to deficiency caused by alcoholism
Wilson disease	Autosomal recessive; **decreased ceruloplasmin**	Copper accumulation, asterixis, dementia, liver cirrhosis, **Kayser–Fleischer ring** in cornea	Hepatolenticular **degeneration of the basal ganglia**

Ach, acetylcholine; CNS, central nervous system; IgA, immunoglobulin A; MPTP, 1-methyl-4-phenyl-1,2,3,6-tetrahydropyridine.

TABLE **2-10** **Antiparkinsonian Agents**

Drug	Mechanism of Action	Side Effects	Notes
Levodopa (L-dopa) (dopamine precursor)	More readily **crosses the blood–brain barrier;** converted to dopamine in the brain by DOPA decarboxylase	Dyskinesias (following dose), akinesia (between doses), postural hypotension, anorexia, depression, psychosis, arrhythmia	Development of tolerance, wildly varying effectiveness **(on–off phenomenon),** often necessitates drug holidays
Carbidopa	Inhibits conversion of L-dopa to dopamine in the periphery by **DOPA decarboxylase**	Decreases systemic side effects of L-dopa such as anorexia and nausea	Given with L-dopa, **does not cross the blood–brain barrier;** inhibition of systemic conversion of L-dopa, which reduces L-dopa dosing approximately 75%
Amantadine	Unclear; may stimulate dopamine receptors, stimulate dopamine release, or inhibit its reuptake	Agitation, restlessness, psychosis, urinary retention	Rapid deterioration of effectiveness over a period of weeks
Selegiline, rasagiline	Selectively and irreversibly **inhibits MAO type B,** which metabolizes dopamine	Dyskinesias, hepatic conversion to amphetamine causes insomnia and anorexia	In high doses, inhibition of MAO type A, which is prevalent in the gut, allowing absorption of ingested amines, which can cause **hypertensive crises**
Entacapone, tolcapone	Inhibits COMT, which metabolizes dopamine	Nausea, dyskinesia, orthostatic hypotension	Administered with levodopa/carbidopa to reduce "wearing off" symptoms at the end of dosing interval
Bromocriptine	Acts as a **dopamine receptor agonist**	Anorexia, nausea, vomiting, postural hypotension, psychosis	Given as an adjuvant with L-dopa, inhibits release of prolactin and growth hormone and is therefore used for **prolactinomas** and **acromegaly**
Pramipexole, ropinirole	Dopamine receptor agonist	Postural hypotension/syncope, dizziness, sedation, fatigue, hallucinations, abnormal dreams	Also used to treat restless leg syndrome
Benztropine	Blocks **muscarinic acetylcholine receptors**	**Atropine-like** side effects, inattention, psychosis	Used in combination with dopamine agonists and L-dopa, **improves tremor and rigidity** but has little effect on bradykinesia

COMT, catechol-*O*-methyltransferase; MAO, monoamine oxidase.

DEMYELINATING DISEASES

Loss of the neuronal sheath can lead to impaired nerve conduction, which, in turn, causes deficits and disease (Table 2-11).

DISEASES THAT CAUSE DEMENTIA

Dementia is a chronic progressive deterioration in cognitive ability in which mental faculties, such as executive function, attention span, judgment, memory, mood, and behavior, are affected (Table 2-12).

ACUTE MENINGITIS

Meningitis is an infection of the meninges resulting in an inflammatory reaction characterized by severe headache, fever, photophobia, and positive Kernig and Brudzinski signs. Meningitis in immunocompetent adults is generally caused by *Streptococcus pneumoniae* or

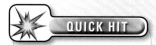

CNS stimulants, which are at the other end of the spectrum from the sedative-hypnotics, usually cause sympathetic stimulation, resulting in increased alertness. They can also lower the seizure threshold. Common drugs of this type are amphetamine, caffeine, cocaine, dextroamphetamine, ephedrine, and methylphenidate.

QUICK HIT

Tay–Sachs disease and Niemann–Pick disease, a deficiency of sphingomyelinase, can both present with a **cherry-red spot** on the macula.

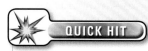

Amantadine, used in the treatment of Parkinson disease, also has antiviral effects and is sometimes used in the prevention and treatment of **influenza A.**

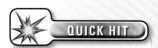

Werdnig–Hoffmann disease is an infantile, autosomal recessive, and lower motor neuron disease similar to ALS.

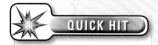

Progressive multifocal leukoencephalopathy is a demyelinating disease caused by JC virus infection of oligodendrocytes. It is seen in patients with immune deficiency.

TABLE 2-11 Demyelinating Diseases of the Nervous System

Disease	Etiology	Clinical Manifestation	Notes
Amyotrophic lateral sclerosis (ALS, Lou Gehrig disease)	No specific pattern of inheritance, although autosomal dominant in 5% of cases (similar symptoms with some heavy metal poisonings, infections, or tumors)	**Both upper and lower motor neuron signs;** loss of lateral corticospinal tracts and anterior motor neurons leading to muscle atrophy	Most common motor neuron disease; rapidly fatal course
Guillain–Barré syndrome	Postviral autoimmune reaction involving peripheral nerves	Muscle weakness and paralysis **ascending upward** from the lower extremities	Young adults; **albuminocytologic dissociation is** pathognomonic (high albumin, low cell count)
Huntington disease	Chromosome 4; **CAG triple-base repeat** with anticipation	Degeneration of **caudate nucleus,** onset at 30–40 years of age, athetoid movements, muscular deterioration, dementia	Usually involves acetylcholine (ACh) and γ-aminobutyric acid (GABA) neurons
Krabbe disease	Autosomal recessive; decrease in β-galactocerebrosidase	Loss of myelin from globoid cells and peripheral nerves, mental retardation, blindness, paralysis, **globoid bodies** in white matter	Usually affects infants; **rapidly fatal**
Metachromatic leukodystrophy	Autosomal recessive defect of arylsulfatase A	Progressive paralysis and dementia, loss of myelin, accumulation of sulfatides, nerves stain **yellow-brown** in color, ataxia	Fatal in first decade
Multiple sclerosis (MS)	Unknown; more common in northern Europe; more common in women	Multiple focal areas of demyelination; variable course; **Triad of MS:** intention tremor, scanning speech, nystagmus	Most common demyelinating disease; increased cerebrospinal fluid (CSF) immunoglobulin

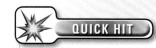

The Nervous System

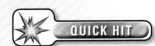

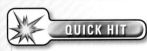

Clinical Vignette 2-2

CLINICAL PRESENTATION: A 28-year-old female presents to the emergency department complaining of numbness in her right leg that lasted several hours, which worsened when she took a **warm** shower. She also complained of feeling fatigued lately and she remembered that 1 year ago she had an episode of **transient unilateral vision loss** that resolved and never recurred. Vital signs: temperature = 97.0° F; blood pressure = 122/75 mm Hg; heart rate = 76 bpm; respiration rate = 18 breaths/min. Physical exam is significant for **nystagmus, scanning speech,** and diminished sensation in the right leg but normal strength.

DIFFERENTIALS: Multiple sclerosis (MS), Guillain–Barré syndrome.

DIAGNOSTIC STUDIES: Order magnetic resonance imaging (MRI) of the brain and a lumbar puncture (LP). MS should be suspected in young adults with relapsing and remitting neurologic signs and symptoms that do not seem associated to the same area of central nervous system (CNS) white matter. MRI shows **demyelinating lesions (plaques)** at the **angles of the lateral ventricles** (which is the classic location of plaques in MS). MS is caused by selective demyelination of the spinal cord and brain, sparing peripheral nervous system (PNS) and gray matter. There are no laboratory tests specific for MS, but LP and cerebrospinal fluid (CSF) analysis will show **oligoclonal bands of IgG in 90%** of patients with MS. Transient sensory deficits are a common presenting feature of MS, as are visual disturbances caused by optic neuritis. Optic neuritis presents as monocular visual loss, pain on movement of eyes, central scotoma (black spot in center of vision), or decreased pupillary reaction to light. Also, be aware of the **Charcot triad:** intention tremor, nystagmus, and scanning speech.

MANAGEMENT: Treat this patient with **high-dose intravenous (IV) corticosteroids,** which can shorten an **acute** attack. After treatment of an acute attack, manage patient with **interferon therapy,** which should be started early in the course of disease. Treat symptoms of muscle spasticity with baclofen and carbamazepine or gabapentin for neuropathic pain.

Neisseria meningitidis. Conditions predisposing an individual to acute bacterial meningitis as a result of pneumococcus include distant foci of infection (such as otitis, sinusitis, or pneumonia), sickle cell disease (secondary to splenic autoinfarction), alcoholism, or trauma with loss of meningeal integrity. Patients with a deficiency of complement components C5 to C8 are at a greater risk of developing meningococcal meningitis. *Haemophilus*

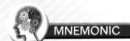

TABLE 2-12 Diseases That Cause Dementia

Disease	Etiology	Clinical Manifestation	Notes
Alzheimer dementia	Unknown; possibly **chromosome 21,** degeneration of nucleus basalis of Meynert, decreased choline acetyltransferase	Progressively worsening memory loss, **neurofibrillary tangles, senile plaques** (amyloid β/A4 protein)	**Most common cause of dementia;** age of onset is usually 65 years (younger in patients with Down syndrome)
Multi-infarct dementia	Cerebral atherosclerosis	Stepwise decline of function, signs of dementia and possible motor deficits	**Second most common cause of dementia**
Primary HIV dementia	Macrophages, infected with HIV, enter CNS	Onset before immunodeficiency, slow thinking, ataxia, *Toxoplasma gondii* on autopsy	**Most common CNS manifestation of HIV**
Frontotemporal dementia (Pick disease)	Unknown; may be familial	Dementia plus personality/behavioral changes; possibly progressive aphasia	
Lewy body dementia	Unknown; combination of genetics and environmental factors	Dementia plus parkinsonian features, visual hallucinations, syncope/falls	More common in men

CNS, central nervous system.

TABLE 2-13 Common Causes of Meningitis in Various Age Groups

Age Group	Causes
Newborns	Group B streptococci *Baby BEL* *Escherichia coli* *Listeria*
Children	*Haemophilus influenzae* b (declining since Hib vaccine introduced) *Streptococcus pneumoniae* *Neisseria meningitidis* *SHIN* Enteroviruses
Adolescents and young adults	Enteroviruses *N. meningitidis* } *sexy bugs* *S. pneumoniae* Herpes simplex virus
Elderly	*S. pneumoniae* Gram-negative rods *Listeria*

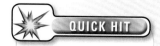
influenzae type B was once a common cause of meningitis in children, although these numbers have decreased because of widespread vaccination (Table 2-13).

Lumbar puncture (LP) is often performed to confirm a suspected diagnosis of meningitis. The LP usually shows increased neutrophils, increased protein, and decreased glucose if bacterial in origin. Also, organisms may be seen on Gram stain. However, if the CSF contains increased lymphocytes and a normal glucose level, viral agents such as enterovirus, HIV, and herpes simplex virus should be considered (Table 2-14). If the LP shows organisms with a thick capsule when stained with India ink, this suggests *Cryptococcus neoformans*; and the infected individual is most likely immunocompromised as a result of HIV infection. Adults who are immunocompromised are also at risk for developing meningitis caused by *Listeria monocytogenes*.

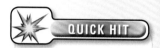
NERVOUS SYSTEM TUMORS

Nearly 50% of the tumors occurring within the nervous system are metastases to the brain from tumors elsewhere in the body. The other 50% are primary nervous system tumors. Tables 2-15 and 2-16 list the most common nervous system tumors in adults and children. Seventy percent of adult brain tumors are supratentorial; 70% of childhood brain tumors are infratentorial.

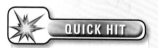
TABLE 2-14 Evaluation of Cerebrospinal Fluid to Determine Cause of Meningitis

Laboratory Test	Bacterial	Viral	Fungal
Opening CSF pressure	↑	N	↑
Lymphocytes	N	↑	↑
Neutrophils	↑	N	N
Glucose	↓	N	↓
Protein	↑	N	↑

↑, Increased; ↓, decreased; CSF, cerebrospinal fluid; N, normal.

QUICK HIT

Psammoma bodies are also seen in papillary adenocarcinoma of the thyroid, serous papillary cystadenocarcinoma of the ovary, and malignant mesothelioma.

P - papillary adenoma
S - serous adenocarcinoma ovary
M - Meningioma
M - Mesothelioma

TABLE 2-15 Nervous System Tumors in Adults

Tumor	Presentation	Significant Features
Metastatic neoplasms	Headache, focal defects, formation of discrete nodules in brain	Nearly half of all intracranial neoplasm; usually bloodborne; commonly from lung, breast, gastrointestinal, thyroid, kidney, genitourinary, and melanoma
Glioblastoma (grade IV astrocytoma)	Cerebral hemisphere tumor, irregular mass with necrotic center surrounded by edema seen on CT	**Most common primary intracranial neoplasm;** poor prognosis; neural tube origin; **pseudopalisading** arrangement of cells; astrocytes stain with GFAP
Meningioma	**Psammoma bodies,** slowly growing, originates in arachnoid cells, follows sinuses hormone receptors	Second most common primary CNS tumor; usually occurs in women; resectable; neural crest origin
Schwannoma	Tinnitus and hearing loss, ataxic gait, positive Romberg sign, increased intracranial pressure, hydrocephalus, benign biphasic neoplasm Verocay bodies - palisading	Third most common primary intracranial tumor; neural crest origin; usually occurs in the cerebellopontine angle and involves CN VIII; seen **bilaterally in neurofibromatosis type 2 (NF-2)**
Oligodendroglioma	Slow-growing frontal lobe tumor -GFAP +1p/19q	Rare; clearing of the cytoplasm around the nuclei **(perinuclear halo)** give tumor cells a **"fried egg" appearance**

CN, cranial nerve; CNS, central nervous system; CT, computed tomography; GFAP, glial fibrillary acidic protein.

TABLE 2-16 Nervous System Tumors in Children

Tumor	Presentation	Significant Features
Pilocytic astrocytoma (grade I astrocytoma)	Benign, usually posterior fossa, good prognosis BRAF mutation	**Most common primary brain tumor in children;** astrocytes stain with GFAP; eosinophilic Rosenthal fibers
Medulloblastoma	Cerebellar mass, may compress the fourth ventricle (**noncommunicating hydrocephalus**), ataxic gait, projectile vomiting	**Most common malignant primary brain tumor of childhood;** neural tube origin; **Homer-Wright rosettes** (circular arrangement of tumor cells around a central tangle of fibrils)
Ependymoma	May compress the fourth ventricle (**noncommunicating hydrocephalus**)	Neural tube origin; **perivascular rosettes** (circular arrangement of tumor cells around a central vessel)
Craniopharyngioma	Endocrine abnormalities, papilledema, **bitemporal hemianopsia** due to compression of optic chiasm	Enlarged sella turcica; **most common supratentorial brain tumor in children; ectodermal origin** (Rathke pouch)

GFAP, glial fibrillary acidic protein.

HEADACHE (Table 2-17)

TABLE 2-17 Primary Headache Syndromes

Type	General Characteristics	Clinical Features	Treatment
Tension	Worsens throughout the day; precipitated by stress, anxiety, and depression; more frequent in women	Tight, **bandlike** pain encircling the entire head; most intense around the neck or back of head; tenderness in posterior neck muscles	Stress reduction, NSAIDs, acetaminophen, and aspirin if mild/moderate; if severe, TCAs or SSRIs
Cluster	Usually occurs in **middle-aged men; episodic**—lasts 2–3 months, with remissions of months to years; occurs around bedtime and lasts 30–90 min	Excruciating periorbital pain ("behind the eye"), **unilateral; stabbing or deep, burning pain;** accompanied by ipsilateral lacrimation, nasal congestion or discharge, facial flushing	Acute: **sumatriptan, oxygen inhalation;** Prophylaxis: **verapamil** taken daily—drug of choice (alternatives: ergotamine, methyllithium, methylsergide, corticosteroids)
Migraine	**Inherited;** caused by serotonin depletion; women > men; family history subtypes: 1. **Classic:** migraine with **aura** (aura usually visual such as flashing lights, scotoma, visual distortions) 2. **Common:** migraine without aura 3. **Menstrual**	Prodromal phase; severe **throbbing or dull achy unilateral headaches,** may be generalized; lasts for 4–72 h; pain is **aggravated by coughing, physical activity, and bending down;** other symptoms include nausea and vomiting, photophobia, and increased sensitivity to smell	Acute: NSAIDs, dihydroergotamine, sumatriptan; Prophylaxis: first line—TCAs and propranolol; second line—verapamil, valproic acid, and methysergide

(handwritten annotation: → serotonin receptor agonist ↳ vasoconstriction)

NSAID, nonsteroidal anti-inflammatory drug; SSRI, selective serotonin reuptake inhibitor; TCA, tricyclic antidepressant.

PSYCHIATRY AND BEHAVIORAL SCIENCE

I. Nonpharmacologic therapeutic modalities (Table 2-18)

TABLE 2-18 Nonpharmacologic Therapeutic Modalities

Therapy	Characteristics	Notes
Biofeedback	Gaining control over physiology via continuous information; motivation and practice required	Used for hypertension, migraine headaches, and tension headaches
Classical conditioning	**A reflexive, natural behavior** is elicited in **response to a learned stimulus** (e.g., ringing of a bell causing salivation)	**Aversive conditioning** pairs an unwanted response to a painful stimulus; stages include acquisition, extinction, and recovery
Cognitive therapy	**Negative thinking** is reorganized into self-affirming, positive thoughts	Short-term psychotherapy used to treat depression and anxiety
Electroconvulsive therapy (ECT)	Electric current introduced into brain to alter neurotransmitter function; improvement seen faster than with pharmacologic regimens	Used for **major depression;** safe; effective; retrograde amnesia is a major side effect
Operant conditioning	Behavior that is not part of the natural repertoire is learned by altering the reward **(reinforcement)**	Reinforcement can be positive or negative; reward schedule includes continuous, fixed, or variable
Psychoanalysis	Intensive treatment based on recovering and integrating past experiences from the unconscious via free association; based on **Freud's theories**	**Id**—sexual drives and aggression; **ego**—controls instinct and interacts with the world; **superego**—morality and conscience
Systematic desensitization	Classical conditioning technique in which relaxation procedures are combined with increasing doses of anxiety-provoking stimuli	Used to **eliminate** phobias
Token economy	Positive reinforcement in which a reward is used to elicit a desired response	Seen often in mental hospitals or parents dealing with children

The Nervous System

II. Eating disorders (Table 2-19)

TABLE 2-19 Eating Disorders

Disorder	Characteristics	Treatment	Notes
Anorexia nervosa	Body weight <85% of ideal, **distorted body image, amenorrhea,** intense fear of gaining weight	Supportive care, counseling, cognitive behavioral therapy, family therapy, **pharmacotherapy is typically ineffective**	Higher incidence in female adolescents, **upper-middle socioeconomic classes;** amenorrhea; decreased libido
Bulimia nervosa	Binge eating, followed by some inappropriate behavior to prevent weight gain (e.g., purging; abuse of laxatives); **normal weight**	Psychotherapy; pharmacotherapy; with **fluoxetine** (first line), other SSRIs, TCAs, or MAOIs; bupropion is contraindicated due to risk of seizures	Normal libido; no amenorrhea (unlike anorexics); erosion of tooth enamel; hypokalemic hypochloremic metabolic alkalosis (due to vomiting); hypertrophy of parotid glands
Binge eating disorder	Binge eating as an expression of deeper psychological problems; no purging; excessive weight gain	Psychotherapy, cognitive behavioral therapy, SSRIs	Patients may have negative attitudes toward food
Compulsive eating	Binge eating; constant preoccupation with and fantasizing about food	SSRIs, SNRIs, cognitive behavioral therapy	A form of obsessive-compulsive disorder
Obesity	BMI >30	Dieting and exercise; strict fad dieting ineffective; bariatric surgery may be useful in selected patients with good dietary compliance	Lower socioeconomic groups; genetics plays a role; increased risk of disease

BMI, body mass index; MAOI, monoamine oxidase inhibitor; SNRI, serotonin-norepinephrine reuptake inhibitor; SSRI, selective serotonin reuptake inhibitor; TCA, tricyclic antidepressant.

III. Drugs of abuse and dependence (Table 2-20)

TABLE 2-20 Drugs of Abuse and Dependence

Drug	Mechanism	Intoxication Effect	Withdrawal Effects
Alcohol	Unknown; possible effect at GABA receptor directly on membranes	Sedation, hypnosis, slurred speech, ataxia, loss of motor coordination, Wernicke–Korsakoff syndrome	Malaise, tachycardia, tremors, seizures, **delirium tremens,** death
Amphetamine	Release of intracellular stores of catecholamines	Insomnia, irritability, tremor, hyperactive reflexes, arrhythmias, anorexia, psychosis	Lethargy, depression, hunger, craving for drug resulting in bizarre psychological behavior, anxiety
Barbiturates	**Potentiation of GABA** action on chloride by **increase of duration** of chloride channel opening	Mental sluggishness, anesthesia, hypnosis	Restlessness, anxiety, tremor, death

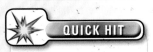

QUICK HIT

Substance abuse is defined as use of psychoactive substances for at least 1 month with interference in the user's life but without meeting the criteria for dependence. Substance dependence involves craving, withdrawal, and tolerance.

QUICK HIT

Alcohol is the most widely used drug, followed by nicotine. Caffeine is the most often used psychoactive substance, followed by nicotine.

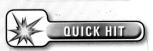

QUICK HIT

Dependence is mediated by **dopamine,** the neurotransmitter linked to the pleasure and reward center.

(continued)

TABLE 2-20 Drugs of Abuse and Dependence (Continued)

Drug	Mechanism	Intoxication Effect	Withdrawal Effects
Benzodiazepines	**Potentiation of GABA** action on chloride by **increase of frequency** of chloride channel opening	Sedation, ataxia, mild respiratory depression	Tremors, anxiety, psychosis, **seizures**
Caffeine	Translocation of Ca^{2+}, inhibition of phosphodiesterase (increase in cAMP, cGMP)	Insomnia, anxiety, agitation	Lethargy, irritability, headache
Cocaine	Blockade of norepinephrine, 5-HT, and dopamine reuptake	Hallucinations, anxiety, arrhythmias, nasal problems, sudden death	Craving, depression, excessive sleeping, fatigue
Lysergic acid diethylamide (LSD)	5-HT agonist action in the midbrain	Pupillary dilation, increased blood pressure and body temperature, piloerection, hallucinations	Flashbacks
Marijuana	Unknown; tetrahydrocannabinol (THC) is active compound; possible endogenous receptors in brain	Increased appetite, visual hallucinations, increased heart rate, decreased blood pressure Impairment of short-term memory and mental activity	Fatigue, hypersomnia, psychomotor retardation
Nicotine	Low doses—ganglionic stimulation; high doses—ganglionic blockade	**Increased heart rate and blood pressure,** irritability, tremors, intestinal cramps	Irritability, anxiety, restlessness, headaches, insomnia, difficulty in concentrating
Opioids (heroin)	Inhibition of adenylate cyclase by opioid receptors within the CNS	Constipation, **pinpoint pupils,** potentially lethal via **respiratory depression,** sedation	Insomnia, diarrhea, sweating, fever, piloerection
Phencyclidine (PCP)	Inhibition of dopamine, serotonin, and norepinephrine reuptake	Hostile, bizarre behavior; nystagmus hypersalivation; anesthesia	Sudden onset of violent behavior

cAMP, cyclic adenosine monophosphate; cGMP, cyclic guanosine monophosphate; CNS, central nervous system; GABA, γ-aminobutyric acid; 5-HT, serotonin.

IV. Schizophrenia

A. Diagnostic features
1. Hallucinations (usually auditory)
2. Delusions
3. Disorganized speech
4. Disorganized or catatonic behavior
5. Negative symptoms: flattened affect, social withdrawal, lack of motivation, thought blocking, poor grooming

B. Neurotransmitters involved: increased dopamine may be implicated

C. Other features
1. Usually first presents in young adulthood
2. Marijuana use during teenage years is a risk factor
3. Enlarged lateral ventricles and third ventricle

D. Subtypes of schizophrenia
1. Paranoid
2. Disorganized

3. Catatonic
4. Undifferentiated
5. Residual

V. Schizophrenia-related disorders

A. Brief psychotic disorder
 1. Symptoms of schizophrenia for <1 month
 2. Usually stress related
B. Schizophreniform disorder—symptoms of schizophrenia for 1 to 6 months
C. Schizoaffective disorder—schizophrenia/psychosis as the primary disorder, in addition to a secondary mood disorder (either bipolar disorder or depression)
D. Delusional disorder
 1. Characterized by non-bizarre delusions that are more than simply overvalued ideas
 2. Absence of hallucinations
 3. Functioning is not impaired, and behavior is not odd

VI. Antipsychotics (Table 2-21)

Experts theorize that an excess of **dopamine** in certain areas of the brain is in some way responsible for psychosis. The development of psychosis as a common side effect of treatment of Parkinson disease with dopamine and dopamine agonists supports this theory. It is thought that most antipsychotics exert their effect by blocking **dopamine** receptors.

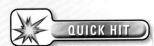
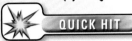
The Nervous System

TABLE 2-21 Antipsychotics

Drug	Clinical Uses	Side Effects	Notes
Typical antipsychotics (traditional neuroleptics) **High potency**			
Haloperidol, fluphenazine	**Schizophrenia, psychosis**; haloperidol is often used off-label for acute agitation and delirium	**EPS** (dystonia, akinesia, akathisia, tardive dyskinesia); toxicity results in **NMS** (rigidity, myoglobinuria, autonomic instability, hyperpyrexia); anticholinergic side effects are less common; **prolonged QT syndrome**	NMS is treated with dantrolene and dopamine agonists
Droperidol	Postoperative nausea and vomiting	*Same as haloperidol*	Rarely used because of QT prolongation and risk of arrhythmia
Trifluoperazine, thiothixene, loxapine, perphenazine	Schizophrenia, psychosis	*Same as haloperidol*; variable QT prolongation	These are sometimes inconsistently classified as "moderate potency" neuroleptics
Typical antipsychotics (traditional neuroleptics) **Low potency**			
Chlorpromazine	Schizophrenia, psychosis	**Anticholinergic side effects** (dry mouth, constipation); weight gain; some alpha blockade (hypotension) and histamine blockade (sedation); EPS and NMS are less common.	
Thioridazine		*Same as chlorpromazine*, plus high risk of QT prolongation and arrhythmias	Not commonly used
Atypical antipsychotics			
Clozapine	Schizophrenia, useful for both positive and negative symptoms	**Agranulocytosis, weight gain, diabetes,** low risk of anticholinergic side effects; EPS and NMS occur at lower rates than with typicals	Second-line agent used for refractory schizophrenia, check weekly blood counts due to risk of agranulocytosis
Olanzapine, quetiapine, risperidone, ziprasidone, paliperidone, sertindole, aripiprazole	**Schizophrenia, bipolar disorder**	**Weight gain, diabetes,** low risk of anticholinergic side effects; EPS and NMS occur at lower rates than with typicals	Of these drugs, olanzapine has the highest risk of weight gain and diabetes

EPS, extrapyramidal symptoms; NMS, neuroleptic malignant syndrome.

Antipsychotic drugs have several particular side effects in common. The side effects may be grouped into the following categories: (1) **extrapyramidal**, (2) **anticholinergic**, (3) **alpha-blocking effect**, and (4) **histamine receptor effects**. Extrapyramidal side effects refer to acute dystonia, akinesia, and akathisia. **Dystonia** presents acutely within a few hours of starting the medication as a muscular spasm, stiffness, and oculogyric crisis. **Akinesia** presents within a few days of starting the medication as parkinsonian symptoms. **Akathisia** presents within a few weeks of starting the medication as restlessness. **Tardive dyskinesia** presents after a few months of starting the medication with stereotypic oral facial movements, likely due to dopamine receptor sensitization. Tardive dyskinesia is often irreversible and is most common in older women who have received long-term treatment with high doses. **Anticholinergic side effects** include dry mouth and constipation. **Alpha-blocking effects** include hypotension. **Histamine receptor effects** include sedation. **Atypical antipsychotics** such as clozapine, olanzapine, risperidone, quetiapine, aripiprazole, and ziprasidone have a lower incidence of extrapyramidal and anticholinergic side effects. Finally, antipsychotics also may be **antiemetic** and have a tendency to **lower the seizure threshold**.

VII. Depression

A. Major depressive disorder (MDD)
1. Diagnostic features (**SIG E CAPS**): sleep disturbances, loss of interest in formerly pleasurable things (anhedonia), guilt, low energy, poor concentration, appetite changes, psychomotor retardation or agitation, suicidal ideation, and depressed mood
2. Symptoms must be present for at least 2 weeks.
3. Neurotransmitters involved: decreased norepinephrine (NE) and 5-HT
4. Decreased REM latency (rapid onset of REM sleep) is commonly seen.
5. Treatment
   a. Pharmacotherapy: selective serotonin reuptake inhibitors (SSRIs), serotonin-norepinephrine reuptake inhibitors (SNRIs), tricyclic antidepressants (TCAs), monoamine oxidase inhibitors (MAOIs)
   b. Nonpharmacologic therapies: cognitive behavioral therapy, electroconvulsive therapy (ECT)
B. Atypical depression
1. Features include hypersomnia, overeating and weight gain, mood reactivity, rejection hypersensitivity
2. Treatment: MAOIs or SSRIs
C. Postpartum depression
1. Depression in the postpartum period that exceeds 2 weeks and may persist for longer than a year
2. Treatment: same as for MDD
D. Dysthymia—A milder form of depression with the same diagnostic features as MDD that lasts at least 2 years
E. Seasonal affective disorder
1. A form of major depression that occurs during the winter season due to a deficiency of retinal stimulation with light
2. Treatment: supplemental light therapy daily

VIII. Antidepressants (Table 2-22)

The "**amine theory**" attributes mood to levels of certain amines such as NE and 5-HT. It is theorized that low levels of these hormones lead to depression, and many of the antidepressants **boost amine levels**. The sites of action of the antidepressants are represented graphically (Figure 2-18).

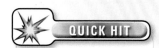

Amitriptyline is somewhat more potent than imipramine and nortriptyline, which means that it often has more significant side effects.

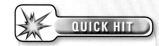

The use of the combination of selective serotonin reuptake inhibitors (SSRIs) and monoamine oxidase inhibitors (MAOIs) may produce a "**serotonin syndrome.**" This constellation of hyperpyrexia, muscle spasm, and mental status changes can be fatal.

The Nervous System

TABLE 2-22 Antidepressants

Class of Antidepressant (Specific Agent)	Mechanism of Action	Clinical Uses	Side Effects	Notes
Selective serotonin reuptake inhibitors (SSRIs) (e.g., fluoxetine, paroxetine, sertraline, citalopram)	Inhibit **reuptake** of 5-HT at neuronal synapses	Major depression, OCD, anxiety disorders, bulimia nervosa	Inhibits liver enzymes, nausea, agitation, **sexual dysfunction** (anorgasmia), dystonic reactions	Contraindicated with **MAOIs** secondary to **serotonin syndrome** (hyperthermia, muscle rigidity, cardiovascular collapse). Allow time for antidepressant effect; usually takes 2–3 weeks
Serotonin-norepinephrine reuptake inhibitors (SNRIs) (venlafaxine, desvenlafaxine, duloxetine, milnacipran, sibutramine)	Inhibit **reuptake** of NE and 5-HT at neuronal synapses	Major depression, anxiety disorders, neuropathic pain (duloxetine), fibromyalgia (milnacipran), obesity (sibutramine)	Sedation, nausea, constipation, hypertension, mild sexual dysfunction	Sibutramine is used only as an appetite suppressant for morbid obesity
Tricyclic antidepressants (TCAs) (amitriptyline, imipramine, nortriptyline, desipramine, clomipramine, doxepin, amoxapine)	Inhibit **reuptake** of NE and 5-HT at neuronal synapses	Major depression, OCD (clomipramine), nocturnal enuresis (imipramine), panic disorder	Sedation, **α-blocking effects** (orthostatic hypotension), **anticholinergic** (tachycardia, dry mouth, urinary retention), hallucinations (in elderly), confusion (elderly) Overdose toxicity results in **convulsions, coma, cardiotoxicity** (arrhythmias), respiratory depression, hyperpyrexia	Desipramine is the least sedating Used off-label for insomnia
Monoamine oxidase inhibitors (MAOIs) (isocarboxazid, phenelzine, tranylcypromine)	Inhibit **degradation** of NE and 5-HT at neuronal synapses	**Atypical depression** (with hypersomnia, anxiety, sensitivity to rejection, hypochondriasis)	**Hypertensive episodes** with ingestion of tyramine-containing foods or beta agonists, hyperthermia, convulsions	Contraindicated with **SSRIs** and **meperidine** secondary to **serotonin syndrome** (hyperthermia, muscle rigidity, cardiovascular collapse)
Other antidepressants				
Bupropion	Inhibits reuptake of NE and dopamine	Major depression, smoking cessation	Tachycardia, insomnia, headache, seizure (especially patients with bulimia)	Does not have sexual side effects
Mirtazapine	α_2-antagonist → increases release of NE and 5-HT	Major depression (especially with insomnia)	**Weight gain**, dry mouth, increased appetite, sedation	
Maprotiline	Blocks NE uptake	Major depression	Sedation, orthostatic hypotension	
Trazodone	Inhibits 5-HT reuptake	Major depression (especially with insomnia), insomnia	Sedation, nausea, **priapism**, postural hypotension	

5-HT, serotonin; OCD, obsessive-compulsive disorder; NE, norepinephrine.

FIGURE 2-18 Antidepressant sites of action

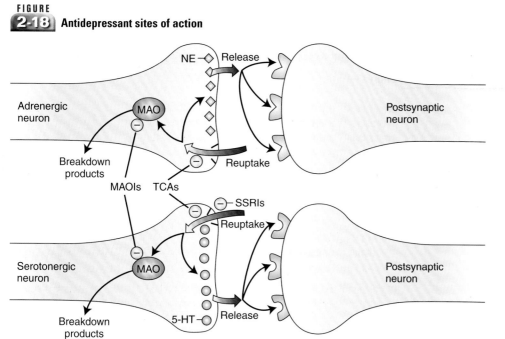

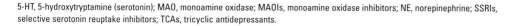

5-HT, 5-hydroxytryptamine (serotonin); MAO, monoamine oxidase; MAOIs, monoamine oxidase inhibitors; NE, norepinephrine; SSRIs, selective serotonin reuptake inhibitors; TCAs, tricyclic antidepressants.

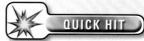

QUICK HIT

An **overdose** of a tricyclic antidepressant (TCA) causes delirium, coma, seizures, respiratory depression, and arrhythmias and is potentially fatal and difficult to treat. The large volume of distribution of a TCA makes dialysis relatively ineffective.

IX. Anxiety disorders (Table 2-23)

TABLE 2-23 Anxiety Disorders

Disorder	Characteristics	Neurotransmitter(s) Involved	Treatment	Notes
Panic disorder	Discrete, episodic periods of intense anxiety or discomfort; palpitations; chest pain; sweating; fear of dying	Decreased serotonin, norepinephrine, GABA	Imipramine; behavioral therapy	Associated with mitral valve prolapse; young women predominantly affected; genetic component
Generalized anxiety disorder	Generalized, persistent anxiety; tension; insomnia; irritability	Decreased serotonin, norepinephrine, GABA	**SSRIs,** buspirone (Table 2-25), benzodiazepines	Anxiety for more than **6 months**
Posttraumatic stress disorder (PTSD)	Result of trauma, hypervigilance, nightmares, flashbacks	Decreased serotonin, norepinephrine, GABA	Counseling, group therapy, benzodiazepines for symptoms	For the first 3 months after the trauma, it is called acute PTSD; symptoms lasting longer than 3 months is chronic PTSD
Obsessive-compulsive disorder	Recurrent thoughts and actions; patients are distressed by repetitive actions	Decreased serotonin	Behavioral therapy, clomipramine, trazodone, SSRIs	
Phobias	Irrational, situational fear	Decreased serotonin, norepinephrine, and GABA	Systematic desensitization; propranolol useful for physiologic manifestations	EEG changes

EEG, electroencephalogram; GABA, γ-aminobutyric acid; SSRI, selective serotonin reuptake inhibitor.

The Nervous System

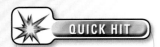

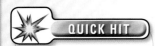

X. Other neuropsychiatric disorders and other psychiatric drugs (*Table 2-24, Table 2-25*)

TABLE 2-24 Other Neuropsychiatric Disorders

Disorder	Characteristics	Treatment	Notes
Bipolar disorder	Rapid speech, decreased need for sleep, hyperenergetic state, impaired judgment followed by a state of depression	**Lithium** (Table 2-25), certain anticonvulsants, atypical antipsychotics	
Cyclothymia	Alternating between dysthymia and hypomania, lasting at least 2 years	Same as bipolar disorder	
Delirium	Impaired cognitive processes, diurnal variation in mood (worse at **night—"sundowning"**), illusions and hallucinations	Treat the underlying cause	**Most common** problem in hospitalized patients with psychiatric disorders
Dissociative disorders	Psychological factors resulting in memory loss and loss of function	Psychotherapy, hypnotherapy, medication for associated symptoms	Includes amnesia, fugue, dissociative identity disorder, depersonalization
Somatoform disorders	Symptoms of disease occur without related pathology	Psychotherapy and therapeutics may help; variable response	Patients truly believe in having illness, whereas factitious disorders are the result of faking illness
Factitious disorder	Patient consciously produces signs or symptoms of illness without a conscious motive or external incentive	Treatment of self-induced illness; avoid unnecessary tests and procedures	
Malingering	Patient consciously produces signs or symptoms of illness for secondary gain (avoiding work, obtaining money, drugs, shelter)	Avoid unnecessary tests and procedures	Patients often leave when confronted
Attention deficit hyperactivity disorder (ADHD)	Hyperactive, poor attention span, highly sensitive to stimuli	Amphetamines (methylphenidate—see Table 2-25)	More common in **male children**
Tourette syndrome	Involuntary **motor and vocal** movements (need both)	Haloperidol, clonidine	Onset occurs in childhood

TABLE 2-25 Other Psychiatric Drugs

Class/Drug	Mechanism of Action	Clinical Uses	Side Effects	Notes
Lithium	Unclear; inhibits regeneration of IP_3 and DAG; important for many second-messenger systems	**Bipolar disorder,** acute mania	Tremor, hypothyroidism, teratogenesis **nephrogenic diabetes insipidus** ↓ Epstein	**Requires close monitoring** of serum levels due to narrow therapeutic window
Buspirone	5-HT receptor agonist	**Generalized anxiety disorder**	Dizziness, drowsiness, headache, nausea	
Varenicline	Partial agonist of nicotinic receptor	Smoking cessation	Nausea, headache, insomnia, abnormal dreams	
Methylphenidate	CNS stimulant—blocks presynaptic reuptake of NE and dopamine	Attention deficit hyperactivity disorder, narcolepsy	Insomnia, restlessness	Contraindicated in patients with heart disease or hypertension

5-HT, serotonin; CNS, central nervous system; DAG, diacylglycerol; IP_3, inositol triphosphate; NE, norepinephrine.

XI. Defense mechanisms *(Table 2-26)*

TABLE 2-26	**Defense Mechanisms**	
Mechanism	**Characteristics**	**Example**
Immature mechanisms		
Acting out	Stress is dealt with through actions	After the death of his brother, a priest breaks all the windows in his church.
Denial	Not accepting the reality of a situation	A woman refuses to consider the possibility of pregnancy after having unprotected intercourse and missing two periods.
Displacement	Feelings for causal source are transferred to another object	A man kicks his dog after getting fired from his job.
Dissociation	Loss of memory or change in personality as a result of stressor	A woman who was sexually abused as a child develops another personality.
Identification	Behavior patterned after another	A teenager smokes pot because his favorite rock star does.
Intellectualization	Reason is used to cope with anxiety	A physician starts reading textbooks and journal articles about her father's cancer.
Isolation of affect	Events are separated from emotion	An airline passenger describes an emergency landing to his family without any emotion.
Projection	One's own characteristics are applied to another	A flirtatious man accuses his wife of cheating.
Rationalization	Analytical reason is used to justify unacceptable feelings	A man claims that his driving under the influence arrest would never have happened if his softball team had won.
Reaction formation	Feelings are denied and opposite actions are performed	A woman who wants to cheat on her husband instead buys him a new car.
Regression	Stress-induced behavior that involves returning to a childlike state	Medical students have a food fight during their lunch break on the day of board examinations.
Repression	Holding back an unacceptable feeling or idea from reaching consciousness	A recent widower feels no sense of loss.
Splitting	Feelings or stressors are placed in distinct, opposite compartments (i.e., either all good or all bad)	A man in a doctor's office describes how much he hates the nurses but loves the receptionist.
Mature mechanisms		
Altruism	One unselfishly assists others	A woman donates her entire estate to her favorite charities upon her death.
Humor	Humor is used to reduce stress	While stuck in an elevator, a young man makes jokes to ease the tension.
Sublimation	Unacceptable impulse is directed into a socially accepted action	A boy who got into a lot of fights as a kid decides to become a professional boxer.
Suppression	Conscious effort to suppress thoughts or feelings	A recent widower actively refuses to think about his deceased wife while packing her things away.

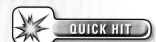

QUICK HIT

Schizotypal is a personality disorder characterized by odd beliefs or magical thinking. **Schizoid** is a personality disorder characterized by voluntary social isolation. Neither of these meets the diagnostic criteria for schizophrenia, but both are risk factors for the development of schizophrenia.

XII. Personality disorders *(Table 2-27)*

TABLE 2-27 **Personality Disorders**		
Disorder	**Characteristics**	**Example**
CLUSTER A		
Paranoid	Hostile, suspicious, mistrustful, usually male	A patient being prepared for surgery yells at the doctors on rounds because he feels they are gossiping about him.
Schizoid	**Voluntarily** socially withdrawn without psychological problems; usually male	A 52-year-old computer programmer lives alone, is not married, has no friends, and is contented.
Schizotypal	Odd behavior, thoughts, and appearance without psychosis	A woman wears many-layered clothing and inappropriately applied makeup and only talks to people with brown-colored hair.
CLUSTER B		
Histrionic	Dramatic, overemotional, sexually provocative, unable to maintain close friendships, usually female	A woman exaggerates her suffering over a mild cold and behaves seductively toward the physician.
Narcissistic	Grandiosity, hypersensitivity to criticism, and lack of empathy	A resident refuses to operate with anyone but the best surgeon in the hospital because he feels it is beneath his talent.
Antisocial	Inability to conform to societal rules; criminal behavior; more often male; requires diagnosis of conduct disorder as child	A multiple rapist has no concern for his victims or the law.
Borderline	Unstable, impulsive, suicide attempts, vulnerable to abandonment, usually female, uses splitting	After an argument with her boyfriend, a woman chases him out of her home and later calls him and tells him she cannot live without him.
CLUSTER C		
Avoidant	Shy, **involuntarily** (compare to schizoid) withdrawn because fears rejection, usually female	A businesswoman defers speaking during presentations to her project partner and has few friends
Obsessive-compulsive	Rigid, perfectionist, stubborn, orderly; found twice as often in males	A businessman works long hours on a project, holding up both the project deadline and his personal life in vain attempts to make it perfect.
Dependent	Defers decision making; not comfortable with an authority position; insecure; has the ability to make long-lasting relationships (unlike avoidant); usually female	A third-year resident often accepts on-call duty for other residents, never speaks up when talked down to by the junior residents, and has trouble writing orders.
Passive–aggressive	Obstinate, inefficient, procrastinating, noncompliant	School student intentionally does poorly on homework because he does not like his teacher.

The Cardiovascular System

DEVELOPMENT

I. Heart

A. The cardiovascular system is derived from the **mesoderm**.

B. Paired endocardial heart tubes form in the **cephalic region** of the embryo.

C. Lateral and cephalocaudal folding causes the heart tubes to join together and lie in a **ventral location** between the primitive mouth and the foregut.

D. The **primitive heart** dilates into five areas, as shown in Figure 3-1. The five embryologic regions and their adult derivatives are as follows:

1. **Truncus arteriosus** → proximal aorta and proximal pulmonary artery
2. **Bulbus cordis** → smooth parts of the right ventricle (conus arteriosus) and left ventricles
3. **Primitive ventricle** → right and left ventricles (trabeculated parts)
4. **Primitive atrium** → right and left atria
5. **Sinus venosus** → smooth part of right atrium, the coronary sinus, and oblique vein

E. The lumen of the truncus arteriosus and bulbus cordis is divided into the aorta and **pulmonary trunk** by the aorticopulmonary septum.

F. The septum primum and septum secundum form the **atrial septum**.

G. The **foramen ovale** is a communication between the right and left atria, which is formed by the walls of the septum primum and septum secundum.

1. It allows blood to flow from the venous side of the circulation to the arterial side without passing through the lungs as a result of **higher pressure on the venous side during gestation**.
2. **After birth**, the foramen ovale closes because of **increased arterial pressure** that pushes the septum primum against the septum secundum.

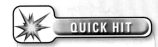

QUICK HIT

In dextrocardia, the heart is located on the right side in the thorax. An isolated, misplaced heart is often accompanied by multiple anomalies. If all of the body's organs are transposed (situs inversus—associated with Kartagener syndrome; immotile cilia caused by a defect in the dynein arms resulting in lung disease and male sterility), the heart is often normal.

FIGURE

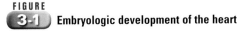
3-1 Embryologic development of the heart

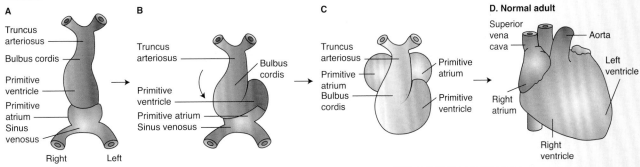

Folding of the developing heart (**A–C**) during weeks 5–8 into the normal adult heart (**D**)

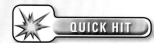

1. maxillary artery
2. stapedial
3. common carotid
4. right subclavian
   aorta
5. —
6. pulmonary artery
   ductus arteriosus

H. The aorticopulmonary septum (also called the spiral septum, derived from neural crest cells), the right and left bulbar ridges, and the AV cushion form the **interventricular septum**.

II. Arterial vessels

A. **Aortic arches (pharyngeal arch arteries):** Initially, there are six paired aortic arches. Arches 3, 4, and 6 play a significant role in the adult. Arch 5 degenerates early in fetal development.
   1. **Arches 1 and 2** give rise to the maxillary artery and stapedial artery, respectively.
   2. **Arch 3** helps form the adult common carotid arteries bilaterally.
   3. **Arch 4** helps form the aorta on the left and the proximal subclavian artery on the right.
   4. **Arch 6** helps form the ductus arteriosus and part of the pulmonary trunk.

B. **Paired dorsal aortae** are paired vessels that run along the length of the embryo. They coalesce to form the **descending aorta**.

III. Venous vessels

A. The paired vitelline, umbilical, and cardinal veins form the definitive adult structures.

B. The **vitelline veins** help form the ductus venosus and hepatic sinusoids, the inferior vena cava, the portal vein, and the superior and inferior mesenteric veins.

C. **Umbilical veins**
   1. No adult vascular structures are formed by these veins.
   2. The left umbilical vein connects to the ductus venosus and carries oxygenated blood from the placenta to the fetus.
   3. **Left umbilical vein** gives rise to ligamentum teres hepatis.
   4. **Right umbilical vein** regresses.

D. **Cardinal veins**
   1. The **anterior cardinal veins** help form the internal jugular vein and the superior vena cava.
   2. The **posterior cardinal veins** help form the inferior vena cava, common iliac veins, azygos vein, and renal veins.

IV. Fetal circulation *(Figure 3-2)*

V. Congenital defects of the heart and great vessels *(Table 3-1)*

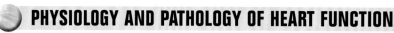

PHYSIOLOGY AND PATHOLOGY OF HEART FUNCTION

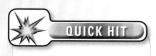

Properly timed and integrated myocyte contraction is essential to normal heart function. Cardiac myocytes have gap junctions that allow for rapid relay of electrical signals between them. Electrical impulses are transmitted via the electrical conduction system composed of the sinoatrial (SA) node, atrioventricular (AV) node, and His–Purkinje cells (Figure 3-3). Normally, the SA node is the pacemaker of the heart. The node exhibits automaticity, in which spontaneous phase 4 depolarization generates rhythmic action potentials (APs). These electrical signals propagate from the SA node through the atrial tissue and cause it to contract. Further propagation leads to excitation of the AV node, the ventricular bundles, and, lastly, the ventricular tissue. The nodal tissues are dependent on Ca^{2+} for their phase 0 depolarization, whereas the cardiac muscular tissue uses Na^+ for phase 0 depolarization. The AV node transmits APs more slowly than do the other cardiac tissues. This feature allows the atria to contract before the ventricles, with time for the ventricles to repolarize, fill with blood, and prepare to receive their next electrical signal. Furthermore, it also prevents excessively rapid beats from reaching and damaging the ventricular tissue. The conduction system of the heart can best be visualized on an

FIGURE 3-2 Fetal circulation

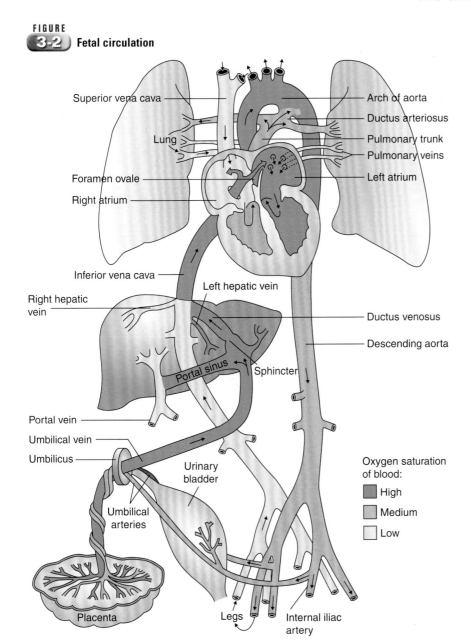

- Superior vena cava
- Lung
- Foramen ovale
- Right atrium
- Inferior vena cava
- Left hepatic vein
- Right hepatic vein
- Portal sinus
- Sphincter
- Portal vein
- Umbilical vein
- Umbilicus
- Umbilical arteries
- Urinary bladder
- Placenta
- Legs
- Arch of aorta
- Ductus arteriosus
- Pulmonary trunk
- Pulmonary veins
- Left atrium
- Ductus venosus
- Descending aorta
- Internal iliac artery

Oxygen saturation of blood:
- High
- Medium
- Low

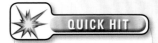

QUICK HIT

The umbilical circulation is one of the only places in the body (along with the pulmonary circulation) where an artery does not carry oxygenated blood. The paired umbilical arteries carry deoxygenated blood to the placenta, whereas the umbilical vein brings oxygenated blood back to the fetus.

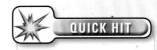

QUICK HIT

The ductus arteriosus closes in the first days of life. Exposure to oxygenated blood alters the production of prostaglandins (PGs). Indomethacin (PG synthesis inhibitor) induces closure of a patent ductus arteriosus (PDA), whereas alprostadil (PGE1) therapy maintains patency.

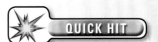

QUICK HIT

Congenital cardiac defects with the **letter D** are initially **left-to-right shunts** (PDA, VSD, AVSD, and ASD), whereas those cardiac defects without the letter D are right-to-left shunts.

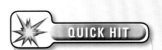

QUICK HIT

The baroreceptor reflex greatly affects total peripheral resistance. The carotid sinus baroreceptors, located at the bifurcation of the carotid arteries, sense arterial pressure. Afferent signals via cranial nerve (CN) IX induce efferent signals via CN X to influence heart rate. Increased arterial pressure causes an increase in vagal output and a reduction of heart rate and blood pressure. A decrease in arterial pressure causes a decrease in vagal output, resulting in an increase in heart rate and blood pressure.

electrocardiogram (ECG). ECG plots can determine disturbances, such as arrhythmias, along the cardiac conduction path.

Multiple mechanisms can affect the intrinsic mechanical properties of the heart. Chronotropic effects on the heart cause a change in heart rate by affecting the rate of depolarization of the SA node. Inotropic effects cause a change in contractility of the heart. Greater contractility allows the heart to squeeze harder and increase cardiac output. Increased intracellular Ca^{2+}, either drug mediated (e.g., cardiac glycosides) or as a result of sympathetic β-receptor stimulation, allows for an increased inotropic effect. The preload and afterload also affect the function of the heart. Increased preload as a result of increased filling of the ventricles lengthens the myocytes, which induces stronger contraction, up to a certain point, after which the myocytes are too stretched to contract effectively. Afterload of the left ventricle is equivalent to aortic pressure. It is influenced by the total peripheral resistance. A higher afterload means the left ventricle must work harder or cardiac output will fall. The cardiovascular system is constantly working to maintain homeostatic equilibrium.

The Cardiovascular System

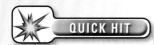

QUICK HIT

The most common type of atrial septal defect (ASD) is a patent foramen ovale.

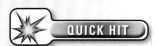

QUICK HIT

Eisenmenger syndrome is the change from a left-to-right shunt to a right-to-left shunt, secondary to increasing pulmonary hypertension; it usually occurs as a result of a chronic, adaptive response to preexisting left-to-right shunts, such as a VSD.

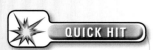

QUICK HIT

Cyanosis occurs in right-to-left shunts: tetralogy of Fallot and transposition of the great vessels (TGA). Cyanosis can lead to clubbing, hypertrophic osteoarthropathy, and polycythemia. Initial left-to-right shunts are not cyanotic: ASD, VSD, PDA, and atrioventricular septal defect (AVSD).

TABLE **3-1** Congenital Defects of the Heart and the Great Vessels

Anomaly	Pathology	Clinical Presentation	Notes
Atrial septal defect (ASD)	**Secundum ASD** (defect of septum primum or septum secundum) Primum ASD (low), sinus venosus ASD (high)	**Left-to-right shunt,** asymptomatic into the fourth decade, murmur, right ventricular hypertrophy	Much higher incidence in females (3:1); 75%–80% are secundum type
Coarctation of the aorta	Infantile (proximal to PDA); adult (constriction at closed ductus arteriosus, distal to the origin of left subclavian artery)	Symptoms depend on the extent of narrowing; infant presents with lower limb cyanosis and right heart failure at birth; adult asymptomatic with upper limb hypertension, rib notching on radiograph from collateral circulation through intercostal arteries, and **weak pulses in lower limbs**	Much higher incidence in males (3:1) and females with **Turner syndrome**
Patent ductus arteriosus (PDA)	Failure of closure of the ductus arteriosus; may be caused by premature birth with **hypoxemia** or structural defects	Continuous **machinery murmur**	Second most common congenital heart defect
Tetralogy of Fallot	Defective development of the infundibular septum; results in **overriding aorta, VSD, pulmonary stenosis, and hypertrophy of the right ventricle**	Cyanosis (may not be present at birth), right-to-left shunt, **"boot-shaped heart"**	Survival to adulthood possible; patient assumes squatting position to relieve symptoms
Transposition of the great vessels	Aorta drains right ventricle; pulmonary artery from left ventricle; **separate pulmonary and systemic circuits**	Incompatible with life unless shunt present; cyanosis (present at birth)	Mother with diabetes
Ventricular septal defect (VSD)	Membranous VSD, Single muscular VSD	Left-to-right shunt; **loud holosystolic murmur means small defect,** large defects can present as heart failure at birth; small defects can close spontaneously	Much higher incidence in males; most common congenital heart defect (33%); 90% are membranous type

FIGURE 3-3 Heart anatomy and signal conduction

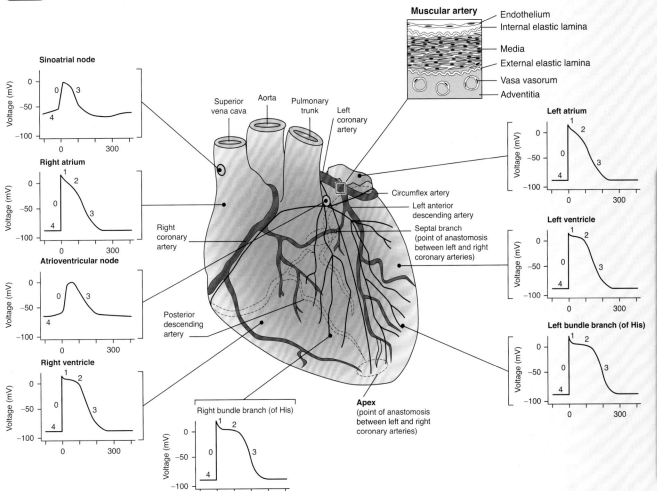

Hormonal systems also respond to changes in homeostasis. A major influence on the cardiovascular system is exerted by the renin-angiotensin-aldosterone (RAA) axis. Whereas the baroreceptors attempt to maintain adequate pressures in the vascular system over a short-term period, the RAA system helps to regulate pressure over a longer period of time. The RAA axis responds to changes in arterial pressure by altering salt and water retention by the kidneys. Low blood pressure causes an increased release of renin, which converts angiotensinogen from the liver to angiotensin I. Angiotensin I travels to the lung, where it is cleaved to angiotensin II (Ang II) by angiotensin-converting enzyme (ACE). Ang II stimulates constriction of arterioles and increases release of aldosterone (salt and water retention; see Chapter 6), both of which increase blood pressure. Atrial natriuretic peptide (ANP) also responds to blood pressure changes. An increase in blood pressure causes stretch of atrial myocytes, which then release ANP. ANP lowers blood pressure by relaxing smooth muscle, increasing salt and water excretion, and inhibiting renin release. Antidiuretic hormone (ADH), also known as arginine vasopressin (AVP), is involved in the response to changes in blood pressure. When released from the pituitary, it acts on the kidney to reduce urine output and retain water while simultaneously constricting arterioles to increase total peripheral resistance (Figure 3-4).

The physiologic function of the heart can be represented in several ways (e.g., pressure–volume loops and the cardiac cycle) (Figure 3-5). The effects of cardiac output, total peripheral resistance, contractility, preload, and afterload are represented on the Frank–Starling curve. Cardiac output is measured using the Fick principle (Figure 3-6), and normal output is approximately 5 L/min.

FIGURE

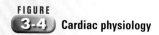

3-4 Cardiac physiology

A. Pressure–volume loop

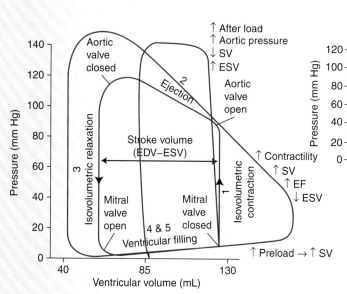

1. **Isovolumetric contraction:** time between mitral valve closure and aortic valve opening; time of highest oxygen consumption

2. **Systolic ejection:** time between aortic valve opening and closing

3. **Isovolumetric relaxation:** time between aortic valve closing and mitral valve opening

4. **Rapid filling:** time after mitral valve opening

5. **Reduced filling:** time right before mitral valve closing

C. Progression of the action potential through cardiac muscle cells

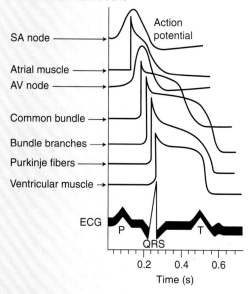

B. The cardiac cycle

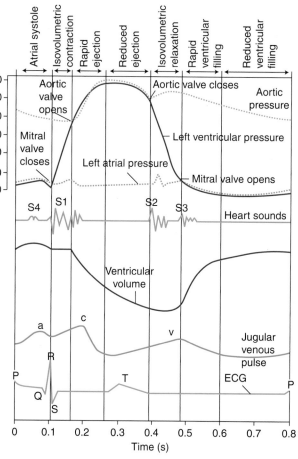

a wave—atrial contraction
c wave—contraction of right ventricle; peak due to tricuspid valve bulging into atrium
v wave—increased atrial pressure secondary to filling against closed tricuspid valve

D. Frank–Starling relationship

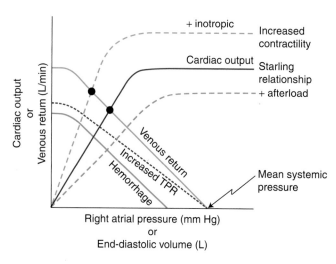

AV, atrioventricular; ECG, electrocardiogram; EDV, end-diastolic volume; ESV, end-systolic volume; SA, sinoatrial; TPR, total peripheral resistance.

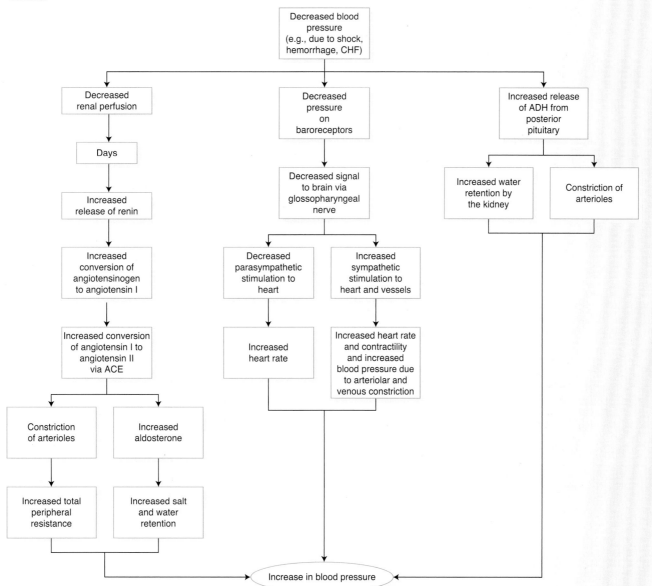

FIGURE 3-5 Physiologic cardiovascular relationships

ACE, angiotensin-converting enzyme; ADH, antidiuretic hormone; CHF, congestive heart failure.

 ## ARRHYTHMIAS *(Figure 3-7) (Table 3-2)*

Arrhythmias can be organized into tachycardias and bradycardias. The ECGs of important arrhythmias can be seen in Figure 3-7, and features of the heart blocks are described in Table 3-2.

ANTIARRHYTHMICS *(Figure 3-8) (Table 3-3)*

Antiarrhythmics work to change different phases of depolarization and repolarization. They also alter the conduction velocity, change the effective refractory period (ERP), and alter the AP duration. The treatment options for arrhythmias are as follows:

I. **Atrial fibrillation**

   A. **Rate control** (with β-blockers, diltiazem, verapamil, or digoxin) is generally preferred over rhythm control.

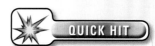

Chronic atrial fibrillation can lead to clots in the atrium that may embolize to the systemic circulation. Treatment is to prevent emboli with anticoagulation such as warfarin.

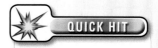

Class IB agents (lidocaine, tocainide, mexiletine, and phenytoin) all have central nervous system (CNS) side effects. Long-term control using tocainide can also cause neutropenia and thrombocytopenia.

The Cardiovascular System

FIGURE 3-6 Important cardiovascular equations

$CO = \dfrac{O_2 \text{ consumption}}{([O_2] \text{ pulmonary artery} - [O_2] \text{ pulmonary vein})}$	**The Fick equation** is used to calculate either cardiac output (CO) or oxygen (O_2) consumption
$CO = SV \times HR$	CO = cardiac output SV = stroke volume HR = heart rate
$R \propto \dfrac{1}{r^4}$	This relationship shows how arteriolar diameter can effectively control systemic resistance. For instance, if the radius (r) is increased by 2, the resistance (R) drops 16-fold.
$\dot{Q} = \dfrac{\Delta P}{R}$	$\dot{Q}$ = flow ΔP = Aortic pressure–right atrial pressure or pressure difference R = resistance
$MBP = CO \times TPR$	MBP = mean blood pressure (equivalent to ΔP) CO = cardiac output (equivalent to $\dot{Q}$) TPR = total peripheral resistance (equivalent to R)
Series resistance: $R_{total} = R_1 + R_2 + R_3 + R_4 \ldots$	
Parallel resistance: $\dfrac{1}{R_{total}} = \dfrac{1}{R_1} + \dfrac{1}{R_2} + \dfrac{1}{R_3} + \dfrac{1}{R_4} \ldots$	This relationship lowers resistance when the body recruits unused parallel vessels (especially in capillary beds)

B. Conversion to sinus rhythm (if indicated) may be achieved with electrical cardioversion or antiarrhythmic drugs (most commonly, amiodarone), although reversion to atrial fibrillation is common.

II. Supraventricular tachycardia
A. Adenosine (diagnostic purposes)
B. Verapamil (long-term control)

III. Ventricular fibrillation
A. Lidocaine or amiodarone

IV. Ventricular tachycardia
A. **Digoxin**

V. Digitalis toxicity
A. Activated charcoal in repeated doses (every 4 to 6 hours for 24 hours)
B. **Digoxin immune Fab** (only if one of the following is present):
  1. Hemodynamic instability
  2. Life-threatening arrhythmias or severe bradycardia (even if responsive to atropine)
  3. Plasma potassium level >5 mEq/L in an acute overdose
  4. Plasma digoxin level >10 ng/mL
  5. Ingestion of >10 mg of digoxin in adults (or >4 mg in children)
  6. Presence of a digoxin-toxic rhythm in the setting of an elevated digoxin level
C. Treat hyperkalemia only if it is causing ECG disturbances and avoid calcium, which can worsen intracellular hyperkalemia in these particular patients.
D. Atropine, if bradycardia is present

VI. Torsades de pointes
A. Intravenous (IV) **Mg^{2+}**

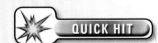

Of the antiarrhythmics, class II and class III agents decrease mortality, whereas other antiarrhythmics can be proarrhythmics, so carefully monitor a patient.

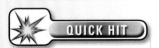

Class II agents (β-blockers) work at nodal tissue, so use these to control ventricular rate affected by atrial fibrillation, atrial flutter, and excess catecholamines.

FIGURE
3-7 ECGs of important arrhythmias

Normal ECG

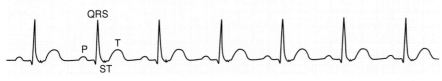

- P wave is atrial depolarization (atrial repolarization usually occurs during the QRS and remains unseen in ECG).
- PR interval (0.12–0.2 s) measures time between atrial and ventricular depolarization.
- QRS interval (normally less than 0.1 s) reflects the duration of ventricular depolarization.
- T wave is ventricular repolarization.

Sustained ventricular tachycardia

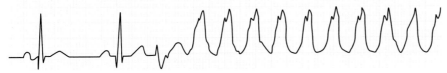

- Constant QRS morphology and fairly regular cycle length
- Initiating beat morphology may differ from ongoing VT
- AV dissociation a hallmark but not always present, nor easy to identify when present

Ventricular fibrillation

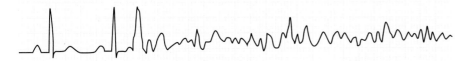

- Undulating baseline, no organized electrical activity
- Incompatible with life
- Atria may be dissociated, still in sinus rhythm

Atrial flutter

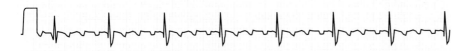

- A regular, saw-toothed pattern of atrial activity, usually very near 300/min
- Discrete, organized atrial activity on intracardiac electrograms
- Usually even-numbered AV conduction ratio (2:1, 4:1)

Atrial fibrillation

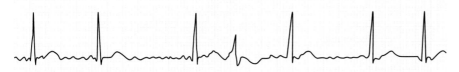

- Undulating, low amplitude atrial activity on ECG
- Intracardiac electrogram shows chaotic rapid spikes
- Variable conduction pattern as AV node is constantly bombarded with impulses; "long-short" sequences yield wide QRS complexes (aberrant, "Ashman" beats)

Wolff–Parkinson–White syndrome

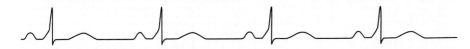

- Accessory atrioventricular conductions
- Anterograde or retrograde conduction
- Tachyarrhythmias
- Blurred QRS (referred to as δ-wave)

AV, atrioventricular; ECG, electrocardiogram; VT, ventricular tachycardia.

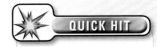

QUICK HIT

Torsades de pointes (twisting of the points): ventricular tachycardia often caused by antiarrhythmic drugs, especially quinidine. It is characterized by a long QT interval and a "short-long-short" sequence before the inception of tachycardia. The ECG shows a series of upward-pointing QRS complexes followed by a series of downward-pointing complexes.

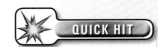

QUICK HIT

Diltiazem can be used to control the ventricular response rate in atrial fibrillation because it slows AV nodal conduction.

The Cardiovascular System

The Cardiovascular System

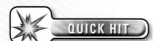
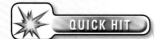
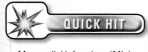
TABLE **3-2** **Conduction Anomalies**

Anomaly	Pathology	Notes	ECG
First-degree heart block	Atrioventricular nodal anomaly **lengthens PR interval** (greater than 0.2 s)	May be caused by drugs (e.g., β-blockers, digitalis, and calcium channel blockers)	
Second-degree heart block: Mobitz type 1 (Wenckebach)	Defect in atrioventricular node; progressively **increasing PR interval until QRS wave is lost**	Relatively common; usually **does not require treatment**	
Second-degree heart block: Mobitz type 2	**Defect in His–Purkinje system;** constant PR interval with random dropped QRS complexes	Less common and more dangerous than Mobitz type 1; **pacemaker**	
Third-degree heart block	No electrical connection between atria and ventricles; **atria and ventricles contract independently**	His–Purkinje system sets the rate of ventricular contraction; pacemaker may be necessary	

FIGURE **3-8** Antiarrhythmic drugs

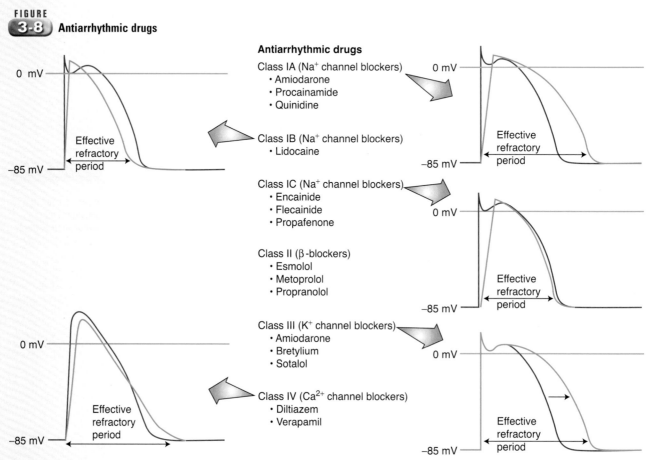

Antiarrhythmic drugs

Class IA (Na+ channel blockers)
• Amiodarone
• Procainamide
• Quinidine

Class IB (Na+ channel blockers)
• Lidocaine

Class IC (Na+ channel blockers)
• Encainide
• Flecainide
• Propafenone

Class II (β-blockers)
• Esmolol
• Metoprolol
• Propranolol

Class III (K+ channel blockers)
• Amiodarone
• Bretylium
• Sotalol

Class IV (Ca2+ channel blockers)
• Diltiazem
• Verapamil

Class IA (slows phase 0, prolongs phase 3); class IB (shortens phase 3); class IC (markedly slows phase 0); class II (suppresses phase 4 depolarization rate); class III (prolongs phase 3); class IV (slows the action potential).

TABLE 3-3 Antiarrhythmics

Therapeutic Agent (common name, if relevant) [trade name, where appropriate]	Class–Pharmacology and Pharmacokinetics	Indications	Side Effects or Adverse Effects	Contraindications or Precautions to Consider; Notes
Digoxin	Inotropic agent—cardiac glycoside; inhibits Na/K/ATPase → indirect inhibition of Na$^+$/Ca^{2+} exchanger → increases Ca^{2+} → increases cardiac contractility	**Severe left ventricular systolic dysfunction** (increases contractility), **atrial fibrillation** (decreases conduction at AV node and depresses SA node)	**Progressive dysrhythmia,** anorexia, nausea, vomiting, headache, fatigue, **confusion, blurred vision, altered color perception, halos around dark objects**	Contraindicated in patients with right-sided heart failure and diastolic failure; **ECG changes: increases PR, decreases QT, depresses ST, and inverts T; toxicities of digoxin are increased by renal failure** (decreases excretion), **hypokalemia** (potentiates the drug's effects), and **quinidine** (decreases clearance and displaces digoxin)
Sodium channel blockers (Class I)				
Quinidine, procainamide, disopyramide	**Class IA—sodium channel blocker; increases AP duration, ERP, QT interval**	**Atrial and ventricular arrhythmia** (especially reentrant and ectopic supraventricular and ventricular tachycardia)	**Torsades de pointes;** reversible lupus-like syndrome (procainamide); **Cinchonism—** headache, tinnitus, thrombocytopenia (quinidine)	Hyperkalemia increases toxicity
Lidocaine, mexiletine, tocainide	**Class IB—sodium channel blocker; decreases AP duration**	**Acute ventricular arrhythmias** (especially post-MI), digitalis-induced arrhythmia; **local anesthesia**	**CNS stimulation and depression, cardiovacular depression**	**Hyperkalemia increases toxicity**
Flecainide, propafenone	**Class IC—sodium channel blocker; no effect on AP duration**	**Ventricular tachycardia progressing to ventricular fibrillation, intractable supraventricular tachycardia,** last resort in ventricular arrhythmias	**Proarrhythmic (especially post-MI), prolongs refractory period in AV node**	**Hyperkalemia increases toxicity**

(continued)

QUICK HIT

Drugs that are used to treat arrhythmias may also cause them, especially when their use is stopped suddenly. This is an important consideration for digoxin, class IA (quinidine, disopyramide, and procainamide), class IC (propafenone, flecainide, and encainide), and class II (propranolol) drugs.

The Cardiovascular System

TABLE 3-3 Antiarrhythmics *(Continued)*				
Therapeutic Agent (common name, if relevant) [trade name, where appropriate]	**Class– Pharmacology and Pharmacokinetics**	**Indications**	**Side Effects or Adverse Effects**	**Contraindications or Precautions to Consider; Notes**
β-blockers (Class II)				
Propranolol, esmolol, metoprolol, atenolol, timolol	β-blocker— decreases cAMP and calcium currents → increases PR interval, suppresses abnormal pacemakers, especially in AV node	**Ventricular tachycardia, supraventricular tachycardia,** slowing the ventricular rate during **atrial fibrillation and atrial flutter**	**Impotence, exacerbation of asthma, bradycardia,** AV block, CHF, sedation, sleep alteration, dyslipidemia (metoprolol)	Esmolol (very short acting)
Potassium channel blocker (Class III)				
Sotalol, ibutilide, bretylium, amiodarone	**Potassium channel blocker— increases AP duration, ERP, and QT interval**	**Wolff– Parkinson– White syndrome; used when other antiarrythmics fail**	**Torsades de pointes,** excessive beta block, and hypotension; amiodarone- **pulmonary fibrosis,** corneal deposits, **hepatotoxicity,** skin deposits, photodermatitis, neurologic effects, constipation, bradycardia, CHF, heart block, and **hypothyroidism/hyperthyroidism**	
Calcium channel blockers (Class IV)				
Verapamil, diltiazem	**Calcium channel blocker— decreases conduction velocity of AV nodal cells, increases ERP, PR interval**	**Prevent nodal arrhythmias (supraventricular tachycardia)**	Constipation, **flushing, edema,** CHF, AV block, sinus node depression, torsades de pointes	
Other				
Adenosine	**Increases potassium efflux → hyperpolarizes the cell**	**Diagnosis and treatment of AV nodal-arrhythmias**	**Flushing, hypotension, and chest pain**	Very short acting
Potassium	**Depresses ectopic pacemaker in hypokalemia**	**Digoxin toxicity**		

AP, action potential; ATPase, adenosine triphosphatase; AV, atrioventricular; cAMP, cyclic adenosine monophosphate; CHF, congestive heart failure; CNS, central nervous system; ECG, electrocardiogram; ERP, effective refractory period; MI, myocardial infarction; SA, sinoatrial.

ATHEROSCLEROSIS

I. **Atherosclerosis** is a disease of large and medium-sized vessels, characterized by the formation of atheromas (i.e., lesions that have a central lipid-rich core surrounded by fibrous tissue) deposited in the intima of arteries. It is the leading cause of mortality in the United States.

II. **Risk factors**
   A. Major risk factors
      1. Dyslipidemia: high blood cholesterol, high low-density lipoproteins (LDLs), high triglycerides, and decreased high-density lipoproteins (HDLs; <45 mg/dL) (Table 3-4)
      2. Diabetes mellitus
      3. Cigarette smoking
      4. Hypertension
      5. Obesity
   B. Minor risk factors
      1. Lack of physical activity
      2. Male sex
      3. Increased age
      4. Family history
      5. Oral contraceptives, decreased estrogens, or premature menopause
      6. Type A personality
      7. Elevated homocysteine level

III. **Pathogenesis**
   A. Atheroma formation
      1. Monocytes adhere to vessel walls, enter tissue, and become macrophages.
      2. Macrophages are transformed into foam cells after engulfing oxidized LDLs.
      3. Foam cells accumulate in the intima.
      4. Foam cells release factors that cause the aggregation of platelets, the release of fibroblast growth factor, and the accumulation of smooth muscle.
      5. After formation of plaque, calcification occurs.
      6. The central core of the plaque consists mainly of cholesterol.
   B. Complications
      1. Plaque rupture
      2. Ischemic heart disease or myocardial infarction (MI)
      3. Stroke
      4. Renal arterial ischemia
      5. Death

 FAMILIAL DYSLIPIDEMIAS (Table 3-4)

TABLE 3-4	Selected Familial Dyslipidemia				
Familial Dyslipidemias	**Elevated**	**Blood Lipid Levels**	**Pathology (see Chapter 5)**	**Clinical Picture**	**Treatment**
Hypercholesterolemia IIa	LDL	↑ Cholesterol	**Decreased LDL receptors**	Greatly increased vascular and heart disease; **xanthomas**	Cholestyramine/ colestipol, lovastatin (and niacin for homozygotes)

(continued)

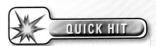

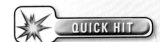

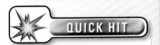

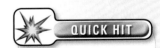

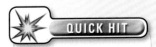

The Cardiovascular System

TABLE **3-4** Selected Familial Dyslipidemia *(Continued)*

Familial Dyslipidemias	Elevated	Blood Lipid Levels	Pathology (see Chapter 5)	Clinical Picture	Treatment
Dysbetalipoproteinemia III	VLDL	↑ TG, ↑ Cholesterol	Altered apolipoprotein E	Increased vascular and heart disease; xanthomas	Niacin and clofibrate or lovastatin
Hypertriglyceridemia IV	VLDL	↑↑ TG, normal to ↑ cholesterol	Hepatic overproduction (with possible decreased clearance) of VLDL	Increased vascular and heart disease; obese, **diabetic, pregnant,** and **alcoholic** patients	Weight loss, low-fat diet, niacin and clofibrate or lovastatin (if necessary)

LDL, low-density lipoproteins; TG, triglycerides; VLDL, very low-density lipoproteins.

 LIPID-LOWERING AGENTS *(Table 3-5)*

TABLE **3-5** Lipid-Lowering Agents

Therapeutic Agent (common name, if relevant) [trade name, where appropriate]	Class–Pharmacology and Pharmacokinetics	Indications	Side Effects or Adverse Effects	Contraindications or Precautions to Consider; Notes
Lovastatin, pravastatin, simvastatin, atorvastatin	**HMG-CoA reductase inhibitors**—inhibits the synthesis of cholesterol precursor mevalonate; **decreases LDL, increases HDL, and decreases TG**	**High LDL, preventative after thrombotic event (e.g., MI, stroke)**	Reversible increase in LFTs, myositis	
Niacin	**Inhibits lipolysis** in fat tissue, **reduces** hepatic **VLDL secretion** into circulation; decreases **LDL, increases HDL, and decreases TG**	**Increased LDL, decreased HDL**	Flushing (decreased by aspirin or long-term use)	
Cholestyramine, colestipol	**Bile acid resin/cholesterol absorption blocker**—binds bile acids → prevents intestinal reabsorption of bile acid and therefore cholesterol; **decreases LDL and increases HDL**	**Increased LDL**	**Tastes like sand, GI irritation,** and decreased absorption of fat-soluble vitamins	
Ezetimibe	**Cholesterol absorption blocker**—prevents cholesterol reabsorption at brush border in the small intestine; **decreases LDL; no effect on HDL or TG**	**Increased LDL**	Increased LFT (rarely)	No proven clinical benefit; may increase plaque thickness
Gemfibrozil, clofibrate, bezafibrate, fenofibrate	**Upregulates lipoprotein lipase (periphery)** → **increases TG clearance; decreases LDL, increases HDL, and decreases TG**	**Increased TG, increased LDL**	Myositis, increased LFTs	Reduces TG more than other agents

GI, gastrointestinal; HDL, high-density lipoprotein; HMG-CoA, 3-hydroxy-3-methylglutaryl-coenzyme A; LDL, low-density lipoprotein; LFT, liver function test; MI, myocardial infarction; TG, triglyceride; VLDL, very low-density lipoprotein.

HYPERTENSION

I. Essential
A. Most common type (95% of cases)
B. Unknown etiology
C. Risk factors
1. Family history
2. Race (more common in Blacks)
3. Obesity
4. Cigarette smoking
5. Physical inactivity
D. Characteristics
1. Blood pressure greater than 140/90 mm Hg on three separate occasions, with the patient comfortably sitting and arm at the level of the patient's heart.
E. Chronic complications
1. Hypertrophy of left ventricle
2. Onion skinning of vessel walls
3. Retinal hemorrhages
F. Essential hypertension predisposes to ischemic heart disease (see next section).

II. Secondary hypertension refers to elevated systemic arterial pressure associated with a condition known to cause hypertension
A. Renal diseases are the most common cause of secondary hypertension.
1. Renal parenchymal disorders (chronic kidney disease)
2. Unilateral renal artery stenosis
a. Atherosclerosis (more common in Black males and older individuals)
b. Fibromuscular dysplasia (more common in White females and younger individuals)
3. Renin–angiotensin axis activated
B. Endocrine causes
1. Primary aldosteronism
2. Pheochromocytoma
3. Hyperthyroidism
4. Acromegaly
5. Cushing syndrome
C. Coarctation of the aorta

III. Malignant hypertension
A. **Hypertensive urgency** is blood pressure ≥180/120 mm Hg without symptoms and without evidence of end-organ damage.
B. **Hypertensive emergency** (malignant hypertension) is blood pressure ≥180/120 mm Hg with evidence of end-organ damage.
1. Cardiovascular—vascular damage, aortic dissection
2. Pulmonary—pulmonary edema
3. Renal—"flea-bitten kidneys," azotemia
4. Ocular—fundal hemorrhages, papilledema
5. Central nervous system—encephalopathy, seizures, coma
C. This type of hypertension causes early death because of cerebrovascular accident (CVA).
D. Young Black males are the usual victims of this type of hypertension.

ANTIHYPERTENSIVE AGENTS (Table 3-6)

I. α-Blockers
A. α-Adrenergic receptors are the primary controllers of vascular tone, blockers are used primarily to lower blood pressure.
1. α_1-Selective agents commonly used in the treatment of hypertension include prazosin, doxazosin, and terazosin.

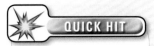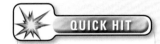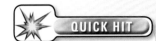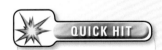

QUICK HIT Hypertrophy of the left ventricle is also caused by left-sided valvular disease such as aortic stenosis and mitral regurgitation.

QUICK HIT Fibromuscular dysplasia of the renal artery causes a "beads-on-a-string" sign on radiograph.

QUICK HIT Treatment for malignant hypertensive emergency (systolic blood pressure greater than 180 mm Hg or diastolic pressure greater than 120 mm Hg) commonly includes IV sodium nitroprusside or IV enalapril. It is dangerous to give pure β-blockers because of unopposed α stimulation. Therefore, an α/β-blocker such as labetalol can be given.

QUICK HIT β-Blockers mask many of the symptoms of hypoglycemia (tremors, sweating, palpitations, etc.) that are mediated by epinephrine. This, as well as the endocrine effects, puts individuals with insulin-dependent diabetes taking β-blockers at increased risk for profound hypoglycemia.

The Cardiovascular System

TABLE 3-6 Antihypertensive Agents

Therapeutic Agent (common name, if relevant) [trade name, where appropriate]	Class—Pharmacology and Pharmacokinetics	Indications	Side Effects or Adverse Effects	Contraindications or Precautions to Consider; Notes
Diuretics				
Hydrochlorothiazide	Thiazide diuretic—inhibits transport of Na⁺ and Cl⁻ into the cells of DCT	**Hypertension, CHF,** idiopathic hypercalciuria, nephrogenic diabetes insipidus	**Hypokalemia, metabolic alkalosis, mild hyperlipidemia, hyperuricemia,** malaise, **hypercalcemia,** hyperglycemia, hyponatremia	Do not give in patients with sulfa drug allergy
Furosemide	Loop diuretic—prevents cotransport of Na⁺, K⁺, and Cl⁻ in **thick ascending limb**	**Hypertension, CHF,** cirrhosis, nephrotic syndrome, **pulmonary edema,** and hypercalcemia	**Potassium wasting, metabolic alkalosis,** hypotension, dehydration, **ototoxicity,** nephritis, and gout	Do not give in patients with **sulfa drug allergy**
RAA system				
Captopril, enalapril, fosinopril, lisinopril, quinapril	ACE inhibitor → inhibits conversion of angiotensin (Ang) I to II → decreases Ang II levels → prevents vasoconstriction from Ang II	**Hypertension, CHF, post-MI agent, prevention/treatment of diabetic nephropathy**	**Cough, angioedema, hyperkalemia,** renal insufficiency (especially in bilateral renal artery stenosis)	Contraindicated in pregnancy (fetal renal malformation)
Losartan, valsartan, irbesartan, olmesartan, candesartan	ARBs → prevents vasoconstriction from Ang II	**Hypertension**	Fetal renal toxicity, **hyperkalemia**	
Sympathoplegics				
Metoprolol, atenolol, acebutolol, esmolol, propranolol, timolol, carvedilol, labetalol	β₁-Blocker (metoprolol, atenolol, acebutolol, esmolol), β₁- and β₂-blocker (propanolol, timolol), carvedilol, and labetalol (α- and β-blocker)	**Hypertension, angina, MI, antiarrhythmic**	**Bronchospasm, bradycardia,** AV block, heart failure, sedation, and sleep alterations	
Prazosin, terazosin, doxazosin	α₁-**Blocker** → vasodilation → decreases total peripheral resistance	**Pheochromocytoma, hypertension, benign prostatic hyperplasia**	**Orthostatic hypotension,** dizziness, and headache	First-dose orthostatic hypotension
Clonidine	Centrally acting sympathetic agent (α₂-agonist) → decreases sympathetic outflow from CNS → decreases peripheral resistance	**Hypertension,** heroin, and cocaine withdrawal	Drowsiness, **dry mouth, and rebound hypertension after abrupt withdrawal**	
Methyldopa	Centrally acting sympathetic agent (α-agonist) → decreases sympathetic outflow from CNS	**Hypertension** (most commonly used in pregnancy)	Sedation and hemolytic anemia	**Positive Coombs test**
Hexamethonium	Nicotinic ganglionic blocker	Hypertensive emergency	Severe orthostatic hypotension, blurred vision, constipation, and sexual dysfunction	
Reserpine	Prevents the storage of monoamines in synaptic vesicle	Hypertension	**Mental depression,** sedation, nasal stuffiness, and diarrhea	

(continued)

The Cardiovascular System

TABLE 3-6 Antihypertensive Agents *(Continued)*				
Therapeutic Agent (common name, if relevant) [trade name, where appropriate]	Class—Pharmacology and Pharmacokinetics	Indications	Side Effects or Adverse Effects	Contraindications or Precautions to Consider; Notes
Guanethidine	Interferes with norepinephrine release	**Severe hypertension**	Orthostatic hypotension, exercise hypotension, impotence, and diarrhea	**Contraindicated in patients taking TCAs**
Vasodilators **Hydralazine**	Increases cGMP → smooth muscle relaxation → vasodilates arterioles → afterload reduction	**Severe hypertension, CHF**	**Compensatory tachycardia**, fluid retention, and **lupus-like syndrome**	**First-line therapy for hypertension in pregnancy**, used with methyldopa; contraindicated in angina/CAD because of compensatory tachycardia
Minoxidil	**K⁺ channel opener** → hyperpolarizes and relaxes vascular smooth muscle	**Severe hypertension**	**Hypertrichosis** and pericardial effusion	
Nifedipine, felodipine, amlodipine	**Dihydropyridine Ca²⁺ channel blockers** block voltage-gated Ca²⁺ channels of **vascular** smooth muscle	**Hypertension, angina pectoris, Prinzmetal angina, Raynaud phenomenon**	Peripheral edema, **flushing, dizziness**, and constipation	
Diltiazem, verapamil	**Non-dihydropyridine Ca²⁺ channel blockers**—block voltage-gated Ca²⁺ channels of **cardiac** smooth muscle	**Hypertension, angina pectoris, arrhythmia**	Cardiac depression, peripheral edema, **flushing, dizziness**, and constipation	
Nitroprusside	Direct release of NO → increases cGMP → vasodilator (arterial dilation)	**Hypertensive emergency, CHF, and angina**	Cyanide toxicity, hypotension	Short acting
Diazoxide	**K⁺ channel opener**— hyperpolarizes and relaxes vascular smooth muscle	**Hypertension**	Hypoglycemia (reduces insulin release) and hypotension	

ACE, angiotension-converting enzyme; ARB, angiotensin II receptor blocker; AV, atrioventricular; CAD, coronary artery disease; cGMP, cyclic guanosine monophosphate; CHF, congestive heart failure; CNS, central nervous system; DCT, distal convoluted tubule; MI, myocardial infarction; NO, nitric oxide; RAA, renin-angiotensin-aldosterone; TCA, tricyclic antidepressant.

   2. They have little impact on the heart, but they do have selective effects that allow them to have other clinical uses (such as treatment for benign prostatic hypertrophy).
  B. Side effects
   1. Postural hypotension with reflex tachycardia (most common)
   2. Nasal congestion and headache
   3. Rebound hypertension if stopped abruptly
  C. Phenoxybenzamine and phentolamine are nonselective α-blockers that can be used in the diagnosis and treatment of the symptoms of pheochromocytoma.

II. β-Blockers
  A. β-Blockers can be divided into four subgroups:
   1. Nonselective β-blockers (β₁ and β₂): propranolol, timolol, and nadolol
   2. β₁-Selective agents: metoprolol, atenolol, acebutolol, and esmolol

3. β_2-Selective agents (discussed in Chapter 4)
4. α/β-Blockers (carvedilol, labetalol)

B. This important class of drugs has many clinical uses:
1. Cardiac uses (most common)
   a. Hypertension
   b. Stable angina
   c. Prophylaxis after an MI
2. Less common uses
   a. Symptomatic treatment of hyperthyroidism
   b. Prophylaxis against migraine headaches
   c. Anxiety disorder

C. Therapeutic effects of β-blockers on various organ systems are listed in Table 3-7.

D. Adverse effects
1. Sexual dysfunction in males
2. Arrhythmias if the drug is stopped abruptly
3. Bronchoconstriction
4. Blocking hypoglycemic response in a diabetic

III. Calcium channel blockers

A. Second-line antihypertensive agents

B. Act by binding to the L-type calcium channel of vascular smooth muscle cells and myocytes

C. Block the entry of calcium into these cells

D. These agents affect both vascular tone and the heart itself. Effects on the heart include negative inotropy and slowing of the conduction system.

E. Calcium channel blockers are often divided into two groups:
1. Dihydropyridines
   a. Examples: nifedipine and amlodipine
   b. Greater effect on vascular smooth muscle than on the heart
2. Non-dihydropyridines
   a. Examples: diltiazem and verapamil
   b. Increasingly greater effects on the myocardium

F. Adverse effects include hypotension, headache, constipation, peripheral edema, and exacerbation of gastroesophageal reflux and bradycardia.

IV. Other antihypertensive agents

A. Clonidine
1. Along with α-methyldopa, a centrally acting antihypertensive agent
2. This agent acts as an agonist at presynaptic α_2 receptors, thereby decreasing central sympathetic tone.

TABLE 3-7 Therapeutic Effects of β-Blockers

Organ System	Effect	Clinical Implication
Cardiac (β_1)	Negative inotropic and chronotropic effects; slowing of SA and atrio-ventricular nodes	Decreases cardiac output; bradycardia can limit dosing; atrioventricular nodal slowing is useful in supraventricular tachycardia
Pulmonary (β_2)	Constriction of airway smooth muscle	β-Blockers are contraindicated in patients with chronic obstructive pulmonary disease
Endocrine	Decreased glycogenolysis, decreased glucagon release	β-Blockers must be used with caution in patients with diabetes taking insulin who are at risk for hypoglycemia
Ocular	Decreased aqueous humor production by processes of ciliary body	β-Blockers, such as timolol, can be used topically for glaucoma

Note: Those effects known to be predominantly caused by either β_1- or β_2-blockers are listed as such. SA, sinoatrial.

3. Adverse effects include sedation and rebound hypertension if the drug is stopped abruptly.

B. Sodium nitroprusside
1. Given intravenously, this agent is the drug of choice for hypertensive emergencies.
2. Given orally, this drug is toxic because it results in cyanide production.
3. It affects both arterial and venous smooth muscle.

C. Vasodilators (hydralazine, minoxidil)
1. Dilate both arteries and veins (predominantly arteries), lowering blood pressure
   a. Reflex tachycardia that results can actually precipitate attacks of angina.
   b. These agents are not first-line agents for hypertension.
   c. These are often used along with β-blockers and diuretics.
2. Adverse reactions to hydralazine include headache, arrhythmias, and a lupus-like reaction.
3. Adverse effects of minoxidil include sodium retention and hypertrichosis.

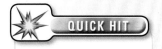

QUICK HIT

Berry aneurysms are commonly associated with adult polycystic kidney disease, an autosomal dominant disease; the gene is located on chromosome 16.

 ANEURYSMS *(Table 3-8)*

TABLE 3-8 **Aneurysms**		
Type of Aneurysm	**Etiology**	**Characteristics**
Arteriovenous fistula	Abnormal communication between arteries and veins; usually secondary to **trauma**	Ischemic changes, aneurysm formation, **high-output cardiac failure**
Atherosclerotic	**Atherosclerotic** disease, coronary artery disease	Usually in the **abdominal** aorta; located between renal arteries and iliac bifurcation
Berry	Congenital medial weakness at the bifurcations of the cerebral arteries	Saccular lesions in cerebral vessels (especially at the **circle of Willis**), hemorrhage into the **subarachnoid** space
Dissecting	**Hypertension,** cystic medial necrosis, **Marfan syndrome**	**Tearing pain;** longitudinal separation of tunica media of aortic wall
Syphilitic	Tertiary syphilis, obliteration of the vasa vasorum, necrosis of the media	Involves **ascending** aorta and aortic root; aortic valve insufficiency
Mycotic (infectious)	Inflammation secondary to bacterial infection; usually salmonella	Involves abdominal aorta

I. Abdominal aortic aneurysm (AAA)

A. Focal dilation of the aorta, generally thought to be due to atherosclerosis

B. The most common location is the infrarenal aorta. Therefore, an AAA may be palpated superior to the umbilicus because the aorta bifurcates at the level of the umbilicus.

C. Presentation
1. Usually asymptomatic until late in the course. May cause some abdominal pain.
2. The most common diagnosis mistaken for AAA in the emergency setting is kidney stones.
3. The most dangerous complication is rupture, which presents as a triad of **hypotension, abdominal pain, and pulsatile mass** in the abdomen. Hypertension increases the risk of rupture of an AAA.

D. All men aged 65 to 75 years with any history of smoking should be screened for AAA with a one-time abdominal sonogram.

E. Treatment is surgical repair for any of the following:
1. Aneurysm diameter ≥5.5 cm
2. Diameter increasing ≥0.5 cm in a 6-month interval
3. Any symptomatic AAA

Clinical Vignette 3-1

CLINICAL PRESENTATION: A 59-year-old male presents to the emergency room with **sudden, severe, and constant low back pain.** Past medical history is significant for **hypertension, hyperlipidemia, emphysema,** coronary artery disease, stable angina, and a 25-pack-year history of **smoking.** The patient was hospitalized for a cerebrovascular accident 7 years ago. Physical examination revealed a 5.8 cm **pulsatile mass** superior to the umbilicus in the abdomen. Temperature = 98.5° F; **blood pressure = 150/90 mm Hg;** heart rate = 80 bpm; and respiration rate = 23 breaths/min.

DIFFERENTIALS: Abdominal aortic aneurysm (AAA), aortic dissection, pyelonephritis/nephrolithiasis, prostatitis, and pancreatitis. Given that this pain developed suddenly and the presence of an abdominal pulsatile mass, this patient most likely has an AAA.

LABORATORY STUDIES: Proper follow-up for this patient would include an **abdominal ultrasound** and/or **computerized tomography (CT) scan with contrast.** The typical diameter for abdominal aorta is **2 cm**; therefore, any size greater than this indicates presence of an aneurysm. Advantages of an ultrasound are that it is quick, easy, and inexpensive; however, it is very operator dependent, less useful in obese individuals, and does not provide information about the iliac arteries, which could also be aneurysmal. **CT angiogram** can also be helpful in describing the anatomy of the aorta prior to surgery, but it is not commonly done in clinical practice. All patients with AAA should also undergo cardiac evaluation because patients with AAA often have underlying vascular pathology. In these patients, **cardiac catheterization** should also be performed to assess cardiac risk and potentially revascularize the patients prior to operation.

MANAGEMENT: As an aneurysm becomes larger than 5.5 cm, the risk of rupture increases exponentially; an aneurysm smaller than 5.5 cm in diameter is less likely to rupture, and risk-to-benefit ratio of surgery is less supportive. Therefore, if an AAA is **smaller than 5.5 cm** in diameter and asymptomatic, the patient can be followed with ultrasound or CT surveillance every 6 months. If the aneurysm is **larger than 5.5 cm** in diameter and symptomatic, the patient should be taken to the operating room. A patient with a ruptured AAA is taken to the operating room.

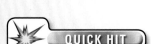

Syphilis is a sexually transmitted disease caused by *Treponema pallidum* (a spirochete) that is characterized initially (primary stage) by a painless, hard chancre. Untreated syphilis progresses to secondary and tertiary stages, which are characterized by rashes, lymphadenopathy, condylomata lata, Argyll Robertson pupils (pupils constrict with accommodation but not with light), and aortic root aneurysms.

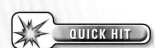

Exercise tolerance testing (stress testing) is a good way to diagnose subacute coronary occlusion. Thallium-201 scans reveal perfusion defects. Technetium (^{99m}Tc) scans are useful for imaging MIs.

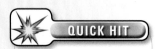

Risk factors for coronary artery disease: smoking; diabetes; ↑ LDL, ↓ HDL; family history; men or postmenopausal women; sedentary lifestyle; hypertension; ↑ age; ↑ homocysteine; obesity.

II. Thoracic aortic dissection

A. A tear in the intima of the aorta, with blood forcing its way into the media and forming a false lumen

B. The most common risk factor is **hypertension**. Other risk factors can include trauma, syphilis aortitis, Marfan syndrome, and Ehlers–Danlos syndrome.

C. Most commonly found in the thoracic aorta
   1. Stanford A dissection involves any part of the ascending aorta and is treated surgically.
   2. Stanford B dissection is confined to the descending aorta (distal to the left subclavian artery).

D. Presentation
   1. Acute, "tearing" chest pain, radiating through to the back
   2. Widened mediastinum on chest x-ray.
   3. Dissections that involve other vessels may cause MI, stroke symptoms or syncope, or decreased peripheral pulses.

E. Management
   1. First, stabilize the blood pressure with β-blockers (labetalol) or nitroprusside.
   2. Surgical repair for Stanford A dissections or Stanford B dissections with rupture or other complications

ISCHEMIC HEART DISEASE

I. It is defined as an inadequate supply of oxygen relative to demand.

II. Ischemic heart disease is most often caused by atherosclerosis.

III. There are four types of ischemic heart diseases.

A. **Angina pectoris**

1. Paroxysmal attacks of retrosternal pain, heaviness, and pressure-like or squeezing chest pain occur and may radiate to the neck, jaw, left shoulder, or arm. Angina pectoris is often associated with diaphoresis and nausea.

2. Imbalance between cardiac perfusion and cardiac demand is characteristic. Ninety percent occlusion of coronary vessel produces symptoms.

3. Three types of angina pectoris:

   a. **Stable angina**
   - Most common form
   - Induced by exercise
   - Relieved by rest
   - Results from chronic stenosis of coronary arteries

   b. **Prinzmetal (variant) angina**
   - Episodic pain occurs at rest.
   - Attacks are unrelated to activity, blood pressure, or heart rate but are related to coronary artery vasospasm.
   - Significant artery stenosis is often present.

   c. **Unstable angina**
   - This type occurs at both rest and activity.
   - It is usually preceded by decreasing physical activity or gradual increase in stable anginal symptoms.
   - It produces pain of increasing duration.
   - It is induced by ruptured atherosclerotic plaque with subsequent platelet-mediated thrombosis, which partially occludes the vessel. This results in ischemia and angina, but there is no myocardial necrosis.

4. Treatment of stable angina

   a. Nitrates
   - These drugs are converted within the cell to nitric oxide, a smooth muscle relaxant.
     (1) The relaxation of vascular smooth muscle causes widespread venous dilation.
     (2) This lowers preload and therefore reduces the workload and oxygen demand of the heart.
     (3) To a lesser extent, the relaxation of coronary arteries provides ischemic myocardium with increased oxygen.
   - Sublingual nitroglycerin is the treatment of choice for acute episodes of angina.
   - A long-acting nitrate such as isosorbide dinitrate can be used for angina prophylaxis.
   - Unwanted side effects of nitrate therapy include headache and tachyphylaxis, postural hypotension, and facial flushing.

   b. Calcium channel

   c. β-Blockers

B. **MI**

1. Lack of adequate perfusion to cardiac tissue leads to myocyte death in affected area.

2. MI is most often caused by atherosclerosis with plaque rupture and thrombus.

3. The subendocardium is most vulnerable to ischemia (because of decreased blood flow during systole) and thus most likely to infarct.

4. In a transmural infarct (see following text), the full thickness of the ventricular wall is affected within 35 hours.

5. Two types of MI are possible:

   a. Non-ST elevation MI (NSTEMI)
   - Formerly called "nontransmural" or "non–Q-wave" infarct
   - As in unstable angina, atherosclerotic plaques rupture.
   - Platelet-mediated thrombosis completely occludes the vessel, resulting in loss of perfusion to inner one-third of muscular wall of ventricle occurs. Clot lysis limits the depth of infarction.

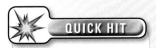

Angina pectoris causes ST depression on ECGs, but this is only observed during the attack, which lasts 2 to 5 minutes.

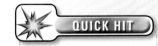

Anticoagulants (heparin, low-molecular-weight heparin, and aspirin), nitrates, and β-blockers can be used to treat unstable angina. Do *not* use calcium channel blockers or tissue plasminogen activator to treat unstable angina.

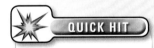

Cocaine use can also result in coronary vasospasm resulting in myocardial ischemia. In general, cocaine works by inhibiting the reuptake of endogenous catecholamines (dopamine, norepinephrine, epinephrine, and serotonin). Conversely, amphetamines stimulate the release of endogenous catecholamines.

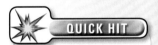

The left anterior descending artery is the most common artery involved in acute MI. Infarcts of this artery affect the left ventricle near its apex or the anterior portion of the interventricular septum.

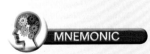

When remembering the sequence of histopathologic changes after an MI, think of the 1-3-1-3 rule: 1 day (**neutrophils** predominate), 3 days (**macrophages** infiltrate), 1 week (**fibroblasts** infiltrate), and 3 weeks (**granulation** tissue most prominent).

The Cardiovascular System

FIGURE 3-9 Myocardial infarction enzyme release and timeline of histologic changes

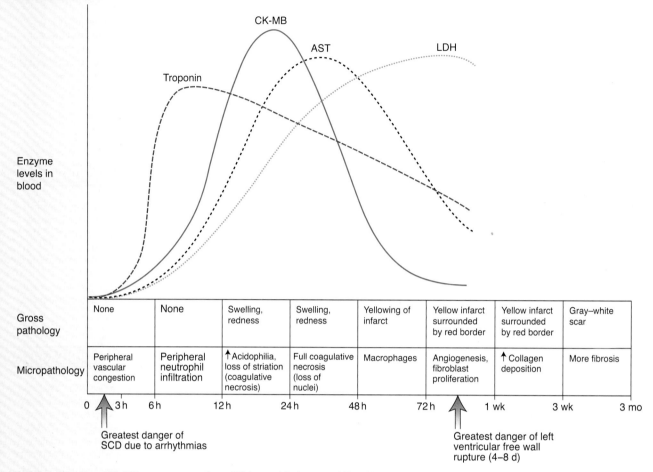

CK-MB, creatine kinase-MB; AST, aspartate transaminase; LDH, lactate dehydrogenase; SCD, sudden cardiac death.

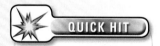

QUICK HIT

Because of state-dependent block, lidocaine works on slightly depolarized or ischemic tissue more so than normal tissue. Therefore, use lidocaine (IV) to suppress acute MI-associated ventricular arrhythmias.

- Tissue infarction and myocardial necrosis lead to release of cardiac enzymes (Figure 3-9).
- ST-segment depression (but no ST elevation) is seen on ECG. Q waves do not develop.

b. ST elevation MI (STEMI)
  - Formerly called "transmural" or "Q-wave" infarct
  - As in NSTEMI, atherosclerotic plaques rupture, and platelet-mediated thrombosis completely occludes the vessel. There is no clot lysis, so the infarction extends to the entire muscular wall.
  - Tissue infarction and myocardial necrosis lead to release of cardiac enzymes (Figure 3-9).
  - ST-segment elevation is seen on ECG, and Q waves eventually develop.

6. Complications
  a. Arrhythmia—especially **ventricular fibrillation** (the primary cause of death in the first hour post-MI) heart block
  b. Papillary muscle rupture—presents as acute mitral regurgitation 2 to 7 days post-MI
  c. Myocardial rupture—rare, occurs most commonly 2 to 7 days post-MI
  d. **Dressler syndrome**—pericardial inflammation occurring **2 to 6 weeks post-MI**; presents with fever, malaise, pleuritic chest pain, pericardial friction rub, and elevated erythrocyte sedimentation rate (ESR)
  e. Ventricular aneurysm—usually due to anterior wall MI

Clinical Vignette 3-2

CLINICAL PRESENTATION: A 45-year-old male was brought to the emergency department complaining of **crushing chest pain of 1-hour duration,** which he described as "a belt closed **tightly** around my chest." He indicated the location of the pain with a closed fist in the substernal region. The morning of admission, the patient was feeling ill and then experienced pain in the chest, which **radiated to his jaw, left shoulder, and down the left arm.** The pain was associated with **nausea;** the patient denied conditions that improved or worsened the pain. The patient's past medical history was significant for **hyperlipidemia** and **hypertension.** The patient stated that **his father recently underwent coronary artery bypass.** Past social history was significant for a 35-pack-year history of **smoking** and social drinking. On physical examination, the patient was found to be in acute distress and diaphoretic. Temperature = 97.6° F; blood pressure = 145/90 mm Hg; **heart rate = 101 bpm; and respiration rate =** 23 breaths/min.

DIFFERENTIALS: Acute myocardial infarction (MI), angina pectoris, aortic dissection, gastroesophageal reflux disease (GERD), pancreatitis and biliary tract disease, pericarditis, and pulmonary embolism (PE). Given the patient's description of pain and family history of coronary artery disease, he most likely has suffered from an acute MI.

LABORATORY STUDIES: An acute MI would be diagnosed via (a) **blood chemistry** showing elevated cardiac enzymes or (b) **ECG** showing ST elevation if transmural or ST depression if subendocardial. With these changes, aortic dissection, GERD, and PE can be ruled out. In an aortic dissection, we would expect a widened mediastinum on **chest radiograph,** confirmed by **CT scan;** also, an **aortogram** showing a double lumen would be diagnostic. Stable angina can be ruled out because it typically lasts a few minutes, and although it can precede an MI, this pain is characteristically **relieved by rest or nitroglycerin.** Other laboratory studies that would be done in this patient include **amylase, lipase, alkaline phosphatase** (elevated in pancreatitis), and **echocardiography** (to rule out pericarditis). Interestingly, pericarditis presents with chest pain that radiates to the trapezoid region, worsens with inspiration, and is relieved by sitting up/leaning forward.

MANAGEMENT: Revascularization, if done early, is beneficial via **thrombolytics** or **angioplasty.** Patients should also receive **morphine** (reduces pain and is a vasodilator), **heparin** (to prevent formation of thrombus), and **nitrates.** This patient should be started and maintained on **aspirin** (shown to decrease mortality), **α-blockers** (prevent remodeling), **ACE inhibitors** (prevent remodeling), and **statins** (lower cholesterol and decrease risk of future coronary events).

  f. Mural thrombus with possible embolization
  g. Progressive ischemic cardiomyopathy and congestive heart failure (CHF)
 7. Remodeling and scar formation occur over a period of 36 months after an infarct (Figure 3-9).
C. Chronic ischemic heart disease (CIHD)
 1. CHF that results from ischemic cardiac damage leads to CIHD.
 2. Hypertrophy of the heart and cardiac decompensation occur as a result of infarction.
 3. CIHD is most often found in the elderly.
D. Sudden cardiac death
 1. This is unexpected death from cardiac failure occurring within 2-hour post-MI.
 2. This is caused less commonly by a congenital anomaly.
 3. Marked atherosclerosis is usually present.
 4. The mechanism of death is almost always because of arrhythmia.

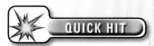

QUICK HIT

Cor pulmonale is right-sided heart failure secondary to lung disorders that lead to pulmonary arterial hypertension.

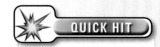

QUICK HIT

Idiopathic dilated cardiomyopathy is the most common form of cardiomyopathy. Treatment includes digitalis, ACE inhibitors, heart transplant, and sometimes chronic anticoagulation.

 CONGESTIVE HEART FAILURE (Table 3-9 and Figures 3-10 to 3-11)

CHF is a clinical diagnosis in which the heart is unable to pump an adequate amount of blood to meet the metabolic needs of the body. A number of factors play a role in CHF, including hormonal changes (RAA and sympathetic activation), peripheral vasoconstriction, and myocardial dysfunction. One of the final common pathways in CHF is

TABLE 3-9 Congestive Heart Failure

	Etiology	Clinical Manifestations
Left-sided congestive heart failure (CHF)	Ischemia (coronary artery disease) Systemic hypertension Left-sided valvular disease Myocarditis Cardiomyopathy Congenital heart disease Pericardial disease	**Pulmonary edema** Dyspnea on exertion/fatigue **Orthopnea** Paroxysmal nocturnal dyspnea Hyperventilation Reduction in renal perfusion (activates renin-angiotensin-aldosterone axis) **S3**
Right-sided CHF	Left-sided heart failure Left-sided lesions **Cor pulmonale** Myocarditis Cardiomyopathy Right-sided valvular disease	Hepatomegaly/ascites **(nutmeg liver)** Splenomegaly **Peripheral edema** (especially pitting edema of the ankles) **Distention of neck veins** Renal hypoxia

hypoperfusion of the kidneys and activation of the RAA axis, which leads to sodium and water retention. Treatment is directed at either blocking the RAA axis or increasing the cardiac performance and, therefore, renal perfusion. Therapeutic agents in CHF treatment include ACE inhibitors, angiotensin II receptor blockers (ARBs), digitalis, diuretics, and dobutamine.

I. ACE inhibitors
A. First-line treatment for CHF
B. ACE inhibitors are able to lower blood pressure (lower afterload), improve cardiac performance, and prevent the aldosterone-mediated salt and water retention typical of CHF.
C. Specific agents:
　1. Enalapril decreases mortality in CHF.
　2. Other ACE inhibitors include captopril and lisinopril.
D. Adverse effects of ACE inhibitors:
　1. Reversible renal failure
　2. Angioedema, hyperkalemia, dry cough, and orthostatic hypotension
　3. ACE inhibitors are fetotoxic and contraindicated in pregnancy.

II. ARBs
A. These agents block the RAA axis at the Ang II receptor, producing the same benefits as ACE inhibitors.
B. Examples of ARBs are losartan and valsartan.
C. These drugs have all the same effects as the ACE inhibitors except that, unlike the ACE inhibitors, they do not increase levels of bradykinin and hence do not cause cough as a side effect.

III. Digitalis
A. Treats CHF by increasing cardiac performance; digitalis treats CHF by increasing the intracellular concentration of calcium in cardiac myocytes, thus increasing contractility.
B. Blocks sodium–potassium pump:
　1. This increases the intracellular sodium concentration.
　2. Activity of a sodium–calcium antiporter is decreased.
　3. Decreased activity of this antiporter raises intracellular calcium levels.
C. Digitalis improves the symptoms of CHF, but unlike ACE inhibitors, it has not been shown to decrease mortality.
D. Digitalis also has a low therapeutic index, which means that the toxic dose is closer to the therapeutic dose.

FIGURE
3-10 **Congestive heart failure**

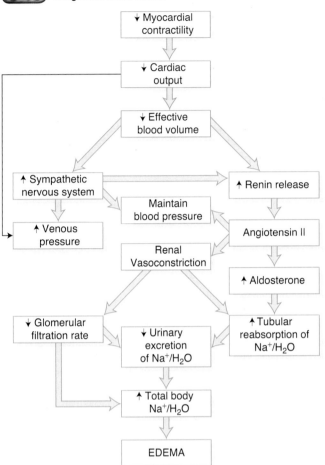

↓ Myocardial
contractility
↓
↓ Cardiac
output
↓
↓ Effective
blood volume

↑ Sympathetic
nervous system
→ ↑ Renin release

↑ Venous
pressure

Maintain
blood pressure ← Angiotensin II

Renal
Vasoconstriction

↑ Aldosterone

↓ Glomerular
filtration rate

↓ Urinary
excretion
of Na+/H2O

↑ Tubular
reabsorption of
Na+/H2O

↑ Total body
Na+/H2O

EDEMA

FIGURE
3-11 **A chest radiograph showing congestive heart failure and pulmonary edema**

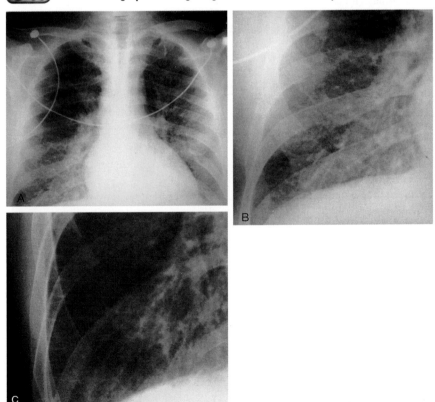

(Reproduced with permission from Daffner RH. *Clinical Radiology: The Essentials.* 2nd ed. Baltimore, MD: Williams & Wilkins; 1999.)

The Cardiovascular System

Clinical Vignette 3-3

CLINICAL PRESENTATION: A 67-year-old female complains to her primary care physician of **easy fatigue** and that each night, she has to **wake up to urinate (nocturia).** She also mentions that each night, her **ankles swell,** and she **sleeps with her head elevated on two to three pillows (orthopnea);** otherwise, she finds herself waking to **catch her breath (paroxysmal nocturnal dyspnea).** Her past medical history is significant for **hypertension;** however, the patient has been noncompliant with medication. Physical examination reveals congestion; **1+ pitting edema,** an **enlarged liver,** and **elevated jugular venous pressure (JVP).** Other findings include **cold and clammy skin and S3 and S4 heart sounds.** Temperature = 98.5° F; **blood pressure = 165/100 mm Hg; heart rate = 92 bpm; and respiration rate = 34 breaths/min.**

DIFFERENTIALS: CHF and renal failure. Given the patient's history and classic presentation, this patient likely has CHF secondary to chronic hypertension.

LABORATORY STUDIES: Proper follow-up for suspect CHF would be (a) **chest radiograph** showing cardiomegaly (Figure 3-11), interstitial edema in the lungs, and pleural effusion; (b) **echocardiogram** (determines the cause of CHF, whether systolic or diastolic; quantifies ejection fraction [EF]); (c) **ECG** showing evidence of chamber enlargement or presence of ischemic disease; (d) **radionuclide ventriculography using** ^{99m}Tc (quantifies EF when echo suboptimal as in chronic obstructive pulmonary disease [COPD]); (e) **cardiac catheterization;** (f) **stress testing;** (g) **urine analysis** (elevated protein would suggest renal failure); and (h) **blood chemistry** (blood urea nitrogen [BUN] and creatinine [Cr] slightly elevated in CHF and markedly elevated in renal failure).

MANAGEMENT: Diastolic dysfunction is treated symptomatically. Systolic dysfunction should be managed by (a) **sodium restriction,** (b) **diuretics** (congestive symptoms), (c) **ACE inhibitors** (decrease preload, afterload, decrease mortality), and (d) **digitalis** (symptomatic relief; use in severe CHF). Note: If the patient cannot tolerate ACE inhibitors, use **ARBs, hydralazine,** and **isosorbide dinitrates.** Also, α-blockers have been proven to decrease mortality in post-MI CHF.

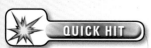

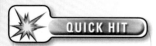

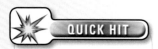

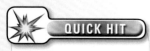

E. Common adverse reactions:
  1. Nausea and headache
  2. Arrhythmias (more serious)

IV. Diuretics, the other major treatment modality for CHF, are not discussed here (see Chapter 6).

INTRINSIC DISEASES OF THE HEART

I. Myocarditis

A. This is defined as inflammation of the cardiac muscle.

B. Etiology
  1. Viral etiology is the most common cause (usually coxsackie B virus, parvovirus B19, and human herpes virus [HHV]-6).
  2. HIV (via toxoplasmosis and metastasis of Kaposi sarcoma) may cause myocarditis.
  3. Bacterial causes include *Staphylococcus aureus, Corynebacterium diphtheriae,* and tuberculosis.
  4. Chagas disease
  5. Lyme disease
  6. Hypersensitivity reactions
  7. Sarcoidosis

C. Physical examination
  1. Muffled S1
  2. Audible S3 heart sound
  3. Murmur of mitral regurgitation
  4. Cardiomegaly

II. Endocarditis

A. Inflammation of the heart lining and connective tissue

B. Causes

1. Rheumatic heart disease—endocarditis may be caused by rheumatic fever (see below).

2. Infective endocarditis

a. Etiology

- Gram-positive cocci are the most common cause. Rarely, the cause is fungi (*Aspergillus* and *Candida*) or gram-negative bacteria.
- Damage, surgical repair, prosthetic heart valves, or congenital abnormalities are predisposing conditions.
- Vegetative growth (usually on atrial surface of valves) can throw septic thrombi to brain or peripheral circulation.
- Endocarditis is complicated by perivalvular abscesses or rupture of chordae tendineae.

b. Clinical features

- Mucosal petechiae
- Janeway lesions (peripheral hemorrhages with slight nodular character)
- Osler nodes (small, tender nodules on fingers and toe pads)
- Splinter hemorrhages (subungual linear streaks)
- Roth spots (retinal hemorrhages)
- Splenomegaly
- The mitral and aortic valves are frequently involved.
- Right-sided valvular lesions (usually of the tricuspid) suggest IV drug abuse and are associated with septic pulmonary emboli.

C. Types

1. Acute endocarditis

a. The cause is most often *S. aureus*.

b. Onset is rapid.

c. Clinical features include fever, anemia, embolic events, and heart murmur.

d. Treatment is with IV antibiotics.

2. Subacute endocarditis

a. The cause is most often the viridans streptococci.

b. It results from poor dentition or oral surgery in patients with preexisting heart disease (and preexisting damage to heart valves).

c. Onset is over a period of 6 months.

d. Treatment is with IV antibiotics.

3. Nonbacterial (marantic) endocarditis

a. This type is associated with metastatic cancer.

b. Sterile fibrin deposits appear on valves.

c. Sterile emboli can cause cerebral infarct.

4. Libman–Sacks endocarditis

a. This is a manifestation of systemic lupus erythematosus (SLE).

b. It is caused by autoantibody damage to valves.

c. Vegetations form on both sides of the valve.

5. Carcinoid syndrome

a. This syndrome is characterized by increased serotonin and other secretory products from a carcinoid tumor.

b. Plaque builds on right-sided valves of the heart.

III. Rheumatic heart disease

A. This is a systemic inflammatory disorder with cardiac manifestations.

B. Pathogenesis

1. Acute rheumatic heart disease usually occurs 2 to 4 weeks after a bout of pharyngitis caused by group A β-hemolytic streptococci.

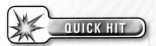

Associate acute endocarditis with Staphylococcal spp., and subacute endocarditis with viridans Streptococci. Associate endocarditis in intravenous drug abuse with *Staphylococcus aureus*.

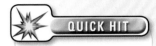

If an endocarditis is caused by *Streptococcus bovis*, look for signs and symptoms for gastrointestinal carcinoma in the patient.

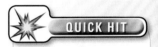

Culture-negative endocarditis can result from the HACEK group of organisms: *Haemophilus aphrophilus*, *Actinobacillus actinomycetem-comitans*, *Cardiobacterium hominis*, *Eikenella corrodens*, and *Kingella kingae*.

The Cardiovascular System

2. Antigenic mimicry occurs between streptococcal antigens and human antigens in the heart.

3. This results in immunologic origin for rheumatic heart disease.

C. Epidemiology

1. Children 5 to 15 years of age have the highest incidence of rheumatic fever.

2. Incidence is decreasing since the advent of penicillin.

D. Cardiac manifestations of rheumatic fever include the following conditions:

1. Pancarditis—inflammation of all structures of the heart

2. Pericarditis with effusions

3. Myocarditis
   a. Leads to cardiac failure
   b. Most common cause of early death in rheumatic fever

4. Endocarditis
   a. Usually afflicts the mitral and aortic valves (areas of high stress and turbulent flow)
   b. Mitral—aortic—tricuspid—pulmonary shows the order in which the valves become involved.
   c. Early nonembolic vegetations occur.
   d. With fibrosis and calcification, valvular damage leads to chronic rheumatic heart disease.

E. Other manifestations of rheumatic fever include:

1. Migratory polyarthritis

2. Sydenham chorea

3. Subcutaneous nodules

4. Erythema marginatum

5. Recent infection by group A streptococci (indicated by elevated antistreptolysin-O titers)

6. Aschoff body
   a. Lesion characterized by focal interstitial myocardial inflammation
   b. Fragmented collagen/fibrinoid material
   c. Anitschkow myocytes: large activated histiocytes
   d. Aschoff cells: granuloma with giant cells

IV. Cardiomyopathies (Table 3-10)

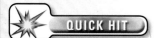

QUICK HIT

Systemic thromboembolism may develop in dilated cardiomyopathy, mitral valve prolapse, or from fragmented vegetations associated with infective endocarditis. Stasis of blood in the ventricle or atria leads to formation of mural thrombi as seen in dilated cardiomyopathy and mitral valve prolapse, respectively.

QUICK HIT

Senile amyloidosis is derived from transthyretin. Primary amyloidosis is caused by the amyloid light chain (AL) protein from immunoglobulin light chains. This is seen in plasma cell disorders (see Chapter 10).

TABLE 3-10	Cardiomyopathies			
	Pathology	Etiology	Clinical Manifestations	Notes
Dilated (systolic or contractile dysfunction)	Dilated ventricles, right and left heart failure, pulmonary edema	**Idiopathic,** alcoholics, thiamine deficiency, peripartum, **coxsackie-virus** B, *Trypanosoma cruzi*, tricyclic antidepressants, lithium, doxorubicin, pregnancy associated	Premature ventricular contractions, **decreased ejection fraction**, JVP, cardiomegaly, hepatomegaly	**Most common** form

(continued)

TABLE 3-10 Cardiomyopathies *(Continued)*

	Pathology	Etiology	Clinical Manifestations	Notes
Restrictive (diastolic dysfunction or loss of compliance)	**Stiffened heart muscle;** may result in right and left heart failure; tricuspid regurgitation	Senile or primary amyloidosis, sarcoidosis, hemochromatosis (associated with systemic diseases)	Peripheral **edema,** ascites, jugular venous distention	Differentiate from hypertrophic cardiomyopathy
Hypertrophic (diastolic dysfunction or loss of compliance)	Ventricular and ventricular septal hypertrophy, mitral regurgitation	Usually **autosomal dominant** (the most common gene affected is β-myosin); young **athletes**	Dyspnea, syncope, **S4,** systolic murmur, cardiomegaly on chest radiograph	Relieved by **squatting, worsened by Valsalva,** exacerbated by physical exertion, sudden death

JVP, jugular venous pressure.

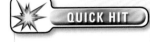

> **QUICK HIT**
>
> Mitral valve prolapse (MVP) is the most frequently occurring valvular lesion, often found in young women and in patients with Marfan syndrome and related to tissue laxity. Characteristics of the heart sound in MVP include midsystolic click, followed by late systolic murmur.

V. Valvular heart diseases *(Table 3-11)*

TABLE 3-11 Valvular Heart Disease and Murmurs

Valvular Disease	Etiology	Physical Examination	Clinical Manifestations
Systolic murmurs Aortic stenosis	**Bicuspid aortic valves, degenerative calcification,** RHD, unicuspid aortic valve, syphilis	Delayed pulses, carotid thrill, **crescendo-decrescendo systolic ejection murmur** at right upper sternal border, decreased intensity with Valsalva	Syncope, angina, dyspnea/CHF, death, treat symptomatic patients with valve replacement
Mitral regurgitation	**RHD** (50% of cases), LV dilation, ischemic heart disease, endocarditis, MVP, papillary muscle dysfunction (secondary to myocardial infarction)	Splitting of S2; S3; **holosystolic** murmur at apex, radiating to the left axilla, increased intensity with squatting or handgrip	Arrhythmias, dilated left atrium, holosystolic murmur
Mitral valve prolapse (MVP)	Myxomatous degeneration of mitral valve leaflets, such that leaflets billow into the left atrium during systole	**Midsystolic click**, often followed by a late systolic murmur; decreased intensity with squatting	Can be associated with chest pain, palpitations, light-headedness, panic attacks
Ventricular septal defect	Congenital defect	Harsh, holosystolic murmur	
Diastolic murmurs Aortic regurgitation	Rheumatic heart disease, syphilitic aortitis, nondissecting aortic aneurysm, Marfan syndrome	Wide pulse pressure, water-hammer-pulse, **S3, blowing, decrescendo diastolic murmur**	Left ventricular enlargement, dyspnea, early diastolic murmur
Mitral stenosis	Usually **rheumatic heart disease**	Cyanosis, **opening snap,** diastolic rumbling murmur	Dyspnea, orthopnea, left atrial enlargement, mid to late diastolic murmur

CHF, congestive heart failure; LV, left ventricular; RHD, rheumatic heart disease.

VI. Peripheral vascular diseases *(Table 3-12)*

TABLE 3-12 Peripheral Vascular Diseases

Disease	Pathology	Vessels Affected	Clinical Manifestations	Notes
Churg–Strauss	Eosinophils, vasculitis, perinuclear antineutro-phil cytoplasmic anti-body (p-ANCA)	Small and medium-sized arteries	**Asthma, elevated plasma eosinophils,** heart disease	May be associated with p-ANCA
Henoch–Schönlein purpura	**IgA** immune complex–mediated acute vasculitis, renal deposits in mesangium	Arterioles, capillaries, venules	Hemorrhagic urticaria, palpable purpura, fever, red blood cell casts in urine, **atopic** patient	Often associated with an **upper respiratory infection;** affects **children**
Kaposi sarcoma	Viral origin, common malignancy in patients with AIDS	Cutaneous and visceral vasculature	Malignant vascular tumor, especially in **homosexual** men	Probably results from reactivation of latent human herpesvirus 8 (HHV-8) infection
Kawasaki disease	Acute necrotizing inflammation	Large, medium, and small vessels	Fever, conjunctival lesions, lymphadenitis, coronary artery aneurysms	Affects **young children**
Rendu–Osler–Weber syndrome	**Autosomal dominant;** hereditary hemorrhagic telangiectasia	Dilation of venules and capillaries	Epistaxis, gastrointestinal (GI) bleeding	Increased occurrence in **Mormon** population
Polyarteritis nodosa (PAN)	Necrotizing degeneration of tunica media, aneurysms	Small and medium-sized arteries	Fever, weight loss, abdominal pain (GI), hypertension (renal)	Associated with **hepatitis B infection**
Takayasu arteritis (pulseless disease)	Inflammation leading to stenosis; **aortic arch** and the origins of great vessels	Medium and large arteries	**Loss of carotid, radial, and ulnar pulses;** fever; night sweats; deficits arthritis; visual; low blood pressure in upper extremities; claudication caused by lack of blood reaching extremities	Pathology referred to as "aortic arch syndrome"; young **Asian females;** corkscrew, widened aorta on angiogram
Temporal arteritis (giant cell arteritis)	Nodular inflammation of branches of carotid (especially **temporal**)	Medium and large arteries	**Headache,** absence of pulse in affected vessels, **visual deficits,** polymyalgia rheumatica	Significant elevation of **sedimentation rate;** affects the **elderly**
Thromboangiitis obliterans (Buerger disease)	Acute, full-thickness inflammation of vessels; may extend to nerves; occlusive lesions in extremities	Small and medium arteries and veins	Cold, pale limb; pain; **Raynaud phenomenon;** gangrene	Typical patient is a young **Jewish** man who **smokes heavily**
Wegener granulomatosis	Antineutrophil antibodies (cytoplasmic antineu-trophil cytoplasmic antibody [**c-ANCA**]) causes necrotizing, **granulomatous lesions** in **kidney, lung,** and upper respiratory tract	Small arteries, small veins of kidneys and respiratory tract	Cough, ulcers of sinuses and **nasal septum,** red blood cell casts in urine, classic triad: (a) necrotizing vasculitis (b) necrotizing granulomas of respiratory tract (c) necrotizing glomerulitis	More common in males

CARDIAC NEOPLASMS

I. Metastatic tumors to the heart are more common than primary tumors

II. Primary tumors
   A. Myxomas
      1. 90% found in atria
      2. Left atrium > right atrium
      3. Cause **ball-valve obstruction**, embolism, and fever
   B. Rhabdomyoma
      1. Most common primary cardiac tumor found in children
      2. Often seen with tuberous sclerosis
      3. Composed of "spider cells" and glycogen vacuoles

 ## DISEASES OF THE PERICARDIUM

I. Cardiac tamponade
   A. This is an accumulation of fluid in the pericardial sac, which causes cardiac filling defects because of compression of the heart.
      1. Blood is usually indicative of a traumatic perforation of the heart or aorta or rupture as a consequence of an MI.
      2. Serous transudate may accumulate as a result of edema or CHF.
   B. The most common causes are neoplasms, idiopathic pericarditis, and uremia.
   C. Principal features of cardiac tamponade include:
      1. Intracardiac pressure is elevated.
      2. Ventricular filling is limited.
      3. Cardiac output is reduced.
      4. Decreased or absent heart sounds on auscultation
   D. Pulsus paradoxus is a greater than normal (10 mm Hg) decline in systolic arterial pressure on inspiration.
   E. Treatment involves pericardiocentesis (removal of fluid from the pericardial cavity).

II. Pericarditis
   A. Pericarditis is defined as an inflammation of the pericardium (fibroserous membrane) covering the heart.
   B. Causes
      1. Usually idiopathic
      2. Coxsackievirus A or B (serous pericarditis)
      3. Tuberculosis (hemorrhagic pericarditis)
      4. Uremia (serofibrinous pericarditis)
      5. SLE (serous pericarditis)
      6. Scleroderma (serous pericarditis)
      7. Post-MI (Dressler syndrome; fibrinous pericarditis)
   C. Physical examination
      1. Jugular venous distention (JVD)
      2. Increase of JVP with inspiration (Kussmaul sign)
      3. Pericardial friction rub
      4. Distant heart sounds
   D. Characteristics
      1. Pain exacerbated by inspiration
      2. Pain relieved by sitting
      3. Cardiomegaly
      4. Hypotension
      5. Diffuse ST elevation on ECG
   E. Persistent, acute pericarditis leads to chronic, constrictive pericarditis.
      1. Both acute and chronic pericarditis mimic right-sided heart failure.
      2. Both acute and chronic pericarditis lead to obliteration of pericardial cavity.
      3. Fibrous tissue proliferation and calcification result.

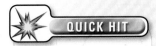

Temporal arteritis is the most common vasculitis in the United States.

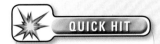

Primary tumors of the heart are very rare. Metastatic (secondary) tumors are more common. Atrial myxomas are the most frequently occurring primary tumors.

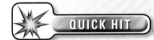

The needle for a pericardiocentesis passes through the skin, superficial fascia, pectoralis major muscle, external intercostal membrane, internal intercostal membrane, fibrous pericardium, and parietal layer of serous pericardium.

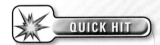

An MI also produces ST elevation. However, in an MI, ST elevation is limited to certain leads (corresponding to anatomical regions) and associated with possible QRS changes.

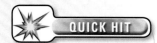

Autoregulation of blood flow in the heart is altered to meet the demands of tissue metabolism via nitric oxide and adenosine. Autoregulation also occurs in the kidney and brain.

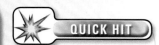

Septic shock is associated with vasodilation, hypotension, and warm extremities.

SHOCK

I. **Shock is defined as a metabolic state in which oxygen delivery is inadequate to meet the oxygen demand.**

II. **Signs and symptoms**
   A. Tachycardia
   B. Hypotension
   C. Oliguria
   D. Mental status changes
   E. Weak pulses
   F. Cool extremities

III. **Types of shock** (*Table 3-13*)

TABLE 3-13 Shock						
Type of Shock	**SVR**	**HR**	**PCWP**	**PCWP After Fluid Challenge**	**Mechanism**	**Clinical Causes**
Cardiogenic	High	Varies	High	Very high	Pump failure	Arrhythmias, heart failure, myocardial infarction
Hypovolemic	High	High	Low	Unchanged or high	Volume loss	Blood/fluid/plasma loss, burns, severe vomiting or diarrhea
Obstructive (tension pneumothorax, massive hemothorax)	High	High	Low or normal	Unchanged or increased	Extracardiac obstruction of blood flow	Tension pneumothorax, massive hemothorax
Obstructive (cardiac tamponade)	High	High	High	High or very high	Extracardiac obstruction of blood flow	Cardiac tamponade
Septic	Low	Low	Low or normal	High	Increased venous capacitance	Gram-negative endotoxemia, direct toxic injury
Neurogenic	Low	Low	Low or normal	high	Massive peripheral vasodilation	Severe cerebral, brain stem, or spinal cord injury
Anaphylactic	Low	High	Low	High	Increased venous capacitance due to histamine release	Type I hypersensitivity reaction to allergen

HR, heart rate; PCWP, pulmonary capillary wedge pressure; SVR, systemic vascular resistance.

The Cardiovascular System

IV. Clinical manifestations of shock
   A. Acute tubular necrosis
   B. Necrosis in the brain
   C. Fatty change in the heart and liver
   D. Patchy hemorrhages in the colon
   E. Pulmonary edema due to acute lung injury

DRUGS THAT CAUSE ADVERSE EFFECTS TO THE CARDIOVASCULAR SYSTEM

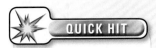

> **QUICK HIT**
>
> Doxorubicin, daunorubicin, and anthracyclines used to treat sarcomas, breast cancer, lung cancer, and acute lymphocytic leukemia result in dose-dependent, irreversible cardiotoxicity.

I. Thrombotic complications: oral contraceptives (estrogen and progestins)

II. Cardiac toxicity: doxorubicin (antineoplastic), daunorubicin (antineoplastic), anthracyclines, tricyclic antidepressants, and lithium

III. Torsades de pointes: class IA (quinidine), class III (sotalol) antiarrhythmics, and tricyclic antidepressants

The Cardiovascular System

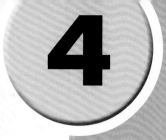

The Respiratory System

 DEVELOPMENT

I. The lung bud forms from the foregut during week 4 of embryologic development.

II. The lining of the lower respiratory tract is derived from endoderm, whereas the connective tissue cartilage and muscle are derived from mesoderm.

III. Normal development causes the lung bud to completely separate from the esophagus at the level of the larynx.

IV. Incomplete separation causes a tracheoesophageal (TE) fistula *(Figure 4-1)*.
   A. In the most common form of TE fistula, the esophagus ends in a blind pouch (esophageal atresia) and air enters the stomach (gastric bubble on radiograph).
   B. Signs and symptoms of esophageal atresia with a TE fistula
      1. Feeding difficulties within the first few days of life
      2. Possible aspiration pneumonia with respiratory distress
      3. Inability to pass nasogastric tube
      4. Copious secretions

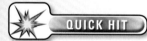

TE fistula is the most common anomaly of the lower respiratory tract.

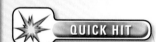

Polyhydramnios is often associated with TE fistula due to the inability of excess amniotic fluid to pass through the stomach and intestine for absorption by the placenta into the mother's circulation.

FIGURE 4-1 Tracheoesophageal fistula

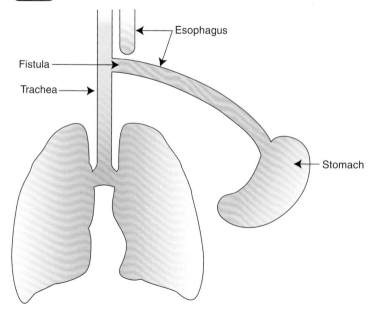

V. Diaphragm muscle

A. This is the primary muscle used for breathing.

B. The diaphragm muscle separates the pleural and peritoneal cavities.

C. It is formed from fusion of the following structures:
1. **Septum transversum**
2. Paired **pleuroperitoneal membranes**
3. **Dorsal mesentery** of the **esophagus**
4. **Body wall**

D. It is innervated by the phrenic nerves (C3, C4, and C5).

E. Improper formation of the pleuroperitoneal membrane or its failure to fuse with the other three parts of the diaphragm can lead to a **congenital diaphragmatic hernia (CDH)**, a condition with serious complications.
1. Abdominal contents are forced into the pleural cavity.
2. Lung hypoplasia results from compression by abdominal viscera.
3. Hernias appear most often on the **left side** (posterolateral).
4. Diaphragmatic hernia is associated with polyhydramnios.
5. Diaphragmatic hernia presents at birth as a flattened abdomen, cyanosis, and inability to breathe.

PHYSICS AND FUNCTION OF THE LUNG

I. Lung volumes

A. **Capacities and volumes in the normal lung** (Figure 4-2)

B. Volumes and pressure during the breathing cycle (Figure 4-3)

C. Spirometry tracing—normal versus diseased (Figure 4-4)

D. Pulmonary function tests—obstructive versus restrictive (Figure 4-5)

II. Compliance

A. Defined as $\Delta V/\Delta P$, where V is volume and P is pressure, compliance describes the ability of the chest wall and lung to expand when stretched.
1. At functional residual capacity (FRC), the lungs have a tendency to collapse.
2. This force is exactly balanced by the chest wall, which has a tendency to expand.
3. Because these forces are in balance at FRC, the airway pressure is 0 mm Hg. Lung volumes above FRC create a positive airway pressure, whereas volumes below FRC create a negative airway pressure.

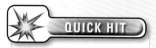

QUICK HIT

The defect of CDH is also known as the foramen of Bochdalek and occurs on the left side in nearly 90% of cases due to the earlier closure of the right pleuroperitoneal opening.

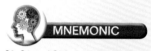

MNEMONIC

C3, C4, and C5 keep the diaphragm phrenically alive.

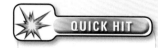

QUICK HIT

The sternocleidomastoid and the internal and external intercostals are accessory muscles of respiration. They are used when there is an increased demand for oxygen (such as in exercise) or in disease states.

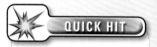

QUICK HIT

Compliance is given by the slope of pressure versus volume curve.

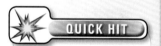

QUICK HIT

Residual volume (RV) or volumes containing RV cannot be directly measured by plethysmography or spirometry but are derived from helium dilution techniques.

The Respiratory System

FIGURE

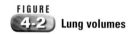

4-2 Lung volumes

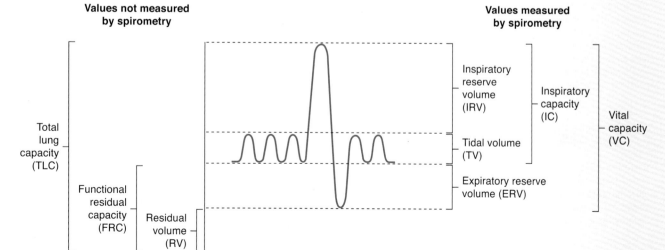

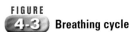

Breathing cycle

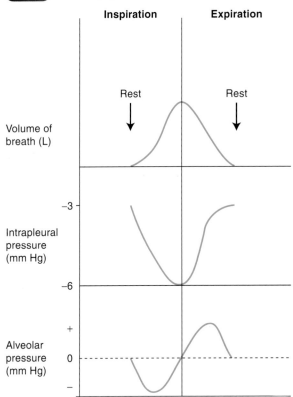

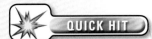

The primary molecule of surfactant is dipalmitoyl-phosphatidylcholine (lecithin). A lecithin-to-sphingomyelin ratio of 2:1 is the normal ratio of surfactant molecules in a newborn. A ratio below 2:1 can result in neonatal respiratory distress, especially in cesarean section delivery.

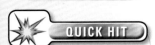

Type II pneumocytes are cuboidal cells with round nuclei, foamy cytoplasm (because of lipid content), and lamellar bodies (secreting granules) containing the surfactant.

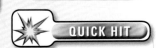

Glucocorticoids administered during pregnancy accelerate fetal lung development by stimulating the production of surfactant-associated proteins and increasing phospholipid synthesis by enhancing phosphatidylcholine activity.

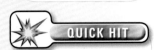

Allergies and allergic asthma release histamine, which is a powerful constrictor of airway smooth muscle and causes increased airway resistance.

4. Low compliance implies a stiff chest wall or lung as seen in:
   a. **Pulmonary fibrosis due to asbestosis, sarcoidosis, and adult respiratory distress syndrome (ARDS)**
   b. **Pulmonary edema**
   c. **Paralysis of the respiratory muscles**
5. High compliance implies a flaccid lung as a result of:
   a. Decreased elastic recoil as seen in **emphysema** and **old age**
   b. Bronchospasm as in **asthma** (Figure 4-4)
B. **Surfactant** plays an important role in lung compliance.
   1. Alveoli have a tendency to collapse.
   2. An alveolus with a small radius has more collapsing pressure than an alveolus with a large radius, according to **Laplace law:**

   $$P \propto T/r$$

   where P is pressure required to prevent alveolar collapse, T is surface tension, and r is alveolar radius.
   3. Surfactant reduces the pressure and prevents collapse by reducing the intermolecular forces between water molecules lining the alveoli.
   4. Surfactant increases compliance and allows the alveoli to expand more easily.
   5. **Neonatal respiratory distress syndrome (NRDS)** occurs in premature infants (<37 weeks' gestation) because **type II (surfactant-producing) pneumocytes** are not yet fully developed and fail to produce sufficient surfactant.
   6. Atelectasis (collapsed alveoli) can result from NRDS.

III. Airway resistance
A. Airway resistance (R) is inversely proportional to the fourth power of the radius (r) (formula: $R \propto 1/r^4$); thus, any mechanism that decreases the radius of the bronchi will greatly affect the airway resistance.

FIGURE
4-4 Spirometry tracings: normal versus diseased

A

Principle of dynamic compression—as effort increases
1) Alveolar pressure increases (↑airflow from lungs)
2) Pressure outside airway increases (↓airflow from lungs)

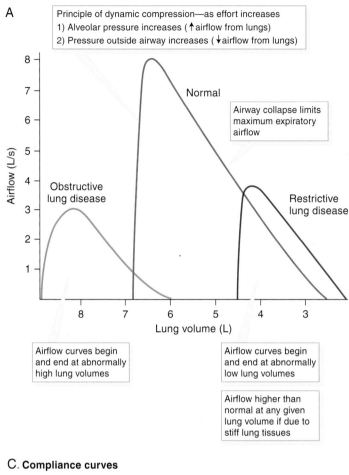

Normal

Airway collapse limits maximum expiratory airflow

Obstructive lung disease

Restrictive lung disease

Airflow curves begin and end at abnormally high lung volumes

Airflow curves begin and end at abnormally low lung volumes

Airflow higher than normal at any given lung volume if due to stiff lung tissues

C. **Compliance curves**

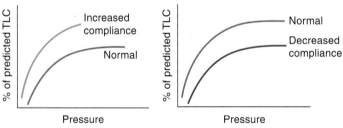

Increased compliance

Normal

Normal

Decreased compliance

B_1. **Normal**

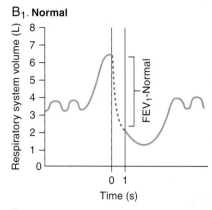

B_2. **Obstructive lung disease**

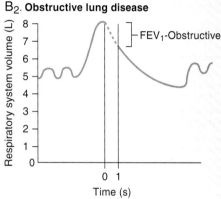

B_3. **Restrictive lung disease**

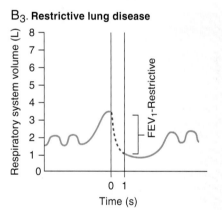

FEV_1, forced expiratory volume at 1 second; TLC, total lung capacity.

B. The **airway radius** is under the control of the parasympathetic and sympathetic nervous systems.
1. **Parasympathetic nervous system**
   a. Causes **constriction** of the airways
   b. Mediated by direct stimulation, airway irritation, and slow-reacting substance of anaphylaxis (SRS-A)
   c. Stimulates mucus secretion
2. **Sympathetic nervous system**
   a. Causes **dilation** of airways
   b. Used as treatment for allergy and asthma (β_2-agonists)
   c. Functions in fight-or-flight autonomic reflexes; dilates airways to help provide oxygen in times of stress

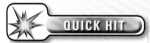

QUICK HIT

SRS-A is a combination of the leukotrienes C_4, D_4, and E_4 (LTC_4, LTD_4, and LTE_4). In the treatment of asthma, zileuton blocks production of leukotrienes by inhibiting the lipoxygenase enzyme, whereas zafirlukast blocks leukotriene receptors. Leukotriene A_4 (LTA_4) is a precursor to leukotriene B_4 (LTB_4), LTC_4, and LTD_4, and LTE_4. LTB_4 is responsible for chemotaxis of neutrophils and adhesion of white blood cells.

The Respiratory System

The Respiratory System

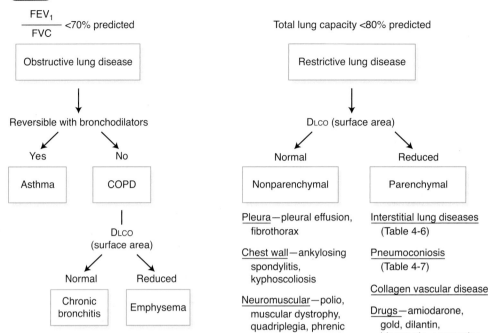

FIGURE
4-5 Interpreting pulmonary function tests: obstructive versus restrictive

COPD, chronic obstructive pulmonary disease; DLCO, diffusing capacity of lung for carbon monoxide; FEV₁, forced expiratory volume at 1 second; FVC, forced vital capacity.

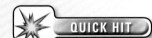

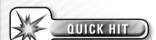

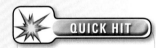

3. Airway radius is also affected by the lung parenchyma, which is bound to the airway and exerts radial traction on it.
   a. In restrictive disorders such as interstitial fibrosis, radial traction of the airway increases → increasing airway diameter → decreasing airway resistance → increasing expiratory airflow. Despite the increased expiratory airflow, the reduced lung compliance will decrease both forced vital capacity (FVC) and forced expiratory volume at 1 second (FEV₁). Therefore, the FEV₁/FVC ratio is normal or increased.
   b. In obstructive disorders such as emphysema, destruction of elastic fibers → decreases radial traction → decreasing airway diameter → increasing resistance → decreasing expiratory airflow and FEV₁/FVC ratios.

IV. **Ventilation and perfusion**
   A. **Ventilation/perfusion (V/Q) ratio**: the ratio of the rate of alveolar ventilation to the rate of pulmonary blood flow
   B. Varies over the entire lung (higher in the apices, lower in the bases in an upright patient), but is 0.8 on average
   C. Dead space
      1. Anatomic dead space is regions of the lung, such as the conducting airways, which are incapable of exchanging oxygen (O_2) and carbon dioxide (CO_2).
      2. Physiologic dead space is the volume of the lungs that does not participate in the elimination of CO_2.

$$V_D = V_T \times [(Pa_{CO_2} - PE_{CO_2})/Pa_{CO_2}]$$

V_D, physiologic dead space (mL); V_T, tidal volume (mL); Pa_{CO_2}, partial pressure of carbon dioxide, arterial blood (mm Hg); PE_{CO_2}, partial pressure of carbon dioxide in expired air (mm Hg).

3. It causes a reduction in ventilation.
4. V/Q is reduced to 0 in complete airway occlusion.
5. A V/Q of 0 is considered a shunt and no gas exchange will occur (areas are perfused but not ventilated).

D. Blood flow obstruction
1. Blockage of a pulmonary artery or smaller vessel causes a reduction in perfusion.
2. A perfusion value of 0 yields an infinite V/Q ratio.
3. A V/Q of infinity is considered **physiologic dead space**.

E. Pulmonary embolism results in increased V/Q ratio (Table 4-1).

F. Blood flow and ventilation vary over the regions of the lung (Figure 4-6) due primarily to gravity.

TABLE 4-1 **Causes of Hypoxemia**				
Cause	Associated Conditions	A–a Gradient	Lab Values	Notes
Right-to-left shunt	Congenital anomaly	Increased		Does not respond to oxygen
Ventilation/perfusion mismatch	Pneumonia, COPD, atelectasis, pulmonary infarction, tumors, granulomatous disease		Increased	Responds to oxygen (A–a gradient corrects)
Decreased diffusion capacity	Thick blood–air barrier (diffuse interstitial fibrosis, sarcoidosis, asbestosis, respiratory distress syndrome), decreased surface area (pneumonectomy, emphysema), decreased hemoglobin (anemia, PE)	Increased	D_{LCO} decreased	Responds to oxygen but A–a gradient remains same
Decreased Po_2 in inspired air	High altitudes, erroneous setting on ventilator	Normal		Responds to oxygen
Hypoventilation of central origin	Opioid or barbiturate overdose	Normal	Elevated P_{CO_2}	Responds to oxygen
Hypoventilation of peripheral origin	Polio, chest trauma (multiple rib fractures → pain with breathing), tetanus, obesity (Pickwickian syndrome), suffocation, drowning, skeletal disease, phrenic nerve paralysis	Normal	Elevated P_{CO_2}	Responds to oxygen

A–a gradient, alveolar–arterial gradient; COPD, chronic obstructive pulmonary disease; D_{LCO}, diffusing capacity of lung for carbon monoxide; PE, pulmonary embolus.

In determining the cause of hypoxemia in a patient, use a three-tier approach: (1) Check whether the A–a gradient is elevated, (2) check whether O_2 administration improved the condition and if the A–a gradient was corrected, and (3) look for other lab findings or associated conditions.

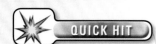

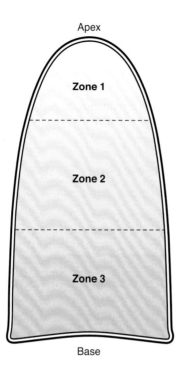

Apex

Zone 1

Zone 2

Zone 3

Base

Zone 1
- Lowest blood flow
- Alveolar pressure > arterial pressure > venous pressure
- Capillaries collapse due to high alveolar pressure
- Ventilation ($\dot{V}$) is decreased less than blood flow [also called perfusion ($\dot{Q}$)]

so: $\dfrac{\dot{V}}{\dot{Q}} = \dfrac{\downarrow}{\downarrow\downarrow} = \uparrow$ (Ventilation in excess of perfusion)

Zone 2
- Blood flow is higher than Zone 1 but lower than Zone 3
- Arterial pressure > alveolar pressure > venous pressure
- Capillaries remain open because arterial pressure is greater than alveolar pressure
- Ventilation ($\dot{V}$) is approximately equivalent to perfusion ($\dot{Q}$)

so: $\dfrac{\dot{V}}{\dot{Q}} \approx 1$

Zone 3
- Highest blood flow
- Arterial pressure > venous pressure > alveolar pressure
- Capillaries remain open because arterial pressure is higher than both alveolar and venous pressure
- Ventilation ($\dot{V}$) is increased less than perfusion ($\dot{Q}$)

so: $\dfrac{\dot{V}}{\dot{Q}} = \dfrac{\uparrow}{\uparrow\uparrow} = \downarrow$ (Perfusion in excess of ventilation)

CONTROL OF BREATHING

I. **Medulla**
   A. Mediates inspiration and expiration
   B. Generates the basic breathing rhythm
   C. Receives input via the vagus and glossopharyngeal nerves
   D. Sends output via the phrenic nerve to the diaphragm and via the spinal nerve to the intercostals and abdominal wall
   E. The cerebral cortex can override the medulla and provide voluntary control of breathing if desired

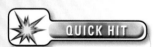

II. **The central nervous system (CNS)** seeks to keep $PaCO_2$ within a narrow range. On the other hand, in the case of oxygen, the nervous system responds only to very low levels of PaO_2.

III. **Depth and rate of respiration control these variables.**
   A. **Central control**
      1. Chemoreceptors in the **medulla** sense the pH of the cerebrospinal fluid (CSF).
      2. CO_2 crosses the blood–brain barrier, where it binds with H_2O to form carbonic acid (H_2CO_3). H_2CO_3 dissociates to hydrogen ion (H^+) and bicarbonate (HCO_3), causing an increase in H^+ (decreasing the pH of the CSF).
      3. Increases in $[H^+]$ (hydrogen ion concentration) directly stimulate the central chemoreceptors, which stimulate breathing.
      4. Decreases in $[H^+]$ reduce stimulation of the receptors and slow respiration.
   B. **Peripheral control**
      1. Chemoreceptors in the **carotid bodies** and at the aortic arch bifurcation sense changes in PaO_2, $PaCO_2$, and $[H^+]$.
      2. Decreases in **PaO_2** below 60 mm Hg stimulate the peripheral chemoreceptors to increase rate and depth of breathing (in the absence of lung disease, decreased PaO_2 is rarely the driving force for respiration).
      3. Increases in **$PaCO_2$** potentiate peripheral chemoreceptor response to PaO_2 (major direct effect of changes in $PaCO_2$ is on the central chemoreceptors).

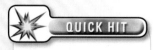

The Respiratory System

4. Increases in arterial $[H^+]$ directly stimulate the chemoreceptors, independent of the Pa_{CO_2} (causes increased respiration in metabolic acidosis).

5. Stimulation of irritant receptors in large airways and stretch receptors in small airways inhibits inspiration.

C. **Abnormal breathing**

1. **Cheyne–Stokes breathing**
   a. Tidal volumes variably increase and decrease and are separated by a period of apnea.
   b. This breathing abnormality is a result of pontine dysfunction and is associated with drug overdose, hypoxia, CNS depression, congestive heart failure (CHF), and increased intracerebral pressure.

2. **Kussmaul breathing**
   a. Deep, labored breathing pattern associated with severe metabolic acidosis (e.g., diabetic ketoacidosis)
   b. Can be either fast or slow

3. **Sleep apnea**
   a. **Obstructive sleep apnea**
   - Risk factors: middle age, male sex, obesity, smoking, hypertension, pharyngeal malformations, use of alcohol and other drugs
   - **Characteristics**
     (1) Ventilatory effort exists.
     (2) Airway is obstructed.
     (3) Apnea is terminated by self-arousal.
     (4) Apnea usually occurs in the nasopharynx or oropharynx when muscles relax during rapid eye movement (REM) sleep.
   b. **Central sleep apnea**
   - Ventilatory effort does not exist.
   - Airway is not obstructed.
   - Patient does not arouse self.
   - Central sleep apnea, like obstructive sleep apnea, occurs in the REM stage of sleep.
   - It is CO_2 threshold–dependent; that is, there is decreased chemoreceptor sensitivity to O_2 and CO_2 concentrations.
   c. **Therapy** includes weight loss (for obstructive sleep apnea) and continuous positive airway pressure (CPAP); multiple drugs have been used in treatment, but none is as effective as CPAP.

IV. Gas exchange

A. Diffusion of gas depends on the **partial pressure difference** between the gas in the alveolus and the gas in the blood (i.e., the difference in pressure across the blood–air barrier).

B. Partial pressure

1. The alveolar partial pressure of oxygen (P_AO_2) can be calculated as follows:

$$P_AO_2 = (760 - 47 \text{ mm Hg}) \, F_iO_2 - (P_ACO_2/0.8)$$

where 760 mm Hg = total atmospheric pressure (at sea level);
47 mm Hg = partial pressure of completely humidified air as found in the alveoli;
F_iO_2 = percentage of air that is oxygen (normally 0.21);
P_ACO_2 = partial pressure of CO_2 in the alveoli (normally 40);
and 0.8 = the ratio of volume of CO_2 produced to the volume of O_2 consumed (respiratory quotient).

2. For O_2, higher pressures will force more oxygen into the blood and allow it to equilibrate more readily.

3. For CO_2, higher partial pressures in the blood (or lower in the alveoli) will force more CO_2 out of the blood and into the lungs, where it can be expired.

4. The amount of O_2 delivered to the tissues is also determined by hemoglobin concentration and red blood cell number (hematocrit) (see Chapter 10).

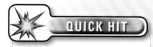

Obstructive sleep apnea causes CO_2 retention, leading to respiratory acidosis and hypoxemia.

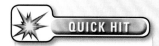

Patients with unexplained daytime sleepiness, arrhythmias, and mood changes should be evaluated for sleep apnea.

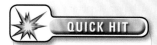

Remember that air contains higher oxygen levels (Po_2 = 160 mm Hg) and virtually no CO_2 (Pco_2 = 0 mm Hg) as compared to arterial gas levels (Po_2 = 100 mm Hg, Pco_2 = 40 mm Hg).

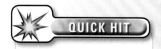

The blood–air barrier is made up of:
(1) Membrane and cytoplasm of type I pneumocytes
(2) Fused basement membrane of type I pneumocytes and endothelial cells
(3) Membrane and cytoplasm of endothelial cells

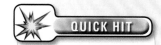

The **right main bronchus** is more vertically oriented than the **left main bronchus** and is therefore the path commonly taken by aspirated particles. If a patient is supine, the object is most likely to enter the **lower lobe**.

The Respiratory System

The Respiratory System

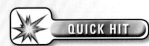

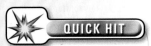

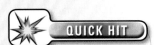

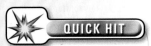

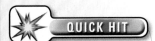

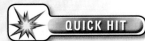

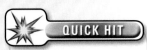

C. Disease affects diffusion capacity of the lung.
  1. Fibrosis causes a thickening of the interstitium, which hinders diffusion across the blood–air barrier.
  2. Emphysema destroys the alveolar walls and decreases the area available for gas exchange.

LUNG DEFENSES

I. Anatomic barriers

A. Impaction
  1. Large particles (**greater than 10 μm in diameter**) fail to turn the corners of the respiratory tract.
  2. Common site: **nasopharynx**
B. Sedimentation
  1. Medium particles (**between 2 and 10 μm in diameter**) settle as a result of weight.
  2. Common site: **small airways**
C. Diffusion
  1. Small particles (**between 0.5 and 2 μm in diameter**) are engulfed by alveolar macrophages (dust cells).
  2. Common site: **alveoli**
D. Suspension: particles **less than 0.5 μm in diameter** remain suspended in air.

II. Nonspecific

A. **Mucociliary escalator**
  1. Particles are trapped in the gel layer of the upper airway.
  2. Ciliary motion removes particles.
B. **Cough**
  1. Cough is a bronchoconstriction that occurs to prevent penetration of particles.
  2. It is also defined as deep inspiration followed by forced expiration.
  3. The cough reflex can be suppressed by antitussive agents such as opioids (see Chapter 9).
  4. Specific mechanisms include secretory immunoglobulin A (IgA) and complement.

ADULT RESPIRATORY DISTRESS SYNDROME AND NEONATAL RESPIRATORY DISTRESS SYNDROME

This group of diseases often leads to respiratory failure and death (Table 4-2).

TABLE 4-2	Adult Respiratory Distress Syndrome (ARDS) and Neonatal Respiratory Distress Syndrome (NRDS)	
	ARDS (Diffuse Alveolar Damage)	**NRDS (Hyaline Membrane Disease)**
Age group	Adults	Premature infants
Causes	**Shock, infection, trauma, or aspiration** resulting in **neutrophil** recruitment and free radical production (oxygen toxicity)	**Lack of surfactant** production
Pathophysiology	Impaired gas exchange caused by pulmonary hemorrhage, pulmonary edema, or atelectasis	Increased work to expand lungs; infant can clear lungs of fluids but cannot fill lungs with air; atelectasis
Features	Respiratory insufficiency; cyanosis; hypoxemia; heavy, wet lungs; diffuse pulmonary infiltrates on radiograph; hyaline membranes in alveoli; pneumothorax may result—may be rapid and fatal	Respiratory insufficiency; cyanosis; hypoxemia; heavy, wet lungs; diffuse pulmonary infiltrates on radiograph; hyaline membranes in alveoli

PNEUMOTHORAX

I. Simple pneumothorax

A. May be caused by **spontaneous** rupture of a bleb (congenital or secondary to paraseptal emphysema) or penetrating trauma causing a loss of negative intrathoracic pressure

B. Is most commonly seen in tall, slender **men 20 to 40 years of age**

C. Presents as sudden chest pain, shortness of breath (SOB), **cough, hyperresonance,** and **decreased breath sounds** over affected lung; chest radiograph shows **radiolucency** and in the case of a **tension pneumothorax,** the **trachea deviates to the side of the pneumothorax**

D. Has a 50% recurrence rate

E. Treatment includes the insertion of a chest tube with suction to create a vacuum for larger defects as well as monitoring for small defects such as air leaks.

II. Tension pneumothorax

A. A flap of tissue allows air to enter pleural space but not to escape, causing an increase in pleural cavity pressure.

B. Pressure builds, the mediastinum is displaced, the **trachea deviates away from the lesion,** jugular venous distention (JVD) occurs, and breath sounds are uneven.

C. Cardiovascular and respiratory compromise may be rapidly fatal.

III. Open sucking chest wound

A. Penetrating trauma to the chest wall and pleura can cause this condition.

B. If the diameter of the lesion approaches the diameter of the trachea, air will preferentially enter through the defect.

PULMONARY VASCULAR DISEASES

A variety of diseases primarily affect the vasculature of the lungs (Table 4-3).

TABLE 4-3 Pulmonary Vascular Diseases

Disease	Etiology	Features	Complications
Pulmonary hypertension	Primary—may be associated with proliferation of vascular smooth muscle	Loud S2	Leads to **cor pulmonale**
	Secondary—owing to COPD or increased pulmonary blood flow (as seen with a left-to-right shunt)	**Left parasternal heave due to right ventricular hypertrophy** Heart failure cells	
Pulmonary embolism	Commonly from proximal **deep vein thrombosis** (usually lower limb such as femoral veins) as a result of **Virchow triad:** blood stasis, endothelial damage (fat, infection, trauma), and hypercoagulable states	**Respiratory alkalosis; increased A–a gradient; hemorrhagic,** red, wedge-shaped infarct Acute-onset dyspnea, chest pain, tachycardia, hypotension *V/Q* ratio approaches infinity saddle embolus—an embolus lodged at the pulmonary artery bifurcation, often fatal	Can lead to cardiovascular collapse and sudden death

(continued)

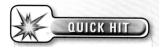

QUICK HIT

Decreased breath sounds and hyporesonance indicate pleural effusion.

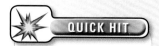

QUICK HIT

Lab values expected in a pneumothorax include increased P_{CO_2}, depressed P_{O_2}, acidotic pH, and compensatory increase in bicarbonate.

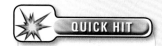

QUICK HIT

Bronchial obstruction can also lead to tracheal deviation with decreased breath sounds; however, in this case, the tracheal deviation is toward the side of the lesion because of the loss of volume. Decreased ventilation to the affected lung also leads to loss of tactile fremitus and hyporesonance.

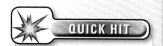

QUICK HIT

Flail chest is caused by multiple fractures of consecutive ribs (each fractured in at least two places), leading to paradoxical movement of the injured area of the chest wall with respiration.

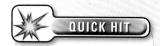

QUICK HIT

The clinical settings in which a pulmonary embolus can occur include cancer, multiple fractures, oral contraceptive use, prolonged bed rest, or CHF.

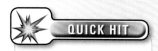

QUICK HIT

Fat emboli are often caused by crush injury with fracture of the long bones and orthopedic surgery.

The Respiratory System

The Respiratory System

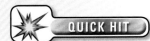

Pulmonary edema caused by heart failure is characterized histologically by hemosiderin-laden macrophages ("heart failure cells") and congested alveolar capillaries.

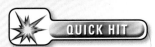

Chronic obstructive pulmonary disease (COPD) is characterized by airflow obstruction. This is in contrast to restrictive pulmonary diseases, which demonstrate defective lung expansion. Obstructive disorders have increased TLC, decreased FEV_1, and decreased FEV_1/FVC. Restrictive disorders show reduced lung volumes and normal or increased FEV_1/FVC. Normal FEV_1/FVC ratio is approximately 80%.

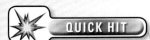

Status asthmaticus is a prolonged asthmatic attack that does not respond to therapy and can be fatal.

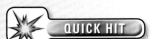

There are many types of asthma, including extrinsic (children), intrinsic (adults), exercise induced, and cold air induced.

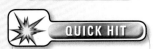

Reid index: Ratio (normally < 0.4) between the thickness of the submucosal mucus-secreting glands and the thickness between the epithelium and cartilage overlying the bronchus.

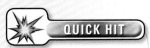

"Blue bloater": Blue refers to cyanosis; bloater refers to the peripheral edema in these patients from pulmonary hypertension and right ventricular overload.

TABLE 4-3 Pulmonary Vascular Diseases (Continued)

Disease	Etiology	Features	Complications
Pulmonary edema	Obliteration of alveoli as a result of intra-alveolar accumulation of fluid	Heart failure or overload leads to **increased hydrostatic pressure** Inflammatory alveolar reactions (caused by drugs, pneumonia, sepsis, and uremia) leads to **increased capillary permeability**	Hypoxia
Wegener granulomatosis	Etiology is unknown but thought to be autoimmune in nature	Focal necrotizing **vasculitis** affecting small-sized to medium-sized vessels Acute necrotizing **granulomas of upper and lower respiratory tract** Bilateral nodular and cavitary infiltrates seen on chest radiograph Mucosal ulceration of nasopharynx seen on examination Associated with c-ANCA	Untreated disease is fatal within several years

A–a gradient, Alveolar–arterial gradient; c-ANCA, cytoplasmic antineutrophil cytoplasmic antibody; COPD, chronic obstructive pulmonary disease; V/Q, ventilation/perfusion.

CHRONIC OBSTRUCTIVE PULMONARY DISEASE

I. **Types of chronic obstructive pulmonary disease (COPD)** *(Table 4-4)*

TABLE 4-4 Types of Chronic Obstructive Pulmonary Disease

Disease	Pathophysiology	Clinical Features and Management
Asthma	**Increased sensitivity** of bronchioles causes bronchoconstriction, muscle hypertrophy, **Curschmann spirals** (twisted, mucus casts of small airways), and **Charcot–Leyden crystals** (enzymes present within eosinophils)	**Cough, wheezing,** dyspnea; common treatment options include inhaled steroids and β_2-agonists
Chronic bronchitis	Caused by persistent irritants and infections; most common cause is smoking; hyperplasia of goblet cells and submucosal glands **(increased Reid index); excess mucus;** possible cor pulmonale	**Productive cough** for at least 3 consecutive months over 2 consecutive years; cyanosis due to decreased O_2 saturation, wheezing; "blue bloater"; chronic respiratory acidosis as mucus plugs block the exhalation of CO_2; **smoking cessation**

(continued)

TABLE 4-4 Types of Chronic Obstructive Pulmonary Disease *(Continued)*

Disease	Pathophysiology	Clinical Features and Management
Emphysema	Dilated alveoli; damaged alveolar walls; **damaged alveolar septae** leads to **enlarged alveolar airspaces;** destruction of structural support to lymphatic vessels leads to heavy pigment deposition; **decreased elastic recoil;** centrilobular (associated with smoking), panacinar (α_1-antitrypsin deficiency), paraseptal (associated with scarred tissue, may lead to spontaneous pneumothorax in young patients), and irregular forms	"Pink puffer"; paraseptal type may lead to pneumothorax; anteroposterior diameter increased ("barrel chested"); hypertrophy of accessory respiratory muscles; episodes of nonproductive cough; **smoking cessation**
Bronchiectasis	**Chronic infection leads to irreversible bronchial dilation;** destruction of bronchial wall; commonly caused by bronchial **obstruction** (e.g., tumor)	Copious amounts of purulent sputum; hemoptysis; possible lung abscess; associated with CF and Kartagener syndrome

CF, cystic fibrosis; CO_2, carbon dioxide; COPD, chronic obstructive pulmonary disease.

II. **Therapeutic agents used in asthma and COPD** *(Table 4-5)*
   A. Inhaled agents
      1. β_2-Agonists
         a. β_2-Agonists are useful for treatment of an acute asthma attack characterized by SOB, chest tightness, wheezing, and cough as a result of bronchoconstriction.
            • The β_2-agonists stimulate adenylyl cyclase, resulting in the conversion of adenosine triphosphate (ATP) to cyclic adenosine monophosphate (cAMP); the increased levels of cAMP result in myriad effects, depending on the cell type in question.
            • β_2-Agonists are potent dilators of the bronchi. They act by relaxing smooth muscle in the airways.
            • Systemic activation of β_2-specific receptors (which is minimal with inhaled β_2-agonists) may result in vasodilation, a slight decrease in peripheral resistance, bronchodilation, increased glycogenolysis in muscle and in the liver, increased release of glucagons, and relaxation of uterine smooth muscle.
         b. Side effects include tachycardia, hyperglycemia, hypokalemia, and hypomagnesemia.
         c. β_2-Agonists have no effect on the inflammation associated with asthma.
         d. Selected β_2-agonists:
            • **Albuterol** or **terbutaline** provides immediate relief of acute attacks without β_1-adrenoceptor stimulation.
            • **Salmeterol** has a longer duration of action and a slower onset of action.
      2. Corticosteroids
         a. In cases of moderate asthma, corticosteroids (inhaled or systemic) can be used to decrease the associated inflammation.
         b. Inhaled corticosteroids such as beclomethasone, triamcinolone, and flunisolide decrease the effect that inflammatory cells (mast cells, eosinophils, macrophages) have on the airway.

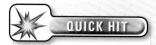

QUICK HIT

Emphysema and bronchitis often coexist in the same patient.

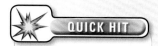

QUICK HIT

Two types of emphysema: Centriacinar primarily affects the respiratory bronchioles, is associated with smoking, and predominantly involves the upper lobes; panacinar is dilation of the entire alveolus, predominantly involves the lower segments, and involves α_1-antitrypsin deficiency.

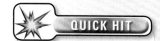

QUICK HIT

In emphysema, smoking attracts neutrophils, which release elastase. α_1-Antitrypsin normally inhibits elastase; however, free radicals caused by smoking inhibit α_1-antitrypsin, allowing elastase to damage the alveolar walls, causing dilation.

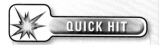

QUICK HIT

"Pink puffer": Pink refers to the lack of cyanosis from the nearly normal arterial oxygen pressures; puffer refers to the severe dyspnea seen in these patients.

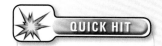

QUICK HIT

Order of β-agonist potency (most potent to least potent): isoproterenol, epinephrine, and norepinephrine. Order of α-agonist potency (most potent to least potent): epinephrine, norepinephrine, and isoproterenol.

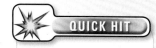

QUICK HIT

β_2-Selective agents such as terbutaline can be used in premature labor to prevent contractions.

The Respiratory System

The Respiratory System

TABLE 4-5 Therapeutic Agents for Asthma and Chronic Obstructive Pulmonary Disease

Therapeutic Agent (common name, if relevant) [trade name, where appropriate]	Class–Pharmacology and Pharmacokinetics	Indications	Side Effects or Adverse Effects	Contraindications or Precautions to Consider; Notes
Epinephrine [Primatene Mist]	Adrenergic agonist (nonselective)—relaxes bronchial smooth muscle through β_2-receptor activity	Asthma	Tachycardia (β_1-receptor activity)	
Isoproterenol [Isuprel]	β-agonist (nonselective)—relaxes bronchial smooth muscle through β_2-receptor activity	Asthma	Tachycardia (β_1-receptor activity)	
Albuterol [Proventil, Ventolin], **levalbuterol** [Xopenex]	**β_2-agonist—leads to relaxation of smooth muscle**	Asthma, **COPD**, bronchitis	**Tremor, tachycardia, arrhythmia,** headache, nausea, vomiting	
Salmeterol [Serevent]	**Long-acting β_2-agonist—leads to relaxation of smooth muscle**	Asthma prophylaxis	**Hand tremor,** headache, nervousness, dizziness, cough, stuffed nose, runny nose, muscle pain/cramps, sore throat	Not for acute asthmatic attacks
Theophylline [Aerolate, Theo-24, Theo-Dur, Theolair, Uniphyl]	Methylxanthines—unknown mechanism; may inhibit phosphodiesterase → decreases cAMP hydrolysis → promotes bronchodilation; stimulates CNS, cardiac muscle; relaxes smooth muscle; produces diuresis; increases cerebral vascular resistance	Asthma	Cardiotoxicity, neurotoxicity	Metabolized by cytochrome P450. Narrow therapeutic window
Ipratropium [Atrovent]	Muscarinic antagonist—competitively blocks muscarinic receptors → prevents bronchoconstriction	Asthma, COPD		
Beclomethasone, dexamethasone, prednisone	Corticosteroids—inhibits leukotriene synthesis → reduces inflammation and leads to bronchodilation	Asthma, COPD	**Osteoporosis, Cushingoid reaction, psychosis, glucose intolerance, infection, hypertension, cataracts, acne**	
Zileuton	Antileukotriene—**5-lipoxygenase inhibitor** → inhibits conversion of arachidonic acid to leukotriene → prevents bronchoconstriction and inflammatory cell infiltration	Asthma		
Zafirlukast [Accolate], **montelukast** [Singulair]	Antileukotriene—**blocks leukotriene receptors** → prevents bronchoconstriction and inflammatory cell infiltration	Asthma (especially Aspirin-induced asthma)		
Cromolyn	Prevents release of mediators from mast cells → prevents bronchoconstriction and inflammation	Asthma prophylaxis		Not for acute asthmatic attacks
Nedocromil [Tilade]	Stabilizes membranes of mast cells and prevents mediator release	Asthma	Unpleasant taste	Not for acute asthmatic attacks

cAMP, cyclic adenosine monophosphate; CNS, central nervous system; COPD, chronic obstructive pulmonary disease.

Clinical Vignette 4-1

CLINICAL PRESENTATION: A 59-year-old woman presents with a chief complaint of **shortness of breath (SOB).** Patient states she has been experiencing worsening SOB with minimal physical exertion. She has been experiencing bouts of **productive cough** every morning for the past 2 years. She has smoked two packs of cigarettes a day for the past 35 years. Patient denies any fevers or bloody sputum. Physical exam reveals an **increased anteroposterior diameter of the chest wall** and **wheezes** and **rhonchi** on inspiration. Temperature = 98.3° F; blood pressure = 142/92 mm Hg; heart rate = 93 bpm; respiration rate = 23 breaths/min.
DIFFERENTIALS: COPD, asthma, CHF. Given the patient's presentation and long-standing history of smoking, this patient most likely has COPD.
LABORATORY STUDIES: Proper follow-up management would include an **arterial blood gas** to provide information regarding the patient's O_2 status because hypoxemia and hypercapnia may be present. **Spirometry** is the next best step in the evaluation process. **Flow volume loops** will assist in identifying restrictive from obstructive pulmonary disease. A forced expiratory volume at 1 second/forced vital capacity ratio in obstructive pulmonary diseases will be below the normal ratio of 0.8.
MANAGEMENT: Initial step in management is smoking cessation. **β-Agonists and anticholinergic agents** provide bronchodilation via nebulizers. Administration of **oxygen** is necessary to correct hypoxemia. **Corticosteroids** can be used in acute exacerbations along with **antibiotics** if there is suspicion of an underlying infection.

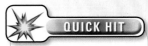

   c. In cases of severe asthma, intravenous methylprednisolone or oral prednisone may be necessary for a short period.
   d. The side effects of inhaled steroids are minimal when compared with systemic steroid use. However, adverse reactions can occur and include oral candidiasis, and, with long-term use, osteoporosis.

B. Other asthma medications
   1. **Cromolyn,** a prophylactic anti-inflammatory agent
   2. **Ipratropium,** a derivative of atropine that blocks the vagal aspect of airway smooth muscle contraction and mucus secretion
   3. **Theophylline,** a bronchodilator, which may result in seizures and arrhythmias
   4. Newer agents
      a. **Zileuton,** a 5-lipoxygenase inhibitor, blocks the conversion of arachidonic acid into leukotrienes, which are responsible for chemotaxis, increased secretion, and bronchospasm.
      b. **Zafirlukast** prevents the chemotactic and bronchospastic effects of leukotrienes C_4, D_4 and E_4 by blocking their receptors.

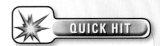

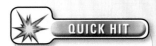

INTERSTITIAL LUNG DISEASE (Table 4-6)

Insterstitial lung disease (ILD) is a noninfectious, nonmalignant condition characterized by inflammation and pathologic changes of the alveolar wall. Differentiation and diagnosis often require histologic evaluation of the lung. It is characterized as having decreased lung volumes and a normal to increased FEV_1/FVC ratio.

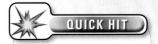

TABLE 4-6 Interstitial Lung Disease

Disease	Pathophysiology	Population Most at Risk	Clinical Features
Eosinophilic granuloma	Presence of Langerhans-like cells and **Birbeck granules;** subset of histiocytosis X	Former **smokers**	Lesions in lung or ribs, pneumothorax
Goodpasture syndrome	Pulmonary hemorrhage, anemia, glomerulonephritis, **antibasement membrane antibodies**	Men, middle-aged people	Hemoptysis, hematuria

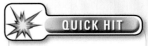

(continued)

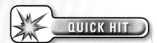

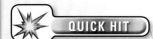

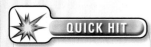

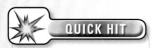

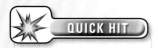

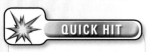

TABLE 4-6 Interstitial Lung Disease *(Continued)*

Disease	Pathophysiology	Population Most at Risk	Clinical Features
Idiopathic pulmonary fibrosis	Chronic **inflammation of alveolar wall;** leukocytes release cytokines that lead to fibrosis; cystic spaces	Sixth decade of life	**Honeycomb lung;** fatal within years
Sarcoidosis	Interstitial fibrosis; diagnosis by exclusion of other causes and biopsy showing **non-caseating granulomatous lesions;** asteroid and Schaumann bodies; increased angiotensin-converting enzyme levels; uveitis; polyarthritis; hypercalcemia; erythema nodosum; cardiomyopathy; central and peripheral neuropathies	**Young Black females**	Dyspnea on exertion, dry cough, fever, fatigue, bilateral hilar lymphadenopathy visible on chest x-ray, increased levels of angiotensin-converting enzyme, hypercalcemia
Hypersensitivity pneumonitis (farmer's lung, pigeon breeder's lung)	Prolonged exposure to organic antigens in atopic individuals; interstitial inflammation; alveolar damage leads to chronic, fibrotic lung	People with an occupational history of farming or bird-keeping	**Dry cough, chest tightness,** general malaise, and fever

ENVIRONMENTAL LUNG DISEASES (PNEUMOCONIOSIS) *(Table 4-7)*

This group of diseases is often caused by workplace exposure to various organic and chemical irritants. A careful history and pulmonary function testing are often important for diagnosis.

Approximately 70% to 80% of newly diagnosed pulmonary tuberculosis (TB) cases in adults are actually a result of reactivation of a clinically unsuspected infection acquired years to decades previously.

TABLE 4-7 Environmental Lung Diseases (Pneumoconiosis)

Disease	Pathophysiology	Clinical Features
Anthracosis	Carbon dust ingested by alveolar macrophages, visible **black deposits seen on gross lung tissue samples**	Usually asymptomatic
Asbestosis	Asbestos fibers ingested by alveolar macrophages, fibroblast proliferation, interstitial fibrosis (lower lobes), **asbestos bodies and ferruginous bodies (hemosiderin laden asbestos fibers),** pleural plaques and effusions *psammoma*	Increased risk of bronchogenic carcinoma and **malignant mesothelioma,** synergistic effect of asbestos and tobacco in causing bronchogenic carcinoma
Coal worker's pneumoconiosis	Carbon dust ingested by alveolar macrophages forms bronchiolar **macules;** may progress to fibrosis	Plaques are asymptomatic; often benign, may progress to fibrosis; may be fatal owing to pulmonary hypertension and **cor pulmonale; no evidence of increased risk for TB or lung cancer**
Silicosis	Silica dust ingested by alveolar macrophages causing release of harmful enzymes; **silicotic nodules** (of collagen that may calcify) and thick pleural scars	Nodules may obstruct air or blood flow; concurrent TB common **(silicotuberculosis)**
Berylliosis	Induction of cell-mediated immunity leads to non-caseating granulomas, several organ systems affected; histologically identical to sarcoidosis	Increases lung cancer

TB, tuberculosis.

RESPIRATORY INFECTIONS

I. **Pneumonia**

A. Pathogenesis

1. Most commonly, pneumonia is caused by **microaspiration** from the oropharynx or **inhalation of infectious droplets or particles**.

2. Alcoholism, nasogastric tubes, and obtunded states increase risk of contracting pneumonia.

3. Normal oral flora consists of gram-positive cocci.

4. Hospitalized patients may be colonized by gram-negative rods (nosocomial infections).

5. Other portals of entry include respiratory droplets, hematogenous spread, contiguous spread, and traumatic inoculation.

B. **Clinical manifestations**

1. **Typical pneumonia** presents with acute fever, purulent sputum, pleuritic pain, and lobar "whited out" infiltrate on chest radiograph (e.g., *Streptococcus pneumoniae*).

2. **Atypical pneumonia** is characterized by slow onset of nonproductive cough, headache, gastrointestinal (GI) symptoms, and diffuse patchy infiltrate on chest radiograph (e.g., *Mycoplasma pneumoniae*).

3. **Nosocomial pneumonia** commonly occurs in the setting of an underlying disease, immunosuppression, or use of a ventilator (e.g., *Pseudomonas aeruginosa, Escherichia coli*).

C. Location of pathology and typical organisms

1. **Lobar** (intra-alveolar infiltrate): *S. pneumoniae*

2. **Bronchopneumonia** (bronchiolar infiltrate): *Staphylococcus aureus, Haemophilus influenzae, Streptococcus pneumoniae*, viral

3. **Interstitial** (diffuse infiltrate in alveolar wall): *M. pneumoniae, Legionella, Pneumocystis jirovecii*, viral

D. Etiology

1. Bacterial and mycoplasmal pneumonias (Table 4-8)

2. Viral pneumonia (Table 4-9)

3. Fungal pneumonia (Table 4-10)

4. Clinical diagnosis of pneumonia (Tables 4-11 and 4-12)

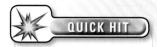

QUICK HIT

The most likely cause for lung abscess formation in a comatose patient is aspiration pneumonia as a consequence of a depressed cough reflex. Other causes of lung abscess formation are septic emboli (from infective endocarditis), spread from adjacent organs, and malignant tumors.

QUICK HIT

Typical pneumonia is characterized histopathologically by intra-alveolar exudation of neutrophils, fibrin, erythrocytes, and bacteria. Sputum is essentially pus consisting of bacteria and neutrophils. However, because organisms causing atypical pneumonia are generally intracellular pathogens, we see the alveolar septae swollen with T cells and macrophages and therefore no sputum production (hence nonproductive cough).

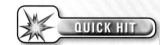

The Respiratory System

TABLE 4-8 Bacterial and Mycoplasmal Pneumonia

Bacteria	Presentation	Population Most at Risk	Clinical Features
Streptococcus pneumoniae	Typical	**Adults**	Most common cause of community-acquired pneumonia
Haemophilus influenzae	Typical	Elderly	Complicates viral infection, chronic respiratory disease
Staphylococcus aureus	Typical	Can cause typical community-acquired pneumonia but also infects immunocompromised and hospitalized patients	Abscesses, complicates viral infection, especially influenza
Streptococcus agalactiae	Typical	**Neonates**	Similar to *Streptococcus pneumoniae*
Klebsiella pneumoniae	Typical	Patients with alcoholism	Aspiration of gastric contents
Mycoplasma pneumoniae	Atypical	**Young adults**	Most common cause of atypical pneumonia; positive cold agglutinin test
Legionella pneumophila	Atypical	Immunocompromised patients	Found in drinking water and air conditioners
Chlamydophila pneumoniae	Atypical	**Young adults**	Upper and lower pulmonary tract infection
Chlamydophila psittaci	Atypical	**Pet bird** owners	Bradycardia, splenomegaly
Chlamydia trachomatis (trachoma)		**Neonates**	Also causes *trachoma* (chlamydial conjunctivitis leading to blindness)

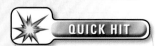

QUICK HIT

Consolidation of lungs in bacterial pneumonia leads to increased fremitus because sounds are better transmitted through consolidation. Bronchial breath sounds may also be appreciated. Conversely, viral pneumonia should not cause lung consolidation, and therefore fremitus should be decreased.

QUICK HIT

Aspirin therapy for the fever of influenza and varicella zoster infections in children is contraindicated because it may cause Reye syndrome. Clinical manifestations of Reye syndrome include encephalopathy and potentially fatal liver damage.

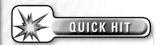

QUICK HIT

Other less common sources of fungal lung infection include *Cryptococcus neoformans* and *Aspergillus* in immunocompromised individuals.

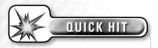

QUICK HIT

Pneumocystis jirovecii is now classified as a fungus but was previously classified as a protozoa.

TABLE 4-9 Viral Pneumonia

Virus	Pathophysiology	Clinical Features
Respiratory syncytial virus (types 1 and 2)	Atypical	Also causes bronchiolitis; more common in winter months; can cause serious respiratory distress in infants
Influenza	Atypical	**Often complicated by secondary bacterial infection**

TABLE 4-10 Fungal Pneumonia

Etiology	Pathophysiology	Clinical Features
Histoplasma capsulatum	Atypical	Most infections are subclinical; tiny yeast forms in macrophages; found in Ohio, Mississippi, and Missouri River Valleys; yeast with a thin cell wall but no true capsule
Coccidioides immitis	Atypical	Most infections are subclinical; nonbudding spherules filled with endospores; "valley fever" found in southwestern deserts of United States
Pneumocystis jirovecii	Atypical	Often fatal common opportunistic infection in immunocompromised patients (such as patients with HIV)
Paracoccidioides brasiliensis	Atypical	Budding yeast resemble spokes of a "captain's wheel"; found in Central and South Americas; yeast with multiple budding
Sporotrichosis	Atypical	Skin nodules that occur along lymphatics in the arms of rose gardeners
Aspergillus	Atypical	Fungal ball of hyphae (aspergilloma) in preexisting lung cavities or invasive pulmonary disease in immunocompromised patients
Blastomyces dermatitidis	Atypical	Yeast forms in body; 5–25-mm yeast with thick refractile wall and broad-based budding; found in Mississippi–Ohio River basins and around the Great Lakes
Candida albicans	Atypical	Yeast and hyphae
Cryptococcus neoformans	Atypical	Yeast with broad capsule

TABLE 4-11 Clinical Diagnosis of Pneumonia

	Bacterial	Viral	Mycoplasma
Age	Any; often younger than 2 years old	Any	Young adults (teenagers)
Fever	>102.28° F	<102.28° F	<102.28° F
Onset	Abrupt	Gradual	Gradual fever, gradual cough
Relatives	Healthy	Sick (concurrent)	Sick (2–3 weeks previous)
Cough	Productive	Dry	Paroxysmal
Pleuritic chest pain	Yes (splinting)	No	No
Physical examination	Tubular breath sounds; dull to percussion	Bilateral, diffuse rales	Rales in one or two segments
Radiographic findings	Consolidated "whited out" lobe	Diffuse, patchy, bilateral	Patchy; one or two lobes; no consolidation

TABLE 4-12 Most Common Causative Agents of Pneumonia by Age

Neonates (Birth–4 weeks)	Children (1 month–20 years)	Young Adults (20–40 years)	Adults (40–60 years)	Elderly (≥60 years)
Group B streptococcus	Viral: RSV, parainfluenza, influenza	Mycoplasma pneumoniae	Streptococcus pneumoniae	S. pneumoniae
Escherichia coli	S. pneumoniae	S. pneumoniae	M. pneumoniae	Anaerobes
	M. pneumoniae	Chlamydophila pneumoniae	Haemophilus influenzae	H. influenzae
	C. pneumoniae		Viruses	Gram-negative rods
			Anaerobes	

RSV, respiratory syncytial virus.

II. Tuberculosis and its treatment (Figure 4-7)

A. Multiple drug therapy is used for the treatment of TB in an effort to combat drug resistance.

B. A common therapeutic regimen includes **isoniazid** (INH), **rifampin**, **ethambutol**, and **pyrazinamide** for a period of 2 months, followed by INH and rifampin for a period of 4 to 7 months.

1. INH

   a. INH, which diffuses into all body fluids, including breast milk, targets the outer layer of the mycobacteria.

   b. A common side effect of INH therapy is paresthesia, which can be corrected by the administration of **pyridoxine** (vitamin B_6).

2. Rifampin

   a. Rifampin inhibits RNA synthesis by blocking the β subunit of bacterial DNA-dependent RNA polymerase.

   b. Rifampin also induces **cytochrome P450 enzymes** in the liver and can decrease the half-lives of other agents in this way.

   c. One side effect of rifampin is the **orange-red color** of bodily fluids.

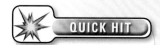
QUICK HIT

Primary TB occurs in the upper part of the lower lobe or lower part of the upper lobe. However, secondary TB occurs in the apical area.

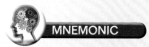
MNEMONIC

Miliary TB—think millet seed to remember multiple seedlike, white-gray lesions.

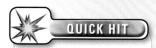
QUICK HIT

Mycobacterium tuberculosis are acid-fast bacteria because they have an envelope that contains large amounts of lipid and even true waxes that prevent the acid-fast stain (carbolfuchsin) from leaking out.

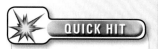
QUICK HIT

Rifampin decreases the half-lives of oral contraceptives as well as warfarin, digitoxin, ketoconazole, propranolol, and prednisone. Consequently, higher doses of these medications may be required to achieve the same therapeutic effect.

The Respiratory System

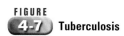
FIGURE 4-7 Tuberculosis

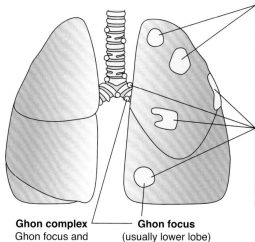

Secondary tuberculosis (TB)
- Reactivation of primary TB, hematogenously spread
- Clinical presentation includes weakness, hemoptysis, weight loss
- Usually located in upper lobe
- Large, cavitary lesions may rupture into bronchi
- May extend beyond lung (miliary TB); common sites include meninges, spine (Pott disease) and psoas major muscle

Primary tuberculosis (TB)
- Subpleural and hilar lymph node granulomas (tubercles) = **Ghon complex**
- **Caseating necrosis** with Langerhans giant cells
- Usually does not become clinically symptomatic
- Heals with calcification seen on chest radiograph

Ghon complex
Ghon focus and hilar lymph nodes

Ghon focus
(usually lower lobe)

III. Upper respiratory infections

A. Otitis externa—most common cause is *P. aeruginosa*

B. Otitis media—most pathogens involved are *S. pneumoniae* and nontypable *H. influenzae*

C. Sinusitis
  1. Results from obstructed drainage outlets of the sinuses
  2. Caused by *S. pneumoniae*, *H. influenzae*, and *Moraxella*

D. Rhinitis
  1. Viral rhinitis
    a. Most commonly caused by rhinoviruses and coronaviruses, also by adenoviruses and parainfluenza viruses
    b. Common cold
  2. Bacterial rhinitis
    a. Often secondary to viral infection
    b. Commonly caused by *Streptococcus*, *Staphylococcus*, and *H. influenzae*
  3. Allergic rhinitis
    a. Type I hypersensitivity reactions
    b. Characterized by eosinophilia

E. Laryngitis
  1. Characterized by edema and inflammation of the vocal cords
  2. Caused by infection (*M. pneumoniae*, parainfluenza virus) or overuse

F. Croup versus epiglottitis (Table 4-13)

IV. Therapeutic agents (*Table 4-14*)

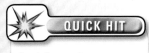

QUICK HIT

Parainfluenza virus causes a disease resembling the common cold in adults and is transmitted via respiratory droplets.

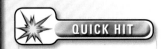

QUICK HIT

The incidence of epiglottitis caused by *Haemophilus influenzae* has decreased dramatically with the introduction of the *H. influenzae* type B vaccine. *H. influenzae* can also cause meningitis in unvaccinated children.

TABLE 4-13 Croup versus Epiglottitis

	Croup	Epiglottitis
Organism	Parainfluenza virus (type 1 or 2)	*Haemophilus influenzae* type B
Pathology	Inflammation of subglottic trachea	Inflamed epiglottis
Age	6 months to 2 years	1–5 years
Fever	<102° F	>102° F
Onset	**Gradual** (barking cough to **stridor**)	**Abrupt; stridor**
Associated symptoms	Rhinorrhea, hoarseness, conjunctivitis	None
Degree of illness	Not toxic, degree of symptoms greater than degree of illness	Toxic
Physical examination	Writhing, anxious, **subglottic edema and "steeple sign"** on radiograph	Quiet, **"sniffing position,"** drooling, **"thumbprint"** epiglottis on radiograph
Outcome	Self-limiting	Medical emergency; 90% of patients require surgery to reestablish airway

TABLE 4-14 Therapeutic Agents for Allergy, Cough, and Cold

Therapeutic Agent (common name, if relevant) [trade name, where appropriate]	Class–Pharmacology and Pharmacokinetics	Indications	Side Effects or Adverse Effects	Contraindications or Precautions to Consider; Notes
Diphenhydramine, dimenhydrinate, chlorpheniramine	H_1 blocker (first generation)	Allergy, motion sickness, insomnia	Sedation, anti-muscarinic, anti-α adrenergic	
Loratadine, fexofenadine, desloratadine, cetirizine	H_1 blocker (second generation)	Allergy	Sedating	Less sedating than first-generation H_1 blocker due to decreased CNS entry

(continued)

Therapeutic Agent (common name, if relevant) [trade name, where appropriate]	Class– Pharmacology and Pharmacokinetics	Indications	Side Effects or Adverse Effects	Contraindications or Precautions to Consider; Notes
Fluticasone [Flonase], beclomethasone, flunisolide [Nasarel], budesonide [Rhinocort], mometasone furoate	Intranasal glucocorti-coids—decrease cyto-kine synthesis, down-regulate inflammatory response in the nasal mucosa	Nasal congestion, allergic rhinitis	Local irritation of nasal mucosa, epistaxis	
Guaifenesin [Robitussin]	Expectorant—thins mucus and lubricates ir-ritated respiratory tract	Cough associated with common cold and minor upper respiratory tract infections		Does not suppress cough reflex
N-acetylcysteine	Mucolytic—loosens mucus plugs	Cough (especially in patients with CF), acetamino-phen overdose		

CF, cystic fibrosis; CNS, central nervous system.

CYSTIC FIBROSIS

I. **Cystic fibrosis (CF) is the most common lethal genetic disease in Caucasians.**

II. **Autosomal recessive mutation occurs on chromosome 7, the CF transmembrane conductance regulator (CFTR) gene. This leads to:**
   A. Deletion of phenylalanine at position 508 in 90% of patients with CF in the United States
   B. Altered chloride and water transport in epithelial cells
   C. High sodium and chloride concentrations on sweat test
   D. Increased mucosal viscosity obstructs exocrine glands, which leads to organ failure
   E. An abnormally high rate of sodium absorption from luminal secretions and a decreased rate of chloride secretion into luminal secretions reduce the salt and water content of bronchiolar secretions.

III. **Chronic pulmonary disease**
   A. Most serious complication and leading cause of death in patients with CF
   B. *P. aeruginosa* infections are the most common in adults, followed by *S. aureus* and *H. influenzae*. In children, *S. aureus* is the most common infection.
   C. Increased residual volume (RV) and increased total lung capacity (TLC) are characteristics of COPD.
   D. Atelectasis
   E. Bronchiectasis

IV. **Pancreatic insufficiency**
   A. Nutritional deficiencies (especially of fat-soluble vitamins A, D, E, and K)
   B. Steatorrhea
   C. β-Cells are initially spared but become functionally inactive with age, leading to an increased need for insulin.

V. **Meconium ileus**
   A. Usually presents in infant with abdominal distention, small bowel obstruction, and emesis

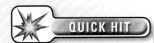

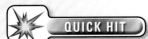

N-acetylcysteine is indicated for the treatment of acetaminophen overdose, as a mucolytic in CF, and is used off-label as prophylaxis against radiocontrast-induced nephropathy.

QUICK HIT

Superior sulcus tumors (**Pancoast tumors**) involve the apex of the lung and result in **Horner syndrome** (ptosis, miosis, anhydrosis). **Superior vena cava (SVC) syndrome** occurs when the SVC is obstructed, resulting in facial cyanosis and swelling.

VI. Treatment of CF includes symptomatic treatment and gene therapy.
   A. Mucolytics: *N*-acetylcysteine lyses the disulfide linkages between mucoproteins, resulting in decreased mucus viscosity.
   B. Inhaled bronchodilators
   C. Corticosteroids: Prednisone has been shown to increase pulmonary function and body weight in patients with CF.
   D. Antibiotics as needed to manage infections

LUNG NEOPLASMS (*Tables 4-15 to 4-17*)

I. Lung neoplasms are the leading cause of cancer death for both men and women in the United States.

II. Lung cancer is the second most common type of cancer (with the first being prostate cancer in men and breast cancer in women).

III. Lung cancer deaths among women are rising rapidly as a result of increased smoking in this population.

IV. Symptoms include cough, hemoptysis, airway obstruction, weight loss, and paraneoplastic syndromes.

TABLE 4-15 Lung Neoplasms

Tumor	Location and Histology	Clinical Features
Adenocarcinoma	**Peripheral;** subpleural; usually on pre-existing parenchymal **scars;** glandular	**Most common type;** may be related to smoking; CEA-positive; K-*ras* oncogenes
Bronchioalveolar	**Peripheral;** subtype of adenocarcinoma; tumor cells line alveolar walls	**Less strongly associated with smoking;** autoantibodies to surfactant may exist
Carcinoid	Major bronchi; spread by direct extension	Increased secretion of **5-HT,** flushing, wheezing, recurrent diarrhea, heart disease, low malignancy
Large cell	**Peripheral;** undifferentiated; giant cells with pleomorphism	Poor prognosis; metastasis to the brain; smoking
Metastasis	**Cannonball** lesions	**Higher incidence than primary lung cancer**
Small cell (oat cell)	**Central;** undifferentiated; **most aggressive;** small, dark blue cells; arise from neuroendocrine (Kulchitsky) cells	Poor prognosis; strongly associated with smoking; ectopic ACTH; ADH secretion
Squamous cell	**Central;** mass from bronchus; keratin pearls; cavitation	Strongly associated with smoking; secretion of **PTH-like peptide**

5-HT, serotonin; ACTH, adrenocorticotropic hormone; ADH, antidiuretic hormone; CEA, carcinoembryonic antigen; PTH, parathyroid hormone.

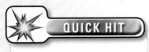

QUICK HIT

Nasopharyngeal carcinoma, common in Southeast Asia and East Africa, is caused by the Epstein–Barr virus.

TABLE 4-16 Other Respiratory Carcinomas

Tumor	Histology	Risk Factors
Nasopharyngeal carcinoma	Lymphoepithelioma (rich in lymphocytes)	Epstein–Barr virus infection; common in Southeast Asia (adult) and East Africa (childhood)
Laryngeal carcinoma	Squamous cell carcinoma	Smoking

TABLE 4-17 Paraneoplastic Syndromes of Lung Cancer

Disorder	Causes and Clinical Presentation
Horner syndrome	Superior sulcus tumors (Pancoast tumors); ptosis, miosis, anhidrosis
Superior vena cava (SVC) syndrome	Insidious compression or obstruction of the SVC; facial cyanosis, facial swelling, headache, venous distention of the neck, upper chest, and arms
Cushing syndrome	**ACTH** secretion; associated with <u>small cell carcinoma</u>; fat deposition of the face (moon faces), upper back (buffalo hump), truncal obesity, muscle weakness, purple striae
Hypercalcemia	Secretion of **PTH-related protein** (PTHrP); associated with **squamous cell lung cancer**
SIADH	Ectopic **antidiuretic hormone (ADH)** production; hyponatremia (Na^+ below 120 mEq/L)
Lambert–Eaton myasthenic syndrome	Proximal muscle weakness with autonomic dysfunction; antibodies produced against presynaptic calcium channels of the neuromuscular junction, no improvement with administration of anticholinesterase agents

ACTH, adrenocorticotropic hormone; PTH, parathyroid hormone; SIADH, syndrome of inappropriate antidiuretic hormone.

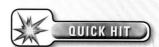

QUICK HIT

Paraneoplastic syndrome is a clinical and biochemical disturbance caused by a neoplasm that is not directly related to the primary tumor or metastases. Secretion of parathyroid hormone (PTH)–like hormone results in hypercalcemia. Ectopic antidiuretic hormone (ADH) production leads to syndrome of inappropriate antidiuretic hormone (SIADH) secretion with urinary retention and high urine osmolality. Adrenocorticotropic hormone (ACTH)–producing tumors lead to Cushing syndrome.

MNEMONIC

To remember the symptoms of Horner syndrome, think "PAM is Horny." P is ptosis, A is anhydrosis, M is miosis.

MNEMONIC

To remember the location, risk factors, and hormone-producing properties for small cell and squamous cell carcinoma, think **s** with **c**entral, **s**moking, and **s**ecretions.

Clinical Vignette 4-2

CLINICAL PRESENTATION: A 74-year-old man presents with shortness of breath, a chronic **bloody cough, increased fatigue, and a weight loss of 20 lb over a 3-month period.** Past medical history is significant for **hypertension, emphysema, coronary artery disease**, and a 26-pack-year history of **smoking.** Physical examination reveals wheezing in the right upper lobe. Temperature = 98.7° F; blood pressure = 140/92 mm Hg; heart rate = 80 bpm; and respiration rate = 25 breaths/min.

DIFFERENTIALS: Lung cancer, TB, pneumonia, left heart failure. Given the patient's presentation and long-standing history of smoking, this patient most likely has lung cancer. The two most common causes of hemoptysis in the United States are bronchitis and lung cancer.

LABORATORY STUDIES: Proper follow-up for this patient would include imaging, such as a chest **CT scan** or a **chest x-ray.** If imaging reveals a mass, **bronchoscopy** can be performed to obtain cells via brushings, bronchoalveolar lavage, or biopsy. **CT-guided fine needle biopsy** can also be performed to gather cells.

MANAGEMENT: Treatments include **surgical resection** and **chemotherapy** independently or in combination with **radiation.** Non–small cell lung cancer should be staged using the TNM (tumor, node, metastasis) system. Patients with stage I or II non–small cell lung cancers can be cured with surgical resection and radiotherapy. Small cell lung cancer often has metastasized at the time of diagnosis, making surgical resection futile and limiting radiotherapy and chemotherapy as the only treatment options.

DRUGS THAT CAUSE ADVERSE EFFECTS TO THE RESPIRATORY SYSTEM

I. **Pulmonary fibrosis:** bleomycin (antineoplastic), amiodarone (antiarrhythmic), busulfan (antineoplastic)

II. **Cough:** angiotensin-converting enzyme inhibitors (versus angiotensin II receptor blockers = no cough)

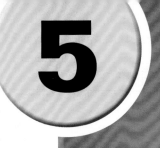

5 The Gastrointestinal System

INNERVATION AND BLOOD SUPPLY OF THE GASTROINTESTINAL TRACT *(Figure 5-1)*

FIGURE 5-1 Innervation and blood supply of the gastrointestinal tract

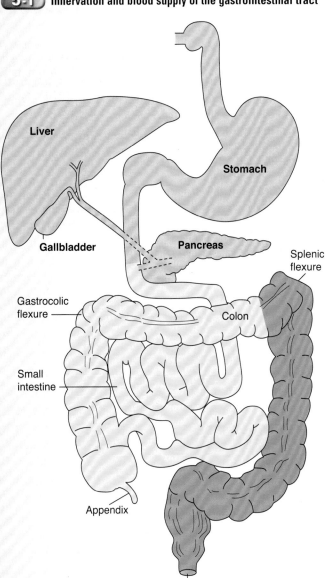

Foregut   Midgut   Hindgut

1) Foregut
   • Derivatives
     – Esophagus
     – Stomach
     – First part of duodenum
     – Liver
     – Gallbladder
     – Pancreas
       (formed from fusion of dorsal and ventral buds)

   • Supplied by celiac trunk

   • Vagal parasympathetic nerve, thoracic nerve, and splanchnic sympathetic nerve

2) Midgut
   • Derivatives
     – Second, third, and fourth parts of duodenum
     – Jejunum
     – Ileum
     – Appendix
     – Proximal two-thirds of colon (up to splenic flexure)

   • Supplied by superior mesenteric artery

   • Vagal parasympathetic nerve, thoracic splanchnic sympathetic nerve

3) Hindgut
   • Derivatives
     – Distal one-third of colon including sigmoid colon and rectum to pectinate line

   • Supplied by inferior mesenteric artery

   • Pelvic splanchnic (S2–S4) parasympathetic nerve and lumbar splanchnic sympathetic nerve

4) Ectoderm
   • Derivatives
     – Oropharynx (anterior two-thirds of tongue, lips, parotid glands, tooth enamel)
     – Anus, distal rectum (from pectinate line outward)

HORMONES OF THE GASTROINTESTINAL SYSTEM (Figure 5-2)

FIGURE
5-2 Hormones of the gastrointestinal system

Motilin
Secreted in upper GI tract to increase smooth muscle contraction in esophageal sphincter, stomach, and duodenum

Nitric oxide
Causes smooth muscle relaxation (e.g., lower esophageal sphincter [LES] relaxation)

Peptide YY
Secreted by endocrine cells of ileum and colon to inhibit gastric H^+ secretion

Glucagon
Secreted by cells of the pancreatic islets to promote glycogenolysis and gluconeogenesis

Gastrin
From antrum of stomach; secreted in response to gastric distention, vagal stimulation, and amino acid entering the stomach; causes gastric H^+ secretion

parietal

Cholecystokinin (CCK)
From cells in duodenum and jenunum and neurons of ileum and colon; secreted in response to amino acids and fatty acids entering the duodenum; causes contraction of gallbladder and pancreatic secretion of enzymes and HCO_3^-

Secretin
From S cells of small intestines; secreted in response to H^+ and fatty acids entering the duodenum; causes pancreatic secretion of HCO_3^- and inhibits gastric H^+ secretion

Somatostatin
Produced by D cells of stomach and duodenum and δ cells of pancreatic islets to inhibit gastric H^+ secretion, pancreatic secretion, and lower bile flow and to promote intestinal SMC contraction

Vasoactive intestinal peptide (VIP)
Secreted by smooth muscle and nerves of intestines; relaxes intestinal smooth muscle, causes pancreatic HCO_3^- secretion, and inhibits gastric H^+ secretion; enteric nervous system (ENS) peptide neurotransmitter, also relaxes lower esophageal sphincter, possibly as part of NO response

Parasympathetic (ACh)
Increases production of saliva; increased gastric H^+ secretion; increases pancreatic enzyme and HCO_3^- secretion; causes gallbadder contraction; allows for gastric receptive relaxation; stimulates enteric nervous system to create intestinal peristalsis; relaxes sphincters

Sympathetic (NE)
Increases production of saliva; decreases splanchnic blood flow in fight-or-flight response; decreases motility; constricts sphincters

Liver

Stomach

Gallbladder
2
Pancreas
1

Duodenum
Colon
3
4
Small intestine

Cecum

Sigmoid

Appendix

Rectum

☐ Retroperitoneal
☐ Partially peritonealized
■ Completely peritonealized

ACh, acetylcholine; GI, gastrointestinal; HCO_3^-, bicarbonate; NE, norepinephrine; NO, nitric oxide; SMC, smooth muscle cells.

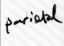

The Gastrointestinal System

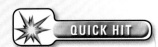

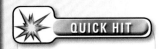

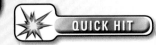

IMPORTANT CONGENITAL MALFORMATIONS OF THE GASTROINTESTINAL SYSTEM (Table 5-1)

With the exception of a Meckel diverticulum, which can remain asymptomatic throughout the life span, congenital malformations of the gastrointestinal (GI) tract will manifest themselves during the neonatal period.

TABLE 5-1 Important Congenital Malformations of the Gastrointestinal System

Malformation	Clinical Features
Hypertrophic pyloric stenosis	Thickening of the pylorus musculature **Projectile vomiting** *(non billious)* Palpable knot "olive" in the pyloric region *, apple core on X-ray*
Extrahepatic biliary atresia	Incomplete recanalization of the bile duct during development Presents shortly after birth Dark urine Clay-colored stool Jaundice
Annular pancreas	Abnormal fusion of ventral and dorsal pancreatic buds, forming a constricting ring around the duodenum Duodenal obstruction (bilious vomiting); presents shortly after birth
Meckel diverticulum	Persistent remnant of the vitelline duct Forms an outpouching (true diverticulum) in the ileum Ulceration and bleeding Fifty percent contain either gastric or pancreatic tissue when symptomatic
Malrotation of the midgut	Normal 270-degree rotation is not completed *Ladd bands* Cecum and appendix lie in upper abdomen Associated with **volvulus** (twisting of intestine), causing an obstruction
Intestinal stenosis or atresia	Results from failure of the normal recanalization of the lumen May produce failure to thrive *(billious vomiting)*
Hirschsprung disease (congenital or toxic megacolon)	Failure of **neural crest cells** to migrate to colon No peristalsis Constipation and abdominal distention in newborn **Bowel movement precipitated by digital rectal examination**
Anal agenesis	Lack of anal opening as a result of improper formation of the urorectal septum May cause rectovesical (anus to bladder), rectovaginal, or rectourethral fistula

THE OROPHARYNX, ESOPHAGUS, AND STOMACH

I. **The digestion of food begins in the oral cavity with salivary enzymes.**

II. **The esophagus transports food to the stomach.**
   A. The upper third of the esophagus is skeletal muscle.
   B. The middle third is both skeletal and smooth muscle.
   C. The lower third is smooth muscle.
   D. The lower esophageal sphincter (LES) relaxes in preparation for the passage of food into the stomach.

III. **The stomach receives and stores food.**
   A. Receptive relaxation—the stomach relaxes to accommodate the entering food (a vagovagal reflex).

B. Three phases of gastric secretion
1. **Cephalic phase**—the sight, smell, taste, or thought of food stimulates secretion.
2. **Gastric phase**—secretion is caused by the entry of food into the stomach.
3. **Intestinal phase**—food entering the intestine causes a feedback stimulation of gastric secretion.
C. Important gastric secretions
1. **Hydrochloric acid (HCl)** is secreted by parietal cells of the fundus.
   a. Stimulated by gastrin, histamine, and vagal stimulation
   b. Inhibited by **omeprazole** (proton pump inhibitor), **cimetidine** (H_2 blocker), chyme in small intestine via gastric inhibitory peptide (GIP), and secretin
2. **Intrinsic factor** is secreted by parietal cells of the fundus.
   a. Binds to vitamin B_{12} (extrinsic factor)
   b. **Vitamin B_{12}–intrinsic factor complex** absorbed in **terminal ileum**
3. **Pepsinogen** is secreted by chief cells.
   a. Pepsinogen is converted to pepsin by the low pH of the stomach.
   b. Pepsin begins the digestion of protein.
4. **Gastrin** secreted by the G cells of the antrum and pylorus stimulates the release of HCl from parietal cells.
5. **Somatostatin is secreted by a variety of cells throughout the GI tract and has a global inhibitory effect.**
D. The stomach grinds food into small particles and forces it into the duodenum.
1. Grinding (trituration) takes place in peristaltic waves occurring at a rate of three to five waves per minute.
2. **Migrating motor complexes (MMCs)**, stimulated by motilin, occur in the interdigestive period and serve to flush undigested food through the GI system.

IV. Nonneoplastic disorders of the oropharynx, esophagus, and stomach (Table 5-2)

TABLE 5-2 Nonneoplastic Disorders of the Oropharynx, Esophagus, and Stomach			
Disorder	**Etiology and Pathology**	**Clinical Features**	**Notes**
Sialolithiasis	Blockage of salivary gland duct preventing release of saliva; follows chronic sialadenitis (inflammation of the salivary glands)	Acute pain; usually in submandibular gland or Stensen duct of the parotid gland	Passage of stone can be induced by stimulating the secretion of saliva (e.g., by sucking on a lemon)
Pleomorphic adenoma	Increased risk with radiation exposure	Benign, recurring, mixed cell tumor of the parotid; may lead to facial nerve injury	Most frequent salivary gland tumor; more common in women 20–40 years of age
Esophageal variceal bleeding	Bleeding from esophageal varices owing to portal HTN	Hematemesis, signs of portal HTN (i.e., caput medusae, ascites)	Usually treated with vasoconstrictors (vasopressin); endoscopy required for diagnosis (to rule out bleeding ulcers)
Boerhaave syndrome	Complete rupture of the esophagus (all layers); caused by severe retching	Often presents as left pneumothorax; surgical correction necessary	Esophageal reflux disease predisposes to this condition
Mallory–Weiss tear	Laceration of the gastroesophageal junction; usually caused by severe retching	Poststretching hematemesis	Alcoholics and bulimics are at an increased risk

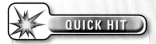

QUICK HIT

Gastroesophageal reflux disease (GERD), a common gastroesophageal disorder, is usually treated with H_2 blockers such as cimetidine or ranitidine or, in more severe cases, with proton pump inhibitors such as omeprazole or lansoprazole.

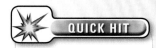

QUICK HIT

Cyclooxygenase-2 (COX-2) inhibitors such as celecoxib and rofecoxib not only reduce the adverse GI side effects and ulcers of normal non-steroidal anti-inflammatory drugs (NSAIDs) but also do not inhibit platelet function.

(continued)

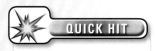

TABLE 5-2	Nonneoplastic Disorders of the Oropharynx, Esophagus, and Stomach *(Continued)*		
Disorder	**Etiology and Pathology**	**Clinical Features**	**Notes**
Acute gastritis	NSAIDs, smoking, alcohol, aspirin, steroids, burn injury (Curling ulcer), brain injury (Cushing ulcer)	Erosive; acute inflammation; necrosis; hemorrhage; **"coffee-ground"** vomitus	Blood in the nasogastric tube
Chronic gastritis	Type A (fundal): autoimmune pernicious anemia, aging Type B (antral): *Helicobacter pylori*	Nonerosive; mucosal inflammation and atrophy of mucosa	Risk factor for gastric carcinoma
Gastric ulcers	***H. pylori*** (70% of cases); bile-induced gastritis; increased permeability of gastric mucosa; associated with the use of aspirin and NSAIDs	Postprandial pain, bleeding, perforation, obstruction	Usually near the lesser curvature; not dependent on increased gastric acid secretion
Dumping syndrome	Postvagotomy; unimpeded passage of hypertonic food to the small intestine, causing distention as a result of osmotic flow of water into the lumen	Nausea, diarrhea, palpitations, sweating, light-headedness, reactive hypoglycemia	Can be prevented by eating only small meals and ingesting solids and liquids separately

HTN, hypertension; NSAIDs, nonsteroidal anti-inflammatory drugs.

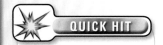

V. Neoplastic disorders of the oropharynx, esophagus, and stomach *(Table 5-3 and Figure 5-3)*

Nonneoplastic and neoplastic disorders originating proximal to the pyloric sphincter often present with hematemesis and dysphagia as a result of alcohol and tobacco abuse.

TABLE 5-3	Neoplastic Disorders of the Oropharynx, Esophagus, and Stomach		
Disorder	**Etiology and Pathology**	**Clinical Features**	**Notes**
Oral cancer	**Smoking,** chewing tobacco, alcohol	Squamous cell carcinoma; may involve tongue	Leukoplakia (white patch on the mucous membrane that cannot be wiped off) is a common precursor lesion
Esophageal adenocarcinoma	**Barrett esophagus;** complication of GERD	**Columnar metaplasia of esophageal squamous epithelium;** distal third of the esophagus	More common in Whites
Esophageal squamous cell carcinoma	Alcohol and tobacco use; esophagitis	Dysphagia, anorexia, pain	More common in Blacks
Gastric carcinoma	***Helicobacter pylori;*** gastritis; low-fiber diet, nitrosamines; blood group A; high-salt diet; increased incidence in Japan owing to greater consumption of smoked foods	Aggressive spread from antrum to nodes and liver; **Virchow node** (enlarged left-sided supraclavicular lymph node); **Krukenberg tumor** (metastatic disease to the ovaries from the stomach characterized by mucinous, signet ring cells)	More common in men older than 50 years; infiltration of stomach walls with tumor cells and subsequent fibrosis leads to linitis plastica (leather-bottle stomach)

GERD, gastroesophageal reflux disease.

FIGURE 5-3 Barium-swallow radiograph of achalasia

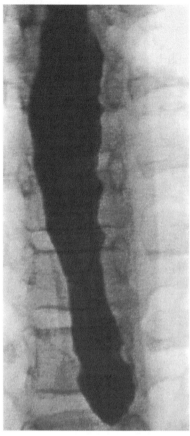

(Reproduced with permission from Humes DH, Dupont HL, Gardner LB, et al. *Kelley's Textbook of Internal Medicine.* 4th ed. Philadelphia, PA: Lippincott Williams & Wilkins; 2000:821.)

Clinical Vignette 5-1

CLINICAL PRESENTATION: During a visit to her primary care physician, a 39-year-old woman complains of **difficulty swallowing.** She also reports some heartburn and weight loss but denies pain on swallowing. She is an otherwise healthy female with no medical problems. Physical examination shows intact cranial nerves, swallowing mechanisms, and motor function of extremities. Vital signs are stable. Barium-swallow radiograph is shown previously.

DIFFERENTIALS: Mechanical obstruction—cancer, strictures, and rings; **oropharyngeal motility disorders**—multiple sclerosis, stroke, poliomyelitis, Parkinson disease, and myasthenia gravis; **esophageal motility disorders**—achalasia, scleroderma, and diffuse esophageal spasm. To remember the differentials for dysphagia, group them according to the phase of swallowing that has been disturbed and the type of pathology present (obstruction or motility disorder). To sort through the differentials, look for three symptoms specific to esophageal pathology: dysphagia (difficulty swallowing), odynophagia (pain on swallowing), and heartburn. Odynophagia would suggest diffuse esophageal spasm, whereas heartburn would suggest gastroesophageal reflux disease (GERD). Determine the type of dysphagia: difficulty with solids indicates mechanical obstruction; trouble with both solids and liquids suggests esophageal motility disorders; and problems in transferring food from the oral cavity suggest oropharyngeal disorders. For oropharyngeal disorders, look for details in the history and physical examination such as aspiration pneumonia, nasal regurgitation, and cranial nerve pathology.

LABORATORY STUDIES: In this case, the **barium-swallow chest radiograph** shows dilation of the esophagus with narrowing at the LES confirming a diagnosis of achalasia. Other significant findings on chest radiograph include pneumonia, thickened esophageal folds, ulcerations, and strictures. **Manometry** is also helpful in esophageal motility disorders, and, in achalasia,

 MNEMONIC

Various emetic substances in the blood stimulate the chemoreceptor trigger zone and area postrema to produce feelings of nausea and vomiting. Remember the extraintestinal causes of vomiting as part of your differential:

Vestibular disturbance/**V**agal
Opiates
Migraine/**M**etabolic (diabetic ketoacidosis, gastroparesis, hypercalcemia)
Infections
Toxicity
Increased intracranial pressure (ICP)/**I**ngested alcohol
Neurogenic, psychogenic
Gestation

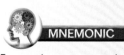 **MNEMONIC**

To remember one cause and treatment of a**CHA**lasia, think **CHA**gas disease and calcium-**CHA**nnel blocker.

(continued)

The Gastrointestinal System

Clinical Vignette 5-1 (Continued)

it would classically show a lack of ordered peristalsis, increased LES pressures, and failure of LES relaxation after swallowing. **Esophagoscopy** is helpful in visualizing and qualifying obstruction and mucosal wall integrity and is important to rule out cancer. **Esophageal pH monitoring** would also be done in this case to rule out GERD. If an oropharyngeal disorder is suspected, a **swallowing electromyography** is indicated and electromyelograms would be abnormal.

MANAGEMENT: Achalasia is treated by calcium channel blockers and nitrates to decrease LES pressure. Patients refractory to medical treatment can undergo endoscopic injection of botulinum toxin at the LES to block the release of acetylcholine locally. Surgical management options include myotomy of the gastroesophageal junction to relieve LES pressure with partial fundoplication to prevent reflux.

THE SMALL INTESTINE, LARGE INTESTINE, AND RECTUM

I.   **Muscular layers of the GI tract is shown in Figure 5-4.**

FIGURE 5-4 Picture of muscular layer of the gastrointestinal tract

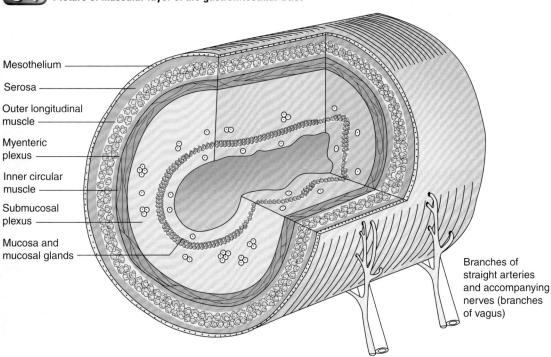

Mesothelium
Serosa
Outer longitudinal muscle
Myenteric plexus
Inner circular muscle
Submucosal plexus
Mucosa and mucosal glands

Branches of straight arteries and accompanying nerves (branches of vagus)

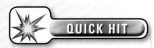

QUICK HIT

Lactose intolerance is caused by a genetic absence or decrease in lactase. Lactose cannot be broken down; it remains in the lumen of the gut and causes **osmotic** diarrhea.

II.   **The small intestine digests and absorbs the food.**
   A. Digestion is mediated by a variety of GI hormones, including cholecystokinin (CCK), secretin, somatostatin, and others (Figure 5-2).
   B. **Carbohydrates**
      1. Pancreatic amylase hydrolyzes glycogen, starch, and most other complex carbohydrates to disaccharides.
      2. Disaccharides are broken down to monosaccharides by intestinal brush border enzymes and absorbed.
      3. Monosaccharides are absorbed by a variety of mechanisms:
         a. Glucose and galactose are absorbed by sodium (Na^+)-dependent transport.
         b. Fructose is absorbed by facilitated diffusion.

C. **Protein**
  1. It is degraded to amino acids, dipeptides, and tripeptides by proteases produced by the pancreas.
     a. Activation of **trypsinogen to trypsin**
        • Autoactivated
        • Activated by intestinal brush border enterokinases
     b. Trypsin degrades the peptide bonds of arginine or lysine.
     c. Trypsin also **activates the other proteolytic pancreatic enzymes**.
  2. Proteins are absorbed by an Na^+-dependent transport.
     a. There are separate carriers for acidic, basic, and neutral amino acids.
     b. Dipeptides and tripeptides are absorbed faster than single amino acids.

D. **Fats**
  1. Lipids are broken into droplets by the mixing action of the stomach.
  2. **Pancreatic lipase** (and to a lesser extent salivary lipase) **hydrolyzes triacylglycerol to fatty acids and 2-monoacylglycerol**. **Chronic pancreatitis** decreases fat digestion and absorption due to decreased lipase release from the exocrine pancreas.
  3. Bile salts (amphipathic molecules) emulsify the hydrolyzed products and form micelles.
  4. Micelles allow for fat absorption (Figure 5-5).
  5. A variety of familial and acquired disorders may disrupt lipid metabolism, resulting in **hyperlipidemia**.
     a. Hyperlipidemia, especially high levels of low-density lipoproteins (LDLs), is associated with coronary artery disease (CAD).
     b. Typically, treatment first involves dietary intervention and then drug therapy, regardless of the cause of the hyperlipidemia.
        • **3-Hydroxy-3-methylglutaryl coenzyme A (HMG-CoA) reductase inhibitors**, also known as **"statins,"** such as atorvastatin, lovastatin, and pravastatin, are an effective and widely used means of lowering LDL.

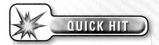

QUICK HIT

Often, the amino acid transporter found in the intestines is identical to the amino acid transporter found in the renal tubules. As such, diseases that affect these transporters have multiorgan system effects. One of these diseases is Hartnup disease, which is a defect in the intestinal and renal tubular absorption of neutral amino acids leading to excretion of tryptophan derivatives and causing pellagra-like symptoms.

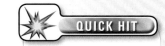

QUICK HIT

Although the statins work well as cholesterol-lowering agents, they can be **hepatotoxic**. Consequently, patients who take them should undergo routine liver function tests.

FIGURE 5-5 Absorption and digestion of fats (lipid metabolism)

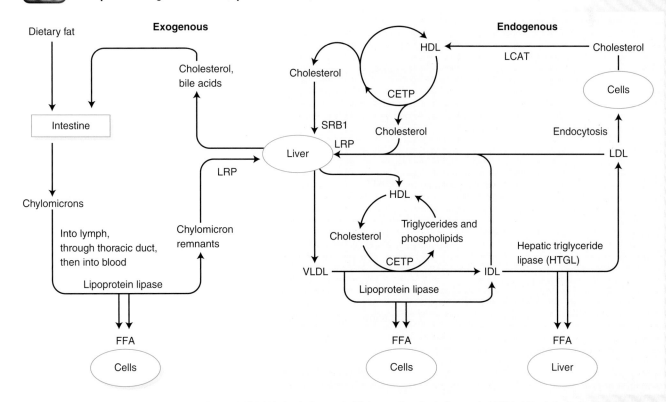

CETP, cholesterol ester transfer protein; FFA, free fatty acid; HDL, high-density lipoprotein; IDL, intermediate-density lipoprotein; LCAT, lecithin-cholesterol acyltransferase; LDL, low-density lipoprotein; LRP, lipoprotein receptor-related protein; SRB1, scavenger receptor class B1; VLDL, very low-density lipoprotein.

The Gastrointestinal System

- **Bile acid-binding resins** such as cholestyramine and colestipol work by binding bile acids in the intestine and promoting their subsequent loss in the stool, which ultimately lowers LDL levels.
- **Nicotinic acid (niacin)** inhibits the release of lipoproteins from the liver, lowering very low-density lipoproteins (VLDLs) and LDL.

III. The large intestine stores and excretes nondigestible material.
  A. Absorbs 2 to 3 L per day of water
  B. **Secretes potassium (K$^+$)**
  C. Mediates defecation of undigested material through both voluntary and involuntary (rectosphincteric reflex) mechanisms

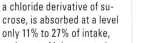

QUICK HIT

The sweetener sucralose, a chloride derivative of sucrose, is absorbed at a level only 11% to 27% of intake, and most of it is excreted, unmetabolized, in feces.

LOCATION OF ABSORPTION OF VITAMINS, MINERALS, AND NUTRIENTS (Figure 5-6)

FIGURE 5-6 Location of absorption of vitamins, minerals, and nutrients

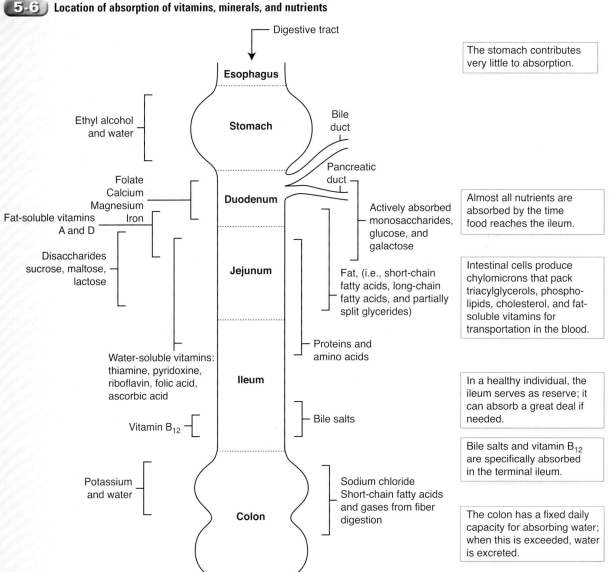

The stomach contributes very little to absorption.

Almost all nutrients are absorbed by the time food reaches the ileum.

Intestinal cells produce chylomicrons that pack triacylglycerols, phospholipids, cholesterol, and fat-soluble vitamins for transportation in the blood.

In a healthy individual, the ileum serves as reserve; it can absorb a great deal if needed.

Bile salts and vitamin B$_{12}$ are specifically absorbed in the terminal ileum.

The colon has a fixed daily capacity for absorbing water; when this is exceeded, water is excreted.

COMMON CLINICAL DISORDERS OF THE SMALL INTESTINE, LARGE INTESTINE, AND RECTUM (Table 5-4)

Common clinical disorders of the GI tract, distal to the pyloric sphincter, will usually present as vague abdominal pain as a result of stimulation of the visceral afferent nerves. If the parietal peritoneum (the abdominal wall), innervated by the somatic afferent nerves, is irritated by the lesion, the pain will become more localized (as is seen in acute appendicitis).

Disorder	Etiology and Pathology	Clinical Features	Notes
TABLE 5-4	**Common Clinical Disorders of the Small Intestine, Large Intestine, and Rectum**		
Hiatal hernia	Saclike herniation of stomach through diaphragm; smoking; obesity	Retrosternal pain (worse in supine position); can lead to **GERD**	Usually occurs in the sliding (versus rolling) form
Duodenal ulcers	***Helicobacter pylori*** (in 90% of cases); hypersecretion of acid; smokers; Zollinger–Ellison syndrome; blood group O; associated with NSAID use	Coffee-ground vomitus; **smooth border;** clean base; black stools; pain at night or 2 h postprandial; perforation may result in acute pancreatitis	Not precancerous
Ischemic bowel disease	Atherosclerosis of celiac artery or mesenteric artery	Abdominal pain, nausea, vomiting, stool positive for blood test	Usually affects watershed areas (splenic flexure or rectosigmoid junction)
Diverticulitis	Outpouchings of the colon obstructed with fecalith leading to inflammation or infection; low-fiber diet	Usually involves the **sigmoid colon;** fever; leukocytosis; colicky pain; usually multiple in number and causes increased risk of perforation	False diverticula: pockets of mucosa and submucosa herniated through muscular layer (not all layers)
Appendicitis	Obstruction (usually fecalith or lymphoid hyperplasia); bacterial proliferation and mucosal invasion	Nausea, vomiting, anorexia, abdominal pain that migrates from epigastrium to right lower quadrant, pain at **McBurney point,** psoas sign or obturator sign, increased WBCs in blood	Differential diagnosis in females includes ectopic pregnancy, ovarian torsion, ruptured ovarian cyst, and pelvic inflammatory disease
Adenocarcinoma	Chronic IBD, low-fiber diet, older age, hereditary polyposis or adenomatous disorders	**Increased CEA** (not diagnostic, used to assess treatment); rectosigmoid tumors present in an **annular manner** producing early obstruction and constipation; **left-sided tumors present with blood in the stool, whereas right-sided tumors typically present with anemia as a result of occult blood loss**	Screen for occult blood in stool and flexible sigmoidoscopy; screening colonoscopy with a positive family history; third most common cause of cancer death (after lung and prostate/breast)
Carcinoid tumor	Arises from **neuroendocrine cells** (Kulchitsky cells); releases vasoactive peptides such as histamine, serotonin, and prostaglandins	**Increased 5-HIAA in urine,** diarrhea, **flushing,** right-sided heart valve lesions, hypotension, bronchospasm	Most common tumor of the appendix but also found in the ileum, rectum, and bronchus

5-HIAA, 5-hydroxyindoleacetic acid; CEA, carcinoembryonic antigen; GERD, gastroesophageal reflux disease; IBD, inflammatory bowel disease; NSAID, nonsteroidal anti-inflammatory drug; WBC, white blood cell.

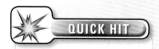

QUICK HIT

Posterior duodenal ulcers are associated with erosion of the gastroduodenal artery and subsequent hemorrhage.

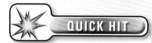

QUICK HIT

Duodenal versus gastric ulcer: In **d**uodenal ulcers, pain *decreases after meals/antacids,* whereas in gastric ulcers, *pain persists after meals/antacids.* Also, duodenal ulcers are associated with *increased acid production,* whereas patients with gastric ulcers have *decreased to normal acid production.* Finally, although all gastric ulcers should be biopsied to rule out gastric *carcinoma,* duodenal ulcers require no such intervention.

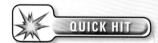

QUICK HIT

Diverticulosis, the most common cause of bleeding from the lower GI tract, can be differentiated from diverticulitis because diverticulitis typically does not cause bleeding but is painful, whereas diverticulosis does cause bleeding but is typically painless.

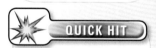

QUICK HIT

Small-bowel obstructions are usually caused by adhesions, whereas large-bowel obstructions are most commonly a result of neoplasms. Ileus, a common cause of temporary small-bowel paralysis, commonly occurs postoperatively.

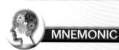

MNEMONIC

Left-sided valvular lesions are not observed in carcinoid syndrome because the lung metabolizes serotonin (5-HT). Remember the symptoms of carcinoid syndrome as "Be FDR": **B**ronchospasm, **F**lushing, **D**iarrhea, and **R**ight-sided valvular lesions.

The Gastrointestinal System

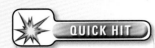

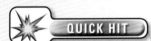

Clinical Vignette 5-2

CLINICAL PRESENTATION: A 21-year-old woman presents to the emergency department with **right lower quadrant pain** of several hours' duration. She reports that the **pain began in the epigastrium** and has since moved to the right lower quadrant. Since the onset of the pain, she reports **no appetite and nausea.** She is otherwise a healthy young female. Physical examination reveals **tenderness at McBurney point.** No peritoneal signs, psoas sign, or obturator sign. Rectal examination gives a negative result. Temperature = 100.3° F; blood pressure = 120/80 mm Hg; heart rate = 95 bpm; and respiration = 20 breaths/min.

DIFFERENTIALS: Appendicitis, mittelschmerz, ovarian cyst rupture, pelvic inflammatory disease, ectopic pregnancy, kidney stones, and Meckel diverticulum. The shift in pain described previously is classic for appendicitis. Also, anorexia, nausea, and vomiting beginning after the onset of pain are typical for appendicitis. Further, gynecologic history is needed on this patient to determine if midcycle pain associated with ovulation (mittelschmerz) was occurring. Also, a pelvic examination is indicated in this patient to further determine the pelvic pathology.

LABORATORY STUDIES: If this were a young man, the history and physical examination would be sufficient to indicate surgery for appendicitis. In a young woman, however, there is a longer differential list and a **computerized tomography (CT) scan** would be helpful in determining the cause of the pain. A **complete blood count (CBC)** often shows a mildly elevated white blood cell (WBC) count, but this is not a consistent finding. A **human chorionic gonadotropin (hCG) pregnancy test** and **pelvic ultrasound** should also be performed on this patient to rule out pelvic pathology.

MANAGEMENT: Laparoscopic or open appendectomy should be performed emergently because of the risk of rupture.

Diarrhea, the passage of abnormal amounts of fluid or semisolid fecal matter, can be mediated by a number of mechanisms. Osmotic diarrhea results when unabsorbed solutes increase intraluminal oncotic pressure, causing an outpouring of water. Surgical resection can lead to an inadequate surface for absorption of nutrients, resulting in a form of **osmotic diarrhea.** Active ion secretion causing obligatory water loss is termed **secretory diarrhea.** Altered intestinal motility, in which there is an alteration of the normally

Clinical Vignette 5-3

CLINICAL PRESENTATION: A 54-year-old woman presents to the emergency department with **severe abdominal pain** of 36 hours' duration. Her past medical history is significant for **CAD, hypertension (HTN),** and **diabetes.** Physical examination reveals a **soft, nondistended, nontender abdomen** with **normal bowel sounds** and no palpable masses. Temperature = 98.9° F; blood pressure = 140/90 mm Hg; heart rate = 99 bpm; and respiration rate = 21 breaths/min.

DIFFERENTIALS: Acute mesenteric ischemia, appendicitis, diverticulitis, colon adenocarcinoma, IBD, and pseudomembranous colitis. Pain disproportionate to the physical findings is strongly suggestive of mesenteric ischemia. As the ischemia progresses, peritonitis, sepsis, and shock may occur.

LABORATORY STUDIES: Mesenteric angiogram is the definitive diagnostic test for mesenteric ischemia. **Plain abdominal radiographs** are obtained to rule out other causes of acute abdominal pain. **Abdominal radiographs with barium enema** often show "thumbprinting" as a result of thickened edematous mucosal folds.

MANAGEMENT: Supportive therapy with intravenous (IV) fluids and broad-spectrum antibiotics should be started. Further treatment depends on the cause of the ischemia. Given the history of CAD in this patient, this is most likely **thrombotic** in nature, and direct **intra-arterial injection of papaverine** (a vasodilator) into the superior mesenteric system during arteriography will relieve the occlusion and vasospasm. An **embolic** occlusion indicates direct **intra-arterial infusion of thrombolytics or embolectomy.** If it is a **venous thrombosis, heparin anticoagulation** should be started. If signs of peritonitis develop, the **nonviable bowel should be resected.**

coordinated control of intestinal propulsion, may also result in diarrhea (often alternating with constipation). Finally, sloughing of colonic mucosa, caused by inflammation and necrosis, often as a result of infection, causes an **exudative form of diarrhea**.

- **Bacterial Causes of Diarrhea** (Table 5-5)
- **Viral Causes of Diarrhea** (Table 5-6)
- **Protozoal Causes of Diarrhea** (Table 5-7)

TABLE 5-5 Bacterial Causes of Diarrhea

Infectious Agent	Clinical Features	Treatment	Notes
Shigella	**Shiga toxin** causes **bloody** diarrhea, mild to severe, 1–2 weeks in duration; fever for 3–4 days; lactose (−)	Bismuth, ampicillin, ciprofloxacin, or trimethoprim-sulfamethoxazole	Fecal leukocytes and stool culture necessary for diagnosis
Salmonella	**Bloody** diarrhea, fever, cramps, nausea, motile, lactose (−)	Supportive therapy only; no opiates; tetracycline may be used if needed, symptoms may be prolonged with antibiotics	Commonly acquired from **eggs, poultry, or turtles**; diagnosis based on stool culture; increased susceptibility in immunocompromised patients
Campylobacter jejuni	**Bloody** diarrhea, fever, crampy abdominal pain, self-limited but may persist for 3–4 weeks	Supportive therapy or possibly erythromycin	**Leading cause of foodborne diarrhea** in United States, spiral (S-shaped), oxidase (+)
Vibrio cholerae	**Watery** diarrhea **(rice-water stools)**, vomiting, and dehydration occur after 12–48 h of incubation	Supportive therapy only; no opiates	Caused by **toxin;** most often occurs in underdeveloped nations; commonly associated with consumption of raw oysters; comma-shaped with flagellum
Clostridium difficile	**Watery** diarrhea caused by antibiotic-induced suppression of normal colonic flora and *C. difficile* overgrowth; **pseudomembranes** on the colonic mucosa	Metronidazole, oral vancomycin	Exotoxin mediated; termed *pseudomembranous colitis* because of the false membranes created on the colon by the bacterial infection
Enterotoxigenic *Escherichia coli* (traveler's diarrhea)	**Watery** diarrhea; 3–6 days' duration; occasional fever and vomiting	Bismuth, trimethoprim-sulfamethoxazole, doxycycline, and ciprofloxacin	Antibiotics reduce duration of infection to 1–2 days
Enterohemorrhagic *E. coli* (O157:H7)	**Shiga-like toxin** causes **bloody** diarrhea	Supportive therapy	Typically, food-borne transmission (e.g., **undercooked hamburger**); diagnosis made by stool culture
Yersinia enterocolitica	**Bloody** diarrhea, fever, cramps, nausea	Supportive therapy only; no opiates	Transmitted by food or contaminated domestic animal feces; clinically indistinguishable from *Salmonella* and *Shigella*

QUICK HIT

Salmonella requires at least 100,000 organisms to be infectious; *Shigella*, however, requires only 100.

QUICK HIT

Vibrio cholerae produces an exotoxin that activates adenylate cyclase in the crypt cells. The increase in cyclic adenosine monophosphate (cAMP) activates chloride secretory channels. Consequently, sodium and water accompany chloride into the lumen, which results in an osmotic diarrhea.

The Gastrointestinal System

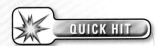

QUICK HIT

Norwalk virus, in contrast to most viruses transmitted via the fecal–oral route, is uncommon in children.

QUICK HIT

The *Giardia* trophozoite has a very characteristic appearance. It is pear shaped, with four pairs of flagella and two nuclei that resemble eyes.

TABLE 5-6 Viral Causes of Diarrhea

Infectious Agent	Clinical Features	Treatment	Notes
Rotavirus	Severe, dehydrating diarrhea; vomiting; low-grade fever	Supportive therapy only	Usually occurs during **winter** months; mainly affects infants
Norwalk virus	Mild diarrhea and vomiting	Supportive therapy only	Epidemics in underdeveloped countries; **affects both children and adults**
Adenovirus (serotypes 40 and 41)	Diarrhea and moderate omiting	Supportive therapy only	Second to rotavirus as the cause of gastroenteritis in children

Handwritten annotations: "RNA ds segment Reo activated by trypsin", "Nonenveloped", "Live vaccine", "DNA", "Noro (calici) dsRNA+ outbreak"

TABLE 5-7 Protozoal Causes of Diarrhea

Infectious Agent	Clinical Features	Treatment	Notes
Entamoeba histolytica	**Bloody** diarrhea, lower abdominal pain, may lead to dysentery with 10–12 bloody and mucous stools per day	Metronidazole	Caused by ingestion of viable cysts via fecal–oral route
Giardia lamblia	**Watery,** foul-smelling diarrhea; nausea; anorexia; cramps lasting weeks to months	Metronidazole	fecal–oral transmission; often contracted while **camping**
Cryptosporidium	**Watery** diarrhea with large fluid loss; symptoms persist in immunocompromised patients; self-limited in healthy individuals	Supportive therapy	Immunocompromised patients (especially **patients with AIDS);** fecal–oral transmission of oocysts

Handwritten annotations: "liver abscess anchovy paste", "ova + PARASITE no mitochondria ANAEROBIC", "public swimming pool", "need cell mediated immunity"

● **Comparison of Inflammatory Bowel Conditions** (Table 5-8)

It is speculated that the pathogenesis of inflammatory bowel disease (IBD) is related to the activation of the immune system and the consequent release of cytokines and inflammatory mediators. The cause of IBD has yet to be discovered; however, there is some suggestion of a genetic component.

TABLE 5-8 Comparison of Inflammatory Bowel Conditions

	Crohn Disease	Ulcerative Colitis
Typical patient	• Young person of Jewish descent • Bimodal age distribution: 25–40 years of age and 50–65 years of age • Female > male	• Person of Jewish descent • Recently quit smoking • Bimodal age distribution: 20–35 years of age and 65+ years of age • Male > female
Clinical findings	• Diarrhea • Abdominal pain • Fever • Malabsorption • Obstruction	• Bloody, mucous diarrhea • Abdominal pain • Fever • Weight loss • Toxic megacolon

(continued)

TABLE 5-8 Comparison of Inflammatory Bowel Conditions *(Continued)*

	Crohn Disease	Ulcerative Colitis
Location	• Small intestine • Colon • "Mouth to anus"	• Colon • Rectum
Histologic findings	• Full-thickness inflammation • **Granulomas**	• Mucosal inflammation • **Crypt abscesses**
Gross findings	• **Cobblestone appearance** • Wall thickening with narrowed lumen • **Skipped areas** • **Fistulas**	• Pseudopolyps • Widened lumen • Toxic megacolon
Diagnostic evaluation	• Colonoscopy • Barium enema • Upper GI series with small-bowel follow-through	• Colonoscopy • Barium enema • Upper GI series with small-bowel follow-through
Risk of malignancy	• Small increase	• Large increase
Associated systemic manifestations	• Arthritis • Eye lesions • Erythema nodosum • Pyoderma gangrenosum • Aphthous ulcers (chancre sores)	• Arthritis • Eye lesions • Erythema nodosum • Pyoderma gangrenosum • Sclerosing cholangitis
Medical treatment	• Sulfasalazine • Steroids • Metronidazole	• Sulfasalazine • Steroids • Metronidazole
Indications for surgery	• Obstruction • Massive bleeding • Perforation • Refractory to medical treatment • Cancer • Toxic megacolon	• Toxic megacolon • Cancer • Massive bleeding • Failure to mature • Refractory to medical treatment

GI, gastrointestinal.

MALABSORPTION SYNDROMES OF THE SMALL INTESTINE
(Table 5-9)

Malabsorption may produce a variety of symptoms ranging from diarrhea to steatorrhea to specific nutrient deficiencies. For example, iron, vitamin B_{12}, fat-soluble vitamins (A, D, E, and K), or protein may be poorly absorbed and lead to systemic manifestations.

TABLE 5-9 Malabsorption Syndromes of the Small Intestine

Syndrome	Pathology	Clinical Features	Notes
Abetalipoproteinemia	Lack of apolipoprotein B; defective chylomicron assembly; enterocytes congested with lipid	Acanthocytes ("burr" cells) in blood; **no chylomicrons, VLDL, or LDL in blood**; retinitis pigmentosa; peripheral neuropathy; mental retardation; ataxia	Autosomal recessive; vitamin E supplements may improve the retinopathy and neuropathy

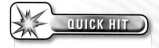

Celiac disease (nontropical sprue) causes decreased absorption of fat and fat-soluble vitamins, leading to skeletal and hematologic conditions due to decreased vitamins D and K.

(continued)

The Gastrointestinal System

The Gastrointestinal System

TABLE 5-9	Malabsorption Syndromes of the Small Intestine *(Continued)*		
Syndrome	**Pathology**	**Clinical Features**	**Notes**
Celiac disease (non-tropical sprue)	Gluten sensitivity	Foul-smelling, pale stool; **villi of small intestine blunted;** stunted growth; symptoms disappear when gluten is removed from diet	Associated with HLA-B8 and HLA-DQW2; predisposes to T-cell lymphoma and GI and breast cancer; if unmanaged, causes vitamin deficiency resulting in skeletal, hematologic, and neurologic symptoms
Disaccharidase deficiency	Enzyme deficiency; bacterial digestion of unabsorbed disaccharide	Diarrhea, bloating	Most commonly lactase deficiency
Tropical sprue	Etiology unclear	Affects small intestine; may cause vitamin deficiencies and megaloblastic anemia	Possible infectious cause; does not improve with gluten removal
Whipple disease	Systemic disease caused by *Tropheryma whipplei*	Diarrhea, weight loss, lymphadenopathy; hyperpigmentation, **macrophages laden with *T. whipplei***	Older White males *PAS+ macrophages in propria lamina*
Bacterial overgrowth	Bacterial overpopulation of small intestine owing to stasis, raised pH, impaired immunity, or **clindamycin** or **ampicillin** therapy	Inflammatory infiltrate in bowel wall	Treat with antibiotics, metronidazole, or oral vancomycin

GI, gastrointestinal; HLA-B8, human leukocyte antigen-B8; LDL, low-density lipoprotein; VLDL, very low-density lipoprotein.

NEOPLASTIC POLYPS *(Table 5-10)*

GI polyps can be very diverse in their presentation. Individuals can be asymptomatic, as is usually the case with tubular adenomas, or can present with serious systemic manifestations such as anemia secondary to invasive cancer.
- **Comparison of Polyposis Conditions** (Table 5-11)

TABLE 5-10	Neoplastic Polyps	
Tubular Adenoma	**Tubulovillous Adenoma**	**Villous Adenoma**
Usually **benign**	Greater potential of malignancy than tubular adenoma	Highly **malignant**
Multiple	Morphologically, shares features of both tubular and villous adenomas	**Sessile** tumors Fingerlike projections
Pedunculated tumors Greater chance of malignancy if genetically predisposed Most common polyp		

TABLE 5-11 **Comparison of Polyposis Conditions**

Disease	Inheritance	Clinical Features
Familial adenomatous polyposis	Autosomal dominant	Colon lined with hundreds of polyps; potential for malignancy approaches 100%
Turcot syndrome	Autosomal dominant	Colonic polyps and **central nervous system (CNS) tumors;** potential for malignancy approaches 100%
Gardner syndrome	Autosomal dominant	Colonic polyps; soft-tissue and **bone tumors;** potential for malignancy approaches 100%
Peutz–Jeghers syndrome	Autosomal dominant	Benign hamartomatous polyps of the gastrointestinal tract (especially the small intestine); **hyperpigmented mouth, hands, and genitalia;** increased incidence of tumors of the uterus, breast, ovaries, lung, stomach, and pancreas
Familial nonpolyposis syndrome	Autosomal dominant	**Defect in DNA repair** causing large number of colonic lesions (especially proximal); potential for malignancy approaches 50%

[handwritten: Lynch]   *[handwritten: after puberty]*

THE HEPATOBILIARY SYSTEM

I. **Microscopic organization of the liver** (*Figure 5-7*)

II. **Enterohepatic cycling and the excretion of bilirubin** (*Figure 5-8*)

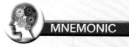
MNEMONIC

Remember the drugs that cause hepatic necrosis by the phrase "**V**ery **A**ngry **H**epatocytes": **V**alproic acid, **A**cetaminophen, and **H**alothane.

FIGURE
5-7 Microscopic organization of the liver

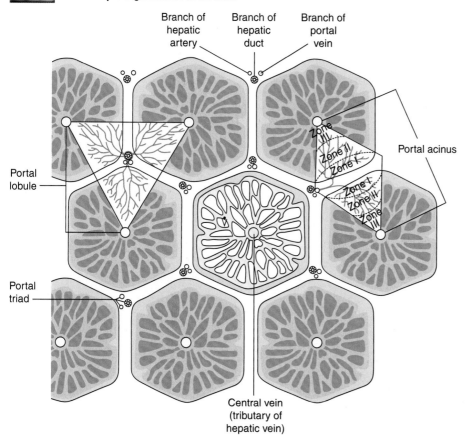

The Gastrointestinal System

FIGURE 5-8 Enterohepatic cycling and the excretion of bilirubin

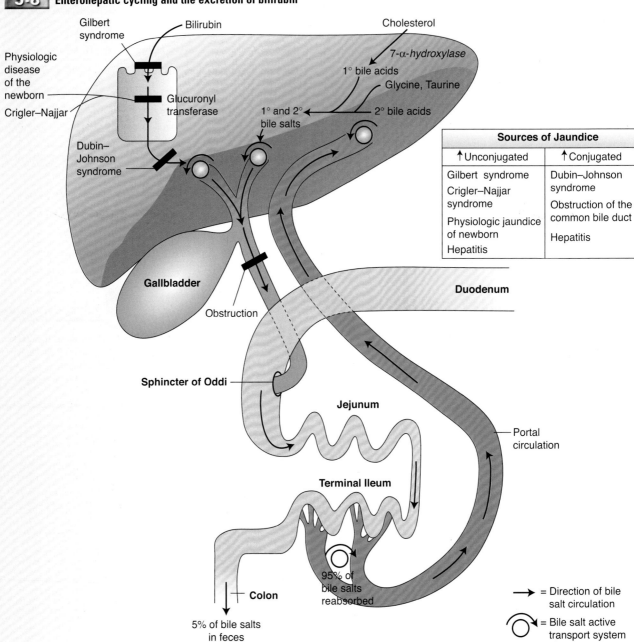

Sources of Jaundice	
↑Unconjugated	↑Conjugated
Gilbert syndrome	Dubin–Johnson syndrome
Crigler–Najjar syndrome	Obstruction of the common bile duct
Physiologic jaundice of newborn	Hepatitis
Hepatitis	

III. Viral hepatitis (Table 5-12 and Figure 5-9)

Viral hepatitis can lead to **direct hyperbilirubinemia**, elevated serum transaminases, icterus, or hepatomegaly, but not ascites. Morphologically, changes range from multifocal hepatocellular necrosis (hepatitis A and hepatitis B) to ballooning degeneration (hepatitis B and hepatitis C) to piecemeal necrosis (hepatitis C).

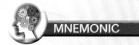

MNEMONIC

To remember that hepatitis A and E are transmitted by the fecal–oral route, think of the phrase **"vowels are bowels."**

TABLE 5-12 Viral Hepatitis

	Hepatitis A	Hepatitis B	Hepatitis C	Hepatitis D	Hepatitis E
Virus family	Picornavirus	Hepadnavirus	Flavivirus	Delta agent	Calicivirus
Viral morphology	Single-stranded RNA	Circular, double-stranded DNA	Single-stranded RNA	Incomplete genome of single-stranded RNA	Single-stranded RNA
Mode of transmission	Fecal–oral	Sexual and parenteral, transplacental	Parenteral; limited sexual; transplacental	Sexual and parenteral, transplacental	Fecal–oral
Diagnostic test	IgM anti-HAV	HBsAg; anti-HBsAg; HBeAg; HBV DNA; IgM anti-HBcAg	Anti-HCV	Anti-sag	None
Severity	Mild	Moderate	Mild	Severe	Mild
Chronic infection	No	10% of adults, 80%–90% of infants, and immunocompromised patients	80%–90%	No increase over hepatitis B alone	No
Carrier state	No	Yes	Yes	Yes	No
Hepatocellular carcinoma	No	Yes	Yes	No	No
Prophylaxis and treatment	Immune globulin; vaccine	Hepatitis B immune globulin; vaccine Interferon and nucleoside analog inhibitors of viral DNA synthesis	Interferon and ribavirin	Hepatitis B immune globulin; vaccine	None
Notes	Incubation period of 14–15 days	**Dane particle:** viral DNA genome, DNA polymerase, HBcAg, HBeAg, HBsAg; has **reverse transcriptase;** incubation period 60–90 days	**Most frequent cause of transfusion-mediated hepatitis**	Defective in replication; **requires coinfection with hepatitis B**	Hepatitis infection in third-world nations; mortality in pregnant females

HAV, hepatitis A virus; HBcAg, hepatitis B core antigen; HBeAg, hepatitis B envelope antigen; HBsAg, hepatitis B surface antigen; HBV, hepatitis B virus; HCV, hepatitis C virus; IgM, immunoglobulin M.

The Gastrointestinal System

The Gastrointestinal System

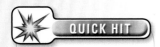

QUICK HIT

Hepatitis B viral DNA, hepatitis B surface antigen (HBsAg), and hepatitis B envelope antigen (HBeAg) are indicators of virus replication. Antibody to hepatitis B surface antigen (HBsAb) is indicative of recovery and immunity. HBsAb is also positive following vaccination. Antibody to hepatitis B core antigen (HBcAb) is positive in early infection; in addition, HBcAb acts as a marker for hepatitis infection during the "window" period, which is the period during acute infection when HBsAg is undetectable and HBsAb has not yet appeared. During the window period, equivalent amounts of surface antigen and antibody neutralize each other and thus are not detectable by testing.

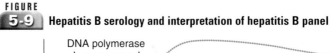

FIGURE 5-9 Hepatitis B serology and interpretation of hepatitis B panel

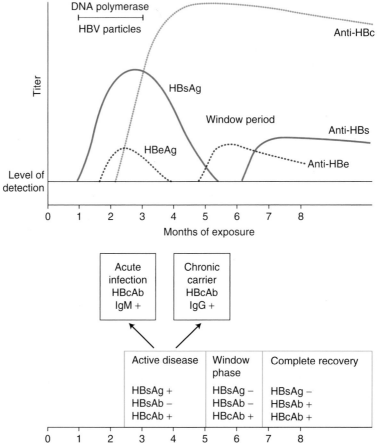

HBcAb, hepatitis B core antibody; HBeAg, hepatitis B envelope antigen; HBsAb, antibody to hepatitis B surface antigen; HBsAg, hepatitis B surface antigen; HBV, hepatitis B virus; IgG, immunoglobulin G; IgM, immunoglobulin M.

IV. Cirrhosis (Table 5-13)

Cirrhosis is a disease of the liver characterized by fibrosis and disorganization of the lobular and vascular structure owing to the destruction and regeneration of hepatocytes.

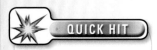

QUICK HIT

Cirrhosis often leads to **portal hypertension.** There are three major collateral circulation pathways that allow blood to return to the heart: (a) left gastric to esophageal plexus to azygous to the superior vena cava (SVC) **(esophageal varices),** (b) inferior mesenteric to superior rectal to inferior rectal to inferior vena cava (IVC) **(hemorrhoids),** and (c) ligamentum teres to superficial abdominals to SVC or IVC **(caput medusae).**

TABLE 5-13	Cirrhosis		
Etiology	**Pathology**	**Clinical Manifestation**	**Notes**
Chronic alcohol abuse	**Micronodular** fatty liver; decreased metabolism of estrogen; decreased synthesis of coagulation factors	**Jaundice,** bleeding, gynecomastia, testicular atrophy, edema, **asterixis,** portal HTN **(esophageal varices,** spider angiomata, and splenomegaly), encephalopathy	**Most common cause of cirrhosis in the United States**
Wilson disease	**Decreased ceruloplasmin**	Copper deposits in liver, basal ganglia (causing extrapyramidal signs), and Descemet membrane of cornea **(Kayser–Fleischer ring)**	Autosomal recessive
Hemochromatosis	Familial; increased total iron; decreased TIBC; increased ferritin; increased transferrin saturation	Iron deposits in liver, diabetes mellitus, increased skin pigmentation, cardiomyopathy	Bronze diabetes; increased risk of hepatocellular carcinoma

(continued)

TABLE 5-13 Cirrhosis (Continued)

Etiology	Pathology	Clinical Manifestation	Notes
Posthepatic cirrhosis	Chronic active hepatitis caused by HBV and HCV infection	Jaundice, pruritus	**Most likely cause of cirrhosis to lead to hepatocellular carcinoma**
α_1-Antitrypsin deficiency	Autosomal recessive; defective α_1-antitrypsin accumulates in hepatocytes	Jaundice, **panacinar emphysema**, pancreatic manifestations	**More severe in homozygous form** (PI*ZZ alleles)
Congestive heart failure	Passive congestion	**Nutmeg liver**	Most often a result of right heart failure

ERCP, endoscopic retrograde cholangiopancreatography; HBV, hepatitis B virus; HCV, hepatitis C virus; HTN, hypertension; TIBC, total iron-binding capacity.

V. Common clinical disorders of the hepatobiliary system (Table 5-14 and Figures 5-10, 5-11, and 5-12)

TABLE 5-14 Common Clinical Disorders of the Hepatobiliary System

Disorder	Etiology and Pathology	Clinical Features	Notes
Cholelithiasis (gallstones)	Very common disease; women older than 40 years of age; obesity; multiparity	Steatorrhea, nausea, vomiting, bile duct obstruction, jaundice, may lead to cholangitis or cholecystitis, malignancy, positive Murphy sign	Cholesterol stones (large); pigment stones (seen in hemolytic anemia or excess bilirubin production); mixed stones (majority)
Primary biliary cirrhosis	**Autoimmune** disease leading to the destruction of intrahepatic bile ducts; middle-aged women	**Pruritus, jaundice, hypercholesterolemia**, RUQ discomfort, portal HTN	Positive **antimitochondrial antibodies;** associated with other autoimmune diseases
Primary sclerosing cholangitis	Fibrosis and stenosis of intrahepatic or extrahepatic bile ducts	Jaundice, pruritus, weight loss	Strong association with **ulcerative colitis;** increased incidence of cholangiocarcinoma
Adenocarcinoma of the gallbladder	Gallstones	Obstructive jaundice, enlarged gallbladder	**Courvoisier law:** obstruction of CBD enlarges the gallbladder, whereas obstructing stones do not; caused by scarring of the gallbladder
Hepatocellular adenoma (hepatoma)	Benign tumor; women 20–30 years of age taking **oral contraceptives**	Usually found incidentally; may cause pain or hemorrhage	10% may become malignant; oral contraceptive use should be stopped, lesion regresses with the cessation of contraceptive
Hepatocellular carcinoma	Cirrhosis, **hepatitis B, hepatitis C**, aflatoxin B (carcinogen in contaminated peanuts)	Increased α-fetoprotein, jaundice, abdominal distention, ascites	**Hematogenous spread**

CBD, common bile duct; HTN, hypertension; RUQ, right upper quadrant.

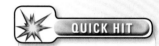

QUICK HIT

Pigment gallstones occurring in children or young adults with no history of pregnancy may be a result of a congenital hemoglobinopathy (e.g., sickle cell disease or thalassemia).

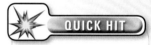

QUICK HIT

Murphy sign: Cessation of inspiration as a result of deep palpation of RUQ by examiner during inspiration; **Charcot triad:** Fever, RUQ pain, and jaundice; **Reynold pentad:** Charcot triad plus hypotension and mental status changes.

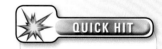

QUICK HIT

Metastatic disease is the most common source of malignancy in the liver.

The Gastrointestinal System

FIGURE
5-10 **Approach to liver studies**

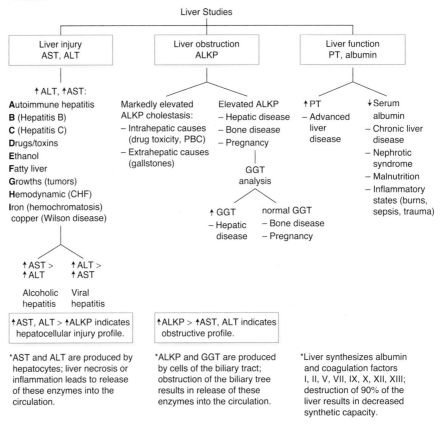

Liver Studies

| Liver injury AST, ALT | Liver obstruction ALKP | Liver function PT, albumin |

↑ALT, ↑AST:
Autoimmune hepatitis
B (Hepatitis B)
C (Hepatitis C)
Drugs/toxins
Ethanol
Fatty liver
Growths (tumors)
Hemodynamic (CHF)
Iron (hemochromatosis)
copper (Wilson disease)

↑AST > ↑ALT — Alcoholic hepatitis
↑ALT > ↑AST — Viral hepatitis

Markedly elevated ALKP cholestasis:
– Intrahepatic causes (drug toxicity, PBC)
– Extrahepatic causes (gallstones)

Elevated ALKP
– Hepatic disease
– Bone disease
– Pregnancy

GGT analysis
↑GGT
– Hepatic disease

normal GGT
– Bone disease
– Pregnancy

↑PT
– Advanced liver disease

↓Serum albumin
– Chronic liver disease
– Nephrotic syndrome
– Malnutrition
– Inflammatory states (burns, sepsis, trauma)

| ↑AST, ALT > ↑ALKP indicates hepatocellular injury profile. | ↑ALKP > ↑AST, ALT indicates obstructive profile. |

*AST and ALT are produced by hepatocytes; liver necrosis or inflammation leads to release of these enzymes into the circulation.

*ALKP and GGT are produced by cells of the biliary tract; obstruction of the biliary tree results in release of these enzymes into the circulation.

*Liver synthesizes albumin and coagulation factors I, II, V, VII, IX, X, XII, XIII; destruction of 90% of the liver results in decreased synthetic capacity.

ALKP, alkaline phosphatase; ALT, alanine aminotransferase; AST, aspartate aminotransferase; CHF, congestive heart failure; GGT, gamma glutamyl transpeptidase; PBC, primary biliary cirrhosis; PT, prothrombin time.

FIGURE
5-11 **Diseases of the gallbladder and biliary tract**

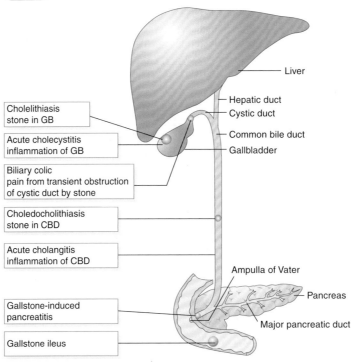

Cholelithiasis
stone in GB

Acute cholecystitis
inflammation of GB

Biliary colic
pain from transient obstruction
of cystic duct by stone

Choledocholithiasis
stone in CBD

Acute cholangitis
inflammation of CBD

Gallstone-induced
pancreatitis

Gallstone ileus

Liver
Hepatic duct
Cystic duct
Common bile duct
Gallbladder
Ampulla of Vater
Pancreas
Major pancreatic duct

CBD, common bile duct; GB, gallbladder.

FIGURE 5-12 Approach to fractionate bilirubin studies

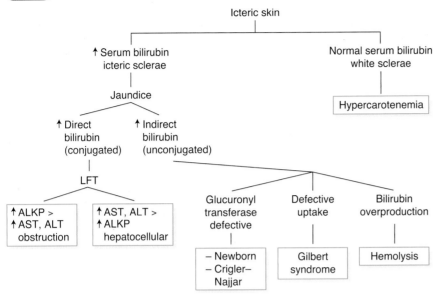

ALKP, alkaline phosphatase; ALT, alanine aminotransferase; AST, aspartate aminotransferase; LFT, liver function test.

Clinical Vignette 5-4

CLINICAL PRESENTATION: A 6-year-old boy presents to the emergency department with multiple episodes of **nausea and vomiting** of 2 days' duration, and today his **"stomach hurts."** The worried mother reports finding the Tylenol bottle half empty this morning. On physical examination, the patient is **jaundiced** and diaphoretic, with **right upper quadrant (RUQ) tenderness.** Temperature = 98.6° F; blood pressure = 110/70 mm Hg; heart rate = 103 bpm; and respiration rate = 22 breaths/min.

DIFFERENTIALS: Acetaminophen-induced liver toxicity and gastroenteritis. The chemical structure of acetaminophen is *N*-acetyl-*p*-aminophenol (APAP). APAP itself is nontoxic but it is metabolized primarily in the liver by cytochrome P450 to a toxic metabolite, *N*-acetyl-*p*-benzoquinoneimine (NAPQI). Glutathione can bind NAPQI and lead to the excretion of non-toxic mercapturate conjugates in the urine. As the glutathione stores are diminished, NAPQI accumulates and covalently binds to the hepatocyte lipid bilayer, causing centrilobular necrosis. Inducers of cytochrome P450, such as ethanol, isoniazid, rifampin, phenytoin, barbiturates, and carbamazepine, can lead to an increased production of NAPQI.

LABORATORY STUDIES: Elevated **serum APAP levels** and **transaminase levels** greater than 1,000 U/L support the diagnosis of APAP hepatotoxicity. **Coagulation studies** should also be obtained to monitor the liver function.

MANAGEMENT: Glutathione stores can be replaced orally or intravenously by sulfhydryl-containing compounds like ***N*-acetylcysteine.** *N*-acetylcysteine also directly detoxifies NAPQI to nontoxic metabolites by acting as a substrate for sulfation. In addition to *N*-acetylcysteine, if the patient presents within hours of the incident, **gastric lavage** and **oral charcoal** could also be performed.

Clinical Vignette 5-5

CLINICAL PRESENTATION: During a visit to her primary care physician, a 42-year-old woman complains of intermittent **right upper quadrant (RUQ) pain** of several months' duration that is worse after **large and fatty meals.** Pain is **steady** and **lasts 1 to 4 hours** and is sometimes associated with nausea and vomiting. Physical exam reveals a soft, nondistended abdomen with mild tenderness in the RUQ, normal bowel sounds, and no palpable masses. No cough tenderness, rebound tenderness, or tenderness to percussion. Temperature = 98.7° F; blood pressure = 130/80 mm Hg; heart rate = 85 bpm; and respiration rate = 20 breaths/min.
DIFFERENTIALS: Biliary colic/cholelithiasis, acute cholecystitis, choledocholithiasis, and acute cholangitis. When differentiating between the various causes of RUQ pain, use these findings to guide your approach: (a) when **obstructive symptoms (jaundice, pruritus, light-colored stools, tea-colored urine, etc.)** are present, consider a stone in the common bile duct (CBD) (e.g., choledocholithiasis or acute cholangitis); (b) **inflammation of the parietal peritoneum** elicited by **cough tenderness, rebound tenderness, tenderness to percussion,** and **still posture** indicates an inflammatory condition (e.g., acute cholecystitis or acute cholangitis); and (c) look for specific signs: **Murphy sign** (acute cholecystitis), **Charcot triad** (acute cholangitis), and **Reynold pentad** (acute suppurative cholangitis).
LABORATORY STUDIES: **Ultrasound** is the most effective imaging study for diagnosing cholelithiasis and is superior to CT and radiography. Relevant findings include stones, a thickened gallbladder wall, and pericholecystic fluid. Dilation of the CBD suggests obstruction. To sort through the differentials, look for an obstructive pattern on **fractionate bilirubin** and **liver enzyme studies** to support choledocholithiasis and acute cholangitis: elevated direct bilirubin and marked increases in alkaline phosphatase in comparison to mild increases in aspartate aminotransferase (AST) and alanine aminotransferase (ALT). **Complete blood count studies** showing an increase in white blood cells with a left shift would support an inflammatory condition (acute cholecystitis or cholangitis).
MANAGEMENT: Uncomplicated cholelithiasis and acute cholecystis are treated surgically with a cholecystectomy. Choledocholithiasis and acute cholangitis are treated by endoscopic retrograde cholangiopancreatography (ERCP); if this fails, surgical exploration of the CBD is attempted. In acute cholecystitis and cholangitis, antibiotics are also given to resolve the underlying infection.

THE PANCREAS

- Common Clinical Disorders of the Pancreas (Table 5-15)

In the United States, alcohol is the most common cause of pancreatic pathology.

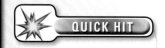
QUICK HIT

Multiple endocrine neoplasia type 1 (MEN 1) involves neoplasia or hyperplasia of the pancreas, the parathyroids, and the pituitary.

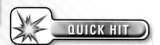
QUICK HIT

Use patient **history** to determine whether the cause of pancreatitis is gallstones or alcohol abuse. The **amylase/ lipase levels** are markedly elevated in gallstone pancreatitis (thousands) in comparison to the increase seen in alcoholic pancreatitis (hundreds); chronic alcohol consumption may lead to less functioning pancreatic tissue.

TABLE **5-15** **Common Clinical Disorders of the Pancreas**

Disorder	Etiology and Pathology	Clinical Features	Notes
Acute pancreatitis	Gallstones (obstructing the ampulla of Vater); alcohol abuse	**Midepigastric pain radiating to the back; increased serum amylase** and lipase; hemorrhage may lead to Cullen or Grey Turner sign; hypocalcemia	Activation of pancreatic enzymes leads to autodigestion
Chronic pancreatitis	**Alcoholism** in adults; cystic fibrosis in children	**Increased serum amylase** and lipase, **pancreatic calcifications,** epigastric pain, steatorrhea	Irreversible; leads to organ atrophy; may lead to formation of pancreatic pseudocyst
Adenocarcinoma of the exocrine pancreas	More common in smokers	Invasive; **Trousseau syndrome** (migratory thrombophlebitis); radiating abdominal pain; obstructive jaundice; **increased carcinoembryonic antigen**	Poor prognosis; over 50% in the head of the pancreas; more common in Blacks, males, patients with diabetes, and people older than 60 years

(continued)

TABLE 5-15 Common Clinical Disorders of the Pancreas *(Continued)*			
Disorder	**Etiology and Pathology**	**Clinical Features**	**Notes**
Insulinoma (endocrine pancreas)	Originates in β cells	**Whipple triad:** hypoglycemia, CNS dysfunction, and reversal of CNS abnormalities with glucose	Most common islet cell tumor
Gastrinoma (Zollinger–Ellison syndrome)	Gastrin-secreting tumor (most commonly, islet cell origin)	Recurrent peptic ulcers	Part of **multiple endocrine neoplasia type 1**

CNS, central nervous system.

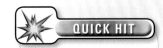

QUICK HIT

The presence of **C-peptide** in the blood distinguishes endogenous insulin secretions (as in an insulinoma) from exogenous insulin administration (as seen in Munchausen syndrome).

 PATHOGENS OF THE GASTROINTESTINAL TRACT

I. Bacterial

Enterobacteriaceae   *Vibrio cholerae*   *Clostridium botulinum*
Salmonella   *Staphylococcus aureus*   *Clostridium difficile*
Shigella   *Campylobacter jejuni*   *Bacillus fragilis*
Escherichia coli   *Helicobacter pylori*

II. Parasitic

Entamoeba histolytica   *Cryptosporidium*   *Ascaris lumbricoides*
Giardia lamblia   *Trichuris trichiura*   *Strongyloides stercoralis*

III. Viral

Adenovirus   Echovirus   Norwalk agent
Coronavirus   Rotavirus   Reovirus

 THERAPEUTIC AGENTS FOR THE GASTROINTESTINAL SYSTEM

Various therapeutic agents have been designed to treat GI diseases such as heartburn (Table 5-16), diarrhea (Table 5-17), nausea (Table 5-18), and constipation (Table 5-19).

TABLE 5-16 Therapeutic Agents for Heartburn				
Therapeutic Agent (common name, if relevant) [trade name, where appropriate]	**Class—Pharmacology and Pharmacokinetics**	**Indications**	**Side Effects or Adverse Effects**	**Contraindications or Precautions to Consider; Notes**
Cimetidine	H_2 blocker—blocks histamine H_2 receptors; reversibly decreases proton secretion by parietal cells	**Peptic ulcer disease, gastritis, esophageal reflux**	**Gynecomastia, impotence,** and decreased libido in males; **dizziness and headaches**	Crosses placenta; decreases renal excretion of creatinine; cytochrome P450 inhibitor
Famotidine [Pepcid], **ranitidine** [Zantac], **nizatidine**	H_2 blocker—blocks histamine H_2 receptors; reversibly decreases proton secretion by parietal cells	**Peptic ulcer disease, gastritis, esophageal reflux**	Confusion, dizziness, and headaches	Crosses placenta; **milder side effect profile** than cimetidine

(continued)

The Gastrointestinal System

| TABLE 5-16 | Therapeutic Agents for Heartburn (Continued) |

Therapeutic Agent (common name, if relevant) [trade name, where appropriate]	Class—Pharmacology and Pharmacokinetics	Indications	Side Effects or Adverse Effects	Contraindications or Precautions to Consider; Notes
Omeprazole [Prilosec], **lansoprazole**, **esomeprazole**	**Proton pump inhibitor— irreversibly inhibits H$^+$/K$^+$- ATPase in gastric parietal cells → decreases proton secretion by parietal cells**	Peptic ulcer disease, gastritis, esophageal reflux, and **Zollinger– Ellison syndrome**		**Inhibits cytochrome P450;** given with clarithromycin and **amoxicillin** for *Helicobacter pylori*
Bismuth [Pepto-Bismol], **sucralfate**	**Cytoprotectant—binds to ulcer base → protection; allows bicarbonate ion secretion to reestablish pH gradient in the mucus layer**	**Traveler's diarrhea,** peptic ulcer disease		
Misoprostol	**Cytoprotectant—PGE$_1$ analog → increased production and secretion of gastric mucosa barrier; decreased acid production**	**Prevents NSAID- induced peptic ulcers;** maintains patent ductus arteriosus	**Diarrhea**	**Abortion-inducing drug,** contraindicated in women of childbearing age
Pirenzepine, propantheline	**Muscarinic antagonist— blocks M$_1$ receptors on ECL cells → decreases histamine secretion; blocks M$_3$ receptors on parietal cells → decreases acid secretion**	Peptic ulcer	**Tachycardia, dry mouth, blurry vision** (difficulty accommodating)	
Aluminum hydroxide	**Antacid**—buffers gastric acid by raising pH	Peptic ulcer, gastritis, esophageal reflux, and diarrhea	**Constipation,** hypophosphatemia, muscle weakness, **osteodystrophy,** seizures, and **hypokalemia**	Can affect the **absorption, bioavailability,** or **urinary excretion** of drugs by changing the **gastric pH, urinary pH,** or **gastric emptying**
Magnesium hydroxide (milk of magnesia)	**Antacid**—buffers gastric acid by raising pH	Peptic ulcer, gastritis, esophageal reflux, and constipation	**Diarrhea, hyporeflexia, hypotension, cardiac arrest, hypokalemia**	Can affect the **absorption, bioavailability,** or **urinary excretion** of drugs by changing **the gastric pH, urinary pH,** or **gastric emptying**
Calcium carbonate [TUMS, Caltrate]	**Antacid**—buffers gastric acid by raising pH	Peptic ulcer, gastritis, esophageal reflux, and calcium deficiency	**Hypercalcemia, rebound acid increase, and hypokalemia**	Can affect the **absorption, bioavailability,** or **urinary excretion** of drugs by changing **the gastric pH, urinary pH,** or **gastric emptying**

ATPase, adenosine triphosphatase; ECL, enterochromaffin-like; PGE$_1$, prostaglandin E$_1$.

TABLE 5-17 Therapeutic Agents for Diarrhea, Ulcerative Colitis, and Crohn Disease

Therapeutic Agent (common name, if relevant) [trade name, where appropriate]	Class—Pharmacology and Pharmacokinetics	Indications	Side Effects or Adverse Effects	Contraindications or Precautions to Consider; Notes
Loperamide [Imodium]	Antidiarrheal—similar to opioid agonist	Oral antidiarrheal		
Aluminum hydroxide	Antidiarrheal—delays gastric emptying	Peptic ulcer, gastritis, esophageal reflux, and diarrhea	Constipation, hypophosphatemia, muscle weakness, osteodystrophy, seizures, and hypokalemia	Can affect the absorption, bioavailability, or urinary excretion of drugs by changing the gastric pH, urinary pH, or gastric emptying
Sulfasalazine	Anti-inflammatory—sulfapyridine (antibacterial) and mesalamine (anti-inflammatory)	Ulcerative colitis, Crohn disease	Malaise, nausea, sulfonamide toxicity, reversible oligospermia	Activated by colonic bacteria
Infliximab	Anti-inflammatory—monoclonal antibody that binds TNF → inhibits proinflammatory effects of TNF	Crohn disease, rheumatoid arthritis	Respiratory infection, fever, and hypotension	

TNF, tumor necrosis factor.

TABLE 5-18 Therapeutic Agents for Nausea

Therapeutic Agent (common name, if relevant) [trade name, where appropriate]	Class—Pharmacology and Pharmacokinetics	Indications	Side Effects or Adverse Effects	Contraindications or Precautions to Consider; Notes
Scopolamine	Anticholinergic—M_1-muscarinic receptor antagonist	Motion sickness; prophylaxis	Dry mouth, drowsiness, and vision disturbances	Delivered transdermally
Promethazine [Phenergan]	Antihistamine—D_2-receptor antagonist; H_1 blocker	Counteracts nausea of migraine; allergies; motion sickness	Sedation, CNS depression, atropine-like effects, allergic dermatitis, blood dyscrasias, teratogenicity, acute antihistamine poisoning	
Prochlorperazine [Compazine]	Dopamine antagonist—D_2-receptor antagonist	Nausea; counteracts nausea of migraine	Teratogenic	
Metoclopramide [Reglan]	Dopamine antagonist—central and peripheral D_2 antagonism at low doses and weak $5-HT_3$ antagonism at high doses; enhances acetylcholine release, prokinetic	Nausea; counteracts nausea of migraine; increases stomach motility	Sleepiness, fatigue, headache, insomnia, dizziness, nausea, akathisia, dystonia, and tardive dyskinesia	
Ondansetron [Zofran]	Serotonin antagonist—$5-HT_3$ blocker	Nausea (caused by cancer therapy or postoperative state)	Headache, constipation, and dizziness	

5-HT, serotonin; CNS, central nervous system.

TABLE 5-19 Therapeutic Agents for Constipation

Therapeutic Agent (common name, if relevant) [trade name, where appropriate]	Class—Pharmacology and Pharmacokinetics	Indications	Side Effects or Adverse Effects	Contraindications or Precautions to Consider; Notes
Methylcellulose [Citrucel] **Psyllium** [Perdiem Fiber]	**Bulk-forming laxative**—dietary fiber	Constipation	Impaction above strictures, fluid overload, gas, and bloating	
Lactulose	**Osmotic laxative**	Decreases ammonia in hepatic encephalopathy; constipation	Abdominal bloating and flatulence	Lowers colon pH so that ammonia is trapped and then excreted
Magnesium hydroxide [Milk of Magnesia]	**Osmotic laxative**	Constipation, peptic ulcer, gastritis, and esophageal reflux	Diarrhea	
Magnesium sulfate, Magnesium citrate	**Osmotic laxative**		Magnesium toxicity (in renal insufficiency)	
Docusate	**Stool softener;** by emulsifying stool, it makes the passage of stool easier	Constipation	Skin rash	
Bisacodyl [Dulcolax]	**Stimulant laxative;** increases peristalsis	Constipation	Electrolyte imbalances (chronic use); gastric irritation	
Senna [Senokot]	**Stimulant laxative;** increases peristalsis	Constipation	Electrolyte imbalances (chronic use); melanosis coli	
Phenolphthalein [Ex-Lax]	**Stimulant laxative**—reduces the absorption of electrolytes and water from the gut	Constipation	Tumorigenic	
Anthraquinones	**Stimulant laxative**—reduces the absorption of electrolytes and water from the gut	Constipation		
Castor oil	**Stimulant laxative**—reduces the absorption of electrolytes and water from the gut; active component is ricinoleic acid	Constipation, labor induction		
Mineral oil [Fleet Mineral Oil Enema]	**Hyperosmolar agent**—draws water into the gut lumen → gut distension → promotes peristalsis and evacuation of bowel	**Preoperative patients;** short-term treatment of constipation		May interfere with the absorption of fat-soluble vitamins
Metoclopramide [Reglan]	**Prokinetic agent**—D$_2$-receptor antagonist; increases resting tone, contractility, LES tone, and motility (does not affect colon transit time)	**Diabetic** and **postoperative gastroparesis**	Sleepiness, fatigue, headache, insomnia, dizziness, nausea, akathisia, **dystonia,** and tardive dyskinesia	Interacts with **digoxin** and **diabetic agents; contraindicated in small bowel obstruction**

LES, lower esophageal sphincter.

The Gastrointestinal System

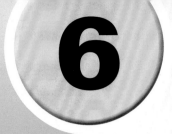

The Renal System

DEVELOPMENT

I. **Intermediate mesoderm**
  A. This forms the urogenital ridges on each side of the aorta.
  B. The **nephrogenic cord** arises from the urogenital ridge and gives rise, wholly or in part, to the pronephros, the mesonephros, and the metanephros.

II. **Pronephros**
  A. Forms in the fourth week
  B. Quickly regresses by the fifth week
  C. Nonfunctional

III. **Mesonephros**
  A. Forms late in the fourth week and is functional until the permanent kidney is able to develop
  B. The **mesonephric duct** forms from the mesonephros.
    1. Forms the ductus deferens, epididymis, ejaculatory duct, and seminal vesicle in the male
    2. Forms the **ureteric bud** from which the **ureter**, **renal pelvis**, **calyces**, and **collecting tubules** in both the male and female are derived
    3. No important genital or reproductive derivatives of the mesonephric duct specific to females are formed.

IV. **Metanephros**
  A. Develops into the **adult kidney**
  B. Formed during the fifth week from the ureteric bud and the metanephric mass (which is induced to form by contact with the ureteric bud) and begins to function in the ninth week
  C. Metanephric mesoderm forms the nephrons.
  D. "Ascends" from sacral levels to low thoracic levels during its development because of longitudinal growth of the fetus
  E. Urogenital sinus forms the **bladder**, which is continuous with allantois. Allantois is equivalent to the median umbilical ligament in the adult.
  F. Urethra
    1. Formed from endoderm and urogenital sinus
    2. Distal portion formed from ectoderm

V. **Congenital anomalies of the renal system** (*Table 6-1*)

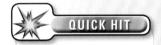

QUICK HIT

The entire collecting system arises from the ureteric bud. The remainder of the renal system arises from the metanephric mesoderm.

TABLE 6-1 **Congenital Anomalies**	
Anomaly	**Characteristics**
Bilateral renal agenesis (Potter syndrome)	• Occurs when the ureteric bud does not form • **Oligohydramnios** • Limb deformities • Facial deformities • **Pulmonary hypoplasia** • Bilateral agenesis is not compatible with life
Accessory renal arteries	• Arise from the aorta • Feed a particular section of the kidney • Are end arteries • **Cutting will produce ischemic infarct** in the area they supply
Congenital polycystic kidney disease	• Multiple small and large cysts causing renal insufficiency • Cysts are "closed"—not continuous with collecting system • Enlarged kidneys palpable on newborn examination • Death within days to weeks
Horseshoe kidney	• Inferior poles of the kidneys are fused • Ascent is arrested at the level of the inferior mesenteric artery • Increases probability of Wilms tumor

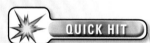

QUICK HIT

In the adult male, the ureter passes posterior to the ductus deferens; in the adult female, the ureter passes posterior to the uterine artery.

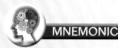

MNEMONIC

To remember the relationship of the arteries to the ureter, think "water under the bridge"; the ureters (which carry water) are posterior to the ovarian/testicular artery and uterine artery.

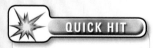

QUICK HIT

The left gonadal (testicular or ovarian) vein drains into the left renal vein; the right gonadal vein drains directly into the inferior vena cava.

The Renal System

GROSS DESCRIPTION OF THE KIDNEY

I. **Paired adult kidneys weigh approximately 150 g each.**

II. **They are located posterior to the peritoneum and at approximately the level of the first lumbar vertebra.**

III. **The right kidney is slightly lower than the left owing to downward displacement by the liver.**

IV. **The left renal vein lies posterior to the superior mesenteric artery and anterior to the abdominal aorta.**

V. **The kidney is highly vascularized; it filters more than 1,700 L of blood per day to produce about 1 L of urine.**

VI. **Kidney and urinary tract** (*Figure 6-1*)

VII. **Distribution of body water** (*Figure 6-2*)

FIGURE 6-1 The kidney and urinary tract

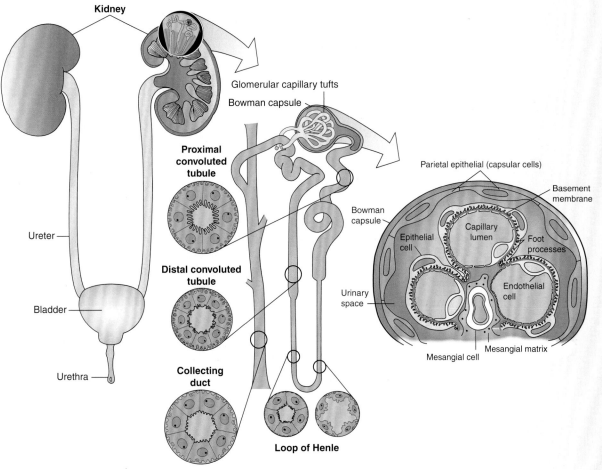

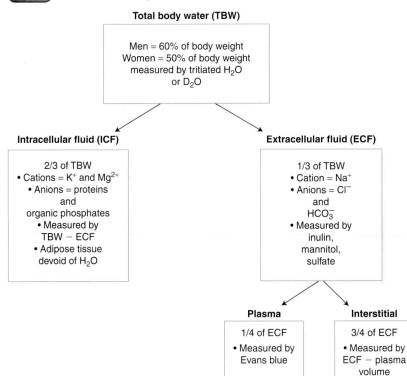

(Adapted with permission from Damjanov I. *A Color Atlas and Textbook of Histopathology*. Baltimore, MD: Lippincott Williams & Wilkins; 1996.)

FIGURE 6-2 Distribution of body water

Total body water (TBW)

Men = 60% of body weight
Women = 50% of body weight
measured by tritiated H_2O
or D_2O

Intracellular fluid (ICF)

2/3 of TBW
• Cations = K^+ and Mg^{2+}
• Anions = proteins and organic phosphates
• Measured by TBW − ECF
• Adipose tissue devoid of H_2O

Extracellular fluid (ECF)

1/3 of TBW
• Cation = Na^+
• Anions = Cl^- and HCO_3^-
• Measured by inulin, mannitol, sulfate

Plasma

1/4 of ECF
• Measured by Evans blue

Interstitial

3/4 of ECF
• Measured by ECF − plasma volume

Cl^-, chloride; D_2O, heavy water; HCO_3^-, bicarbonate; H_2O, water; K^+, potassium; Mg^{2+}, magnesium; Na^+, sodium.

The Renal System

NORMAL KIDNEY FUNCTION

I. Renal blood flow (RBF)
A. 25% of cardiac output

B. **RBF = renal plasma flow (RPF)/[1 − hematocrit (Hct)]**

C. Renal vasculature **autoregulates** RBF, keeping it constant even when arterial pressure varies from 100 to 200 mm Hg.

II. Renal plasma flow
A. Effective RPF is measured by clearance of para-aminohippuric acid (**PAH**), which is filtered and secreted.

B. This measurement underestimates by 10%.

III. Glomerular filtration rate (GFR)
A. Normal GFR is 90 to 125 mL/min based on creatinine.

B. It is measured by **inulin** clearance. Inulin is an ideal marker for the measurement of GFR because it is a substance that is **filtered** by the kidney but **not reabsorbed or secreted**. Therefore, urine levels of inulin vary directly with GFR. However, inulin clearance is not practical for clinical use.

C. GFR is clinically measured with **creatinine** clearance. Endogenous creatine is the most common clinical marker because it is **filtered, minimally secreted,** and **not reabsorbed** by the kidneys. Although creatinine excretion is generally 10% to 20% greater than filtration, this discrepancy is cancelled by the overestimation of plasma creatinine. Therefore, creatinine is relatively accurate for GFR calculation.
  1. Decreases in GFR cause a rise in blood urea nitrogen (BUN) and creatinine levels.
  2. GFR decreases with age.

D. GFR is driven by Starling forces (filtration is always favored) (Figure 6-3).

E. Renal clearance
  1. Removal of a substance from the blood by renal excretion
  2. Determined by the following equation:

$$\text{Clearance} = [U \times V]/P \text{ (in mL/min)}$$

where U = concentration of substance in urine in mg/mL

V = urine volume (urine flow rate) in mL/min

P = plasma concentration of substance in mg/mL

FIGURE 6-3 Starling forces on the glomerular capillary

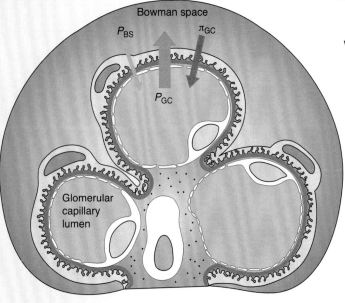

The Starling forces influence the glomerular filtration rate (GFR)

$$\text{GFR} = K_F \left[(P_{GC} - P_{BS}) - (\pi_{GC} - \pi_{BS}) \right]$$

where K_F: The filtration coefficient of the glomerular capillaries

P_{GC}: The hydrostatic pressure exerted by the fluid in the glomerular capillary. A dilated afferent arteriole increases P_{GC}, as does a constricted efferent arteriole.

P_{BS}: The hydrostatic pressure exerted by the fluid in Bowman space. Blockage or constriction of the ureters increases P_{BS}.

π_{GC}: The oncotic pressure of the glomerular capillary. The value of π_{GC} increases along the length of the capillary because the protein concentration in the capillary increases as water is forced into Bowman space.

π_{BS}: The oncotic pressure in Bowman space. This value is usually zero.

The Renal System

Note: One common pitfall to using creatinine is muscle mass. Plasma creatinine varies directly with muscle mass, so individuals with lower **muscle mass** (e.g., emaciated, elderly) may have an artificially higher GFR and individuals with high muscle mass (e.g., bodybuilders) may have an artificially lower GFR. Similarly, with age and loss of muscle mass, GFR may remain stable when in fact there is a decline in glomerular function and a decrease in GFR.

   3. Factors that determine clearance
      a. Highly cleared substances (e.g., PAH) are those that are filtered and secreted and not reabsorbed.
      b. Poorly cleared substances are those that are either not filtered (e.g., protein) or are completely reabsorbed (e.g., glucose).
      c. Reabsorption
         • Limited by the number of transporters for certain compounds (e.g., glucose) in various segments of tubule
         • Transport maximum (T_m) is the maximum rate of reabsorption at which the transporters are saturated.
         • At concentrations above T_m, excess is excreted.

IV. Filtration fraction (FF)

   A. **FF = GFR/RPF**
   B. The normal FF is 20%.
   C. Variables that change FF:
      1. Ureteral obstruction decreases FF.
      2. Increased plasma proteins decrease FF (e.g., multiple myeloma).
      3. Decreased plasma proteins increase FF (e.g., liver failure).
      4. Constriction of efferent arteriole increases FF (e.g., angiotensin II).
      5. Dilation of efferent arteriole decreases FF (e.g., ACE inhibitors).
      6. Constriction of afferent arteriole (e.g., nonsteroidal anti-inflammatory drugs [NSAIDs]) and dilation of afferent arteriole (e.g., prostaglandins) changes GFR and RPF, but the FF remains constant.

V. Innervation and hormones

   A. Juxtaglomerular apparatus (JGA) produces renin and is stimulated by the β-sympathetic adrenergics in the kidney and by a fall in pressure of the afferent arteriole.
   B. **Renin** cleaves angiotensinogen to **angiotensin I**.
   C. Angiotensin I is cleaved to **angiotensin II** by angiotensin-converting enzyme (**ACE**) in the lung.
      1. Functions of angiotensin II
         a. Stimulates aldosterone release from the zona glomerulosa
         b. Stimulates secretion of antidiuretic hormone (ADH, also known as arginine vasopressin [AVP]) and adrenocorticotropic hormone (ACTH) from the pituitary
         c. Acts as a potent local vasoconstrictor of the renal arterioles at low plasma levels
         d. Acts as a general systemic vasoconstrictor at high plasma levels
         e. Stimulates thirst
         f. Stimulates epinephrine and norepinephrine release from adrenal medulla
      2. Angiotensin II is inactivated to angiotensin III, a potent stimulator of aldosterone secretion but not an effective vasoconstrictor.

VI. Hormones and the nephron *(Figure 6-4)*

VII. Effects of volume change on fluid levels *(Table 6-2)*

A variety of hormones, such as ADH, aldosterone, and atrial natriuretic factor, regulate extracellular and intracellular volumes. Intake and output, as well as hormonal imbalance, can significantly alter the homeostatic fluid balance in the body.

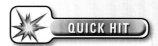

QUICK HIT

The T_m for glucose is reached at approximately 350 mg/dL. Greater concentrations result in an osmotic diuresis, such as that seen in diabetics with hyperglycemia.

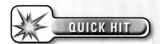

QUICK HIT

Fanconi syndrome is a **hereditary** or **acquired** dysfunction of the proximal renal tubules. As a result of impaired glucose, amino acid, phosphate, and bicarbonate reabsorption, it manifests clinically as glycosuria, hyperphosphaturia, aminoaciduria, and acidosis.

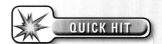

QUICK HIT

ACE inhibitors, such as **captopril** and **enalapril**, reduce hypertension by inhibiting the conversion of angiotensin I to angiotensin II, thereby decreasing the release of aldosterone. Angiotensin II receptor blockers, such as losartan and valsartan, prevent angiotensin II from interacting with its receptor. This prevents angiotensin II from causing constriction of efferent arterioles.

The Renal System

FIGURE 6-4 Hormones and the nephron

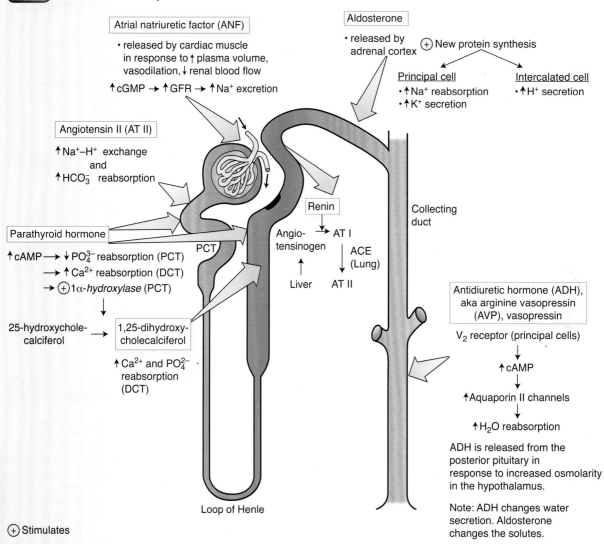

Atrial natriuretic factor (ANF)
- released by cardiac muscle in response to ↑ plasma volume, vasodilation, ↓ renal blood flow

↑cGMP → ↑GFR → ↑Na⁺ excretion

Angiotensin II (AT II)
↑Na⁺–H⁺ exchange and ↑HCO₃⁻ reabsorption

Aldosterone
- released by adrenal cortex

⊕ New protein synthesis

Principal cell
- ↑Na⁺ reabsorption
- ↑K⁺ secretion

Intercalated cell
- ↑H⁺ secretion

Parathyroid hormone

↑cAMP → ↓PO₄³⁻ reabsorption (PCT)
→ ↑Ca²⁺ reabsorption (DCT)
→ ⊕ 1α-hydroxylase (PCT)

PCT

Renin

Angio-tensinogen → AT I

ACE (Lung)

Liver   AT II

Collecting duct

25-hydroxychole-calciferol → 1,25-dihydroxy-cholecalciferol

↑Ca²⁺ and PO₄²⁻ reabsorption (DCT)

Antidiuretic hormone (ADH), aka arginine vasopressin (AVP), vasopressin

V₂ receptor (principal cells)
↓
↑cAMP
↓
↑Aquaporin II channels
↓
↑H₂O reabsorption

ADH is released from the posterior pituitary in response to increased osmolarity in the hypothalamus.

Note: ADH changes water secretion. Aldosterone changes the solutes.

Loop of Henle

⊕ Stimulates

ACE, angiotensin-converting enzyme; AT I, angiotensin I; Ca²⁺, calcium; cAMP, cyclic adenosine monophosphate; cGMP, cyclic guanosine monophosphate; DCT, distal convoluted tubule; GFR, glomerular filtration rate; H⁺, hydrogen ion; HCO₃⁻, bicarbonate; H₂O, water; K⁺, potassium; Na⁺, sodium; PCT, proximal convoluted tubule; PO₄³⁻, phosphate; V2, vasopressin receptor type 2.

TABLE 6-2 Effects of Volume Change on Fluid Levels

Type	Key Examples	ECF Volume	ICF Volume	ECF Osmolarity	Hct and Serum [Na⁺]
Isosmotic volume expansion	Isotonic fluid infusion (e.g., normal saline or lactated Ringer solution)	↑	No change	No change	↓ Hct − [Na⁺]
Isosmotic volume contraction	Diarrhea	↓	No change	No change	↑ Hct − [Na⁺]
Hyperosmotic volume expansion	High NaCl intake	↑	↓	↑	↓ Hct ↑ [Na⁺]
Hyperosmotic volume contraction	Sweating, fever, diabetes insipidus	↓	↓	↑	− Hct ≠ [Na⁺]
Hyposmotic volume expansion	SIADH	↑	↑	↓	− Hct ↓ [Na⁺]
Hyposmotic volume contraction	Adrenal insufficiency	↓	↑	↓	↑ Hct ↓ [Na⁺]

−, no change; ECF, extracellular fluid; Hct, hematocrit; ICF, intracellular fluid; Na⁺, sodium; SIADH, syndrome of inappropriate secretion of antidiuretic hormone.
Reproduced with permission from Costanzo LS. *BRS Physiology*. 2nd ed. Baltimore, MD: Lippincott Williams & Wilkins; 1998.

VIII. Electrolyte balance in the nephron (Figure 6-5)

Acidosis or alkalosis is determined by evaluating blood pH, arterial partial pressure of carbon dioxide (Pa_{CO_2}), and bicarbonate (HCO_3^-) concentration. Anion gap (AG) is calculated using the following equation: $AG = Na^+ - (Cl^- + HCO_3^-)$. A normal AG is between 10 and 16 mEq/L. Certain acidotic conditions result in an elevated AG by altering the concentration of anions not considered in the above formula (lactate, β-hydroxybutyrate, formate). Table 6-3 compares acidosis with alkalosis. Table 6-4 outlines the effects of metabolic and respiratory acid–base disturbances.

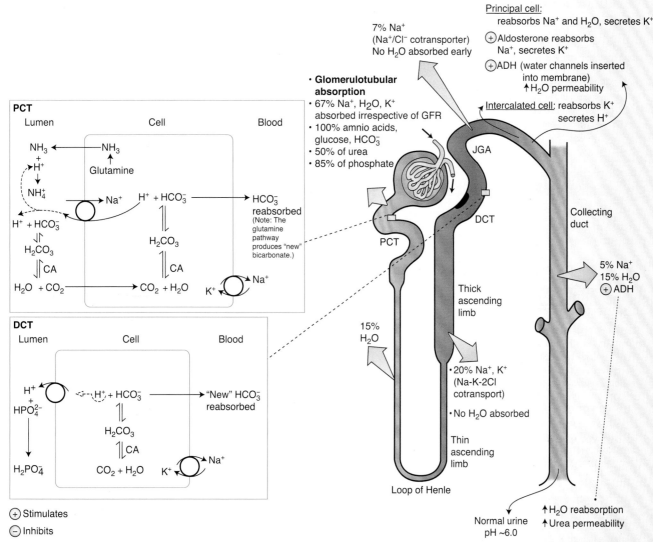

FIGURE 6-5 Electrolyte balance in the nephron

ADH, antidiuretic hormone; CA, carbonic anhydrase; Cl⁻, chloride; CO₂, carbon dioxide; DCT, distal convoluted tubule; GFR, glomerular filtration rate; H⁺, hydrogen ion; HCO₃⁻, bicarbonate; H₂CO₃, carbonic acid; H₂O, water; HPO₄²⁻, H₂PO₄⁻, two forms of phosphate ions; JGA, juxtaglomerular apparatus; K⁺, potassium; Mg²⁺, magnesium; Na⁺, sodium; NH₃, ammonia; NH₄⁺, ammonium; PCT, proximal convoluted tubule.

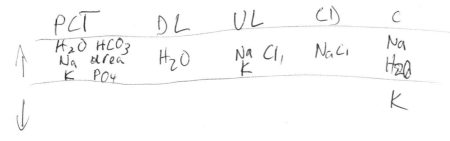

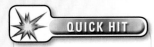

MNEMONIC

To remember the causes of increased anion gap metabolic acidosis, think **MUDPILES**: **M**ethanol, **U**remia, **D**iabetic keto-acidosis, **P**araldehyde, **I**soniazid or **I**ron tablets, **L**actic acidosis, **E**thylene glycol, **S**alicylates.

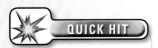

QUICK HIT

Renal tubular acidosis (RTA) is characterized by a normal anion gap. Type 1 (distal) RTA is caused by a failure to excrete titratable acid and NH_4^+. Type 2 RTA is caused by renal loss of HCO_3^-. Type 4 RTA is caused by hypoaldosteronism, which leads to poor excretion of NH^{4+} and hyperkalemia.

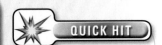

QUICK HIT

Emphysema and bronchitis often cause chronic respiratory acidosis.

QUICK HIT

A patient's respiratory status affects and is affected by his or her acid–base status. This is because of the reversible conversion of CO_2 to H^+ in the following way: $H_2O + CO_2 \leftrightarrow H_2CO_3 \leftrightarrow HCO_3^- + H^+$. The first reaction is catalyzed by the enzyme carbonic anhydrase.

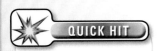

QUICK HIT

Salicylate (aspirin) overdose causes respiratory alkalosis initially, followed by an increased anion gap metabolic acidosis.

TABLE **6-3** **Acidosis and Alkalosis**

Metabolic Disturbance	Presentation	Causes
Metabolic acidosis	• Fatigue • Shortness of breath • Abdominal pain • Vomiting • **Kussmaul respirations** • Hypotension • Tachycardia	• Chronic renal failure • Lactic acidosis • Uremia • **Ketoacidosis** • Intoxication (aspirin, methanol, ethylene glycol) • **Diarrhea**[a] • **Renal tubular acidosis**[a] • Acetazolamide[a]
Respiratory acidosis	• **Hypercapnia** • Confusion • Blunted sensation and pain • **Asterixis** • Papilledema	• Respiratory depression by drugs • Cerebral disease • Cardiopulmonary arrest response • Neuromuscular disease (e.g., myasthenia gravis) • Poor ventilation secondary to disease (e.g., asthma, pneumonia, bronchitis, emphysema)
Metabolic alkalosis	• No specific signs or symptoms • Can cause apathy, stupor, and confusion • If coupled with low calcium, can cause tetany	• Diuretics (loop and thiazide) • Vomiting • Milk alkali syndrome • Large intake of alkaline substance • **Cushing syndrome** • Primary aldosteronism
Respiratory alkalosis	• **Hyperventilation** • Numbness • Tingling • Paresthesia • Tetany, if severe	• Asthma • Pneumonia • Pulmonary edema • Heart disease with cyanosis • Pulmonary fibrosis • Aspirin intoxication • **Gram-negative sepsis** • Fever • Anxiety • Pregnancy • Drugs • Conditions that stimulate the medullary respiratory center (e.g., altitude) • Aspirin intoxication (via stimulation of respiratory center)

[a]Normal anion gap acidosis (other acidosis items have an increased anion gap).

TABLE 6-4 Effects of Metabolic and Respiratory Acid–Base Disturbances

Primary Disorder	pH	[H⁺]	[HCO₃⁻]	PCO₂	Respiratory Compensation	Renal Compensation
Metabolic acidosis	$\downarrow$	$\uparrow$	$\downarrow^a$ (lost by buffering)	$\downarrow$	Hyperventilation	$\uparrow$ H⁺ excretion (NH₃) $\uparrow$ "New" HCO₃⁻ reabsorption
Metabolic alkalosis	$\uparrow$	$\downarrow$	$\uparrow^a$	$\uparrow$	Hypoventilation	$\uparrow$ HCO₃⁻ excretion
Acute respiratory acidosis	$\downarrow$	$\uparrow$	$\uparrow$	$\uparrow^a$	None	Not yet
Chronic respiratory acidosis	$\downarrow$ (more normal)	$\uparrow$	$\uparrow\uparrow$	$\uparrow^a$	None	$\uparrow$ H⁺ excretion (NH₄⁺) $\uparrow$ "New" HCO₃⁻ reabsorption
Acute respiratory alkalosis	$\uparrow$	$\downarrow$	$\downarrow$	$\downarrow^a$		Not yet
Chronic respiratory alkalosis	$\uparrow$ (more normal)	$\downarrow$	$\downarrow\downarrow$	$\downarrow^a$		$\downarrow$ H⁺ excretion $\downarrow$ HCO₃⁻ reabsorption

^{a}Primary disorder.

$\uparrow$, increased; $\downarrow$, decreased; H⁺, hydrogen ion; HCO₃⁺, bicarbonate; NH₄⁺, ammonium.

Clinical Vignette 6-1

CLINICAL PRESENTATION: A 24-year-old male medical student is brought to the emergency department after being found **unconscious** in his apartment by his roommate. It is unknown whether he suffered any trauma, but the roommate tells you that they just finished exam week at the medical school. There are no signs of injury on examination. The roommate tells you that the patient has no other medical problems. The patient cannot be aroused in the emergency department but does respond to pain. Vital signs: temperature = 100.8° F; **respiration rate (RR) = 35 breaths/min;** blood pressure = 150/90 mm Hg; heart rate = 104 bpm. Pupils are round and reactive to light bilaterally. Laboratory tests reveal the following: WBC = 8.4; Hgb = 14.2; Hct = 30.9; Na = 140; K = 3.8; Cl = 102; **HCO₂ = 13;** BUN = 16; Cr = 0.8; Gluc = 110. Arterial blood gasses are obtained and reveal the following: **pH = 7.19; Paco₂ = 26; Pao₂ = 95.**

DIFFERENTIAL: This patient has metabolic acidosis. In approaching a patient with metabolic acidosis, the **first step is the calculation of the AG:** AG = Na⁺ − (Cl⁻ + HCO₃⁻). This patient has an increased AG metabolic acidosis (AG >15) for which differentials are diabetic ketoacidosis (DKA), alcoholic ketoacidosis, lactic acidosis, starvation, renal failure, and overdose of salicylate, methanol, or ethylene glycol. Given that the patient is not diabetic and has a glucose of 114 mg/dL, DKA is unlikely. Also, renal function is not impaired. Because the cause is unclear, further testing is necessary.

LABORATORY STUDIES: To determine the cause of the AG metabolic acidosis in this patient, **serum ketone, salicylate, lactate, blood alcohol, methanol,** and **ethylene glycol levels** should be obtained. Next, determine whether this is a primary acid–base disorder or mixed disorder. Using **Winter's formula** [1.5 (measured HCO₃) + 8 ± 2], the expected Paco₂ level in this patient is 25.5 to 29.5 mm Hg. With a Paco₂ of 26 mm Hg, this patient has an appropriate respiratory compensation response (RR of 35 breaths/min). If actual Paco₂ is higher than expected, there is an additional acidotic process occurring. If actual Paco₂ is lower than expected, then there is an additional alkalotic process occurring.

MANAGEMENT: Management depends on the cause of metabolic acidosis. **Sodium bicarbonate** may be needed in cases of severe acidemia, and **mechanical ventilation** may be required if patient is fatigued from hyperventilation.

The Renal System

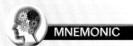

GLOMERULAR DISEASES

I. Nephrotic syndrome
    A. Features
        1. **Proteinuria** of >3.5 g of protein per 24 hours
        2. Hypoalbuminemia
        3. Edema
        4. Hyperlipidemia
    B. Etiology
        1. Idiopathic—75%
        2. Systemic disease—25%
    C. Common types (Table 6-5)

II. Nephritic syndrome
    A. Features
        1. **Hematuria**
        2. Hypertension
        3. Oliguria
        4. Azotemia
    B. Common types of nephritic glomerular diseases (Table 6-6)

III. Glomerular deposits in disease (*Figure 6-9*)

TABLE 6-5 **Nephrotic Glomerular Diseases**

Glomerular Disease	Etiology	Clinical Features	Notes
Minimal change disease (lipoid nephrosis)	Fusion of foot processes on the basement membrane leads to loss of negative charge and changes in the protein selectivity; altered appearance of villi on epithelial cells	Electron microscopy shows **fusion of podocyte foot processes** (Figure 6-6) and lipid-laden renal cortices	**Common in young children** (usually younger than 5 years of age); responds well to steroids; albumin usually selectively secreted
Membranous nephropathy	Idiopathic; secondarily caused by SLE, hepatitis B, syphilis, gold, penicillamine, malignancy	Basement membrane thickening; **"spike and dome"** with **subepithelial IgG and C3 deposits**	Common in young adults
Diabetic nephropathy	Microangiopathy leading to thickening of basement membrane	Basement membrane thickening	Two types: diffuse and nodular glomerulosclerosis; nodular glomerulosclerosis has **Kimmelstiel–Wilson nodules** (Figure 6-7); usually leads to renal failure
Renal amyloidosis	Subendothelial or mesangial amyloid deposits; associated with multiple myeloma	Stains: periodic acid-Schiff (PAS) (−); **Congo Red (+)**	Increasing severity leads to renal failure
Focal and segmental glomerulosclerosis	Has four possible etiologies: idiopathic; superimposed on preexisting pathology; associated with loss of renal mass; secondary to other disorders (e.g., heroin abuse or HIV)	Sclerosis of some glomeruli; only capillary tuft is involved in affected glomeruli	Clinically similar to minimal change disease but affects older population

C3, third component of complement; IgG, immunoglobulin G; SLE, systemic lupus erythematosus.

FIGURE
6-6 **Minimal change disease**

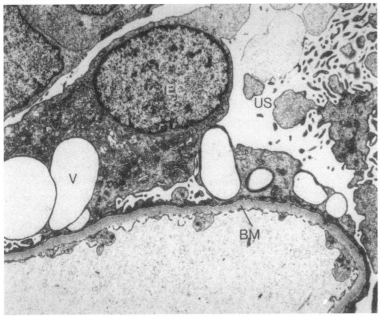

Electron micrograph showing effacement of the podocyte foot processes. BM, basement membrane; EC, endothelial cell; US, urinary space; V, vacuole. (Reproduced with permission from Rubin E, Farber JL. *Pathology.* 3rd ed. Philadelphia, PA: Lippincott Williams & Wilkins; 1999.)

FIGURE
6-7 **Diabetic nodular glomerulosclerosis**

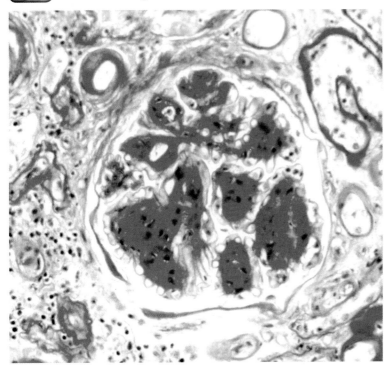

A periodic acid-Schiff stain demonstrates nodular Kimmelstiel–Wilson lesions at the periphery of the glomerulus, which are pathognomonic of diabetic glomerulosclerosis. (Reproduced with permission from Rubin E, Farber JL. *Pathology.* 3rd ed. Philadelphia, PA: Lippincott Williams & Wilkins; 1999.)

TABLE 6-6 Nephritic Glomerular Diseases

Disease	Etiology	Special Features	Notes
Poststreptococcal glomerulonephritis	Poststreptococcal pharyngitis or impetigo, hepatitis B, high ASO titer, low C3, type III hypersensitivity	**"Lumpy bumpy"** deposits of antigen-antibody-C3 complexes, subepithelial humps on electron microscopy	Common in children, self-resolving, most common organisms are group A hemolytic streptococci, red cell casts in urine
Rapidly progressive **(crescentic)** glomerulonephritis	**ANCA positive**, poststreptococcal etiology 50%, renal failure within weeks or months	Accumulation of fibrin, macrophages, and PMNs in Bowman capsule; wrinkling of basement membrane on electron microscopy **(crescents)**	If it also involves upper respiratory system, then it is termed **Wegener granulomatosis**
Goodpasture syndrome	**Antiglomerular basement membrane and alveolar basement membrane antibodies** (type II hypersensitivity)	**Linear pattern** of IgG on fluorescence microscopy; may be associated with hemoptysis and pulmonary hemorrhage	Usually **males in their mid-20s**
Alport syndrome	Hereditary structural defect in collagen IV leads to leaky basement membrane	Glomerular basement membrane splitting on electron microscopy	Appears before age 20 years; associated with deafness and ocular problems
Lupus nephropathy	**Anti-dsDNA**	WHO classifications: ● WHO I: normal ● WHO II: mesangial proliferation; little clinical relevance ● WHO III (focal proliferative): <50% of glomeruli affected ● **WHO IV (diffuse proliferative): worst prognosis; wire-loop lesions** (Figure 6-8) (subendothelial immune complex deposition of IgM and IgG + C3) ● WHO V: membranous glomerulonephritis	Degree of kidney involvement correlates to SLE prognosis; may have nephritic qualities
IgA nephropathy (Berger disease)	IgA deposits in mesangium; hematuria usually follows infection	Mesangial cell proliferation on electron microscopy	Minimal clinical significance; common
Membranoproliferative glomerulonephritis	Type 2 has IgG autoantibody; C3 is reduced in all three types	Basement membrane thickens and appears as two layers; **"train-track"** appearance on electron microscopy	Three types: type 1, type 2 (dense deposit disease), and type 3; may lead to either nephrotic or nephritic syndromes

ANCA, antineutrophil cytoplasmic antibody; ASO, antistreptolysin-O; C3, third component of complement; dsDNA, double-stranded DNA; Ig, immunoglobulin; PMN, polymorphonuclear leukocyte; SLE, systemic lupus erythematosus; WHO, World Health Organization.

FIGURE
6-8 Diffuse proliferative lupus nephritis

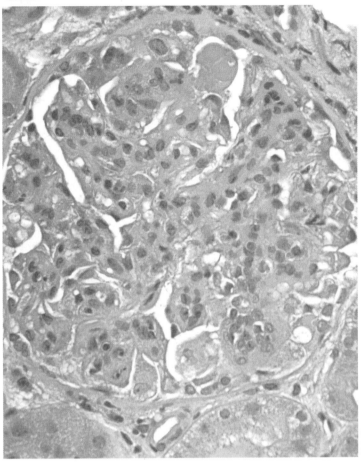

There is a diffuse increase in the cellularity of the glomerulus and thickening of basement membrane. Wire-loop thickening occurs as a result of subendothelial immune complex deposition. (Reproduced with permission from Rubin E, Farber JL. *Pathology.* 3rd ed. Philadelphia, PA: Lippincott Williams & Wilkins; 1999.)

 URINARY TRACT INFECTIONS

I. **Cystitis**
    A. Characteristic clinical features
       1. **Dysuria**
       2. **Frequency**
       3. **Urgency**
       4. Suprapubic pain
    B. Etiology and pathogenesis
       1. Bacteria gain access to the urinary tract via the urethra.
       2. Cystitis most frequently involves normal colonic flora.
          a. *Escherichia coli* is the most common cause (approximately 80%).
          b. *Proteus, Klebsiella,* and *Enterobacter* are also implicated.
          c. *Staphylococcus saprophyticus* causes 10% to 15% of infections in young women.
          d. Nosocomial cystitis is frequently caused by *Pseudomonas* or *Staphylococcus aureus.*
       3. **Women** have a higher incidence of infection because they have shorter urethras.
       4. Other risk factors include sexual activity, pregnancy, urinary obstruction, neurogenic bladder, and vesicoureteral reflux.

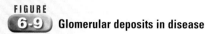

FIGURE 6-9 Glomerular deposits in disease

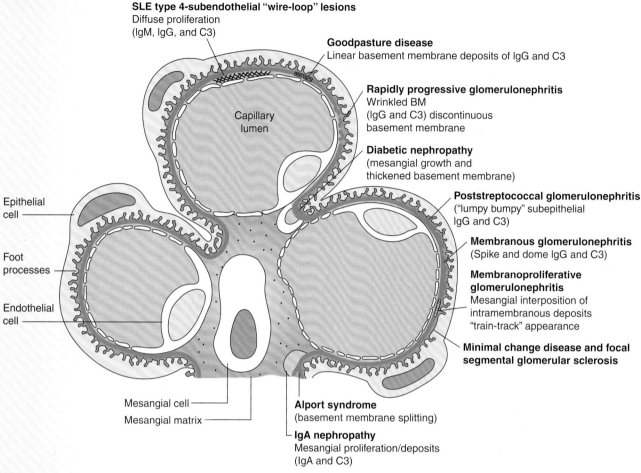

SLE type 4-subendothelial "wire-loop" lesions
Diffuse proliferation
(IgM, IgG, and C3)

Goodpasture disease
Linear basement membrane deposits of IgG and C3

Rapidly progressive glomerulonephritis
Wrinkled BM
(IgG and C3) discontinuous
basement membrane

Diabetic nephropathy
(mesangial growth and
thickened basement membrane)

Poststreptococcal glomerulonephritis
("lumpy bumpy" subepithelial
IgG and C3)

Membranous glomerulonephritis
(Spike and dome IgG and C3)

**Membranoproliferative
glomerulonephritis**
Mesangial interposition of
intramembranous deposits
"train-track" appearance

**Minimal change disease and focal
segmental glomerular sclerosis**

Capillary
lumen

Epithelial
cell

Foot
processes

Endothelial
cell

Mesangial cell
Mesangial matrix

Alport syndrome
(basement membrane splitting)

IgA nephropathy
Mesangial proliferation/deposits
(IgA and C3)

BM, basement membrane; C3, third component of complement; Ig, immunoglobulin; SLE, systemic lupus erythematosus.

Clinical Vignette 6-2

CLINICAL PRESENTATION: A 6-year-old girl presents to her pediatrician with **puffy eyes** of 2 weeks' duration. The mother tells you that the patient has been taking **more naps than usual** and that the pants they had bought recently no longer fit her around the waist. The parents deny any recent upper respiratory infections (URIs). Physical examination shows **periorbital edema, pedal edema, ascites,** and **weight gain.** Cardiothoracic and pulmonary exam is negative, and vital signs are normal.

DIFFERENTIALS: Nephrotic syndrome, glomerulonephritis, congestive heart failure, sinusitis, allergic reaction, hepatic failure. Generalized edema and fatigue are expected in nephrotic syndrome, glomerulonephritis, congestive heart failure (CHF), and hepatic failure. The absence of murmur/gallops/crackles makes CHF less likely. The absence of jaundice makes hepatic failure less likely. A recent URI would suggest glomerulonephritis. Sinusitis is more likely to produce edema localized to periorbital region. Abrupt onset periorbital edema along with conjunctivitis, urticarial rash, wheezing, and rhinorrhea is expected in an allergic reaction. Minimal change disease is the most common cause of nephrotic syndrome in the patient's age group.

LABORATORY STUDIES: **Urinalysis** shows **proteinuria** in both nephrotic and nephritic syndromes but is more severe in nephrotic syndrome. **Hematuria** is seen in nephritic syndrome. **Blood studies** would reveal **hypoalbuminemia** and **hyperlipidemia** in nephrotic syndrome and **azotemia** in nephritic syndrome.

MANAGEMENT: Nephrotic syndrome is best treated by **albumin infusion** followed by **diuretics** and **corticosteroids.** Many children grow out of minimal change disease.

C. Diagnostic findings
    1. Characteristic clinical features are present.
    2. Pyuria (more than 8 leukocytes/high-power field)
    3. Bacterial culture yields $>10^5$ organisms/mL.
D. Treatment
    1. Cystitis is treated with antibiotics.
    2. Recurrent cystitis may require prophylactic antibiotics.

II. Acute pyelonephritis

A. Characteristic clinical features
    1. **Flank pain** or **costovertebral angle tenderness**
    2. **Dysuria**
    3. **Fever**
    4. Chills
    5. Nausea and vomiting
    6. Diarrhea
B. Etiology and pathogenesis
    1. Bacteria **ascend** from an infected urinary bladder to the kidney via the **vesicoureteral reflux**.
    2. Infection may also spread **hematogenously** to the kidney (may not necessarily be preceded by acute cystitis).
    3. Causative organism is usually *E. coli*.
C. Diagnostic findings
    1. Characteristic clinical features are present.
    2. Bacteriuria, pyuria, and **white blood cell casts** are seen on urine microscopy.
    3. Urine and blood cultures are performed to determine infection.
D. Treatment
    1. Treatment is with **antibiotics**, often **intravenously**.
    2. Recurrent infection can lead to chronic pyelonephritis. This condition has several complications:
        a. **Scarring and deformity of the renal pelvis and calyces**
        b. Interstitial fibrosis and tubular atrophy
        c. Ischemia of the tubules leading to microscopic "**thyroidization**" of the kidney

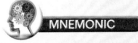

To remember the most common pathogens of UTIs, think **KEEPS**: *Klebsiella, Enterobacter, E. coli, Proteus, S. saprophyticus.*

MAJOR CAUSES OF ACUTE RENAL FAILURE (*Figure 6-10*)

I. Prerenal failure is defined as oliguria and an increase in BUN and creatinine with inherently normal renal function.

A. Hypovolemic states
    1. Hemorrhage
    2. Burns
    3. Dehydration
    4. Vomiting
    5. Diarrhea
    6. Diuretics
    7. Pancreatitis
B. Low cardiac output states
    1. Arrhythmias
    2. Pulmonary embolus
    3. Myocardial or valvular disease
    4. Cardiac tamponade
    5. Pulmonary hypertension
C. **Renal vasoconstrictive states** resulting in ischemia may be caused by the following:
    1. Cirrhosis with ascites
    2. Vasoconstrictive drugs: epinephrine, norepinephrine, cyclosporine, amphotericin B
D. Intrinsic decrease of renal perfusion
    1. Cyclooxygenase (COX) inhibitors, NSAIDs
    2. ACE inhibitors

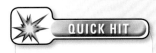

Cyclooxygenase is inhibited by aspirin and other nonsteroidal anti-inflammatory drugs (NSAIDs).

FIGURE
6-10 Etiology of acute renal failure

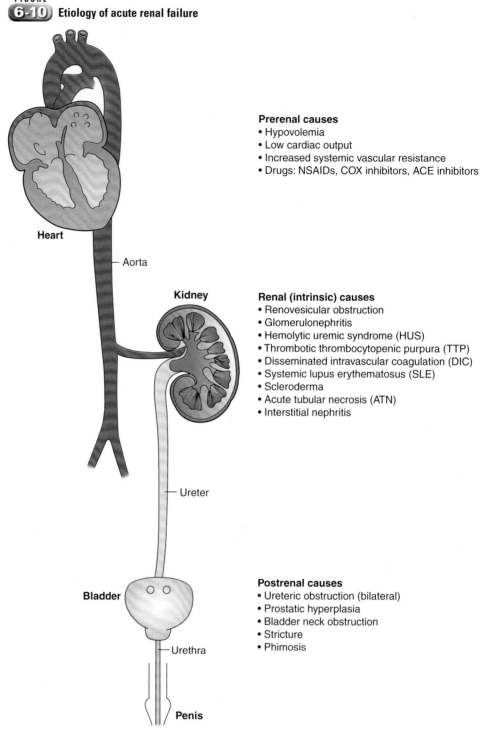

Prerenal causes
- Hypovolemia
- Low cardiac output
- Increased systemic vascular resistance
- Drugs: NSAIDs, COX inhibitors, ACE inhibitors

Heart

Aorta

Kidney

Renal (intrinsic) causes
- Renovesicular obstruction
- Glomerulonephritis
- Hemolytic uremic syndrome (HUS)
- Thrombotic thrombocytopenic purpura (TTP)
- Disseminated intravascular coagulation (DIC)
- Systemic lupus erythematosus (SLE)
- Scleroderma
- Acute tubular necrosis (ATN)
- Interstitial nephritis

Ureter

Bladder

Postrenal causes
- Ureteric obstruction (bilateral)
- Prostatic hyperplasia
- Bladder neck obstruction
- Stricture
- Phimosis

Urethra

Penis

ACE, angiotensin-converting enzyme; COX, cyclooxygenase; NSAIDs, nonsteroidal anti-inflammatory drugs.

TABLE 6-7 Prerenal versus Intrinsic Renal Failure

	Prerenal Renal Failure	Intrinsic Renal Failure
Fractional excretion of Na$^+$	<1	>1
Urine sodium concentration	<10 mg/dL	>20 mg/dL
Urine creatinine to plasma creatinine	>40	>20
Urine casts	Hyaline	Muddy brown and granular
Plasma blood urea nitrogen–to–creatinine ratio	>20	<10–15

Na$^+$, sodium.

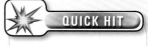

QUICK HIT

Fractional excretion of sodium (FENa$^+$) is calculated using the formula:

$$FENa^+ = 100 \times \frac{\frac{urine\ [Na^+]}{serum\ [Na^+]}}{\frac{urine\ [Cr]}{serum\ [Cr]}}$$

II. **Acute intrinsic renal failure is the inherent malfunction of the renal tissue. It may be glomerular, tubular, or interstitial. Table 6-7 compares prerenal failure with intrinsic renal failure.**
  A. **Acute tubular necrosis** (ATN)
    1. Drugs that may lead to ATN are exogenous toxins (contrast, cyclosporine, aminoglycosides, ethylene glycol, acetaminophen, heavy metals) or endogenous toxins (myoglobin, uric acid, oxalate).
    2. Ischemia can result in ATN via causes related to prerenal failure.
  B. Obstruction of renal vasculature from atherosclerosis, vasculitis, or other factors may also cause acute intrinsic renal failure.
  C. Diseases that affect the glomeruli or microvasculature
    1. Disseminated intravascular coagulation (DIC)
    2. Glomerulonephritis
    3. Hemolytic uremic syndrome (HUS)
    4. Thrombotic thrombocytopenic purpura (TTP)
    5. Pregnancy
    6. Scleroderma
    7. Systemic lupus erythematosus (SLE)
  D. **Interstitial nephritis** can have many causes.
    1. β-Lactams
    2. Sulfonamides
    3. Trimethoprim (TMP)
    4. Rifampin
    5. COX inhibitors
    6. Diuretics
    7. Captopril
    8. Infection
    9. Idiopathic
  E. Acute renal transplant rejection is a cause of ATN.

III. **Postrenal failure is bilateral obstruction of the ureters or obstruction of the urethra. It accounts for less than 5% of acute renal failure (ARF) and has a variety of causes.**
  A. Urolithiasis (see section on stone formation)
  B. Prostatic hyperplasia
  C. Tumor obstructing the bladder or the ureters bilaterally
  D. Neurogenic bladder

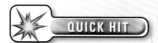

QUICK HIT

Exogenous toxins causing acute tubular necrosis include contrast, cyclosporine, ethylene glycol, and acetaminophen. Endogenous toxins include myoglobin, uric acid, and oxalate.

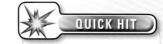

QUICK HIT

The most **common** cause of acute renal failure (ARF) is therapeutic drugs.

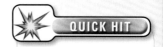

QUICK HIT

HUS and TTP cause a "flea-bitten" kidney.

QUICK HIT

Renal transplant rejection rates can be decreased by administration of cyclosporine and muromonab-CD3 (OKT3).

CHRONIC RENAL FAILURE AND UREMIA (*Figure 6-11*)

I. **Major causes of chronic renal failure (CRF)**
  A. **Hypertension**
  B. **Diabetes mellitus**

The Renal System

FIGURE
6-11 Manifestations of chronic renal failure and uremia

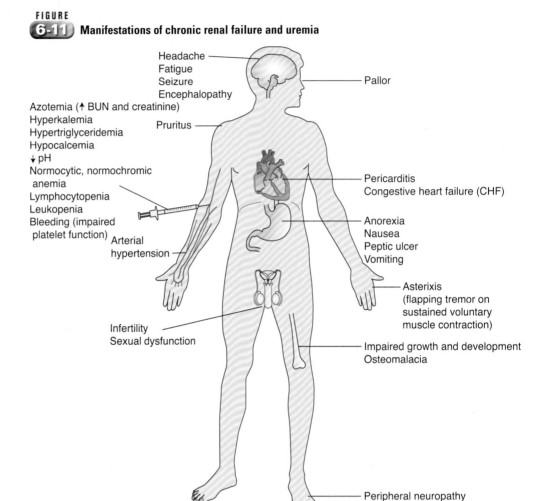

BUN, blood urea nitrogen.

II. Profound loss of renal function leads to uremia.

A. GFR is reduced to 50% to 65% of normal.

B. Byproducts of amino acid and protein metabolism (especially urea) cause a variety of signs and symptoms.

1. **Endocrine and electrolyte findings**
   a. Hyperkalemia
   b. Hyperphosphatemia
   c. Hypertriglyceridemia
   d. Hyperuricemia
   e. Hypocalcemia and osteomalacia as a result of decreased 1,25-dihydroxy-cholecalciferol levels
   f. Impaired growth and development
   g. Infertility and sexual dysfunction
   h. Metabolic acidosis

2. **Gastrointestinal findings**
   a. Anorexia
   b. Nausea
   c. Peptic ulcer
   d. Vomiting

3. **Renal findings**: azotemia

4. **Cardiovascular and pulmonary findings**
   a. Arterial hypertension
   b. Congestive heart failure
   c. Pericarditis

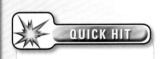

QUICK HIT

Uremia causes burr cells. Burr cells are misshapen red blood cells (RBCs) with irregular fingerlike projections from their surface.

The Renal System

5. Dermatologic findings
   a. Pallor
   b. Pruritus
   c. "Uremic frost" (crystallized urea on the skin)
6. Neuromuscular findings
   a. Asterixis
   b. Headache and fatigue
   c. Peripheral neuropathy
7. Hematologic findings
   a. Increased susceptibility to infection
   b. Lymphocytopenia and leukopenia
   c. Normocytic, normochromic anemia

Clinical Vignette 6-3

CLINICAL PRESENTATION: A 55-year-old woman presents to her primary care physician with the chief complaint of **nausea, vomiting,** and **feeling "out of it"** over the past 2 days. She also reports **urinating less frequently** and **weight gain,** although she does not have much of an appetite. Her past medical history is significant for **CHF.** Physical examination reveals generalized edema and a 10-lb weight gain since her last visit 1 month ago.

DIFFERENTIALS: Acute renal failure (ARF), chronic renal failure (CRF), acute tubular necrosis. ARF is defined as rapid, progressive decrease in renal function characterized by elevation in blood urea nitrogen/creatinine (BUN/Cr) and possibly oliguria. Renal failure can be prerenal, intrinsic renal, or postrenal. Prerenal failure is caused by insufficient renal perfusion as in CHF, whereas postrenal failure is caused by obstructed renal outflow. Intrinsic renal failure is caused by parenchymal damage to the glomerulus, tubules, interstitium, or vasculature. There are a number of causes for each type of renal failure (Figure 6-10). In this patient, hypovolemia from CHF is the cause of insufficient renal perfusion. Acute tubular necrosis causes 85% of intrinsic renal failure, but we would expect some history of renal ischemia or toxin exposure (see Quick Hit). CRF has lab findings in common with ARF, but we would expect clinical manifestations of uremia and multiple instances of abnormal BUN, Cr, and urinalysis.

LABORATORY STUDIES: A urinalysis would be obtained looking for the presence of casts. Presence of muddy brown casts (seen in acute tubular necrosis), red blood cell (RBC) casts (glomerular disease), or white blood cell (WBC) casts (pyelonephritis, acute interstitial nephritis) would not be expected in ARF. **Urine chemistry** consisting of BUN/Cr, fractional excretion of sodium (FENa$^+$), and urine osmolality would also be obtained. In prerenal and postrenal failure, the **BUN:Cr ratio** is typically greater than 20:1 because of increased urea absorption as compared to intrinsic renal failure. In prerenal failure, the FENa$^+$ is less than 1% because the decreased glomerular filtration rate causes massive reabsorption of sodium and water, whereas in intrinsic renal failure, the FENa$^+$ is greater than 2% to 3% because Na is poorly reabsorbed. Similarly, we expect increased **urine osmolality** in prerenal failure because the kidney is able to reabsorb water, whereas we see decreased urine osmolality in intrinsic renal failure because renal water reabsorption is impaired. Also, **renal ultrasound** would be obtained to rule out obstruction. Renal ultrasound showing small, echogenic kidneys are pathognomonic of CRF.

MANAGEMENT: The most important part of therapy is to follow urinary output: Patients with ARF first experience an **oliguric phase** followed by a **diuretic phase.** Approximately 40% of patients go on to a **recovery phase** with normalization of urine output. **Correct fluid imbalance**—some patients with ARF are dehydrated, whereas others are volume overloaded. Correct any **electrolyte abnormalities** and **optimize cardiac output.** Order **dialysis** if symptomatic uremia, acidemia, hyperkalemia, or volume overload develops.

The Renal System

KIDNEY STONE FORMATION (Figure 6-12)

FIGURE

6-12 **Comparison of different types of kidney stones**

Calcium stones
A. Calcium oxalate (CO)   B. Calcium phosphate (CP)

80% of stones
Men
20–30 years of age
Multiple (every 2–3 years)
Familial predisposition
Radiopaque
May be caused by primary hyperthyroidism
CP stones form more readily in alkaline urine pH >6

Struvite
12% of stones
Women
Risk factors:
Catheter, UTIs (especially *Proteus*)
May fill renal pelvis and calyces ("staghorn")
Radiopaque

Uric acid
7% of stones
Men
Risk factors:
50% have gout
Strong negative birefringence
Radiolucent
Associated with cell lysis (e.g., chemotherapy, leukemia)
Uric acid increases urine acidity to pH <5.5

Cystine
1% of stones
Uncommon
Hereditary
Radiopaque (because of sulfur component)
Natural inhibitors of stone formation are (1) citrate,
(2) nephrocalcin, (3) Tamm-Horsfall protein (aka uromodulin), and
(4) uropontin.

Clinical manifestations of kidney stones include hematuria and flank pain. UTI, urinary tract infection.

AUTOSOMAL DOMINANT POLYCYSTIC KIDNEY DISEASE (Figure 6-13)

FIGURE
6-13 **Autosomal dominant polycystic kidney disease (ADPKD) versus normal kidney**

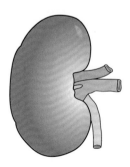
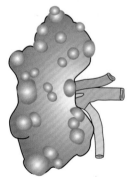

Normal kidney   Kidney with ADPKD

I. Etiology of autosomal dominant polycystic kidney disease (ADPKD)
   A. Autosomal dominant
   B. Occurs in midlife

II. Clinical features of ADPKD
   A. Bilateral
   B. Kidney parenchyma is partially replaced with cysts
   C. **Hematuria**
   D. Hypertension
   E. **Large palpable kidneys**
   F. Progressively worsening renal function leading to renal failure

III. ADPKD is associated with berry aneurysms of circle of Willis and cystic disease in other organs, especially the liver.

RENAL CANCERS (Table 6-8)

I. The classic triad of hematuria, flank pain, and a flank mass is seen only in 10% to 20% of patients with renal cancer. Most are sporadic; however, smoking accounts for 20% to 30% of the cases.

TABLE 6-8 Renal Cancers

Malignancy	Etiology	Clinical Features	Notes
Renal cell carcinoma	**Smoking;** alteration of chromosome 3 (as seen in **von Hippel–Lindau disease**)	Afflicts men 45–65 years of age; hematuria; mass; pain; fever; **secondary polycythemia;** paraneoplastic syndrome; usually extends from renal poles, with **clear cells**	Most common renal malignancy; may be associated with increased erythropoietin (EPO)
Wilms tumor (nephroblastoma)	Chromosome 11 abnormality, **WAGR**	**Palpable flank mass** in children 2–5 years old; hematuria	Most common renal malignancy of childhood (see following)
Transitional cell carcinoma	Cyclophosphamide treatment, **smoking,** aniline dye exposure	Hematuria	Most common tumor of the collecting system

WAGR, Wilms tumor, aniridia, genitourinary abnormalities, and mental retardation.

II. Nephroblastoma (Wilms tumor)
   A. **Most common malignant renal tumor in children**
   B. Malignant tissue is derived from embryonic nephrogenic tissue.
   C. Peak incidence is between 2 and 4 years of age.
   D. The **two-hit theory** of oncogenesis, which explains the etiology of Wilms tumor, requires a mutation of both copies of the Wilms tumor-1 (WT-1) tumor-suppressor gene on chromosome 11p.
   E. **Characteristic clinical features**
      1. Hematuria
      2. Hypertension
      3. Large abdominal mass
      4. Intestinal obstruction
   F. Part of **WAGR syndrome** (Wilms tumor, Aniridia, Genital anomalies, mental Retardation)

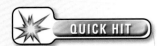

QUICK HIT

In altitude sickness, in order to get enough oxygen, hyperventilation occurs, which causes respiratory alkalosis. Carbonic anhydrase inhibitors speed metabolic compensation by increasing urinary excretion of HCO_3^-, causing metabolic acidosis.

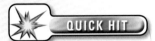

QUICK HIT

Mannitol and other osmotic diuretics also "pull" fluid into the bloodstream, thus decreasing pressure in glaucoma, in cases of **increased intracranial pressure**, and in surgery.

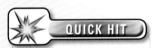

QUICK HIT

Loop diuretics, which have direct **pulmonary vasodilatory** properties, are particularly useful in the treatment of pulmonary edema.

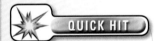

QUICK HIT

Thiazide diuretics are sulfa derivatives and should be used with caution in patients with sulfa drug allergies.

DIURETICS AND FLUID BALANCE

I. Diuretics

A. The diuretics in Figure 6-14 can be grouped into five main categories, each with a different mechanism of action (Table 6-9). The side effects of each type of diuretic are also different, which means that certain diuretics are better suited for certain patients.

FIGURE 6-14 Effects of diuretics on the nephron

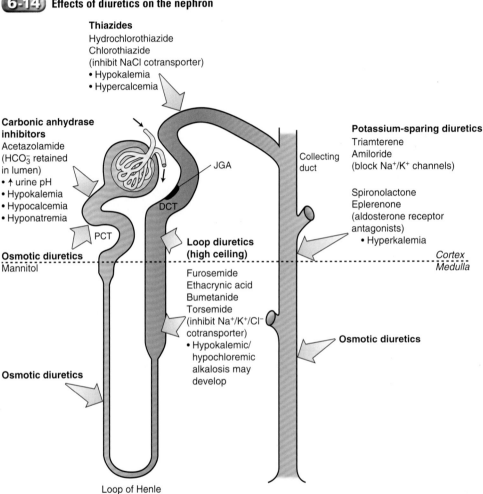

Thiazides
Hydrochlorothiazide
Chlorothiazide
(inhibit NaCl cotransporter)
• Hypokalemia
• Hypercalcemia

Carbonic anhydrase inhibitors
Acetazolamide
(HCO_3^- retained in lumen)
• ↑ urine pH
• Hypokalemia
• Hypocalcemia
• Hyponatremia

JGA

DCT

PCT

Osmotic diuretics
Mannitol

Collecting duct

Potassium-sparing diuretics
Triamterene
Amiloride
(block Na^+/K^+ channels)

Spironolactone
Eplerenone
(aldosterone receptor antagonists)
• Hyperkalemia

Cortex
Medulla

Loop diuretics (high ceiling)
Furosemide
Ethacrynic acid
Bumetanide
Torsemide
(inhibit $Na^+/K^+/Cl^-$ cotransporter)
• Hypokalemic/ hypochloremic alkalosis may develop

Osmotic diuretics

Osmotic diuretics

Loop of Henle

Cl^-, chloride; DCT, distal convoluted tubule; HCO_3^-, bicarbonate; JGA, juxtaglomerular apparatus; K^+, potassium; Na^+, sodium; PCT, proximal convoluted tubule.

The Renal System

TABLE 6-9 Diuretics

Therapeutic Agent	Mechanism of Action	Electrolytes Lost in Urine	Indications	Side Effects	Notes
Acetazolamide	Carbonic anhydrase inhibitors—inhibit carbonic anhydrase in **PCT,** which prevents HCO_3^- reabsorption	Na^+ HCO_3^-, K^+	Glaucoma, urinary alkalinization, metabolic alkalosis, altitude sickness	**Hyperchloremic metabolic acidosis, sulfa drug allergy,** neuropathy, ammonium toxicity	Causes decreased secretion of HCO_3^- in aqueous humor
Loop diuretics					
Furosemide, torsemide, bumetanide, ethacrynic acid	Prevents cotransport of Na^+, K^+, and Cl^- in **thick ascending limb** of loop of Henle	Na^+, Cl^-, Ca^{2+}, K^+	**Congestive heart failure,** cirrhosis, nephrotic syndrome, pulmonary edema, hypertension, hypercalcemia	**Ototoxicity, hypokalemic metabolic alkalosis, dehydration, sulfa drug allergy** (not ethacrynic acid), nephritis, gout	Has rapid onset and short duration of action, which is ideal for relieving acute edema
Mannitol	Osmotic diuretic—prevents isosmotic reabsorption of filtrate in **PCT, loop of Henle,** and **collecting tubule**	Na^+ and all other filtered solutes	Shock, drug overdose, decrease intracranial or intraocular pressure; maintenance of urine flow in rhabdomyolysis	Pulmonary edema, dehydration; contraindicated in anuria and congestive heart failure	Results in increased urine volume; readily filtered and not reabsorbed
Potassium-sparing diuretics					
Spironolactone, eplerenone	Binds to intracellular aldosterone steroid receptors in **collecting tubules**	Na^+, Cl^-	Hyperaldosteronism, potassium depletion, congestive heart failure, post-MI	**Hyperkalemic metabolic acidosis, gynecomastia,** and antiandrogen effects (spironolactone only)	Results in decreased secretion of K^+ and H^+, which can lead to **hyperkalemic metabolic acidosis**
Triamterene, amiloride	Blocks Na^+ channels in **collecting tubules**	Na^+, Cl^-	Hypertension, potassium depletion	**Hyperkalemic metabolic acidosis**	Often given in combination with a thiazide
Thiazides					
Hydrochlorothiazide (HCTZ), chlorthalidone,	Inhibit transport of Na^+ and Cl^- into cells of the **DCT**	Na^+, Cl^-, K^+	Hypertension, idiopathic hypercalciuria, nephrogenic diabetes insipidus	**Hypokalemic metabolic alkalosis,** hyponatremia, **hyperglycemia, hyperlipidemia,** hyperuricemia, hypercalcemia, **sulfa drug allergy**	Causes decreased Ca^{2+} excretion, can lead to K^+ wasting with chronic therapy

Ca^{2+}, calcium; Cl^-, chloride; DCT, distal convoluted tubule; HCO_3^-, bicarbonate; K^+, potassium; MI, myocardial infarction; Na^+, sodium; PCT, proximal convoluted tubule.

The Renal System

II. Antidiuretic hormone

A. ADH causes an increase in the expression of **water channels** in the collecting tubule, which results in an increase in the reabsorption of water. Urine output drops, and concentration increases.

B. In the syndrome of inappropriate secretion of antidiuretic hormone (SIADH), **lithium** or **demeclocycline**, which blocks the effects of ADH, can be administered to prevent excessive water retention.

C. In central diabetes insipidus, either **desmopressin** (an ADH analog) or ADH can be given to prevent the excessive loss of dilute urine. These drugs are not useful in the nephrogenic (also known as the peripheral) form of diabetes insipidus, in which the kidneys do not respond to ADH.

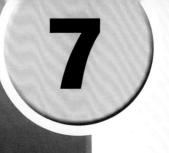

The Endocrine System

 DEVELOPMENT

I. Hypothalamus
A. A division of the **diencephalon**
B. Forms from the embryologic forebrain (see Chapter 2)

II. Pituitary gland consists of two lobes
A. Anterior lobe: forms from **Rathke pouch**, an ectodermal diverticulum of the primitive mouth that invaginates upward
B. Posterior lobe: forms from an evagination of the **hypothalamus**

III. Thyroid gland
A. It forms from the endoderm of the floor of the pharynx.
B. It begins as a diverticulum that migrates caudally.
C. Thyroid follicular cells are derived from endoderm.

IV. Parathyroid glands
A. **Inferior parathyroid glands** develop from the **third pharyngeal pouch**.
B. **Superior parathyroid glands** develop from the **fourth pharyngeal pouch**.
C. The parathyroid glands migrate caudally and come to lie on the dorsal surface of the thyroid gland.

V. Adrenal glands
A. **Gross description**
   1. Paired adult adrenal glands weigh 4 g each.
   2. They are located immediately anterosuperior to the superior renal poles.
   3. They are enclosed in renal fascia.
B. **Adrenal cortex**
   1. Forms from the mesoderm
   2. Includes three major parts
      a. Zona glomerulosa and zona fasciculata are present at birth.
      b. **Zona reticularis** is not completely formed until 3 years of age.
C. Medulla of adrenal gland
   1. **Chromaffin cells** form from neural crest cells that invade the adrenal glands during development.
   2. These cells are in essence postganglionic neurons of the sympathetic nervous system.

VI. Pancreas
A. It forms from a ventral and dorsal bud of endoderm from the foregut.
   1. The ventral bud forms the uncinate process and part of the pancreatic head.
   2. The dorsal bud forms part of the head, body, and tail.

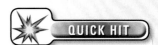

QUICK HIT

DiGeorge syndrome is a malformation of the third and fourth pharyngeal pouches caused by a mutation of 22q11, leading to a spectrum of disorders including thymic hypoplasia, T-cell deficiency, absent parathyroids, and hypocalcemia.

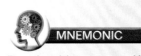

MNEMONIC

Thyroglossal duct cysts are **midline** cysts of the neck. **B**ranchial cleft cysts lie **l**aterally anywhere along the **a**nterior border of the sternocleidomastoid muscle.

B. Exocrine pancreas: Acinar cells and ducts form from endoderm surrounded by mesoderm.
C. Endocrine pancreas: Mesodermal cells aggregate to form **pancreatic islet cells**.

VII. Gonads (*see Chapter 8*)

CONGENITAL MALFORMATIONS (*Table 7-1*)

There is a wide spectrum of developmental abnormalities involving the endocrine system. Some of these malformations are anatomic, whereas others are biochemical.

TABLE 7-1 **Congenital Malformations**	
Malformation	**Description**
Craniopharyngioma	Cystic tumor of the pituitary that forms from the remnants of the **Rathke pouch**; may cause diabetes insipidus
Thyroglossal duct cysts	A remnant of the descending migratory path of the thyroid that persists into adult life Most are asymptomatic, but an infection may cause swelling and produce a progressively enlarging movable mass
Absence of parathyroid glands	Occurs in **DiGeorge syndrome** (thymic aplasia) (see Chapter 10) Inability to produce parathyroid hormone leads to hypoparathyroidism and hypocalcemia
Congenital adrenal hyperplasia	Figure 7-9
Annular pancreas	Ventral and dorsal pancreatic buds form a ring around the duodenum; may cause **duodenal obstruction**
Accessory pancreatic tissue	Normal pancreatic tissue found within the wall of the stomach; most common type of choristoma (normal tissue found misplaced within another organ)

HORMONES (*Table 7-2*)

Hormones are biologically active chemicals formed in an organ and carried through the blood to act on adjacent cells of the same organ or on a different body part. Hormone function can be localized or systemic. Hormones can alter the activity or structure of the target organ(s) depending on the specificity of the hormone's effects. Hormones play an essential role in homeostasis, reproductive function, and metabolism, and they are vital in nearly every other body system as well.

The Endocrine System

TABLE 7-2 Hormones

Hormone	Secreted by	End-Organ Effects of Hormones	Stimulated by	Inhibited by
GnRH	Hypothalamus	LH/FSH secretion	Puberty	Progesterone, testosterone
FSH	Anterior pituitary gland	Growth of follicles and estrogen secretion (acts on granulosa cells); maturation of sperm (acts on Sertoli cells)	Pulsatile release of GnRH	Constant GnRH release; inhibin
LH	Anterior pituitary gland (basophils)	Ovulation; formation of corpus luteum; estrogen/progesterone synthesis (acts on theca lutein cells); synthesis/secretion of testosterone (acts on Leydig cells)	Pulsatile release of GnRH	Constant GnRH release; progesterone, testosterone
Estrogen	Ovary (granulosa cells)	Proliferative phase of menstrual cycle; development of female reproductive organs	FSH	Estrogen
Progesterone	Ovary (granulosa lutein cells)	Breast development; secretory activity during luteal phase	LH	Progesterone
Testosterone	Testes (Leydig cells)	Spermatogenesis; conversion of testosterone to dihydrotestosterone via 5α-reductase stimulates development of secondary male sex characteristics	LH	Testosterone
hCG	Placenta (syncytiotrophoblast)	Increased estrogen/progesterone synthesis; maintains corpus luteum secretion of estrogen and progesterone	Trophoblast differentiation after implantation of fertilized egg	
ACTH	Anterior pituitary	Synthesis and secretion of adrenal cortical hormones	CRH, stress	Cortisol
Cortisol (glucocorticoids)	Adrenal cortex (zona fasciculata)	Anti-inflammatory effects (via inhibition of phospholipase A2); immunosuppressive effects; stimulation of gluconeogenesis; increased blood sugar	ACTH	Cortisol
Aldosterone	Adrenal cortex (zona glomerulosa)	Increased renal sodium reabsorption and potassium secretion; increase in blood volume	Decrease in blood volume; angiotensin II; hyperkalemia; hyponatremia	Hypernatremia, hypokalemia, fluid overload
TSH	Anterior pituitary	Synthesis and secretion of thyroid hormone (T_4, T_3)	TRH	T_4, T_3

(continued)

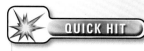

QUICK HIT

Luteinizing hormone (LH), follicle-stimulating hormone (FSH), human chorionic gonadotropin (hCG), and thyroid-stimulating hormone (TSH) are hormones consisting of two subunits: α and β. The α subunits in these hormones are identical, whereas the β subunit is unique for each.

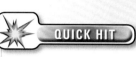

QUICK HIT

Finasteride, a 5α-reductase inhibitor, is used in the treatment of benign prostatic hyperplasia. Flutamide, a competitive androgen receptor blocker, is used to treat prostatic carcinoma.

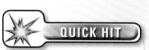

QUICK HIT

Antibodies specific for β-hCG are used in pregnancy tests. Increased β-hCG can be detected 1 to 2 weeks after conception.

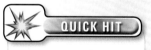

QUICK HIT

The hormone hCG is increased in normal pregnancy, hydatidiform moles, choriocarcinomas, gestational tumors, ectopic pregnancy, and pseudocyesis.

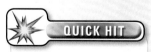

QUICK HIT

The anti-inflammatory effect of cortisol is mediated by its induction of **lipocortin**, which inhibits phospholipase A2 and prostaglandin synthesis. Cortisol also inhibits the production of interleukin-2 (IL-2).

The Endocrine System

TABLE 7-2 Hormones (Continued)

Hormone	Secreted by	End-Organ Effects of Hormones	Stimulated by	Inhibited by
T$_4$, T$_3$	Thyroid	Growth; maturation of CNS; increased basal metabolic rate, cardiac output, and nutrient use	TSH, estrogen	Somatostatin, dopamine
Somatostatin (somatotropin-inhibiting hormone)	Hypothalamus	Inhibited secretion of growth hormone	Growth hormone, somatomedins (IGF)	
GH (somatotropin)	Anterior pituitary (acidophils)	Decreased glucose uptake; increased protein synthesis, growth, organ size, and lean body mass	GHRH, exercise, sleep, puberty, hypoglycemia, estrogen, stress, endogenous opiates	Somatomedins (IGF), somatostatin, obesity, pregnancy, hyperglycemia
Prolactin	Anterior pituitary (acidophils)	Stimulation of milk production and secretion, breast development, inhibition of ovulation	Prolactin-stimulating factor, TRH	Prolactin-inhibiting factor (dopamine)
Oxytocin	Hypothalamus via posterior pituitary	Milk ejection from breast (milk letdown), uterine contraction	Suckling, sex, dilation of the cervix	Alcohol, stress
PTH	Parathyroid gland (chief cells)	Increased serum calcium, increased renal calcium absorption, inhibition of phosphate reabsorption, activates vitamin D to increase intestinal calcium absorption	Decreased serum calcium, mild decreased serum magnesium	Severe decrease in serum magnesium
Vitamin D 1,25-dihydroxycho-lecalciferol	Kidney (active form produced by activity of 1α-hydroxylase), sun-exposed skin	Increased intestinal calcium and phosphorus absorption, increased bone calcium resorption, increased kidney phosphate and calcium reabsorption	Decreased serum calcium, increased PTH, decreased serum phosphate	
ADH (vasopressin)	Hypothalamus via posterior pituitary	Increased water permeability in distal tubules and collecting duct to regulate osmolarity (V2 receptor), constriction of vascular smooth muscle (V1 receptor)	Volume contraction, nicotine, opiates, increased serum osmolarity	Ethanol, ANF, decreased serum osmolarity
ANF	Atrial myocytes	Vasodilation to decrease systemic BP, increase urinary Na$^+$ and H$_2$O excretion	Atrial stretch due to blood volume increase	ANF
Glucagon	Pancreatic islet cells (α cells)	Increased blood glucose, increased glycogenolysis and gluconeo-genesis in the liver, increased lipolysis and ketone production	Decreased blood glucose; increased amino acids, ACh	Increased blood glucose; insulin; somatostatin
Insulin	Pancreatic islet cells (β cells)	Decreased blood glucose caused by increased uptake into muscle and fat, decreased glycogenolysis and gluconeogenesis, increased protein synthesis, increased fat deposition, inhibition of lipolysis	Increased blood glucose, amino acids; glucagon; ACh	Decreased blood glucose; somatostatin
Leptin	Fat cells	Reduced food intake (satiety); inhibits the arcuate nucleus and lateral nucleus of the hypothalamus, stimulates the ventrome-dial nucleus of the hypothalamus	Obesity, overeating, pregnancy	Fasting

ACh, acetylcholine; ACTH, adrenocorticotropic hormone; ADH, antidiuretic hormone; ANF, atrial natriuretic factor; BP, blood pressure; CNS, central nervous system; CRH, corticotropin-releasing hormone; FSH, follicle-stimulating hormone; GH, growth hormone; GHRH, growth hormone–releasing hormone; GnRH, gonadotropin-releasing hormone; hCG, human chorionic gonadotropin; IGF, insulin-like growth factor; LH, luteinizing hormone; PTH, parathyroid hormone; T$_3$, triiodothyronine; T$_4$, thyroxine; TRH, thyrotropin-releasing hormone; TSH, thyroid-stimulating hormone.

I. Hormones of the hypothalamic–pituitary axis (*Figure 7-1*)

II. Hormones of the adrenal gland (*Figure 7-2*)

III. Hormone second-messenger system

The second-messenger system is the process by which extracellular signals are translated into cellular responses. Biologically active chemicals, such as hormones, bind to receptor sites on the cell membrane, resulting in phosphorylation of intracellular proteins or changes in ion channel conductivity and subsequent cellular modulation (Table 7-3 and Figure 7-3).

FIGURE 7-1 Hormones of the hypothalamic–pituitary axis

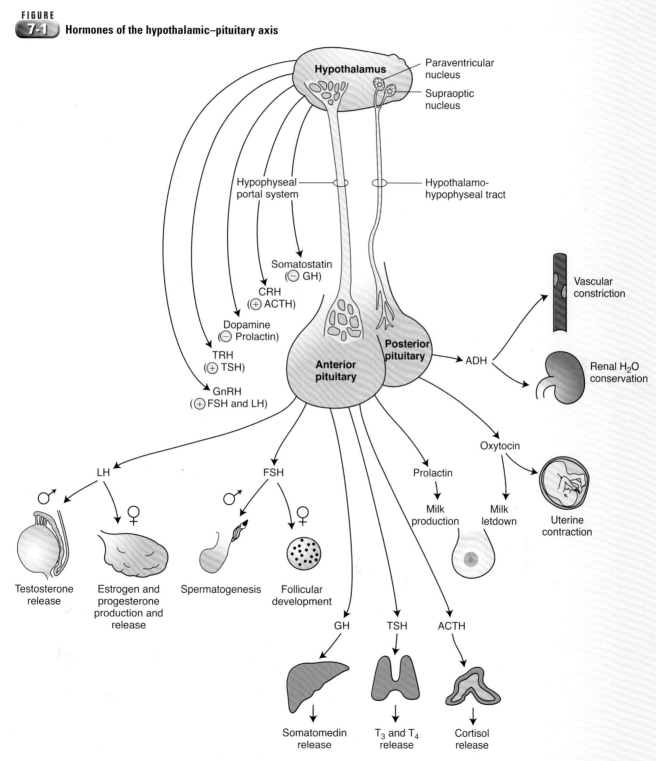

ACTH, adrenocorticotropic hormone; ADH, antidiuretic hormone; CRH, corticotropin-releasing hormone; FSH, follicle-stimulating hormone; GH, growth hormone; GnRH, gonadotropin-releasing hormone; LH, luteinizing hormone; T$_3$, triiodothyronine; T$_4$, thyroxine; TRH, thyrotropin-releasing hormone; TSH, thyroid-stimulating hormone.

The Endocrine System

MNEMONIC

To remember the anatomic layers of the adrenal cortex, think **GFR: G**lomerulosa, **F**asciculata, and **R**eticularis. To remember the hormones produced by each layer, think **"the deeper you go, the sweeter it gets"**: aldosterone (**salt** hormone), glucocorticoid (**sugar** hormone), and androgens (**sex** hormone).

FIGURE
7-2 Hormones of the adrenal gland

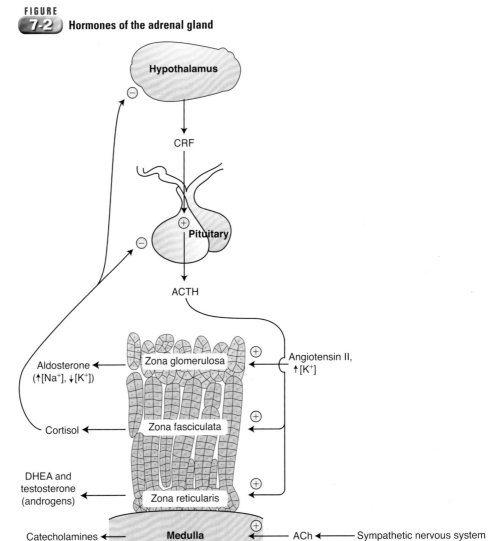

ACh, acetylcholine; ACTH, adrenocorticotropic hormone; CRF, corticotropin-releasing factor; DHEA, dehydroepiandrosterone; Epi, epinephrine; NE, norepineprine.

TABLE **7-3** **Hormone Second-messenger Systems**

cAMP	cGMP	IP₃	Steroid	Tyrosine Kinase
β₁-agonists	ANF	α₁-agonists	Aldosterone	Insulin
β₂-agonists	EDRF	GnRH	Estrogen	IGF-1
LH		TRH	Glucocorticoids	Prolactin
FSH		GHRH	Testosterone	GH
TSH		Angiotensin II	Progesterone	
ADH (V₂)		ADH (V₁)	Thyroid	
hCG		Oxytocin	Vitamin D	
CRH				
PTH				
Calcitonin				
Glucagon				

ADH, antidiuretic hormone; ANF, atrial natriuretic factor (also known as ANP, atrial natriuretic peptide); cAMP, cyclic adenosine monophosphate; cGMP, cyclic guanosine monophosphate; CRH, corticotropin-releasing hormone; EDRF, endothelium-derived relaxing factor; FSH, follicle-stimulating hormone; GH, growth hormone; GHRH, growth hormone–releasing hormone; GnRH, gonadotropin-releasing hormone; hCG, human chorionic gonadotropin; IGF, insulin-like growth factor; IP₃, inositol triphosphate; LH, luteinizing hormone; PTH, parathyroid hormone; TRH, thyrotropin-releasing hormone; TSH, thyroid-stimulating hormone.

The Endocrine System

FIGURE 7-3 Hormone second-messenger systems

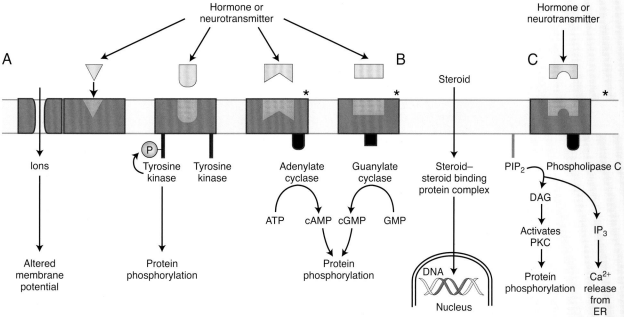

A. Peptide mechanism. Peptide binds to hormone receptor site and influences various second-messenger systems. These hormones are typically short acting and do not involve gene regulation, in contrast to steroid hormones, which have a slower onset of action.

B. Steroid mechanism. Lipid-soluble steroid penetrates cell membrane and binds to steroid-binding protein. This complex enters the nucleus and influences DNA synthesis.

C. Phospholipase C mechanism

D. G-protein mechanism.

1. Messenger system before hormone binding
2. After hormone binding, GTP replaces GDP on G protein.
3. GTP, attached to α subunit, dissociates from the β–γ complex and converts ATP to cAMP.
4. Hormone is released from binding site and complex returns to inactive state when GTPase cleaves GTP to GDP.

*Mechanism using a G protein, as shown in D.

ATP, adenosine triphosphate; cAMP, cyclic adenosine monophosphate; cGMP, cyclic guanosine monophosphate; DAG, diacylglycerol; ER, endoplasmic reticulum; GDP, guanosine 5′-diphosphate; GMP, guanosine monophosphate; GTP, guanosine triphosphate; IP₃, inositol triphosphate; PIP₂, phosphatidylinositol 4,5-bisphosphate; PKC, protein kinase C.

G-Protein Class	Action	Examples
G_q	Activates phospholipase C → cleaves phospholipids to form PIP_2, which is subsequently cleaved into DAG and IP_3. DAG activates protein kinase C. IP_3 increases intracellular calcium, which also has downstream effects (including activating protein kinase C).	H_1, α_1, V_1, M_1, M_3
G_s	Stimulates adenylyl cyclase → converts ATP to cAMP, which activates protein kinase A	β_1, β_2, D_1, H_2, V_2
G_i	Inhibits adenylyl cyclase → decreased cAMP production → decreased activity of protein kinase A	M_2, α_2, D_2

ATP, adenosine triphosphate; cAMP, cyclic adenosine monophosphate; DAG, diacylglycerol; IP₃, inositol triphosphate; PIP₂, phosphatidylinositol 4,5-bisphosphate.

CALCIUM HOMEOSTASIS (Figure 7-4)

FIGURE 7-4 Calcium homeostasis

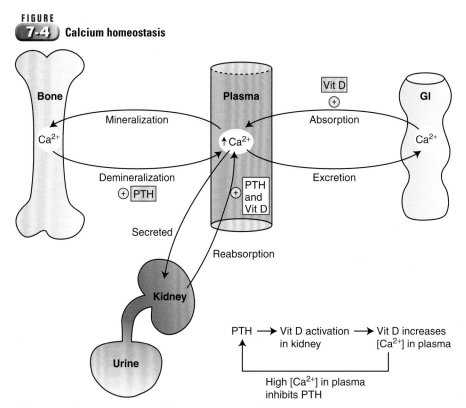

Ca²⁺, calcium; GI, gastrointestinal tract; PTH, parathyroid hormone; Vit D, vitamin D.

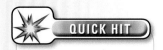

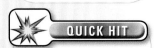

INSULIN AND GLUCAGON

Insulin is a polypeptide hormone that serves to regulate several physiologic processes. Its primary role, in conjunction with the polypeptide hormone glucagon, is to **maintain blood glucose levels.** When blood glucose levels rise after a meal, insulin is released from the β cells of the pancreatic islets of Langerhans in proportion to the glucose concentration of blood. Innervation of pancreatic islets by a branch of the vagus nerve helps coordinate insulin release with digestion. Insulin interacts with surface receptors on muscle and adipose tissue and stimulates glucose absorption and triacylglycerol synthesis. In the liver, insulin inhibits gluconeogenesis and glycogen breakdown.

Insulin is formed by two polypeptides linked by disulfide bridges (Figure 7-5). The insulin receptor is **tyrosine kinase** linked; binding of insulin to the α subunit causes phosphorylation of the tyrosine kinase connected to the β subunit. This stimulates recruitment of glucose transporters (GLUTs) to the cell membrane (GLUT-4 in skeletal muscle) and increases the uptake of glucose (Figure 7-6). Glucagon counteracts the actions of insulin. It is a single polypeptide secreted by the α cells of the islets of Langerhans. Glucagon is secreted in response to low blood glucose, increased amino acids in the blood, and epinephrine. Glucagon secretion leads to a rise in blood glucose concentration via **gluconeogenesis** and **glycogenolysis.** Release of glucagon is inhibited by insulin. Glucagon is also responsible for the formation of ketone bodies, and increased uptake of amino acids by the liver muscle is not responsive to glucagon.

- **Blood Levels of Glucose, Insulin, and Glucagon after a High-Carbohydrate Meal** (Figure 7-7)

FIGURE 7-5 Formation of insulin

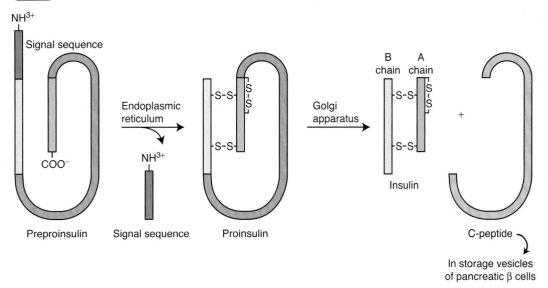

FIGURE 7-6 Insulin recruitment of glucose transporters

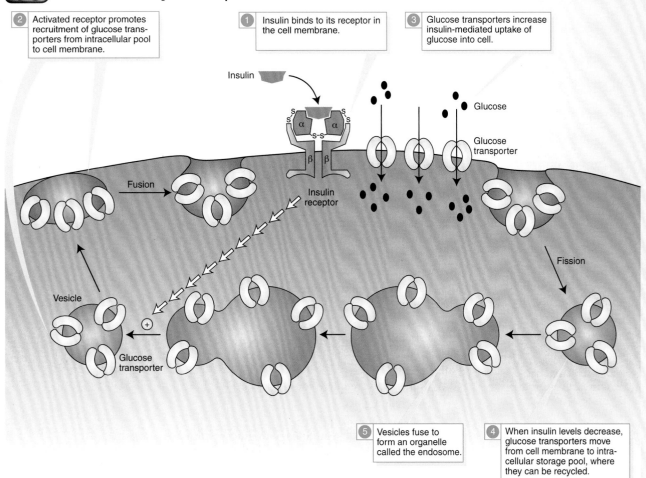

2. Activated receptor promotes recruitment of glucose transporters from intracellular pool to cell membrane.

1. Insulin binds to its receptor in the cell membrane.

3. Glucose transporters increase insulin-mediated uptake of glucose into cell.

5. Vesicles fuse to form an organelle called the endosome.

4. When insulin levels decrease, glucose transporters move from cell membrane to intracellular storage pool, where they can be recycled.

(Adapted with permission from Champe PC, Harvey RA. *Lippincott's Illustrated Reviews: Biochemistry.* 2nd ed. Philadelphia, PA: Lippincott-Raven; 1994.)

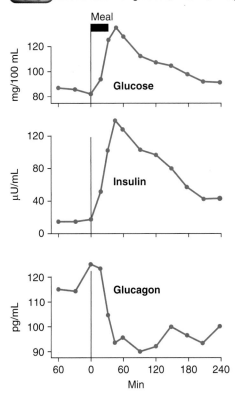

FIGURE
7-7 Blood levels of glucose, insulin, and glucagon after a high-carbohydrate meal

(Adapted with permission from Champe PC, Harvey RA. *Lippincott's Illustrated Reviews: Biochemistry.* 2nd ed. Philadelphia, PA: Lippincott-Raven; 1994.)

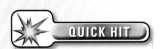

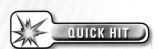

BLOOD GLUCOSE LEVELS

I. Hypoglycemia

A. Causes
   1. Excess insulin administration (in a patient with diabetes)
   2. Sulfonylurea administration
   3. Alcohol ingestion
   4. Insulinoma
   5. Factitious hyperinsulinism

B. **Symptoms**
   1. Sweating
   2. Palpitations
   3. Anxiety
   4. Tremor

C. **Whipple triad** (required for diagnosis)
   1. Low blood glucose
   2. Hypoglycemic symptoms
   3. Improvement of symptoms with glucose administration

D. In patients with diabetes, these symptoms may not be present, and blood glucose may be allowed to drop to dangerous levels; coma or death may result.

E. Therapy
   1. Glucose or intravenous (IV) dextrose should be given after measuring blood glucose levels.
   2. Glucagon should be administered.
   3. Epinephrine is sometimes appropriate therapy.

Clinical Vignette 7-1

CLINICAL PRESENTATION: A 4-year-old boy presents to the emergency department having woken up this morning feeling **lethargic** and **confused**. The child's past medical history is significant for two prior episodes of hypoglycemia. The patient's parents also report **resting tremor**. Mother denies **seizure activity**, **loss of consciousness**, and recent trauma. Mother did urine dipstick, which showed glucose level of 42 mg/dL (low). Parents administered glucose orally and brought the patient to the emergency department. Physical examination revealed an **anxious, diaphoretic** child with **slurred speech**. No hepatomegaly. Vital signs: Temperature = 97.5° F; heart rate = 119 bpm; respiration rate = 30 breaths/min; blood pressure = 109/55 mm Hg; oxygen saturation = 99% on room air.

DIFFERENTIALS: Hyperinsulinism, fatty acid oxidation defect, glycogen storage disease, glycogen synthesis defect, gluconeogenesis defect, glucagon deficiency, cortisol deficiency, and growth hormone deficiency. Figure 7-8 groups the various causes of hypoglycemia in the child by pathophysiology.

LABORATORY STUDIES: **Urine ketones** should be assessed via urinalysis. If urine ketones are low, it indicates the presence of a hyperinsulinemic state or a defect in fatty acid oxidation (resulting in an inability to produce ketones). These are best differentiated by obtaining an **insulin level**. If urine ketones are high, further workup is necessary to differentiate liver metabolism from endocrine defects. Consequently, **serum lactate**, **pyruvate**, **liver function tests**, and **uric acid** levels should be obtained to help rule out possibilities such as maple syrup urine disease, glycogenolysis defect, glycogen storage disease, and gluconeogenesis defect. Also, **serum cortisol** levels should be obtained to rule out cortisol deficiency. Eventually, the patient should be screened for **growth hormone** and **pituitary hormones**.

MANAGEMENT: Key point is to **treat first** and evaluate lab studies later. After blood samples are drawn, a quick bedside glucose reading should be done. If hypoglycemia is mild and the patient is able to tolerate oral dosing, treat with **oral glucose**. If severe hypoglycemia occurs and/or if the patient is unable to tolerate oral dosing, provide dextrose bolus followed by appropriate **maintenance infusion**.

FIGURE 7-8 Causes of hypoglycemia

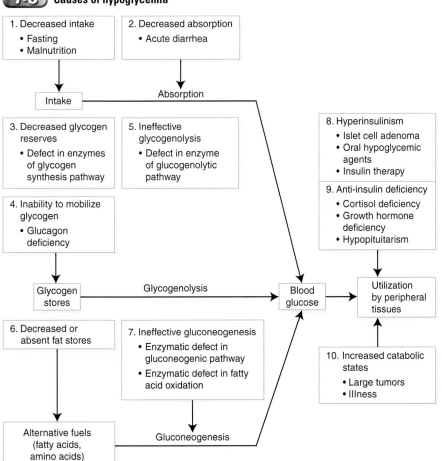

II. Hyperglycemia

A. Causes
   1. Diabetes mellitus
   2. Chronic pancreatitis
   3. Acromegaly
   4. Cushing syndrome
   5. Adverse drug reactions
      a. Furosemide
      b. Glucocorticoids
      c. Growth hormone
      d. Oral contraceptives
      e. Thiazides
B. Acute symptoms
   1. Ketoacidosis or hyperosmolar hyperglycemic nonketotic syndrome (see Table 7-6)
   2. Polyuria
   3. Polydipsia
   4. Polyphagia
   5. Weight loss
   6. Encephalopathy
      a. Tremulousness
      b. Convulsions
      c. Coma

The chronic symptoms of hyperglycemia mimic the chronic complications of diabetes (see Table 7-7).

DIABETES MELLITUS

Diabetes mellitus (or, simply, diabetes) refers to a group of disorders that are characterized by hyperglycemia and affect 1% to 2% of the U.S. population. Although the pathogenesis of these disorders is varied, individuals with diabetes lack the ability to produce sufficient insulin or respond to secreted insulin in order to meet their metabolic needs. Furthermore, all patients with diabetes are vulnerable to complications such as nephropathy, neuropathy, and retinopathy. Monitoring and control of blood sugar, insulin replacement, proper diet, and exercise can significantly reduce the morbidity and mortality of this disease.

I. Diagnosis of diabetes mellitus (Table 7-4)

TABLE 7-4 Diagnosis of Diabetes Mellitus

	Normal	IFG	IGT	DM
Random blood glucose (mg/dL)	<200			≥200 (with symptoms)
Fasting blood glucose (mg/dL)	<100	100–125		≥126 (on two occasions)
Blood glucose after oral glucose tolerance test (mg/dL)	<140		140–199	≥200
Hemoglobin A$_{1c}$ (%)	<5.7	5.7–6.4	5.7–6.4	≥6.5

DM, diabetes mellitus; IFG, impaired fasting glucose; IGT, impaired glucose tolerance.

II. Type 1 versus type 2 diabetes mellitus (Table 7-5)

TABLE 7-5 Type 1 versus Type 2 Diabetes Mellitus

	Type 1 Diabetes (15%)	Type 2 Diabetes (85%)
Cause	Possible **autoimmunity** to β cells triggered by viral cause	Increased **insulin resistance**, decreased receptors, or decreased conversion of proinsulin to insulin
Chromosomal association	6 (HLA-DRQ, HLA-DR3/DR4)	Unknown
Family history	Weak predictor	Strong predictor
Age of onset	Younger than 25 years of age	Older than 40 years of age
Body habitus	Normal to thin	Obese
Plasma insulin	Low	Normal to high
Plasma glucagon	High but suppressible	High and resistant to suppression
Pancreas morphology	Atrophy and fibrosis; β-cell depletion	Atrophy and amyloid deposits; variable β-cell population
Acute complication (Table 7-6)	Ketoacidosis	Hyperosmolar hyperglycemic state (HHS)
Common symptoms	**Polydipsia, polyuria, polyphagia (symptoms of hyperglycemia)**	Variable: from asymptomatic to polydipsia, polyuria, and polyphagia
Response to insulin therapy	Responsive	Variable
Response to oral therapy	Unresponsive	Responsive

HLA-DQ, human leukocyte antigen-DQ.

III. Diabetic ketoacidosis and hyperosmolar hyperglycemic state (Table 7-6)

TABLE 7-6 Diabetic Ketoacidosis and Hyperosmolar Hyperglycemic State

	DKA	HHS
Pathology	Increased serum **ketones**; anion gap metabolic acidosis (pH <7.2); **hyperglycemia** (glucose 300–800 mg/dL because of increased production and decreased uptake)	**Hyperglycemia** (>600 mg/dL); **hyperosmolarity** (>320 mg/dL); pH >7.3
Patient	Type 1 diabetes	Type 2 diabetes
Precipitating event	**Infection, insufficient insulin** (new-onset diabetes, medication reduction/omission), severe medical illness (MI, stroke, trauma), dehydration, alcohol or drug abuse, corticosteroids	**Infection, dehydration**, medication noncompliance, severe illness (MI, stroke, trauma), alcohol or drug abuse, corticosteroids
Clinical presentation	Nausea and vomiting, **Kussmaul respiration**, abdominal pain, fruity breath odor, osmotic diuresis, shock, coma	Confusion, possibly seizures or coma, nausea and vomiting, osmotic diuresis
Mortality	10%	17%
Treatment	Insulin, saline, K⁺ replacement	Saline (essential), insulin

DKA, diabetic ketoacidosis; HHS, hyperosmolar hyperglycemic state; MI, myocardial infarction.

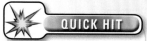

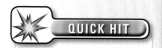

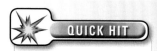

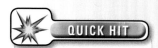

QUICK HIT

The ketone bodies (**acetoacetate, β-hydroxybutyrate**) are produced by the liver from acetyl coenzyme A (CoA) in the fasting state. The body (including the brain after 4 to 5 days) uses the ketone bodies for energy instead of glucose and amino acids. Red blood cells (RBCs), however, can only use glucose.

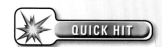

The Endocrine System

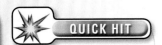

QUICK HIT

Kussmaul respirations are deep and labored but may be either rapid or slow.

IV. Chronic symptoms of diabetes (Table 7-7)

TABLE 7-7	**Chronic Symptoms of Diabetes Mellitus**
Anatomic Location	**Clinical Features**
Red blood cells	**Glycation (HbA$_{1c}$)**; measure of long-term control of diabetes (reflects past 3 months)
Blood vessels/cardiovascular system	**Atherosclerosis**, dyslipidemia, coronary artery disease, gangrene, peripheral vascular disease
Eyes	**Retinopathy**, hemorrhage, hard exudates, cotton-wool spots, cataracts, glaucoma
GI tract	Constipation, **gastroparesis**
Kidneys	Nephropathy, **nodular sclerosis**, **Kimmelstiel–Wilson nodules**, chronic renal failure, azotemia
Penis	**Erectile dysfunction** as a result of autonomic neuropathy
Extremities	**Stocking-glove peripheral neuropathy**, nonhealing ulcers

GI, gastrointestinal; HbA$_{1c}$, hemoglobin A1c.

V. Treatment of diabetes mellitus (Tables 7-8 and 7-9)

The goal of treatment of both type 1 and type 2 diabetes mellitus is steady control of blood glucose levels. However, because the pathogenesis underlying these two disease processes is different, the therapy is also different.

Type 1 diabetes mellitus, which can be viewed simply as a total deficiency of insulin, may be treated with careful administration of exogenous insulin. This agent has been the only treatment option for type 1 diabetes mellitus for many years and remains so today. However, advances have been made in both the type of insulin and the method of delivery. To maintain steady glucose levels, different preparations of human insulin have been designed, each with a characteristic rate of onset and duration of action (Table 7-8). Insulin, a peptide hormone, cannot be given orally. It is typically administered subcutaneously and, in emergencies, intravenously.

Some combination of these types of insulin usually can be found that provides adequate glucose control during both the fed and fasting states. Treatment of type 1 diabetes mellitus is essentially a balancing act—too much insulin causes hypoglycemia, and too little leads to hyperglycemia, which, over time, leads to the long-term complications of diabetes mellitus.

TABLE 7-8	**Commonly Used Insulin Preparations**		
Insulin Preparation	**Onset of Activity**	**Time of Peak Activity**	**Duration of Action**
Insulin lispro	5–15 min	1–2 h	3–4 h
Insulin aspart	5–15 min	1–2 h	3–4 h
Insulin glulisine	5–15 min	1–2 h	3–4 h
Regular insulin	30 min	2–4 h	6–8 h
NPH (neutral protamine Hagedorn) insulin	1–2 h	4–12 h	18–24 h
Insulin detemir	3–4 h	3–9 h	6–24 h
Insulin glargine	3–4 h	No peak	24 h or longer

TABLE **7-9** **Therapeutic Agents for Diabetes**

Therapeutic Agent (common name, if relevant) [trade name, where appropriate]	Class—Pharmacology and Pharmacokinetics	Indications	Side Effects or Adverse Effects	Contraindications or Precautions to Consider; Notes
Insulin				
Lispro [Humalog], **aspart** [Novolog], **glulisine** [Apidra]	**Rapid-acting insulin—** see *mechanism for regular insulin*	**Diabetes mellitus** (typically **type 1**), **hyperkalemia, stress-induced hyperglycemia**	**Hypoglycemia** (diaphoresis, vertigo, tachycardia), insulin allergy, insulin antibodies, lipodystrophy	
Regular insulin [Humulin R, Novolin R]	**Short-acting insulin—liver:** promotes glucose storage as glycogen, increases triglyceride synthesis **Muscle:** facilitates protein and glycogen synthesis **Adipose tissue:** improves triglyceride storage by activating plasma lipoprotein lipase; reduces circulating free fatty acids	**Diabetes mellitus** (typically **type 1**), **hyperkalemia, stress-induced hyperglycemia**	**Hypoglycemia** (diaphoresis, vertigo, tachycardia), insulin allergy, insulin antibodies, lipodystrophy	
NPH [Humulin N, Novolin N]	**Intermediate-acting insulin—** *see mechanism for insulin*	**Diabetes mellitus** (typically **type 1**)	**Hypoglycemia** (diaphoresis, vertigo, tachycardia), insulin allergy, insulin antibodies, lipodystrophy	
Glargine [Lantus], **detemir** [Levemir]	**Long-acting insulin—***see mechanism for regular insulin*	**Diabetes mellitus** (typically **type 1**)	**Hypoglycemia** (diaphoresis, vertigo, tachycardia), insulin allergy, insulin antibodies, lipodystrophy	
Sulfonylureas				
Tolbutamide, chlorpropamide	**First-generation sulfonylureas**—closes potassium channel in β-cell membrane → reduces K^+ efflux, increases Ca^{2+} influx → increases secretion of insulin	Oral treatment for **type 2 diabetes**	**Hypoglycemia**, GI disturbances, muscle weakness, mental confusion	Rarely used due to toxicity
Glyburide [DiaBeta, Micronase], **glimepiride** [Amaryl], **glipizide** [Glucotrol]	**Second generation sulfonylureas**—closes potassium channel in pancreatic β-islet cell membrane → reduces K^+ efflux, increases Ca^{2+} influx → increases secretion of insulin	Oral treatment for **type 2 diabetes**	**Hypoglycemia**, GI disturbances, muscle weakness, mental confusion, weight gain	Not useful in type 1 diabetes mellitus because it requires some β-cell function.
Biguanides				
Metformin [Glucophage]	**Biguanide—decreases hepatic gluconeogenesis**, increases glycolysis → decreases serum glucose levels	**First-line** oral treatment for **type 2 diabetes**	**Lactic acidosis**, GI upset (diarrhea, nausea, abdominal pain), metallic taste; decreased vitamin B_{12} absorption	Stop drug in patients undergoing studies or procedures involving contrast; **contraindicated in patients with renal dysfunction**
Thiazolidinediones				
Pioglitazone [Actos], **rosiglitazone** [Avandia]	**Glitazones—bind PPARγ receptors; improve target cell sensitivity to insulin**	Oral treatment for **type 2 diabetes**	**Weight gain, edema**, rare hepatotoxicity, increases LDL and triglycerides; rosiglitazone may increase the risk of MI	Contraindicated in CHF

(continued)

The Endocrine System

TABLE 7-9	**Therapeutic Agents for Diabetes** (Continued)			
Therapeutic Agent (common name, if relevant) [trade name, where appropriate]	**Class—Pharmacology and Pharmacokinetics**	**Indications**	**Side Effects or Adverse Effects**	**Contraindications or Precautions to Consider; Notes**
Other				
Sitagliptin [Januvia], **saxagliptin** [Onglyza], **linagliptin** [Tradjenta]	**DPP-IV inhibitors**—prevents degradation of incretin hormones → decreased glucagon, increased insulin, delays gastric emptying	Oral treatment for **type 2 diabetes**	Diarrhea, constipation, edema	
Exenatide [Byetta]	**Incretin mimetic**—agonizes GLP-1 receptors → decreases glucagon, increases insulin, delays gastric emptying	Injectable treatment for **type 2 diabetes**	Mild weight loss, nausea, hypoglycemia, constipation, slight risk of pancreatitis	Derived from exendin, a hormone found in Gila monster saliva
Liraglutide [Victoza]	**Incretin mimetic**—synthetic GLP-1 analog → decreases glucagon, increases insulin, delays gastric emptying	Injectable treatment for **type 2 diabetes**	Mild weight loss, nausea, vomiting, diarrhea, slight risk of pancreatitis	Increased incidence of medullary thyroid cancer in animal models
Pramlintide [Symlin]	**Analog of amylin**, a pancreatic hormone secreted with insulin that decreases glucagon and delays gastric emptying	Injectable treatment for **type 2 diabetes**	Nausea, vomiting, hypoglycemia	
α-Glucosidase inhibitors				
Acarbose [Precose] **miglitol**	**α-Glucosidase inhibitor**—inhibit intestinal brush border enzyme α-glucosidase → delays sugar hydrolysis and glucose absorption from gut → decreases **postprandial hyperglycemia**	Oral treatment for **type 2 diabetes** postprandially	**GI effects** (flatulence, cramps, diarrhea); may reduce absorption of iron	

CHF, congestive heart failure; DPP-IV, dipeptidyl peptidase-IV; GI, gastrointestinal; GLP-1, glucagon-like peptide-1; LDL, low-density lipoprotein; NPH, neutral protamine Hagedorn; PPARγ, peroxisome proliferator-activated receptor gamma.

Type 2 diabetes mellitus, which is more complex than type 1 disease, is characterized primarily by insulin resistance. In some cases, a strict regimen of diet and exercise completely reverses the course of the disease. In many cases, however, drugs are required to control blood sugar levels. The most commonly used drugs in type 2 diabetes mellitus are metformin and the insulin sensitizers. **Metformin**, in the biguanide class of agents, is considered by many to be the first-line drug of choice in type 2 diabetes mellitus and acts primarily by decreasing hepatic glucose production. Advantages include the very low risk of hypoglycemia as well as the weight loss and improvement in lipid profiles in many patients. The one feared adverse reaction is lactic acidosis, a rare but serious complication. Also, nausea and diarrhea are side effects of this medication.

Pioglitazone and **rosiglitazone**, of the thiazolidinedione class, are the two most common insulin sensitizers. Like metformin, these agents can be used alone or as part of a multidrug regimen for diabetic blood sugar control. Both drugs have a low risk of hypoglycemia. However, they have been known to exacerbate congestive heart failure, and frequent monitoring of liver function is required. Rosiglitazone may increase the risk of myocardial infarction (MI) and cardiovascular events.

Sulfonylureas were once the mainstay of treatment for type 2 diabetes, but they are used less frequently today. These drugs, which include agents such as glipizide and glyburide, act by increasing the release of insulin from the pancreas. To a lesser extent, these agents also decrease glucagon levels and increase insulin binding at target sites in the periphery. The primary side effect of these drugs is hypoglycemia.

The Endocrine System

Clinical Vignette 7-2

CLINICAL PRESENTATION: An 8-year-old female child presents to the emergency department with complaints of several days of **vomiting** and **thirst**. The mother also reports that the patient has **not been acting like herself** lately and has been **urinating** more than usual. The patient recently recovered from an **upper respiratory infection** with high fevers. On examination, the patient is breathing rapidly and deeply (**Kussmaul respirations**), and a **sweet smell** is noticed on her breath. Her **skin and oral mucosa are dry**.

DIFFERENTIALS: Diabetic ketoacidosis (DKA), hyperosmolar hyperglycemic state (HHS), gastroenteritis, hypoglycemic coma, metabolic acidosis (from causes other than DKA).

LABORATORY STUDIES: A **urinalysis** should be obtained with interest in glucose and ketone levels—high glucose and ketone levels suggest DKA. **In HHS, the glucose levels are elevated but there is no ketosis.** HHS is more often seen in patients with type 2 diabetes, and DKA is more often seen in patients with type 1 diabetes. A **blood chemistry** would also be key in differentiating causes; in DKA, it would show high glucose, high ketones, and an acidotic profile with low pH, low bicarbonate, and elevated anion gap from the ketones (organic acids). Also in DKA, serum potassium is high because the acidosis causes a shift of serum hydrogen ions into cells in exchange for intracellular potassium ions. Serum sodium appears decreased because hyperglycemia increases serum osmolality shifting water out of cells. Blood glucose and serum osmolality are significantly higher in HHS than in DKA, and ketones are not found because there are sufficient levels of insulin to prevent lipolysis, thereby preventing ketogenesis. HHS usually presents with a nonacidotic profile. Metabolic acidosis can also cause vomiting, Kussmaul respirations, a low blood pH, and bicarbonate. Causes of metabolic acidosis with a normal anion gap include diarrhea, renal tubular acidosis, or acetazolamide overdose. Causes of metabolic acidosis with an elevated anion gap include chronic renal failure, lactic acidosis, DKA, uremia, salicylate overdose, methanol ingestion, and ethylene glycol ingestion. To determine the cause of the metabolic acidosis in this patient, **salicylate**, **lactate**, **blood alcohol**, **methanol**, and **ethylene glycol levels** should be obtained. Finally, in gastroenteritis, a metabolic alkalosis from the vomiting is expected. In hypoglycemic coma, the glucose levels are low.

MANAGEMENT: Three-tiered approach: (1) **Rehydration**—a fluid bolus is indicated because the patient is severely dehydrated. Monitor rehydration status by noting resolution of mental status changes. The most common complication of this treatment is **cerebral edema** from too rapid a change in serum osmolality. (2) **Insulin**—to facilitate peripheral uptake of glucose, decrease ketone body formation. (3) **Potassium replacement**—although blood studies show high serum potassium levels, that is misleading because the acidosis caused the potassium to shift out of cells and the body is actually potassium starved.

 OBESITY

Obesity is a multifactorial disease with a variable genetic component and is associated with diet, lifestyle, drugs, and endocrine disorders. Multiple therapeutic strategies including diet, exercise, bariatric surgery, and drugs can be attempted. Table 7-10 summarizes pharmacologic agents available in treating obesity.

TABLE 7-10 Therapeutic Agents for Obesity

Therapeutic Agent (common name, if relevant) [trade name, where appropriate]	Class—Pharmacology and Pharmacokinetics	Indications	Side Effects or Adverse Effects	Contraindications or Precautions to Consider; Notes
Orlistat	**Inhibits pancreatic lipases** → alters fat metabolism	**Obesity** (long term)	**Steatorrhea**, GI irritation, reduced absorption of fat-soluble vitamins, and headache	**Used in conjunction with modified diet**
Phentermine	**Sympathomimetic—** stimulates the release of norepinephrine	Obesity (short term)	Hypertension, tachycardia, euphoria, tremor	Contraindicated in patients with cardiovascular disease or with history of drug abuse

GI, gastrointestinal.

PITUITARY DISORDERS (Table 7-11)

The pituitary gland sits in the sella turcica. The anterior portion is regulated by the hypothalamus. The posterior portion contains extensions of hypothalamic neurons. Excess prolactin can result from estrogen therapy or drugs, such as antipsychotics, that interfere with dopamine (prolactin-inhibiting hormone).

TABLE 7-11 Pituitary Disorders

Disorder	Etiology	Clinical Features	Laboratory Diagnosis	Treatment
Prolactinoma	Lactotrophic (chromophobic) anterior pituitary tumor; **most common** pituitary tumor	Decreased libido, vision changes, amenorrhea, gynecomastia, galactorrhea, virilization	Minimal or no increase in serum prolactin after TRH given	Bromocriptine or surgery
Acromegaly (adults)/ gigantism (children)	Somatotrophic (acidophilic) anterior pituitary adenoma	Prominent forehead, jaw; **large hands, feet; enlargement of viscera**; hyperglycemia; renal failure; hypertension; mental disturbances	Excess growth hormones and somatomedins (IGF-1)	Transsphenoidal surgery, bromocriptine, radiation, or octreotide
Cushing disease	Hypersecretion of ACTH from basophilic adenoma of pituitary	(Table 7-13)	Suppression of ACTH secretion during high-dose dexamethasone test	Surgery or pituitary irradiation
Panhypopituitarism (Simmonds disease, Sheehan syndrome)	Pituitary tumors, ischemia, trauma; DIC; sickle cell anemia	Marked wasting, **panhypopituitarism**, headache, vomiting	Decreased levels of FSH, LH, ACTH, TSH	Hormone replacement
SIADH	Pituitary hypersecretion; ectopic production of ADH **(small cell lung cancer)**	Decreased urinary output, fatigue, mental disturbances	Hyponatremia, high urine osmolality	Fluid restriction
Diabetes insipidus	**Central** (neurogenic): ADH insufficiency **Nephrogenic**: lack of end-organ (kidney) response	Dehydration, thirst, polyuria, recent trauma to the head or anoxia	(Table 7-12), hypernatremia	Central: desmopressin (DDAVP) replaces ADH Nephrogenic: fluid restriction and thiazide response diuretics (works by a paradoxical effect)

ACTH, adrenocorticotropic hormone; ADH, antidiuretic hormone (vasopressin); DDAVP, 1-deamino-8-D-arginine vasopressin; DIC, disseminated intravascular coagulation; FSH, follicle-stimulating hormone; IGF-1, insulin-like growth factor-1; LH, luteinizing hormone; SIADH, syndrome of inappropriate secretion of antidiuretic hormone; TRH, thyrotropin-releasing hormone; TSH, thyroid-stimulating hormone.

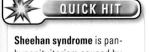

QUICK HIT

Sheehan syndrome is panhypopituitarism caused by postpartum pituitary necrosis resulting from blood loss and ischemia during childbirth.

DIABETES INSIPIDUS *(Table 7-12)*

Diabetes insipidus is a disease characterized by excessive low-osmolality urine output. There are two forms: central and nephrogenic.

TABLE 7-12 Diabetes Insipidus

	Urine Osmolality Greater than 280 mOsm/kg with Dehydration	Response to Antidiuretic Hormone after Dehydration
Normal	+	−
Central diabetes insipidus	−	+
Partial diabetes insipidus	+	+
Nephrogenic diabetes insipidus	−	−
Primary polydipsia	+	+

THE ADRENAL GLANDS

I. Congenital adrenal hyperplasia *(Figure 7-9)*

The adrenal glands are anatomically divided into a medulla and a cortex. The cortex itself is divided into three anatomic layers. The four anatomic layers of the adrenal glands are responsible for various metabolic functions in the body.

II. Adrenal cortex pathology *(Table 7-13)*

TABLE 7-13 Adrenal Cortex Pathology

Disease	Etiology	Clinical Features
Cushing syndrome	Excess cortisol as a result of **iatrogenic corticosteroid therapy (most common cause)**, adrenal adenoma (more common than carcinoma); ectopic ACTH from neoplasm (especially **small cell lung carcinoma**)	Peripheral muscle wasting and weakness; **central obesity** with rounds facies and increased fat deposition at upper back, easy bruising with abdominal striae; bone demineralization, osteoporosis, psychosis, acne; hirsutism; hyperglycemia; hypertension
Cushing disease	Excess cortisol as a result of **pituitary hypersecretion of ACTH**; bilateral hyperplasia of adrenal cortex	Identical to Cushing syndrome
Conn syndrome (primary hyperaldosteronism)	Adrenal cortex **adenoma** (more common than hyperplasia, which is more common than carcinoma), sodium retention, **low plasma renin**	**Hypertension**, hypokalemic alkalosis
Secondary hyperaldosteronism	Renal tumors, renal ischemia, edematous conditions (cirrhosis, nephrotic syndromes, congestive heart failure), **increased plasma renin**	**Hypertension**, hypokalemic alkalosis

(continued)

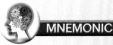

MNEMONIC

Both nephrogenic and central diabetes insipidus present with dilute urine after dehydration. In diagnosing these subtypes of diabetes insipidus, think after administering antidiuretic hormone: **C**oncentrated urine = **C**entral; **N**o effect = **N**ephrogenic.

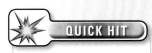

QUICK HIT

Surprisingly, diabetes insipidus can be treated with hydrochlorothiazide (a diuretic).

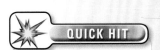

QUICK HIT

Primary polydipsia, a psychological condition of drinking excess water, causes a decrease in plasma osmolality, and thus can be differentiated from diabetes insipidus, which causes an increase in plasma osmolality. Patients who present with primary polydipsia are generally young or middle-aged women with a history of neurosis.

QUICK HIT

Diabetes insipidus may be transiently induced during pregnancy due to greater metabolism of vasopressin (ADH).

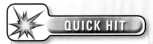

QUICK HIT

21-Hydroxylase deficiency is the **most common** adrenal enzyme deficiency.

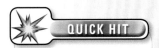

QUICK HIT

Small cell lung carcinoma is a potential source for ectopic ACTH production resulting in paraneoplastic syndrome.

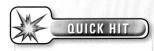

The Endocrine System

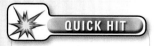

TABLE **7-13** **Adrenal Cortex Pathology** (Continued)

Disease	Etiology	Clinical Features
Addison disease	Most commonly **idiopathic** cortisol deficiency; possibly autoimmune; may be caused by tumor, infections (i.e., tuberculosis)	**Hypotension**, low serum sodium, **hyperpigmentation**, increased serum potassium
Waterhouse–Friderichsen syndrome	***Neisseria meningitidis*** infection leads to disseminated intravascular coagulation (**DIC**); hemorrhagic adrenal **necrosis** and circulation collapse	Acute hypotension and salt wasting; **shock**; more common in children; death within hours if not treated

ACTH, adrenocorticotropic hormone.

FIGURE **7-9** Congenital adrenal hyperplasia

Congenital adrenal hyperplasias (CAH)

Steroid hormone synthesis

Cholesterol (C27)

NADPH, O₂ → *Desmolase*

Pregnenolone (C21)

3-β-*Hydroxysteroid dehydrogenase*

Progesterone (C21)

17-α-*Hydroxylase*

17-α-Hydroxyprogesterone (C21)

21-α-*Hydroxylase*

11-Deoxycorticosterone (C21)   11-Deoxycortisol (C21)   Androstenedione (C19)

11-β-*Hydroxylase*

Corticosterone   Testosterone (C19)   Testosterone (C19)

Aldosterone   Cortisol (C21)   Estradiol (C18)

17-α-Hydroxylase deficiency
- Sex hormones and cortisol not produced
- Increased production of mineralocorticoids causes sodium and fluid retention and, therefore, hypertension.
- Patient is phenotypically female but is unable to mature (amenorrhea and lack of secondary sexual characteristics).

21-α-Hydroxylase deficiency
- Most common form of CAH
- Usually a partial deficiency
- ACTH levels elevated, causing an increased flux to sex hormones and, therefore, masculinization.
- Lack of mineralocorticoid production leads to inadequate Na⁺ retention and, therefore, hypotension.

11-β-Hydroxylase deficiency
- Decrease in serum cortisol, aldosterone, and corticosterone
- Increased production of deoxycorticosterone causes fluid retention and hypertension.
- Masculinization as with 21-α-hydroxylase deficiency

ACTH, adrenocorticotropic hormone; NADPH, reduced nicotinamide adenine dinucleotide phosphate.

III. Adrenal medulla pathology (Table 7-14)

TABLE 7-14 Adrenal Medulla Tumors

Tumor	Pathology	Clinical Manifestation
Neuroblastoma	**Malignant;** excess catecholamine secretion; N-*myc* (oncogene) amplification	**Children;** degree of N-*myc* amplification related to prognosis; abdominal pain, constipation, possibly some hypertension
Pheochromocytoma	**Benign** (10% malignant); tumor of chromaffin cells; seen in MEN 2a and 2b	**Adults;** hypertension (usually paroxysmal); palpitations, sweating, and headache; increased urinary vanillylmandelic acid **(VMA)**

MEN 2a and 2b, multiple endocrine neoplasia types 2a and 2b.

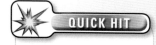

QUICK HIT

The pheochromocytoma rule of 10s: 10% are malignant, 10% multiple, 10% bilateral, 10% familial, 10% extra-adrenal, and 10% children.

Clinical Vignette 7-3

CLINICAL PRESENTATION: A 37-year-old woman presents to her primary care physician with a chief complaint of **weight gain, fatigue, acne,** and **hirsutism.** After further questions, the patient reports that she has not had her period for 3 months. Her past medical history is significant for a bone marrow transplantation, for which the patient is currently on medication. Patient denies a family history of diabetes or hypertension. Physical examination reveals **central obesity, abdominal striae, bruising** on thighs and buttocks, and **muscle weakness.** Vital signs: Temperature = 97.5° F; heart rate = 80 bpm; respiration rate = 20 breaths/min; **blood pressure = 140/90 mm Hg.**

DIFFERENTIAL: Iatrogenic Cushing syndrome, adrenocorticotropic hormone (ACTH)–producing pituitary adenoma (Cushing **disease**), adrenal adenoma, ectopic ACTH production, and obesity. This patient is exhibiting signs and symptoms of high cortisol termed *Cushing syndrome*. Some findings (i.e., **obesity, hypertension, osteoporosis, diabetes mellitus**) are nonspecific and less helpful in diagnosis of Cushing syndrome. **Easy bruising, striae, virilization,** and **myopathy** are more helpful in the diagnosis. Also, patients with **Cushing disease** can have **hyperpigmentation** as a result of elevated ACTH levels, whereas patients with **Cushing syndrome** due to other causes will not have hyperpigmentation. The most common cause of Cushing syndrome is an unfavorable response to prescribed steroids; patient's recent transplantation history suggests the possibility that she received immunosuppressive steroids.

LABORATORY STUDIES: Figure 7-10 outlines the approach. The first step is to determine whether cortisol levels are elevated in this patient, which can be done via a **urine 24-hour free cortisol level** or an **overnight dexamethasone suppression test.** In this latter test, dexamethasone is given at night, and serum cortisol levels are measured in the morning. In normal individuals, dexamethasone should suppress the pituitary–adrenal axis, resulting in decreased cortisol in the morning. In Cushing syndrome, the serum cortisol remains elevated. The next step is to determine the cause of the cortisol elevation, which could be from (a) **increased ACTH production** at the level of the pituitary or ectopically, (b) **increased cortisol production** at the level of the adrenal gland, or (c) **exogenous cortisol** in the form of prednisone. To determine the cause, measure **ACTH levels,** which would be low in the case of exogenous cortisol and adrenal adenoma, because cortisol feedback inhibits the pituitary from secreting ACTH. Knowing which medications the patient is using helps in differentiating these causes. ACTH levels are high in patients with obesity, patients with ectopic ACTH production, or pituitary ACTH adenoma. The key differentiating factor is that **low-dose dexamethasone** will suppress ACTH production in obese individuals, **high-dose dexamethasone** will suppress ACTH production in pituitary adenoma cases, and nothing will suppress ACTH levels in the patients with ectopic ACTH production.

MANAGEMENT: This patient most likely has iatrogenic Cushing syndrome, which is remedied by **tapering of the glucocorticoid.** Pituitary or adrenal adenoma requires **surgical removal of the neoplasm.**

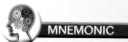

MNEMONIC

To remember the side effects of glucocorticoids, think CUSHINGOID:

Cataract
Ulcers
Skin: striae, thinning, bruising
Hypertension/**H**irsutism/**H**yperglycemia
Infections
Necrosis (avascular necrosis of the femoral head)
Glycosuria
Osteoporosis/**O**besity
Immunosuppression
Diabetes

The Endocrine System

FIGURE
7-10 Approach to Cushing syndrome

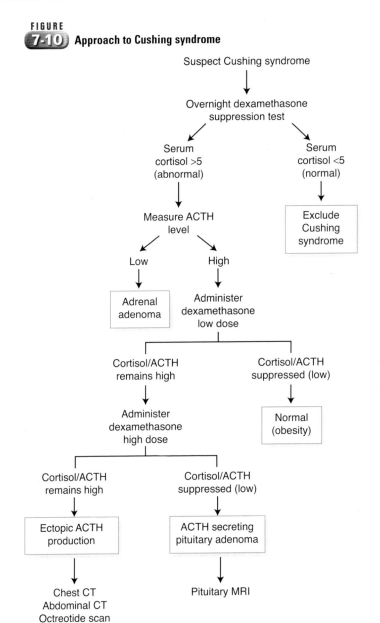

ACTH, adrenocorticotropic hormone; CT, computed tomography; MRI, magnetic resonance imaging.

THERAPEUTIC AGENTS FOR THE HYPOTHALAMUS, PITUITARY, AND ADRENAL GLANDS (Table 7-15)

TABLE 7-15 Therapeutic Agents for Hypothalamic, Pituitary, and Adrenal Conditions

Therapeutic Agent (common name, if relevant) [trade name, where appropriate]	Class—Pharmacology and Pharmacokinetics	Indications	Side Effects or Adverse Effects	Contraindications or Precautions to Consider; Notes
Growth hormone (somatropin, somatrem)	Synthetic analog of growth hormone—causes liver to produce insulin-like growth factors (somatomedins)	Replacement therapy in children with **growth hormone deficiency, Turner syndrome; burn victims**		Should not be used in patients with closed epiphyses
Growth hormone–releasing hormone (GHRH)	Synthetic analog of GHRH—stimulates release of GH	**Dwarfism**	**Pain at injection**	
Octreotide [Sandostatin]	Synthetic analog of somatostatin—decreases release of GH, gastrin, secretin, VIP, CCK, glucagon, insulin	**Acromegaly, glucagonoma, insulinoma, carcinoid syndrome**	Nausea, cramps, gallstones	
Oxytocin [Pitocin, Syntocinon]	Synthetic analog of oxytocin—stimulates uterine contraction and contraction of breast myoepithelial cells; milk letdown reflex	**Induces labor; control uterine hemorrhage**		
Desmopressin (DDAVP)	Synthetic analog of ADH—recruits water channels to luminal membrane in collecting duct	Central diabetes insipidus, nocturnal enuresis, von Willebrand disease	Overhydration; allergic reaction; larger doses result in pallor, diarrhea, hypertension; coronary constriction; chronic rhinopharyngitis	**Synthetic analog to vasopressin; intranasal administration**
Prednisone, hydrocortisone, triamcinolone, dexamethasone, beclomethasone	Glucocorticoid—inhibits protein synthesis; reduces lymph node and spleen size; inhibits cell cycle activity of lymphoid cells; lyses T cells; suppresses antibody, prostaglandin, and leukotriene synthesis; blocks monocyte production of IL-1	Addison disease, rheumatic arthritis, autoimmune disorders, allergic reaction, asthma, organ transplantation (especially during rejection crisis)	**Osteoporosis, Cushingoid reaction, acne, psychosis, glucose intolerance, infection, hypertension, cataracts, peptic ulcers**	

ADH, antidiuretic hormone; CCK, cholecystokinin; GH, growth hormone; IL-1, interleukin 1; VIP, vasoactive intestinal peptide.

THYROID

I. Formation of thyroid hormone (*Figure 7-11*)

FIGURE 7-11 Formation of thyroid hormone

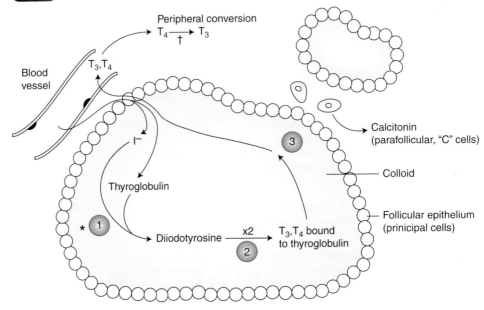

1. Oxidation of I⁻ by peroxidase followed by iodination of thyroglobulin
2. Condensation
3. Proteolytic release of hormone from follicle
* Inhibited by propylthiouracil and methimazole
† Inhibited by propylthiouracil

T$_3$, triiodothyronine; T$_4$, thyroxine.

II. Myxedema

A. Can be described as hypothyroidism of the adult

B. Causes
1. Hashimoto thyroiditis (see the following)
2. Idiopathic causes
3. Iodine deficiency
   a. A problem in geographic areas with poor nutrition
   b. Deficiency in pregnant women can lead to cretinism in the child (see the following).
4. Paradoxically, high doses of iodine lead to a decrease in thyroid hormone production.
5. **Overirradiation** of the thyroid using iodine-131 for treatment of hyperthyroidism.

C. Clinical features of the hypothyroid state
1. Cold intolerance
2. Weight gain
3. Constipation
4. Lowering of voice
5. Menorrhagia
6. Slowed mental and physical function
7. Dry skin with coarse and brittle hair
8. Reflexes showing slow return phase ("hung reflex")

D. Treatment is usually with levothyroxine (T$_4$)

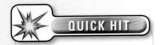

III. Cretinism

A. Can be describe as **hypothyroidism** of the **fetus or child**
B. Causes
  1. **Iodine-deficient diet** in the mother or during the early life of the child
  2. Thyroid-related enzyme deficiency
  3. Thyroid developmental defect
  4. Failure of thyroid descent during development
  5. Transfer of antithyroid antibodies from the mother with an autoimmune disease to the fetus
C. Clinical features
  1. Impaired physical growth
  2. Mental retardation
  3. Enlarged tongue
  4. Enlarged, distended abdomen

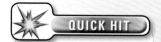

QUICK HIT

Because of the devastating effects that hypothyroidism can have on children (**cretinism**), thyroid hormone levels (along with galactosemia and phenylketonuria) are routinely evaluated at birth in the United States.

IV. Hashimoto thyroiditis

A. An **autoimmune** disorder causing **hypothyroidism** and a **painless goiter**
  1. Dense infiltrate of lymphocytes into the thyroid gland
  2. Antithyroglobulin and antithyroid peroxidase (formerly antimicrosomal) antibodies
  3. **5:1 female predominance**
  4. Incidence increases with age.
  5. Associated with human leukocyte antigen-DR5 (**HLA-DR5**) and **HLA-B5**
B. Is the **most common form of hypothyroidism in those with adequate iodine** intake
C. Clinical features
  1. Slowly progressing course with stages of euthyroid state, hyperthyroid state, and hypothyroid state
  2. May lead to a scarred and shrunken gland in hypothyroid state
  3. Microscopically, thyroid resembles lymph node
D. Associated with other autoimmune disorders
  1. Diabetes mellitus
  2. Pernicious anemia
  3. Sjögren syndrome

V. Subacute (de Quervain) thyroiditis

A. Transient hyperthyroidism with painful goiter
  1. Focal destruction of thyroid
  2. Granulomatous inflammation
  3. 3:1 female predominance
  4. Associated with HLA-B35
B. Causes—possibly as a result of recent viral infection with coxsackie virus, echovirus, adenovirus, measles, or mumps
C. Clinical features
  1. Acute febrile state
  2. Rapid, painful enlargement of the thyroid
  3. Transient hyperthyroidism owing to gland destruction
D. Self-limited disease

VI. Graves disease

A. **Autoimmune** disorder causing **hyperthyroidism** and **goiter**
  1. Thyroid-stimulating immunoglobulin (**TSI**) is an immunoglobulin G (IgG) antibody to the thyroid-stimulating hormone (TSH) receptor.
  2. Binding of TSI to the TSH receptor stimulates thyroid hormone production and hyperplasia of the thyroid gland.
  3. It is associated with **HLA-DR3** and **HLA-B8**.
  4. It has a **4:1 female** predominance.

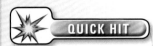

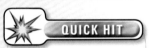

B. Clinical features of Graves disease
1. Hyperthyroidism and goiter caused by autoimmune immunoglobulins
   a. Increased total thyroxine (T_4)
   b. Increased triiodothyronine (T_3)
   c. Decreased TSH level
   d. Increased resin radioactive T_3 uptake
   e. Increased radioactive iodine
2. Exophthalmos, proptosis
3. Warm, moist, and flushed skin
4. Thin, fine hair
5. Cardiovascular system
   a. Increased heart rate and cardiac output
   b. **Palpitations and fibrillations**
6. Muscle atrophy
   a. Weakening of skeletal muscles occurs.
   b. Vital capacity of lungs decreases owing to weakened respiratory muscles.
7. **Weight loss** occurs despite an increased appetite.
8. Diarrhea is common.
9. Menstrual flow may decrease or stop.
C. Treatment (Table 7-16)
1. Antithyroid drugs (e.g., propylthiouracil or methimazole)
2. A β-**blocker** to reduce the cardiac effects
3. Radioactive iodine (iodine-131)
4. Surgery

TABLE 7-16 Therapeutic Agents for Thyroid Disorders

Therapeutic Agent (common name, if relevant) [trade name, where appropriate]	Class—Pharmacology and Pharmacokinetics	Indications	Side Effects or Adverse Effects	Contraindications or Precautions to Consider; Notes
Propylthiouracil (PTU)	Antithyroid agent—inhibits peroxidase enzyme in thyroid → decreases synthesis of thyroid hormone; also blocks peripheral conversion of T_4 to T_3	**Hyperthyroidism**	**Agranulocytosis**	**Crosses the placenta and can cause fetal goiter and hypothyroidism;** preferred to methimazole in treating pregnant females with moderate to severe hyperthyroidism
Methimazole [Tapazole]	Antithyroid agent—inhibits peroxidase enzyme in thyroid → decreases synthesis of thyroid hormone	**Hyperthyroidism**	**Agranulocytosis**	**Crosses the placenta;** can cause fetal goiter, hypothyroidism, and aplasia cutis (fetal scalp defect).
Levothyroxine (T_4) [Synthroid, Levothroid]	Synthetic analog of thyroxine (T_4)	**Hypothyroidism**	Tachycardia, heat intolerance, tremors, arrhythmia	
Triiodothyronine (T_3) [Triostat]	Synthetic analog of thyroid hormone T_3	**Hypothyroidism**	Tachycardia, heat intolerance, tremors, arrhythmia	

Clinical Vignette 7-4

CLINICAL PRESENTATION: A 40-year-old woman presents to your office with a 20-lb **weight loss** over the past 2 months despite **eating more**. She also reports **irregular menses, diarrhea,** and **difficulty sleeping and concentrating**. She denies chest pain and palpitations. Physical examination reveals **warm, moist skin** and **resting hand tremor**. Neck examination shows a **diffusely enlarged, nontender thyroid gland**. Vital signs: Temperature = 99.0° F; respiration rate = 20 breaths/min; **heart rate = 99 bpm; blood pressure = 140/90 mm Hg.**

DIFFERENTIALS: Hyperthyroidism (Graves disease, factitious hyperthyroidism, subacute thyroiditis, multinodular goiter, thyroid adenoma), Hashimoto thyroiditis, menopause, panic disorder, and pheochromocytoma. The patient's symptoms are indicative of thyrotoxicosis. Of all the causes of thyrotoxicosis listed previously, **exophthalmos** and **thyroid bruit** occur only in Graves disease. Also, although Hashimoto thyroiditis eventually results in hypothyroidism, early findings in the disease are consistent with hyperthyroidism.

LABORATORY STUDIES: Figure 7-12 outlines the approach to determining a cause of hyperthyroidism in a patient. **Serum thyroid-stimulating hormone (TSH) and triiodothyronine (T_3)/thyroxine (T_4)** should be obtained. These tests would show elevated T_3/T_4 and suppressed TSH in hyperthyroidism and would be normal in menopause, panic disorder, and pheochromocytoma. A **thyroid scan with radioactive iodide uptake** is useful for distinguishing between the various causes of hyperthyroidism listed previously. A negative scan would be expected for subacute thyroiditis and factitious hyperthyroidism. These can be further differentiated by a thorough history and physical examination. The patient with subacute thyroiditis has a tender thyroid, systemic flulike symptoms, and possible history of recent viral infection. Factitious hyperthyroidism is more often seen in healthcare workers with access to T_3/T_4 who are abusing it for weight loss purposes. A positive scan of different types would be observed in Graves disease, multinodular goiter, and thyroid adenoma. In Graves disease, a diffuse hot scan would be seen, whereas in multinodular goiter, several nodules—both hot and cold—would be visualized. In thyroid adenoma, only one such hot nodule would be seen. Graves disease can be further supported by presence of **thyroid-stimulating immunoglobulin G,** which binds to thyrotropin receptors on the thyroid gland. These lab studies would be normal in menopause and panic disorder. Normal **urine metanephrines** and **vanillylmandelic acid** would rule out pheochromocytoma.

FIGURE 7-12 Approach to thyrotoxicosis

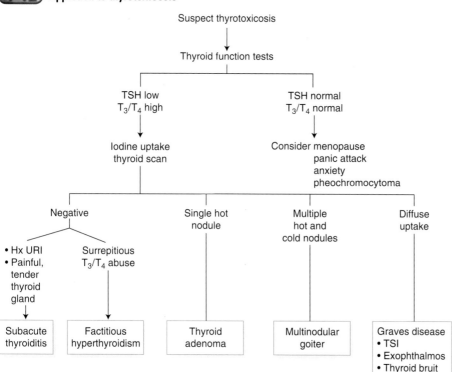

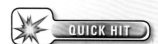

QUICK HIT

Thyrotoxicosis factitia is a factitious disorder in which the patient intentionally self-administers excess thyroid hormone (levothyroxine) to simulate the symptoms of hyperthyroidism.

Hx, history; T_3, triiodothyronine; T_4, thyroxine; TSH, thyroid-stimulating hormone; TSI, thyroid-stimulating immunoglobulin; URI, upper respiratory infection.

The Endocrine System

VII. Thyroid neoplasms (*Table 7-17*)

TABLE 7-17 Thyroid Carcinomas

Tumor	Description
Papillary carcinoma	• **Most common** thyroid cancer • **Best prognosis** of the thyroid cancers • **3:1 female predominance** • Usually occurs in third to fifth decade of life • **Associated with radiation exposure** in childhood, associated with *RET* oncogene mutation • "Ground glass" nuclei of neoplastic cells, also called "Orphan Annie eyes" due to the way the chromatin disperses • **Psammoma bodies** may be present • Forms pàpillary projections covered with cuboidal epithelium within glandular spaces
Follicular carcinoma	• Good prognosis, although worse than papillary • **3:1 female predominance** • More common in iodine-deficient areas • **Associated with *RAS* oncogene mutation** in 40% of cases • Uniform cuboidal cells lining follicles • Lacks the distinctive nuclear features of papillary carcinoma
Medullary carcinoma	• Parafollicular (C) cell neoplasm • **Secretes calcitonin,** no hypercalcemia or hypocalcemia • Associated with MEN 2a and MEN 2b • **Associated with *RET* oncogene mutation**
Anaplastic thyroid carcinoma	• Anaplastic, undifferentiated neoplasm • More common in older patients • Rapidly fatal

MEN 2a and 2b, multiple endocrine neoplasia types 2a and 2b.

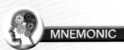

MNEMONIC

To remember the symptoms of hypercalcemia, think:
Bones: pain in bones
Stones: renal stones
Groans: abdominal pain
Psychiatric overtones: confused state

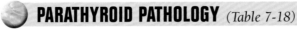

PARATHYROID PATHOLOGY (*Table 7-18*)

TABLE 7-18 Parathyroid Disorders

Condition	Etiology	Clinical Features
Primary hyperparathyroidism	**Adenoma** (most common); hyperplasia more common than carcinoma; seen in **MEN 1** and **MEN 2a;** excess parathyroid hormone (PTH); **hypercalcemia**	**Osteitis fibrosa cystica** (cystic "brown tumors" of bone); **renal calculi** and nephrocalcinosis; duodenal ulcers
Secondary hyperparathyroidism	**Hypocalcemia** caused by **chronic renal failure** (loss of vitamin D activation); parathyroid hyperplasia; excess PTH; high alkaline phosphatase	Cystic bone lesions; metastatic **calcification** of organs
Hypoparathyroidism	Most commonly secondary to **thyroidectomy;** seen in DiGeorge syndrome; **hypocalcemia**	Tetany; positive **Chvostek** and **Trousseau** signs
Pseudohypoparathyroidism	Autosomal recessive; deficient organ response to PTH	**Short stature;** underdeveloped fourth and fifth digits

MEN 1 and 2a, multiple endoplasmic neoplasia types 1 and 2a.

MULTIPLE ENDOCRINE NEOPLASIA SYNDROMES (Table 7-19)

TABLE 7-19 Multiple Endocrine Neoplasia Syndromes

Type 1 (Wermer)	Type 2a (Sipple)	Type 2b
Parathyroid hyperplasia, pituitary adenomas, pancreatic tumors, angiofibromas	**Medullary thyroid carcinoma, parathyroid hyperplasia, pheochromocytoma**	**Mucosal neuromas** (particularly of the GI tract), **medullary thyroid carcinoma, pheochromocytoma**, marfanoid body habitus

GI, gastrointestinal.

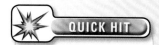

The multiple endocrine neoplasia (MEN) syndromes are autosomal dominant conditions in which more than one endocrine organ is affected by either hyperplasia or neoplasia.

MNEMONIC

MEN 1 is a disease of **3 Ps**: **P**ituitary, **P**arathyroid, and **P**ancreas.

MNEMONIC

MEN 2a is a disease of **1 M and 2 Ps**: **M**edullary thyroid carcinoma, **P**arathyroid, and **P**heochromocytoma.

MNEMONIC

MEN 2b is a disease of **2 Ms and 1 P**: **M**ucosal neuromas, **M**edullary thyroid carcinoma, and **P**heochromocytoma.

The Endocrine System

8 The Reproductive System

 DETERMINATION OF SEX

Before the seventh week of gestation, the fetal gonads are not differentiated into either the male or female genotype. Primordial germ cells migrate into the genital ridge mesoderm to form testes and ovaries. The presence or absence of the Y chromosome and the sex-determining region of the Y chromosome (SRY) determine gonadal differentiation. Therefore, the "default" gender is female if there is no SRY region on an active Y chromosome. Gender determination, which occurs after the seventh week, depends on the type of gonads present.

 FEMALE REPRODUCTIVE SYSTEM DEVELOPMENT

I. **Ovaries and other female reproductive structures**
   A. Primordial follicles contain primary **oocytes (XX genotype)** and follicular (granulosa) cells, which form the ovaries.
   B. As the upper abdomen grows, the ovaries "descend" toward the perineum.
   C. The gubernaculum assists in this descent and then becomes the ovarian ligament and the round ligament of the uterus.
   D. The **paramesonephric ducts** develop into the fallopian tubes and eventually into the uterus.

II. **Vagina and uterus** (Figure 8-1)

III. **Breasts**
   A. Only the main lactiferous ducts develop during the fetal life.
   B. Glands enlarge during puberty owing to the increased levels of estrogens, progestins, prolactin, and growth hormone.

FIGURE
8-1 Development of the female genital tract

B. Stages of development of the female external genitalia

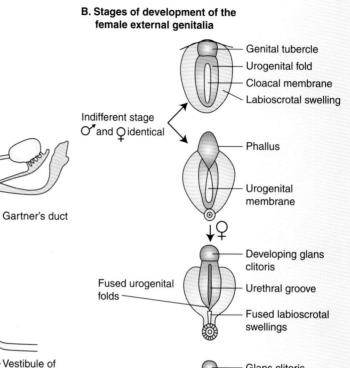

- Genital tubercle
- Urogenital fold
- Cloacal membrane
- Labioscrotal swelling

Indifferent stage ♂ and ♀ identical

- Phallus
- Urogenital membrane

↓ ♀

- Developing glans clitoris
- Urethral groove

Fused urogenital folds

- Fused labioscrotal swellings

- Glans clitoris
- Labium minora
- Labium majora

A. Reproductive system of the newborn female

- Ovary (after descent)
- Ovarian ligament
- Uterine tube
- Gartner's duct
- Round ligament of uterus
- Inguinal canal
- Vagina
- Labium majus
- Hymen
- Vestibule of vagina

Structures arising from:
- ☐ Paramesonephric duct
- ☐ Urogenital sinus
- ☐ Mesonephric duct

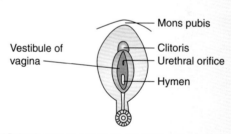

- Mons pubis
- Vestibule of vagina
- Clitoris
- Urethral orifice
- Hymen

(Adapted with permission from Moore KL, Persaud TVN. *The Developing Human: Clinically Oriented Embryology.* 6th ed. Philadelphia, PA: WB Saunders; 1998.)

MALE REPRODUCTIVE SYSTEM DEVELOPMENT

I. Testes and other male reproductive organs

A. Primary sex cords contain primordial germ cells of **XY genotype**. The Y chromosome codes for the testes-determining factor that allows for male gonadal differentiation (i.e., formation of medullary cords and seminiferous tubules).

B. Müllerian-inhibiting factor (**MIF**) is secreted by **Sertoli cells**. MIF causes regression of the Müllerian (paramesonephric) ducts and their associated female genital structures (uterine tubes and uterus).

C. The mesonephric ducts, under the influence of testosterone, become the ductus deferens, the seminal vesicles, and the ejaculatory ducts in the adult male.

II. The prostate gland forms from the urogenital sinus (Figure 8-2)

FIGURE 8-2 Development of the male genital tract

B. Stages of development of the male external genitalia

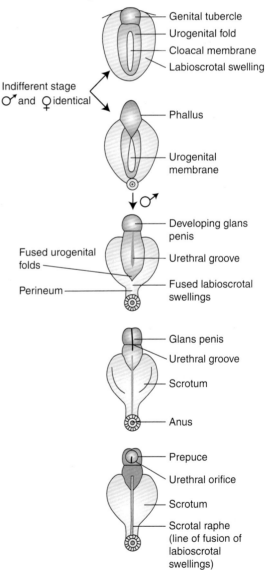

Indifferent stage ♂ and ♀ identical

- Genital tubercle
- Urogenital fold
- Cloacal membrane
- Labioscrotal swelling

- Phallus
- Urogenital membrane

♂

Fused urogenital folds

Perineum

- Developing glans penis
- Urethral groove
- Fused labioscrotal swellings

- Glans penis
- Urethral groove
- Scrotum
- Anus

- Prepuce
- Urethral orifice
- Scrotum
- Scrotal raphe (line of fusion of labioscrotal swellings)

A. Reproductive system of the newborn male

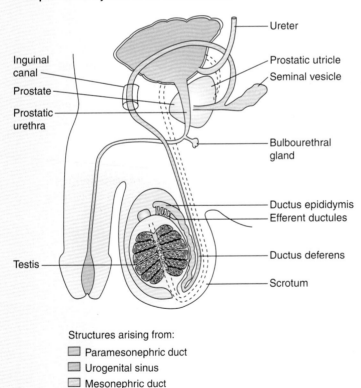

- Ureter
- Prostatic utricle
- Seminal vesicle

Inguinal canal

Prostate

Prostatic urethra

- Bulbourethral gland

- Ductus epididymis
- Efferent ductules

- Ductus deferens

Testis

- Scrotum

Structures arising from:

 Paramesonephric duct
☐ Urogenital sinus
☐ Mesonephric duct

(Adapted with permission from Moore KL, Persaud TVN. *The Developing Human: Clinically Oriented Embryology.* 6th ed. Philadelphia, PA: WB Saunders; 1998.)

III. External genitalia

A. Dihydrotestosterone (DHT) is responsible for the masculinization of genitalia.

B. The genital tubercle enlarges to become the glans penis.

C. The urogenital fold becomes the shaft of the penis.

D. The labioscrotal swellings fuse in the midline and become the scrotum.

- **Spermatogenesis versus Oogenesis** (Figure 8-3)
- **Important Anatomic Features of the Perineum** (Figure 8-4)

FIGURE
8-3 Spermatogenesis versus oogenesis

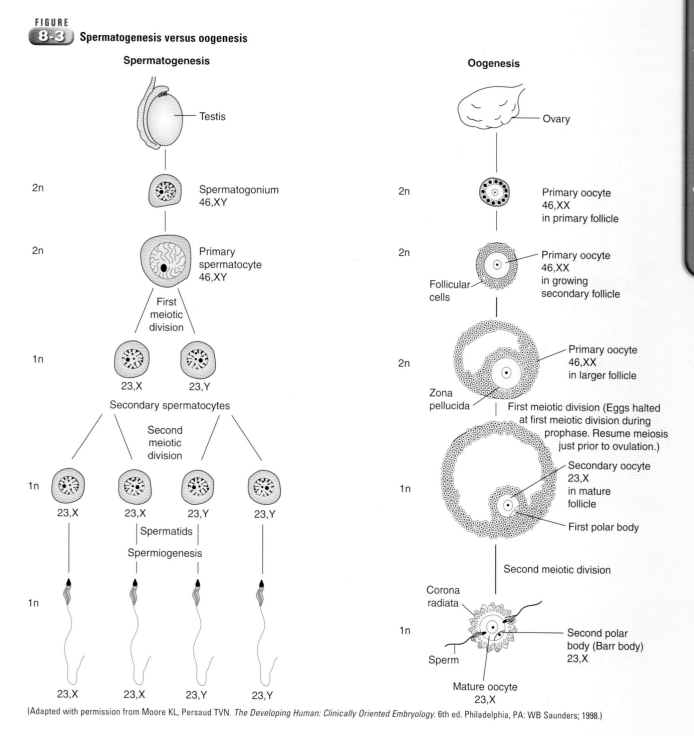

(Adapted with permission from Moore KL, Persaud TVN. *The Developing Human: Clinically Oriented Embryology.* 6th ed. Philadelphia, PA: WB Saunders; 1998.)

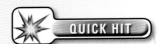

QUICK HIT

Puberty in males, usually occurring at age 15 years, is marked by an increased testosterone, leading to a greater hair distribution, growth of genitalia, nocturnal emissions, deepening of the voice, and increased muscle mass. Precocious puberty in males has a similar pathology to that in females, with the exception that it has a later age of onset.

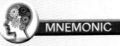

MNEMONIC

To remember the path of the sperm through the male reproductive system, think of the phrase "SEVEN UP": **S**eminiferous tubules, **E**pididymis, **V**as deferens, **E**jaculatory duct, **N**othing, **U**rethra, **P**enis.

FIGURE 8-4 Important anatomic features of the perineum

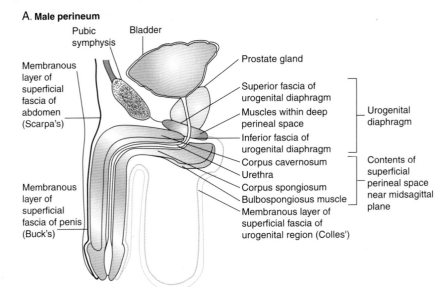

A. Male perineum

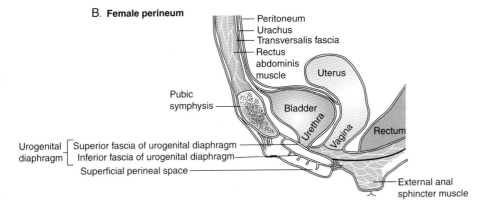

B. Female perineum

CONGENITAL MALFORMATIONS

Congenital malformations are most often caused by exposure to teratogens during the third to eighth weeks of pregnancy, which is the period of organogenesis (Table 8-1).

TABLE 8-1 Congenital Malformations	
Malformation	**Clinical Features**
Hypospadias	• Urethra opens on the **ventral** side of the penis • Spongy urethra does not form properly or the **urogenital folds** do not fuse • Paucity of hormone receptors or too little hormone produced from the testes may play a role • More common than epispadias
Epispadias	• Urethra opens on the **dorsum** of the penis
Undescended testis (cryptorchidism)	• Most are of unknown cause • May be unilateral or bilateral • Most testes descend before 1 year of life • If testes remain undescended, **sterility or testicular cancer** can result
Congenital inguinal hernia (indirect hernia)	• A communication is formed between the **tunica vaginalis** (adjacent to the testis) and the peritoneal cavity • A loop of intestine may herniate into the opening and become entrapped, resulting in obstruction
True hermaphroditism	• **Both testicular** and **ovarian tissue** are present • External genitalia are ambiguous • Usually 46,XX
Female pseudohermaphroditism	• XX genotype with **virilization** of the external genitalia is present • The cause is **excess androgen exposure** • This malformation is most often caused by congenital adrenal hyperplasia, a **21-hydroxylase deficiency** (autosomal recessive disease with low cortisol and high ACTH)
Male pseudohermaphroditism	• XY genotype with varying ambiguities of the external genitalia • The cause is a **lack of MIF and testosterone**
Androgen insensitivity syndrome (testicular feminization)	• **XY** genotype with female phenotype • Caused by a **defective androgen receptor** • Vagina ends blindly (no uterus) • Normal female pubertal development occurs but pubic hair is scant and there are no menses
Double uterus completely	• The cause is failure of the **paramesonephric ducts** to fuse • The condition may appear in two forms: uterus divided internally by a thin septum or a division of only the superior part of the uterus (bicornuate uterus)
Kallmann syndrome	• A deficiency of GnRH results in decreased FSH and LH • No secondary sexual characteristics are present • Associated with hypoplasia of the olfactory bulbs **(anosmia)**

ACTH, adrenocorticotropic hormone; FSH, follicle-stimulating hormone; GnRH, gonadotropin-releasing hormone; LH, luteinizing hormone; MIF, müllerian-inhibiting factor.

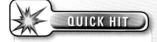

Epispadias is associated with exstrophy of the bladder.

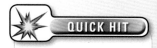

Congenital inguinal hernia is associated with cryptorchidism.

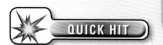

In androgen insensitivity syndrome (AIS), affected individuals have normal testes with normal production of testosterone and normal conversion to DHT, which differentiates this condition from 5α-reductase deficiency. Because the testes produce normal amounts of MIF, affected individuals do not have fallopian tubes, a uterus, or a proximal (upper) vagina. In AIS, the external female genitalia and breasts develop by default because of the **lack of responsiveness of androgen receptors to DHT** during development. In 5α-reductase deficiency, **lack of DHT** results in a female genotype. At puberty in these individuals, a testosterone surge results in adequate levels of DHT, resulting in growth of male genitalia and "penis at 12" syndrome.

The Reproductive System

GENETIC ABNORMALITIES

The incidence of genetic abnormalities as a result of aberrant chromosomes significantly increases when the mother is older than 35 years of age. In these patients, additional consideration should be given to genetic testing.

- Genetic Abnormalities Caused by Abnormal Somatic Chromosomes (Table 8-2)
- Genetic Abnormalities Caused by Abnormal Sex Chromosomes (Table 8-3)

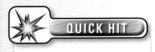

QUICK HIT

There is an increased incidence of trisomy 21 in women older than 35 years of age. The incidence of the Robertsonian translocation type of Down syndrome is familial and does not increase with the age of the mother.

QUICK HIT

Down syndrome is the most common genetic cause of mental retardation in males; fragile X is the second most common.

TABLE 8-2	Genetic Abnormalities Caused by Abnormal Somatic Chromosomes	
Syndrome	**Genotype**	**Description**
Down syndrome	Trisomy 21 (95%) or Robertsonian translocation of 14 and 21	• **Mental retardation** • Epicanthal folds • Large tongue • Brushfield spots on iris • Simian crease in hands • Increased incidence of congenital heart disease, acute leukemia, and dementia of the Alzheimer type later in life
Edwards syndrome	Trisomy 18	• Duodenal atresia • Mental retardation • Micrognathia • **Rocker bottom feet** • Second digit overlaps third and fourth • Increased incidence of congenital heart disease
Patau syndrome	Trisomy 13	• Mental retardation • Microphthalmia • Polydactyly • Cleft lip and palate
Cri du chat syndrome	Deletion of 5p (5p−)	• Catlike cry • Mental retardation • Microcephaly • Hypertelorism

MNEMONIC

To remember that fragile X is due to trinucleotide repeat **CGG**, think: "**S**ee **G**iant **G**onads."

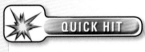

GAA   FA
CAG   HD
CGG   FX
CTG   MD

TABLE 8-3	Genetic Abnormalities Caused by Abnormal Sex Chromosomes	
Syndrome	**Genotype**	**Description**
Turner syndrome	45,XO	• **Monosomy** of the X chromosome • Absence of Barr body • Short stature • Webbed neck • Widely spaced nipples • Wide, "shield-like" chest • Wide carrying angle of arms • Lack of sexual maturity • Amenorrhea • Coarctation of the aorta
Klinefelter syndrome	47,XXY	• Tall with long limbs • Often presents with gynecomastia • Hyalinization of seminiferous tubules • Hypogonadism, lack of spermatogenesis leading to sterility • One Barr body

(continued)

TABLE 8-3 Genetic Abnormalities Caused by Abnormal Sex Chromosomes
(Continued)

Syndrome	Genotype	Description
XYY syndrome	47,XYY	• Normal-appearing male, often tall • Often associated with **aggressive behavior** • May be overrepresented in the population of incarcerated males
XXX syndrome	47,XXX	• Usually asymptomatic • Rarely associated with **menstrual irregularities** and mild mental retardation • Two Barr bodies
Fragile X syndrome	46,XY	• The end of the X chromosome appears delicate • **Macroorchidism** • Common cause of **mental retardation** • Long face • Low-set, large ears
Prader–Willi syndrome	−15q12 (no paternal contribution, imprinting disorder)	• Obesity • **Hyperphagia** • **Hypogonadism** • Short stature • Mental retardation
Angelman syndrome	−15q12 (no maternal contribution, imprinting disorder)	• Ataxia • Mental retardation • **Inappropriate laughter** • Patient appears to act like a **"happy puppet"**

(handwritten margin notes: "paternal" next to Prader–Willi; "ho"; "maternal" next to Angelman)

MENARCHE, MENSTRUATION, AND MENOPAUSE

I. Menarche

A. First menstruation; usually occurs between **11 and 14 years of age**

B. Follows thelarche (development of breast buds) by 2 years

C. Precocious puberty

1. Pubertal changes before 9 years of age in boys and 8 years of age in girls

2. True precocious puberty

a. Early but normal pubertal development

b. Precocious puberty is **usually familial and not pathologic.**

c. May cause emotional and social adjustment problems

3. Incomplete precocious puberty

a. Premature development of a single pubertal characteristic

b. Types

- Premature thelarche: breast budding before 8 years of age
- Premature adrenarche: growth of axillary hair
- Premature pubarche: growth of pubic hair

c. Generally self-limited

4. Etiology

a. Central—increased follicle-stimulating hormone (FSH) and luteinizing hormone (LH) (from the pituitary) lead to sex steroid production by the gonads.

b. Peripheral—caused by increased sex steroids not driven by pituitary gonadotropins (gonadal tumors, adrenal pathology, exogenous estrogens, etc.)

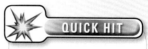

QUICK HIT

Breast surgery should not be performed in girls with precocious puberty because the excision of a "lump" in premature thelarche leads to the loss of an entire breast.

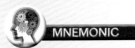

The Reproductive System

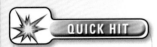

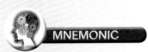

II. Menstruation and fertilization

FIGURE 8-5 Hormone function within the menstrual cycle

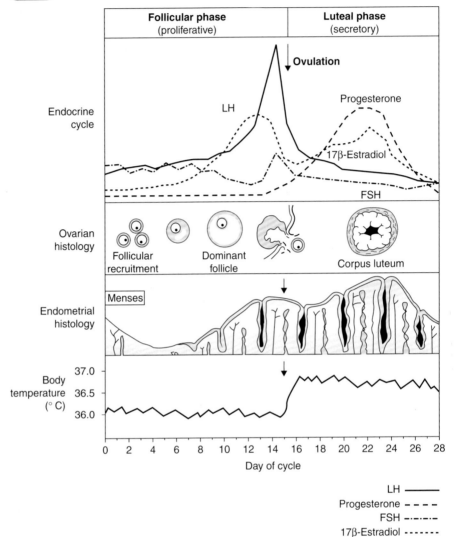

FSH, follicle-stimulating hormone; LH, luteinizing hormone.

A. Hormone formation and function (Figure 8-5)
1. Ovarian **steroids** are synthesized from **cholesterol**.
2. LH from the pituitary regulates the conversion of cholesterol to pregnenolone (the first step in estrogen synthesis) in the theca cells.
3. FSH from the pituitary regulates the final step in estrogen synthesis in the granulosa cells.
4. Estrogen
   a. Secreted by the follicular cells of the **ovary**
   b. Induces development of the secondary sex characteristics
   • Binds to the estrogen receptor
   • Activated estrogen-receptor complex interacts with nuclear chromatin.
   • Initiates hormone-specific RNA synthesis
   • Results in protein synthesis
   c. Stimulates uterine growth and development
   d. Induces proliferation of endometrium
   e. Causes thickening of the vaginal mucosa

     f. Induces development of the breast ductal system

     g. Causes bone growth (increased osteoblastic activity and decreased osteoclastic activity)

   5. Progesterone

     a. Secreted by the **corpus luteum** produced in response to LH

     b. Converts proliferative endometrium to secretory endometrium

     c. Inhibits uterine contractions

     d. Increases the viscosity of cervical mucus

     e. Increases the basal body temperature

     f. Induces the development of breast glandular system

B. Menstrual cycle (Figure 8-6)

   1. One cycle is defined as the time from the onset of one menses to the next, with an average of **28 days**.

   2. Characteristic changes in the ovary lead to ovulation and hormone production (Figure 8-7).

FIGURE 8-6 The menstrual cycle

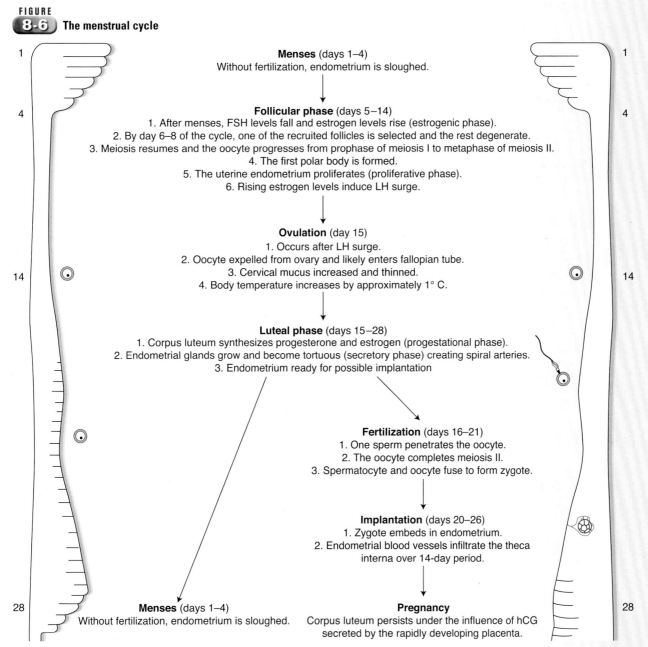

Menses (days 1–4)
Without fertilization, endometrium is sloughed.

Follicular phase (days 5–14)
1. After menses, FSH levels fall and estrogen levels rise (estrogenic phase).
2. By day 6–8 of the cycle, one of the recruited follicles is selected and the rest degenerate.
3. Meiosis resumes and the oocyte progresses from prophase of meiosis I to metaphase of meiosis II.
4. The first polar body is formed.
5. The uterine endometrium proliferates (proliferative phase).
6. Rising estrogen levels induce LH surge.

Ovulation (day 15)
1. Occurs after LH surge.
2. Oocyte expelled from ovary and likely enters fallopian tube.
3. Cervical mucus increased and thinned.
4. Body temperature increases by approximately 1° C.

Luteal phase (days 15–28)
1. Corpus luteum synthesizes progesterone and estrogen (progestational phase).
2. Endometrial glands grow and become tortuous (secretory phase) creating spiral arteries.
3. Endometrium ready for possible implantation

Fertilization (days 16–21)
1. One sperm penetrates the oocyte.
2. The oocyte completes meiosis II.
3. Spermatocyte and oocyte fuse to form zygote.

Implantation (days 20–26)
1. Zygote embeds in endometrium.
2. Endometrial blood vessels infiltrate the theca interna over 14-day period.

Menses (days 1–4)
Without fertilization, endometrium is sloughed.

Pregnancy
Corpus luteum persists under the influence of hCG secreted by the rapidly developing placenta.

FSH, follicle-stimulating hormone; hCG, human chorionic gonadotropin; LH, luteinizing hormone.

FIGURE 8-7 Developmental changes in the ovary

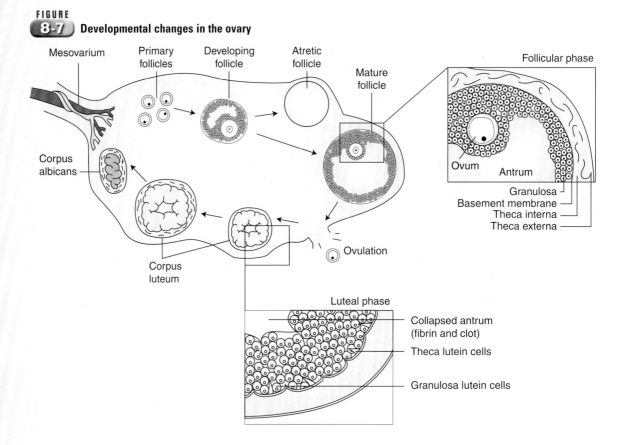

C. **Disorders**

1. **Abnormal uterine bleeding**

a. Functional menstrual disorders, characterized as excessive bleeding either during ("menorrhagia") or between ("metrorrhagia") menstrual periods

b. Most common gynecologic problem during reproductive years

c. Causes

- Organic lesions (polyps, fibroids)
- Hormonal dysregulation (anovulatory cycles, polycystic ovary syndrome, functional ovarian cysts)
- Neoplasia (endometrial hyperplasia, cancer)
- Abnormal pregnancy (ectopic pregnancy, abortion)

2. **Polycystic ovary syndrome** (Stein–Leventhal syndrome)

a. Triad of

- **Androgen excess** (hirsutism, acne)
- **Ovulatory dysfunction** or anovulation (causing secondary amenorrhea)
- Characteristic **appearance of the ovaries on ultrasound** (stromal fibrosis and small follicular cysts)

b. Also associated with obesity and insulin resistance

c. Increased LH and testosterone, increased estrogen (from aromatization of testosterone in adipose tissue), decreased FSH

d. Endometrial hyperplasia is common; increased risk of endometrial adenocarcinoma

e. Treat with weight loss; clomiphene or metformin for infertility/anovulation; oral contraceptives or progesterone; spironolactone for androgen excess

3. **Endometriosis**

a. Nonneoplastic endometrial tissue located outside the uterus

b. Responds to hormonal variations of menstrual cycle

c. Most commonly occurs on the ovaries (bilateral)

d. Presents as pain before and during menstruation

e. Multiple, small, hemosiderin-filled endometrial implants; "powder burns"; scarring; adhesions; endometriomas (large, blood-filled sacs called "**chocolate cysts**")

f. May result in infertility

g. Treat with oral contraceptive pills (OCPs), leuprolide, and/or surgical excision. Danazol, a mild androgen, is rarely used anymore because of side effects.

4. **Amenorrhea** (Figures 8-8 and 8-9)

a. **Primary amenorrhea**: absence of menarche in a woman by age 16 years
   • Genetic (Turner syndrome, androgen insensitivity syndrome)
   • Structural (imperforate hymen, Müllerian duct agenesis)
   • Delayed puberty

b. **Secondary amenorrhea**: cessation of menstruation for >3 months in a woman of reproductive age with cyclic periods or >6 months in a woman with irregular periods
   • Pregnancy
   • Ovarian failure
   • Polycystic ovary syndrome
   • Thyroid disorders
   • Athleticism
   • Anorexia
   • Stress

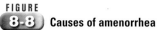

FIGURE 8-8 Causes of amenorrhea

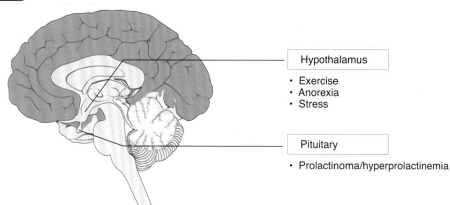

Hypothalamus
• Exercise
• Anorexia
• Stress

Pituitary
• Prolactinoma/hyperprolactinemia

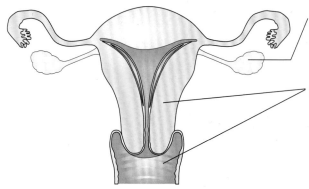

Ovary
• Turner syndrome (streak gonads)
• Ovarian failure
• PCOS

Uterus/Vagina
• Müllerian duct agenesis (absence of uterus, upper 2/3 vagina)
• Androgen insensitivity syndrome (absence of ovaries, uterus, upper 2/3 vagina) (presence of undescended testes, normal breast and external female genitalia)
• Imperforate hymen
• Transverse vaginal septum

In approaching the various causes of amenorrhea, it is easiest to conceptualize them within the hypothalamic-pituitary-ovarian-uterine framework. It is postulated that stress, exercise, and anorexia act at the level of the hypothalamus to stop the menstrual cycle. Prolactin tumors at the pituitary level disrupt the neuroendocrine regulation of gonadotropin-releasing hormone, resulting in an abnormal menstrual function. At the ovarian level, ovarian failure, polycystic ovary syndrome (PCOS), and streak gonads of Turner syndrome result in menstrual dysfunction. Müllerian duct agenesis, imperforate hymen, and androgen insensitivity syndrome are abnormalities at the uterine and vaginal level.

The Reproductive System

FIGURE
8-9 Approach to amenorrhea

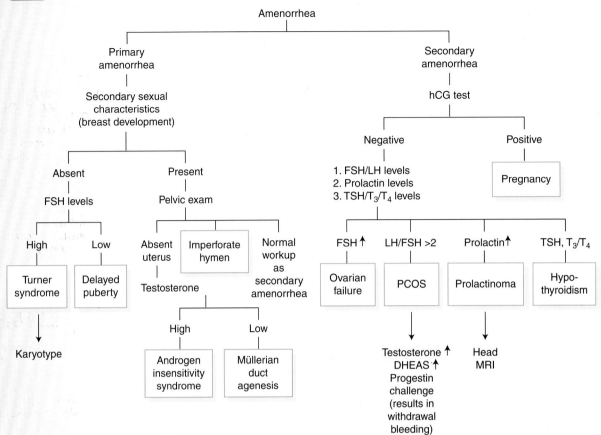

DHEAS, dehydroepiandrosterone sulfate; FSH, follicle-stimulating hormone; hCG, human chorionic gonadotropin; LH, luteinizing hormone; MRI, magnetic resonance imaging; PCOS, polycystic ovary syndrome; T_3, triiodothyronine; T_4, thyroxine; TSH, thyroid-stimulating hormone.

III. Menopause

A. Last physiologic menstrual cycle usually occurs in the **early 50s** (mean age is 51½ years).

B. Estrogen levels fall (because of the reduced ovarian function) and FSH levels increase.

C. Early signs
1. Anxiety
2. Mood swings
3. Irritability
4. Depression
5. **Hot flashes**: bouts of flushing and sweating

D. Late signs
1. Vaginal dryness
2. Painful intercourse
3. Urinary tract infections
4. Atrophy of breast tissue because of lack of estrogen stimulation
5. **Osteoporosis**
6. **Decreased high-density lipoprotein (HDL)**, leading to an increased risk of **coronary artery disease**

E. Management of patients who are menopausal or postmenopausal may involve estrogen replacement therapy.
1. Effects
a. Decreases sleep disturbances
b. Increases HDL and decreases low-density lipoprotein (LDL)
c. Decreases postmenopausal vaginal atrophy

d. Decreases bone resorption and osteoporosis
e. Decreases frequency of "hot flashes" by reestablishing hypothalamic control of norepinephrine secretion
2. Risks and contraindications
a. History of estrogen-dependent cancer
b. Increased risk of breast and endometrial cancer
c. In women with an intact uterus, estrogen increases the risk of developing endometrial carcinoma. Therefore, estrogen is combined with progestin to decrease the effects of unopposed estrogen.
d. Women's Health Initiative showed that estrogen increased the absolute risk of stroke by 0.13% when compared to placebo.

IV. Oral contraceptives

A. Agents that interfere with ovulation to prevent pregnancy
B. Combination pills contain progestin and estrogen.
1. The estrogen component suppresses ovulation.
2. The progestin component thickens the cervical mucus, reducing the passage of sperm.
C. Other agents
1. Progestin-only
a. Available as pills, intramuscular (IM) injection, or progestin implants
b. Progestin-only pills have higher failure rates; injections and implant devices have lower failure rates than combination oral contraceptives.
c. Increased rate of menstrual irregularities
2. Mifepristone (RU-486), a progestin antagonist
a. Results in fetal abortion when given early in pregnancy (within first 6 weeks)
b. Interferes with progesterone and decreases human chorionic gonadotropin (hCG)
D. Side effects
1. Cardiovascular disease
a. Women older than 35 years of age who smoke are at greatest risk from thromboembolism.
b. Progestin-predominant preparations can lead to an increase in the LDL:HDL ratio.
2. Benign liver hepatomas and hemangiomas
3. Gallbladder disease
4. Emotional changes

PREGNANCY AND ITS ASSOCIATED COMPLICATIONS

I. Normal pregnancy

A. For clinical purposes, assume that a **woman of childbearing age is pregnant** unless proven otherwise.
B. Normal gestation is **40 weeks**.
C. Clinical signs include missed periods, swollen breasts, fatigue, nausea, and **elevated β-human chorionic gonadotropin (β-hCG)** (serum).
D. Hormonal regulation
1. During fertilization, **β-hCG** produced by the placenta **prevents corpus luteum regression**.
2. During the first trimester, the corpus luteum produces estrogen and progesterone.
3. Second and third trimesters
a. Progesterone is produced by the placenta.
b. Estrogen production is regulated by the interplay among the fetal adrenal gland, fetal liver, and placenta.
4. The initiating event in parturition is unknown, but delivery can be induced by oxytocin.

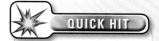
QUICK HIT
Clomiphene interferes with the negative feedback provided by estrogen to the brain and causes an increase in gonadotropin-releasing hormone (GnRH). This leads to stimulation of ovulation and can be used to treat infertility associated with anovulatory cycles.

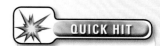
QUICK HIT
Taking oral contraceptives provides other benefits, such as decreased risk of dysmenorrhea, iron deficiency anemia, ectopic pregnancy, benign breast disease, endometrial cancer, ovarian cysts, ovarian cancer, and postmenopausal hip fracture.

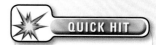
QUICK HIT
A pudendal nerve block can be performed to alleviate the pain of childbirth. One hand is inserted into the vagina to locate the ischial spine, which is used as a landmark, while the other hand inserts a needle, which contains anesthetic for the pudendal nerve, which crosses the ischial spine at this level, thus anesthetizing the skin lateral to the vaginal opening.

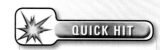
QUICK HIT
The narrowest diameter that the fetus must transverse during birth is the pelvic outlet, from ischial spine to ischial spine (interspinous distance).

Clinical Vignette 8-1

CLINICAL PRESENTATION: A 17-year-old girl presents to her primary care physician with the chief complaint that she has not **had her period for several months.** She previously had fairly regular menses, with menarche at age 13 years. She is the daughter of a **middle class family,** an **excellent student,** and **active in track** outside of class. Physical examination shows a well-developed female with **normal external female genitalia.** Pelvic examination is deferred.

DIFFERENTIALS: Pregnancy, anorexia nervosa, exercise, pituitary prolactinoma, polycystic ovary syndrome, ovarian failure, Turner syndrome, and hypothyroidism. **Any female who reports missing her period should be evaluated for pregnancy.** The first step in approaching amenorrhea is to determine whether the patient has had periods in the past (secondary amenorrhea) or has never experienced menstruation (primary amenorrhea). There are four diagnoses unique to primary amenorrhea: Turner syndrome, Müllerian duct agenesis, imperforate hymen, and androgen insensitivity syndrome. These disorders can be ruled out in this case because the patient has a history of periods. (*Note:* Mosaic Turner syndrome can have some menstrual bleeding prior to the cessation of periods.) Figure 8-8 shows the various causes of amenorrhea. On the USMLE, look for certain symptoms that suggest some disorders over others: hirsutism (polycystic ovary syndrome [PCOS]), obesity (PCOS), galactorrhea (prolactinoma), webbed neck (Turner), widely spaced nipples (Turner), presence of abdominal masses (testes in androgen insensitivity syndrome), and renal anomalies (Müllerian duct agenesis). Pelvic examination would be helpful in assessing imperforate hymen, androgen insensitivity syndrome (blind-ending short vaginal canal and absence of uterus and ovaries), and Müllerian duct agenesis (blind-ending short vaginal canal and absence of uterus).

LABORATORY STUDIES: In approaching secondary amenorrhea (Figure 8-9), first obtain a **pregnancy test.** If negative, a battery of tests would be performed, including **follicle-stimulating hormone (FSH), luteinizing hormone (LH), thyroid-stimulating hormone (TSH)/triiodothyronine (T$_3$)/levothyroxine (T$_4$), and prolactin levels** to rule out hypothyroidism and prolactinoma, respectively. FSH and LH levels are expected to be high in cases of ovarian defects (Turner syndrome, ovarian failure, and PCOS) and low to normal in defects at the hypothalamic/pituitary level (pituitary tumors, anorexia, and athleticism). To further differentiate among these, if LH/FSH >2, it suggests PCOS, and **testosterone** and dehydroepiandrosterone sulfate **(DHEAS) levels** should be measured (will likely be elevated). Also, progestin challenge should induce withdrawal from menstrual bleeding. Turner syndrome with ovarian failure can be distinguished by karyotype. In cases of suspected anatomical abnormalities, a pelvic ultrasound should be performed.

MANAGEMENT: Most treatments of secondary amenorrhea are directed to correct the underlying disease process via surgery or restore ovulatory cycle via estrogen–progestin therapy. PCOS is treated based on the reproductive desire of the female—**spironolactone** with **clomiphene citrate** is used if the patient is interested in conceiving; otherwise, **oral contraception** may be used.

5. Lactation
    a. Estrogen and progesterone block the effect of prolactin on the breast.
    b. Prolactin levels rise throughout pregnancy and suppress ovulation.
    c. Estrogen/progesterone levels fall after delivery.
E. Prenatal diagnostic procedures
    1. **Amniocentesis** is an aspiration of fluid from the amniotic sac at ≥15 weeks' gestation.
        a. α-Fetoprotein (**AFP**) assay for neural tube defects
        b. **Spectrophotometry** to determine hemolytic disease of the newborn (see Chapter 10)
        c. Sex chromatin studies for X-linked disease
        d. **Cell culture** studies for chromosomal abnormalities
        e. Enzyme and DNA analysis
        f. Infection testing (cytomegalovirus [CMV] or *Toxoplasma* DNA)
    2. Maternal serum AFP
        a. Elevated in neural tube defects
        b. Reduced in Down syndrome

MNEMONIC

Remember the causes of **I**ncreased **M**aternal **S**erum **A**lpha Feto**P**rotein: **I**ntestinal obstruction, **M**ultiple gestation/**M**yeloschisis, **S**pina bifida cystica, **A**nencephaly/**A**bdominal wall defects, **F**etal deaths, and **P**lacental abruption.

3. Chorionic villus sampling
   a. It can be performed at 10 weeks of pregnancy.
   b. Cells are aspirated from the chorionic villus.
   c. Cells are evaluated for genetic abnormalities.
4. **Ultrasound**
   a. Measures fetal size, determines sex, and diagnoses fetal malformations
F. Apgar score
1. It is used for physical assessment of child 1 minute and 5 minutes after birth.
2. Five categories are scored 0, 1, or 2, with 2 being indicative of better performance.
   a. Color (blue = 0, trunk pink = 1, all pink = 2)
   b. Heart rate (0 = 0, <100 = 1, 100+ = 2)
   c. Reflexes (none = 0, grimace = 1, grimace and irritable = 2)
   d. Muscle tone (none = 0, some = 1, active = 2)
   e. Respiration (none = 0, irregular = 1, regular = 2)

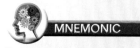

II. Abnormal placental attachment
A. **Abruptio placentae** *abrupt detachment*
1. Placenta separates from the uterine wall before parturition.
2. It is associated with painful bleeding in the third trimester.
3. It usually leads to fetal **death**.
4. It may result in hemorrhage and disseminated intravascular coagulation (DIC) in mother.
B. **Placenta accreta** *creeping in*
1. Direct connection of the myometrium to placenta after loss of decidua basalis
2. Caused by prior surgery or trauma during pregnancy
3. Improper separation results in massive **hemorrhage**
C. **Placenta previa** *preview the cervix*
1. Placenta attaches to the lower uterus and blocks the cervical os.
2. It is associated with **painless bleeding** in the third trimester.

III. Ectopic pregnancy
A. Risk factors
1. **Pelvic inflammatory disease (PID)** (e.g., chronic salpingitis)
2. Previous surgery
3. Endometriosis
4. Previous ectopic pregnancy
B. Clinical features
1. Amenorrhea
2. Pelvic pain and cervical tenderness
3. Tissue mass (usually in the fallopian tubes)
4. Elevated β-hCG levels without intrauterine pregnancy

IV. Preeclampsia
A. Diagnosis requires only **hypertension** and any **proteinuria** during pregnancy. It is often associated with **edema**.
B. Most common in the last trimester of first pregnancy
C. May result in eclampsia if untreated
1. Eclampsia has manifestations similar to preeclampsia, but it also includes seizures and possibly DIC.
2. **HELLP syndrome** is a severe, atypical variant of eclampsia, characterized by Hypertension, Elevated Liver enzymes, and Low Platelets.

V. Hydatidiform mole
A. A benign placental tumor resembling a "**cluster of grapes**," with a marked increase in β-hCG
B. Manifests as vaginal bleeding and an increase in uterine size
C. "Snowstorm" pattern seen on ultrasound

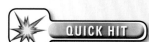

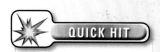

D. Two types
 1. **Complete mole**
  a. Diploid XX karyotype
  b. No embryo present
  c. Completely paternal in origin
 2. **Partial mole**
  a. Triploid karyotype (XXX, XXY, or XYY)
  b. Embryonic parts may be present

VI. Gestational diabetes

A. Insulin resistance occurs in normal pregnancy.
B. The diagnosis is made using a 3-hour 100-g oral glucose tolerance test, if the patient's serum glucose exceeds two of the four following criteria (exact cutoffs may vary by institution):
 1. Fasting >105 mg/dL
 2. 1 hour >190 mg/dL
 3. 2 hours >165 mg/dL
 4. 3 hours >145 mg/dL
C. High blood glucose leads to hyperglycemia in the fetus, macrosomia (enlarged body), increased risk of birth trauma, and increased likelihood of cesarean section because of the large size of fetus.
D. Neonatal hypoglycemia can occur because the infant's increased insulin production is too great.

VII. Infections causing birth defects (TORCHES)

A. The **TORCHES** are Toxoplasmosis, Other infections, Rubella, Cytomegalovirus infection, HErpes simplex, and Syphilis.
B. This group of infectious organisms can cause birth defects if the mother is infected during pregnancy, especially in the first trimester.
 1. Infection with herpes simplex more commonly occurs during the passage through the birth canal.
C. Important agents in the "other" category are HIV, hepatitis B, and parvovirus B19.

GYNECOLOGIC DIAGNOSTIC TESTS

I. Wet mount

A. Vaginal epithelial scrapings placed on a glass slide with a drop of saline
B. Microbes detected
 1. *Trichomonas* appears as a pear-shaped, flagellated organism with sporadic movement.
 2. Bacterial vaginosis appears as vaginal epithelium with spotting and stippling (**clue cells**).

II. Potassium hydroxide (KOH) preparation

A. KOH is added to a microscope slide prepared with vaginal epithelial scrapings.
B. Epithelium is dissolved with KOH.
C. Microbes detected
 1. *Candida*, which is resistant to KOH, remains on the slide and is identified by its **budding cells with short hyphae**.
 2. KOH reacts with bacterial amines, producing a "fishy odor" characteristic of bacterial vaginosis (whiff test).

III. Papanicolaou (Pap) smear

A. Cells from the cervix are scraped and fixed onto a glass slide.
B. Human papillomavirus (HPV) is characterized by **koilocytes** (large epithelial cells with perinuclear clearing).
C. Precancerous lesions detected: cervical intraepithelial neoplasia (**CIN**) 1, 2, and 3

D. Cancers detected
1. Invasive **squamous cell carcinoma** (most common)
2. Cervical adenocarcinoma

SEXUALLY TRANSMITTED DISEASES

Between 20% and 50% of those patients with one sexually transmitted disease (STD) will have a coexisting infection with another. The sexual partners of those diagnosed with an STD should be treated. Physicians should encourage their patients to make partners aware of potential STD risk and urge them to seek diagnosis and treatment (Table 8-4).

TABLE 8-4 Sexually Transmitted Diseases

Microbe	Disease
Klebsiella granulomatis	Granuloma inguinale; biopsy shows **Donovan bodies**
Chlamydia trachomatis	Urethritis; **acute pelvic inflammatory disease**; cervicitis; serotypes L1, L2, and L3 cause lymphogranuloma venereum, with ulcerative lesions of the genitalia
Haemophilus ducreyi	Chancroid, **painful** ulcerative lesions of the genitalia
Herpes simplex virus-2	Genital herpes, urethritis, **painful** ulcerative lesions of the genitalia
HIV types 1 and 2	**AIDS**
Human papillomavirus (especially serotypes 6 and 11)	**Genital or anal warts** (condyloma acuminatum) of vulva
Human papillomavirus (especially serotypes 16, 18, 31, and 45)	**Squamous cell carcinoma** of cervix, vagina, anus, or penis; CIN
Neisseria gonorrhoeae	Urethritis, **acute pelvic inflammatory disease**, cervicitis, pharyngitis, monoarticular **arthritis**
Treponema pallidum	Syphilis: Primary syphilis—chancres (**painless** ulcerative lesions of the genitalia) Secondary syphilis—gray, wartlike lesions on the genitalia (condyloma lata); rash on palms and soles Tertiary syphilis—neurologic manifestations such as tabes dorsalis and ascending aortic aneurysm
Trichomonas vaginalis	Vulvovaginitis, male urethritis

CIN, cervical intraepithelial neoplasia.

FEMALE GYNECOLOGIC NEOPLASMS

Tumors of the gynecologic organs may manifest themselves as abnormal uterine bleeding and, as such, a heightened level of suspicion must be maintained with this presentation. Many of these neoplasms can be detected, and even prevented (as is the case with cervical cancer), by routine gynecologic examinations.

I.   Ovarian neoplasms of epithelial cell origin (*Table 8-5*)

II. Ovarian neoplasms of germ cell origin (*Table 8-6*)

III. Tumors of the uterus (cervix and body) (*Table 8-7*)

IV. Tumors of the vulva and vagina (*Table 8-8*)

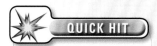

QUICK HIT

Chlamydia is the most common bacterial sexually transmitted disease (STD) in the world in part because of the fact that it goes undetected so frequently. If a person is diagnosed with gonorrhea, treatment for gonorrhea should be supplemented with chlamydia therapy for both the patient and his or her partner.

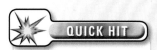

MNEMONIC

To remember the painful ulcers of the genitalia, think in *H. ducreyi* "you do cry," and HSV**2** is painful, **too**. Syph**ilis** is pain**less**.

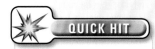

QUICK HIT

Some nonsexually transmitted infections of the genitourinary tract include *Candida albicans*, which causes vulvovaginitis; *Staphylococcus aureus*, which can result in toxic shock syndrome; bacterial vaginosis; and *Escherichia coli* and *Staphylococcus saprophyticus*, both of which can cause urinary tract infections (UTIs).

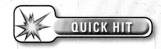

QUICK HIT

Salpingitis, often associated with PID, can lead to infertility if left untreated.

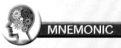

QUICK HIT

PID can be diagnosed via bimanual pelvic examination eliciting **"the chandelier sign"** (exquisite cervical motion tenderness).

MNEMONIC

Remember the features of *Trichomonas* with the four Fs: **F**lagella, **F**rothy discharge, **F**ishy odor, and **F**lagyl (treatment).

The Reproductive System

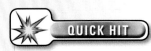

QUICK HIT

Toxic shock syndrome can result from bacterial (*Staphylococcus aureus*) overgrowth on tampons. The enterotoxin involved acts as a superantigen, causing excess activation of T-helper cells, resulting in an increased cytokine production and septic shock.

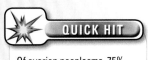

QUICK HIT

Of ovarian neoplasms, 75% are epithelial in origin. These tumors are usually seen in middle-aged to elderly women.

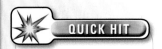

QUICK HIT

Cancer antigen 125 (CA-125) is elevated in more than 80% of ovarian carcinomas.

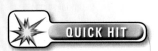

QUICK HIT

Germ cell tumors account for only 25% of ovarian neoplasms, but they are the most common ovarian tumors found in women younger than 20 years of age.

Vessels to the ovary suspensory (infundibulopelvic) ovarian mass can cause torsion

TABLE 8-5 Ovarian Neoplasms of Epithelial Cell Origin

Neoplasm	Morphology	Clinical Presentation
Serous cystadenoma	Cystic *psammoma*	Benign; frequently bilateral *Post menopause, BRCA, Lynch, OCP protective*
Serous cystadenocarcinoma	Cystic *shaggy appearance*	Malignant; frequently bilateral; most common (50% of ovarian neoplasms)
Mucinous cystadenoma	Mucin-filled cysts	Benign
Mucinous cystadenocarcinoma	Mucin-filled cysts	Malignant; **pseudomyxoma peritonei** (diffuse peritoneal metastasis secreting mucin)
Endometrioid adenocarcinoma	Resembles endometrium	Malignant
Brenner tumor	Resembles **transitional epithelium** *Bladder like*	Benign; rare tumor
Clear cell cancer	Abundant **clear cytoplasm**	Usually unilateral; rare

TABLE 8-6 Ovarian Neoplasms of Germ Cell Origin

Neoplasm	Morphology	Clinical Features
Dysgerminoma *(Most common)*	Large cells with clear cytoplasm *PLAP, bHCG, LDH* *Fried egg appearance*	Malignant; **equivalent of seminoma;** occurs in children
Endodermal sinus (yolk sac) *premenopausal but also children*	Resembles yolk sac *primative glomeruli* *schiller-Duval bodies*	Malignant; produces **AFP**
Immature teratoma	Elements from multiple embryonic layers; poorly differentiated; resembles fetal or embryonic tissue	Malignant
Mature teratoma (dermoid cyst)	Elements from multiple embryonic layers, including hair, bone, tooth, and nervous tissue; duplication of maternal genetics; resembles adult tissue	**Most common germ cell neoplasm** (90%); **benign** (versus malignant in males)
Monodermal teratoma	Elements from multiple embryonic layers; one tissue type develops, most commonly thyroid tissue **(struma ovarii)**	Benign; hyperthyroidism
Choriocarcinoma	Usually seen in combination with other germ cell tumors *cyto-/syncytiotrophoblasts*	Malignant; produces (β-hCG)
Granulosa-theca tumor	Lipid-laden cells; fibroblast proliferation; cuboidal cells in cords; eosinophilic follicles **(Call–Exner bodies)** *coffeebean nuclei*	Benign; may secrete estrogen, leading to precocious puberty or endometrial hyperplasia or carcinoma
Thecoma fibroma	Fibroblast proliferation	Benign; rare; in combination with ascites and hydrothorax, referred to as **Meigs syndrome**
Sertoli–Leydig cell tumor	Tubules containing Sertoli and Leydig cells *Reinke crystals*	Produces testosterone; virilization
Metastasis	Most commonly from gastrointestinal tract, breast, or ovary; **Krukenberg tumor**, primary from stomach with signet-ring cells bilaterally	Only 5% of ovarian neoplasms

AFP, α-fetoprotein; hCG, human chorionic gonadotropin.

TABLE 8-7 Tumors of the Uterus (Cervix and Body)

Neoplasm	Clinical Features
Cervical intraepithelial neoplasia (CIN)	• May be classified as CIN I, CIN II, or CIN III • Neoplastic changes in the endometrium beginning at the **squamocolumnar junction** • CIN I: mild dysplasia extending less than one-third the thickness of the epithelium • CIN II: cells appear more malignant with increased mitotic figures and variation in nuclear size; approximately two-thirds of the epithelium involved • CIN III: also called carcinoma in situ; involves the full thickness of the cervical epithelium • Associated with HPV 16, 18, 31, 33, and 45 infection
Squamous cell carcinoma of the cervix	• Evolves from a progression of CIN • Increased incidence is associated with **early sexual activity** and **multiple sex partners**, smoking, and immunosuppression
Leiomyoma	• Benign tumor of the uterine body • The **most common tumor of women** (the most common malignancy in women is breast cancer) • Often multiple • Size increases with pregnancy and decreases with menopause
Leiomyosarcoma	• Uncommon • Does not arise from a preexisting dysplastic or neoplastic condition (fibroids)
Endometrial carcinoma	• The **most common malignancy** of the female genital tract • Associated with nulliparity • More often found in older women • Exogenous **estrogen** administration or estrogen-producing tumors may be the predisposing factors • Other risk factors are diabetes, tamoxifen, hypertension, and obesity • Usually presents as vaginal bleeding

HPV, human papillomavirus.

TABLE 8-8 Tumors of the Vulva and Vagina

Tumor	Description
Papillary hidradenoma	• **Most common** benign tumor of the vulva • Often presents as an ulcerated and bleeding nodule • Originates from apocrine sweat glands • Can easily be surgically removed
Squamous cell carcinoma of the vulva	• Similar to squamous cell carcinoma of the cervix • Highest occurrence in **older women** • Vulvar dystrophy precedes carcinoma • Associated with the infections of HPV 16, 18, 31, 33, and 45
Paget disease of the vulva	• Noninvasive intraepithelial adenocarcinoma, similar to Paget disease of the breast • Not always associated with underlying adenocarcinoma (unlike Paget disease of the breast)
Malignant melanoma	• Similar to malignant melanoma of the skin • 10% of malignant tumors of the vulva
Squamous cell carcinoma of the vagina	• The vagina is rarely a primary site of cancer formation • Usually an extension of squamous cell carcinoma of the cervix
Clear cell adenocarcinoma	• A rare malignant tumor • Occurs in the daughters of women given **diethylstilbestrol (DES)** during pregnancy
Sarcoma botryoides	• A type of rhabdomyosarcoma • Usually occurs in **girls younger than 5** years of age • **"Bunch of grapes"** that protrude from the vagina

HPV, human papillomavirus.

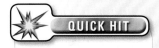

QUICK HIT

Estrogens can be synthesized by adipose tissue. This may be partially responsible for predisposing obese women to endometrial carcinoma.

The Reproductive System

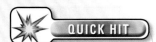

QUICK HIT

Male breast cancer represents 1% of all breast cancers.

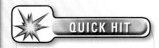

QUICK HIT

Breast cancer is the **most common cancer** of women but the second leading cause of cancer death after lung cancer. The most common location is the upper outer quadrant.

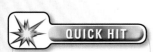

QUICK HIT

The presence of estrogen or progesterone receptors on breast cancer reflects a good prognosis because of the ability to use hormonal (antiestrogen) therapy.

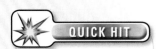

QUICK HIT

Gynecomastia (enlargement of the breast tissue in males) can be caused by marijuana, alcoholism, cimetidine, ketoconazole, spironolactone, and digitalis.

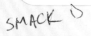

SMACK

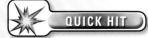

QUICK HIT

Tamoxifen, a selective estrogen receptor modulator, can be used to treat advanced breast cancer in postmenopausal women. It can lead to the regression of estrogen-stimulated tumors in some cases.

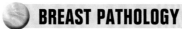

BREAST PATHOLOGY

Risk factors for breast cancer include being older than 45 years of age, nulliparity, early menarche, late menopause, high-fat diet, *HER*-2/neu oncogene activation, first-degree relative with positive history, and a history of breast cancer in the contralateral breast (Table 8-9).

TABLE 8-9 Breast Pathology

Condition	Pathology	Clinical Features
Acute mastitis	Entry of ***Staphylococcus aureus*** through nipple; focal cellulitis versus abscess	Most often occurs during **nursing**; may be caused by eczema
Fibrocystic changes	Breast mass; tender during menstruation; usually **bilateral; "blue-domed"** cysts	**Most common breast disorder**; nonneoplastic hypertrophy of breast tissue that is hormonally mediated; predisposition to cancer only if there is evidence of cellular atypia
Fibroadenoma	Painless; rubbery mass	Benign; **most common tumor in patients younger than 25 years of age**; not a precursor to malignancy
Intraductal papilloma	Tumor of the lactiferous ducts	May present as **serous discharge** or bloody discharge; benign, small risk of cancer
Phyllodes tumor	Large, bulky mass; cysts; leaflike projections; ulceration of the skin	Malignant potential, although most are benign; may recur
Ductal carcinoma in situ (DCIS)	Tumor cells fill the ducts but do not penetrate basement membrane; **comedocarcinoma** associated with caseous necrosis and cheesy discharge	Malignant; may progress to invasive
Lobular carcinoma in situ (LCIS)	Tumor cells do not penetrate basement membrane; estrogen-receptor (ER) and progesterone-receptor (PR) positive	Malignant; no palpable lesion— **usually found incidentally** on breast biopsy; associated with infiltrating ductal cancers arising from other lesions
Infiltrating ductal carcinoma	Firm mass; cells may form glands; fibrous stroma	Malignant; **most common** carcinoma of the breast; may be progression of ductal carcinoma in situ
Infiltrating lobular carcinoma	Cells line up **"single file"; inactivation of E-cadherin**	Malignant; often multiple and bilateral; **bloody discharge**
Paget disease	Superficial lesion of nipple or areola; **Paget cells** in epidermis (large cell with marginal clearing seen)	Malignant; indicative of **underlying ductal carcinoma**
Medullary carcinoma	Soft, fleshy tumor; characterized by lymphocytic infiltrate	Malignant
Inflammatory breast cancer	Inflammatory changes superimposed on any histologic type of breast cancer	Findings may include peau d'orange, dimpling of the breast, nipple retraction

PROSTATE PATHOLOGY *(Figure 8-10)*

FIGURE
8-10 The prostate

Prostatic carcinoma
- Most common male cancer
- Enlarged, firm, nodular prostate on DRE
- Elevated serum PSA and alkaline phosphatase
- Frequent metastasis is to bone (especially the spine)
- Effects on the lateral lobe

Benign prostatic hyperplasia
- Most common cause of male urinary tract obstruction
- Bladder distention or hypertrophy
- UTIs
- Increased residual volume and frequency
- Nocturia, difficulty initiating stream
- Caused by age-related increase in testosterone and estrogen
- Common after 40 years of age
- Effects on middle lobe

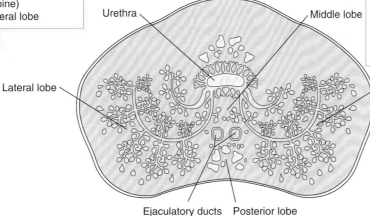

Urethra — Middle lobe

Lateral lobe — Lateral lobe

Ejaculatory ducts   Posterior lobe

DRE, digital rectal examination; PSA, prostate-specific antigen; UTI, urinary tract infection.

The Reproductive System

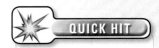

QUICK HIT

Benign prostatic hyperplasia (BPH) develops in the transition zone of the prostate surrounding (and potentially obstructing) the urethra.

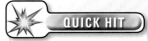

QUICK HIT

BPH is not a precancerous disorder, and it cannot be accurately diagnosed by measuring prostate-specific antigen (PSA).

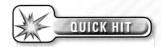

QUICK HIT

Prostate cancer is the second most common cause of cancer death in males. The leading cause is lung cancer.

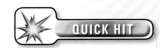

QUICK HIT

The digital rectal examination is essential because many of the male pelvic organs can be assessed. When the examining finger is introduced into the rectum, anal tone (S_2S_4 innervation) can be evaluated. Anteriorly, from inferior to superior, lies the lower border of the prostate, the posterior aspect of the prostate, and the bladder, if distended.

Clinical Vignette 8-2

CLINICAL PRESENTATION: A 55-year-old man presents to his primary care physician with the chief complaint of **frequent urination** that has increased over the past few months. Although he feels an **urgent need to urinate immediately,** the patient finds that he has a **weak urinary stream** with **intermittent flow** and that he is **straining to urinate,** with resulting feeling of **incomplete emptying.** Also, the patient reports **waking to urinate** at night and has noted **some blood in his urine** lately. Rectal examination deferred reveals an enlarged prostate with no nodules palpable. Otherwise, the physical examination is benign and the vital signs are stable.

DIFFERENTIAL: Benign prostatic hyperplasia (BPH), urethral strictures, urinary tract infection, bladder cancer, bladder stone, and bladder trauma. Lower urinary tract symptoms can be best remembered by the mnemonic **WISE FUN. WISE** refers to the obstructive symptoms: **W**eak urinary stream, **I**ntermittent flow, **S**training to urinate, and incomplete **E**mptying. **FUN** refers to the irritative symptoms: **F**requency, **U**rgency, and **N**octuria. BPH can present with any of these lower urinary tract symptoms and also hematuria. Urethral strictures can also result in obstructive symptoms, urinary tract infection (UTI) in irritative symptoms, and bladder cancer/stones/trauma in hematuria.

LABORATORY STUDIES: Urinalysis and **urine culture** should be obtained to rule out urinary tract infection. Also, **ultrasound** is useful for determining the bladder and prostate size but is not commonly used in initial evaluation of uncomplicated cases. More precise measurements of prostate can be made via **transrectal ultrasound,** which is indicated in select patients.

MANAGEMENT: An **α-blocker** relaxes the prostatic smooth muscle and is the first-line treatment for BPH. The most common side effect is dizziness. A **5α-reductase** inhibitor (finasteride) reduces symptoms by reducing the volume of the prostate. If pharmacologic therapy is unsuccessful, **transurethral resection of the prostate** is the gold standard surgical procedure for the treatment of BPH. Open radical prostatectomy is a cancer operation and is **not** indicated for benign prostatic obstruction.

TESTICULAR PATHOLOGY

Anatomic disorders of the testis occur more often in young children, whereas the infectious and neoplastic diseases are more likely to occur in the young adult, sexually active population. Routine testicular examinations can often prevent and detect serious complications. When detected early, testicular neoplasms are one of the most curable cancers.

I.   Testicular disorders *(Table 8-10)*

II. Testicular neoplasms *(Table 8-11)*

MNEMONIC

To remember the layers of the scrotum, consider the phrase "Some Darn Englishman Called It The Testis"; from superficial to deep: **S**kin, **D**artos, **E**xternal spermatic fascia, **C**remaster, **I**nternal spermatic fascia, **T**unica vaginalis, and **T**estis.

TABLE 8-10	Testicular Disorders
Disorder	**Clinical Features**
Hydrocele	• **Serous fluid** collects in the tunica vaginalis • Caused by **patency** between the peritoneal cavity and the tunica vaginalis
Hematocele	• **Blood** collects in the tunica vaginalis • Usually caused by **trauma**
Varicocele	• **Engorgement of the veins** of the spermatic cord • Most noticeable when patient is standing
Spermatocele	• Epididymal cyst containing **sperm**
Cryptorchidism	• **Failure** of one or both of the testes to **descend** • Increased incidence of **germ cell testicular cancer** such as seminoma and embryonal carcinoma (see testicular neoplasms [Table 8-11]) • Failure of descent leads to testicular **atrophy**, **sterility**, and increased risk of **germ cell neoplasia**
Testicular torsion	• **Twisting** of the spermatic cord • If untreated, will result in **testicular** necrosis
Orchitis	• Testicular infection and inflammation • May be viral or bacterial in origin • Can lead to **sterility if bilateral**
Epididymitis	• **Inflammation and infection** of the epididymis • Most often caused by ***Neisseria gonorrhoeae***, ***Chlamydia trachomatis***, *Escherichia coli, and Mycobacterium tuberculosis*

The Reproductive System

TABLE 8-11 Testicular Neoplasms

Neoplasm	Site of Origin; Morphology	Clinical Features
Seminoma	Germ cell; arranged in lobules or nests	Malignant; incidence highest in 35–40-year-olds; painless enlargement of testis; **most common germ cell tumor**; similar to dysgerminoma of the ovary; radiosensitive and curable
Embryonal carcinoma	Germ cell; variable morphology with papillary convolutions	Malignant; highest incidence in men in their 20s; more aggressive than seminomas; very common in mixed tumors
Yolk sac tumor (endodermal sinus tumor)	Germ cell; anastomosing cords; malignant; presents with pain or metastasis; similar to ovarian tumor; peak incidence in childhood (infants to 3 years of age); increased **AFP**	
Teratoma	Two or more embryonic layers; **multiple tissue types** such as cartilage, epithelium, liver, and muscle	Malignant; occurs at any age but more common in children; mature: heterogeneous tissue in organoid fashion; immature: incompletely differentiated
Mixed germ cell tumor	Variable	Malignant; aggressive; more than one neoplastic pattern; **most common**
Leydig cell tumor (interstitial)	Testicular stroma; intracytoplasmic **Reinke crystals**	Benign; produces androgens, estrogens, or corticosteroids; often seen with **precocious puberty** or gynecomastia; similar to ovarian Sertoli–Leydig cell tumor
Sertoli cell tumor	Testicular stroma; forms cordlike structures	Benign; minor endocrine abnormalities; similar to ovarian Sertoli–Leydig cell tumor
Choriocarcinoma	Trophoblastic cells; villous structures resembling placenta	Malignant; hemorrhagic; **β-hCG** elevated; peaks in early adulthood

AFP, α-fetoprotein; hCG, human chorionic gonadotropin.

PSYCHOSOCIAL DEVELOPMENT (Figure 8-11)

FIGURE 8-11 Stages of development

	Infancy (0–1 year old)	Toddler (1–3 years old)	School age (3–11 years old)	Adolescence (11–20 years old)	Early adulthood (20–40 years old)	Middle adulthood (40–60 years old)	Late adulthood (60–80 years old)
Freud	Oral	Anal	Phallic-oedipal (3–6 years old), latency (6–11 years old)	Genital			
Erikson	Trust versus mistrust	Autonomy versus shame and doubt	Initiative versus guilt (3–6 years old), industry versus inferiority	Identity versus role confusion	Intimacy versus isolation	Generativity versus stagnation	Ego integrity versus despair
Piaget	Sensorimotor (0–2 years old)	Preoperational (2–7 years old)	Concrete operations (7–11 years old)	Formal operations			
Characteristics	Reflexes: • Palmar grasp (0–2 months old) • Rooting (0–3 months old) • Babinski (0–12 months old) Milestones: • Turn over (5 months old) • Sit (6 months old) • Walk (12 months old)	Terrible two's ("no"); band-aid, parallel play (2–4 years old); balance on one foot (2 years old); climb stairs (3 years old)	Cooperative play (4–7 years old); conservation of mass (7–11 years old); button clothes, throw a ball (4 years old)	First menstruation (11 years old), first ejaculation (13 years old), peer pressure	New family, children, role in society solidified, period of reassessment	Height of career, midlife crises, menopause (45–55 years old)	Depression (ECT), women outlive men by 6–8 years, Kübler-Ross (stages of grief and dying) • Denial • Anger • Bargaining • Depression • Acceptance

ECT, electroconvulsive therapy.

THE FAMILY UNIT AND RELATED CONCEPTS

I. Postpartum depression

    A. Up to 50% of all women develop a short-lived depression after giving birth (postpartum blues).

    B. Etiology

        1. Change in hormone levels

        2. Increased responsibility

        3. Fatigue

    C. Major depression is seen in 5% to 10% of all women after childbirth.

II. Attachment of the child to the mother

    A. **Anaclitic depression**: sustained absence of mother when child is between 6 and 12 months of age leads to a withdrawn and unresponsive infant.

    B. **Harlow** showed that monkeys raised in **isolation** do not develop normally.

        1. Males are more affected than females.

        2. Recovery is not possible if isolation lasts longer than 6 months.

    C. **Bowlby** showed that **physical contact** between the mother and the child is crucial to development.

    D. **Spitz** observed that children **without proper mothering** are slow to develop and have a greater number of medical problems.

    E. **Mahler** documented the development as a process in which the infant **separates** from the mother.

        1. Normal autistic phase (0 to 1 month): infant has little interaction

        2. Symbiotic phase (15 months): infant is close to mother

        3. Separation–individuation phase (5 to 16 months): child realizes individuality and begins to explore the environment.

III. Child abuse

    A. It includes physical abuse, sexual abuse, and emotional neglect.

    B. Risk factors

        1. Substance abuse by parents

        2. Poverty

        3. Marital problems or single-parent home

    C. Physical abuse is marked by numerous fractures, bruises, subdural hematomas, or burns (at various stages of healing).

    D. Sexual abuse of children is marked by trauma to the genitalia, STDs, or urinary tract infections.

    E. Abuse predisposes the child to posttraumatic stress disorder (PTSD), dissociative disorders, depression, anorexia, phobias, and personality disorders.

    F. Physician intervention is necessary and obligatory.

IV. Family therapy

    A. Involves all members of a family even though only one person might have a problem

    B. Identifies dysfunctional behavior and encourages communication and problem solving

    C. Based on the concept that the family system is composed of subsystems in which boundaries are established and mutual accommodation occurs

SEXUALITY

I. Gender

A. **Gender identity** is an individual's sense of being male or female, whereas **gender role** is the expression of one's gender.

B. Sexual orientation is a physical preference for one or both genders (heterosexual, homosexual, and bisexual).

C. Psychological factors play a role in gender identity and sexual orientation.

1. **Transsexual:** a person who has the sense of being in the wrong-sex body and has a strong desire to correct it

2. **Homosexual:** a person who has a sexual preference for same-sex individuals

3. **Transvestite:** a man who dresses in women's clothing for pleasure, usually heterosexual

II. Sexual dysfunction

A. Premature ejaculation (early climax without reaching plateau phase) is the **most common** male sexual disorder.

B. The most common sexual dysfunction in women is **sexual arousal disorder,** in which lubrication cannot be maintained throughout the sexual act.

C. Impotence (in men)

1. Failure to achieve erection or ejaculation

2. Usually has an organic component but may be psychogenic (e.g., caused by stress or anxiety)

   a. It is often related to alcohol abuse.

   b. It may also result from medical problems such as diabetes or illicit drug use.

   c. Psychogenic cause can be confirmed by observing erections during rapid eye movement (REM) sleep.

D. Vaginismus (in women)

1. Spasm in the outer third of the vagina

2. Difficulty during intercourse or pelvic examination

3. Often results from rape, incest, or abuse

E. Paraphilias (Table 8-12)

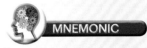

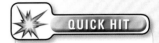

The Reproductive System

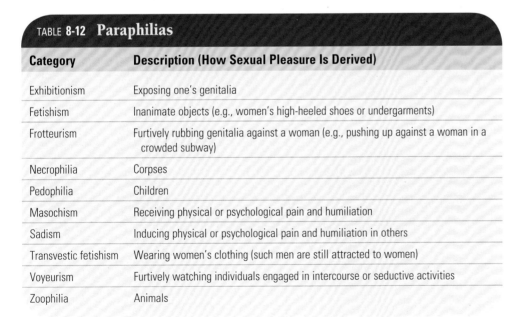

TABLE 8-12 Paraphilias	
Category	**Description (How Sexual Pleasure Is Derived)**
Exhibitionism	Exposing one's genitalia
Fetishism	Inanimate objects (e.g., women's high-heeled shoes or undergarments)
Frotteurism	Furtively rubbing genitalia against a woman (e.g., pushing up against a woman in a crowded subway)
Necrophilia	Corpses
Pedophilia	Children
Masochism	Receiving physical or psychological pain and humiliation
Sadism	Inducing physical or psychological pain and humiliation in others
Transvestic fetishism	Wearing women's clothing (such men are still attracted to women)
Voyeurism	Furtively watching individuals engaged in intercourse or seductive activities
Zoophilia	Animals

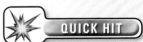

Clinical Vignette 8-3

CLINICAL PRESENTATION: A 45-year-old man presents to his primary care physician for his yearly physical examination. His past medical history is significant for **diabetes, hypertension,** and **hypercholesterolemia.** He has been keeping physically fit with **lengthy bike rides**. He has not cut back on his tobacco usage and smokes 0.5 pack per day for 5 years. As you review the systems, he tells you that he has had **increasing difficulty achieving a firm erection**. He denies any **recent penile or perineal trauma, surgery, or radiation**. Vital signs: temperature = 97.4° F; respiration rate = 20 breaths/min; blood pressure = 150/90 mm Hg; and heart rate = 85 bpm.

DIFFERENTIALS: Erectile dysfunction (ED) from vascular, neurologic, iatrogenic, traumatic, or psychogenic origin. It is important to note that the bolded items in this patient's history are the risk factors for ED.

LABORATORY STUDIES: Direct injection of prostaglandin E_1 into the corpora should result in a normal erection within minutes if the penile vasculature is normal. **Nocturnal penile tumescence testing** is useful in distinguishing psychogenic from organic impotence. Inadequate nocturnal erections suggest organic dysfunction, whereas normal erection during rapid eye movement (REM) sleep suggests psychogenic etiology. Given his diabetic history, formal **neurologic testing** may be needed.

MANAGEMENT: All patients with ED should be given an empiric trial of **sildenafil** as long as they do not have any contraindications. Contraindications include use of nitrates, active cardiac disease, or hypertension. **Phosphodiesterase inhibitors** such as sildenafil increase cyclic guanosine monophosphate (cGMP), which relaxes the smooth muscle surrounding the penile arterioles with resulting dilation of vasculature and erection. Patients with ED refractory to therapy with oral phosphodiesterase inhibitors should be referred to urology for other therapies such as **vacuum constriction device, prostaglandin E_1 injections,** and surgical placement of a **penile prosthesis.**

THERAPEUTIC AGENTS FOR THE REPRODUCTIVE SYSTEM (Table 8-13)

Table 8-13

Therapeutic Agent (common name, if relevant) [trade name, where appropriate]	Class—Pharmacology and Pharmacokinetics	Indications	Side Effects or Adverse Effects	Contraindications or Precautions to Consider; Notes
Hormone antagonists				
Finasteride [Proscar]	**Antiandrogen—5α-reductase inhibitor** → decreases the conversion of testosterone to dihydrotestosterone	**Benign prostatic hyperplasia**; male-pattern baldness	Decreased libido, decreased ejaculate volume	
Flutamide [Eulexin]	**Antiandrogen**—nonsteroidal, competitive androgen receptor blocker	**Metastatic prostate cancer**		
Ketoconazole [Nizoral]	**Antiandrogen**—inhibits ergosterol (steroid) synthesis → inhibits adrenal and gonadal steroid synthesis; also prevents cell membrane formation	**Prostate carcinoma, fungal infections**	Nausea, vomiting, diarrhea, rash, headache, anorexia, thrombocytopenia, gynecomastia, hepatotoxic	**Inhibits cytochrome P450**
Spironolactone [Aldactone]	**Antiandrogen**—inhibits steroid binding	**Hirsutism in women, acne in women**; hyperaldosteronism, hypokalemia, hypertension, edema, and CHF	Gynecomastia, breast pain, hyperkalemia, impotence, menstrual irregularities	
Mifepristone (RU-486)	**Antiprogesterone**—synthetic steroid, progesterone receptor blocker → blocks the effects of progesterone → myometrium contraction	**Termination of intrauterine pregnancy**	**Heavy bleeding, uterine cramping**, GI effects (nausea, vomiting, and anorexia)	Controversial "morning after" drug
Anastrozole [Arimidex]	Aromatase inhibitor	**Breast cancer** in postmenopausal women; endometriosis	Hot flashes, nausea, vomiting	Can be used in ER-positive or hormone receptor–unknown breast cancer
Hormone agonists				
Methyltestosterone [Android, Virilon]	**Androgen**—androgen receptor agonist	**In males: hypogonadism, delayed puberty** (promotes secondary sex characteristics), impotence; **In females: estrogen receptor positive breast cancer**	**Masculinization (hirsutism), testicular atrophy**, prostate hyperplasia, prostate cancer, impotence, **stunted growth** (premature epiphyseal plate closure), hyperlipidemia	Decreased testicular testosterone leading to Leydig cell inhibition and gonadal atrophy

(continued)

The Reproductive System

TABLE 8-13 Therapeutic Agents for the Reproductive System (Continued)

Therapeutic Agent (common name, if relevant) [trade name, where appropriate]	Class—Pharmacology and Pharmacokinetics	Indications	Side Effects or Adverse Effects	Contraindications or Precautions to Consider; Notes
Ethinyl estradiol, diethylstilbestrol (DES), mestranol	**Estrogen**—bind estrogen receptor	In women: **hypogonadism, ovarian failure**, menstrual abnormalities; **contraception** In men: androgen-dependent prostate cancer	**Endometrial cancer**, endometrial bleeding, hypertension, **thrombosis** (stroke, cardiovascular disease)	Used in combination with progestin in patients with intact uterus; increased risk of endometrial cancer with unopposed estrogen therapy; females exposed to DES in utero have an increased risk of **vaginal clear cell adenocarcinoma**
Progesterone, norethindrone, levonorgestrel [Plan B], **norgestimate, desogestrel, gestodene**	**Progesterone**—bind progesterone receptors	**Endometrial cancer**, amenorrhea, abnormal uterine bleeding, **prevention of pregnancy**		Also used to prevent endometrial hyperplasia in postmenopausal women taking estrogen

Partial agonists and antagonists

Clomiphene [Clomid]	**Selective estrogen receptor modulator**—binds estrogen receptors in pituitary → prevents normal feedback inhibition, increases LH and FSH release from the pituitary → stimulates ovulation	Infertility—stimulates ovulation; **PCOS**	**Hot flashes, ovarian enlargement, multiple gestation pregnancy, visual disturbances**	
Tamoxifen	**Selective estrogen receptor modular**—competitively binds estrogen receptors; breast **(estrogen antagonist)**: prevents proliferation of estrogen receptor positive tumor cells; **endometrium (partial agonist); bone (agonist)**: decreases bone turnover, increases bone density	**Treats estrogen-dependent breast cancer in postmenopausal women**; reduces contralateral breast cancer	**May increase the risk of endometrial cancer; hot flashes**; flushing; increased risk of blood clots	
Raloxifene [Evista]	**Selective estrogen receptor modulator**—breast **(estrogen antagonist); endometrium (estrogen antagonist)**: prevents the proliferation of endometrium; **bone (estrogen agonist)**: decreases bone turnover, increases bone density; **cardiovascular (estrogen agonist)**: decreases LDL	**Osteoporosis, breast cancer**	**Hot flashes**, sinusitis, weight gain, muscle pain, leg cramps, **increased risk of blood clots**	Unlike estrogen, raloxifene **does not decrease HDL**

(continued)

TABLE 8-13 **Therapeutic Agents for the Reproductive System** *(Continued)*

Therapeutic Agent (common name, if relevant) [trade name, where appropriate]	Class—Pharmacology and Pharmacokinetics	Indications	Side Effects or Adverse Effects	Contraindications or Precautions to Consider; Notes
Other				
Leuprolide [Lupron]	**GnRH analog**—agonist (when given pulsatile), antagonist (when given continuously)	**Infertility** (given pulsatile), **prostate cancer** (given continuous), **uterine fibroids**, endometriosis, precocious puberty	Nausea, vomiting, antiandrogen effects (testicular atrophy), menopausal symptoms	
Sildenafil [Viagra], **vardenafil** [Levitra], **tadalafil** [Cialis]	**Phosphodiesterase type 5 inhibitor (cGMP-specific)**— increased cGMP → smooth muscle relaxation → increased blood flow in the corpus cavernosum → penile erection	**Erectile dysfunction**	**Abnormal vision** (impaired blue-green color vision), UTIs, **cardiovascular events, priapism, dyspepsia**, headache, flushing	Risk of hypotension (fatal) in a patient taking nitrates
Misoprostol [Cytotec]	**Prostaglandin—PGE$_1$ analog** → cervical dilation, uterine contractions	**Induction of labor**, termination of pregnancy		
Dinoprostone	Prostaglandin—PGE$_2$ analog → cervical dilation, uterine contraction	Induction of labor, termination of pregnancy		
Ritodrine, terbutaline	β-agonist → uterine relaxation	Inhibits preterm labor; used to treat uterine hyperstimulation in labor		
Combination oral contraceptives	**Combination of estrogen and progesterone—estrogen** → inhibits midcycle surge of gonadotropin secretion → prevents ovulation; **progesterone** → alters endometrium cervical mucus, tube motility, and peristalsis → less suitable for sperm penetration and implantation	**Contraception, acne, hirsutism, PCOS**		Contraindicated in patients with stroke or prior thromboembolic event, estrogen-dependent tumor, pregnancy, hypertriglyceridemia, **heavy smokers**; avoid use in women with migraines with aura and poorly controlled hypertension
Hormone replacement therapy	**Combination of estrogen and progesterone**	**Menopause** (relief of symptoms), osteoporosis, vulvar/vaginal atrophy, hypoestrogenism (hypogonadism)	Possible increased risk of **stroke**	Combination of progesterone and estrogen is used because **unopposed estrogen increases the risk of endometrial cancer**

cGMP, cyclic guanosine monophosphate; CHF, congestive heart failure; ER, estrogen receptor; FSH, follicle-stimulating hormone; GI, gastrointestinal; GnRH, gonadotropin-releasing hormone; HDL, high-density lipoprotein; LDL, low-density lipoprotein; LH, luteinizing hormone; PCOS, polycystic ovary syndrome; PGE, prostaglandin E; UTI, urinary tract infection.

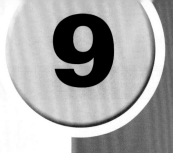

9 The Musculoskeletal System

DEVELOPMENT

I. Bone formation

A. **Endochondral bone**
   1. Forms over a cartilage frame
   2. Becomes the **long bones** of the skeleton (e.g., **femur**)

B. **Membranous bone**
   1. Forms without a cartilage frame
   2. Becomes the **flat bones** of the skeleton (e.g., bones of the cranium)

II. Skeletal muscle

A. It derives from **somites**.

B. Each somite produces its own **myotome**.

C. Each somite produces its own **dermatome**.

III. Pharyngeal arches

Begin to develop in the **fourth week** and originate from **neural crest cells**.

A. Arch 1   *(cleft lip, palate)*
   1. Innervated by the mandibular branch of the trigeminal nerve (**cranial nerve [CN] V**)
   2. Gives rise to the following muscles:
      a. Muscles of mastication (temporalis, masseter, lateral pterygoid, medial pterygoid)
      b. Two tensor muscles (tensor veli palatini, tensor tympani)
      c. Two other muscles (mylohyoid, anterior belly of the digastric)
   3. Gives rise to the following skeletal structures:
      a. Malleus
      b. Incus
   4. Gives rise to the following ligamentous structures:
      a. Anterior ligament of malleus
      b. Sphenomandibular ligament

B. **Arch 2**
   1. Innervated by the facial nerve (**CN VII**)
   2. Gives rise to the following muscles:
      a. Muscles of facial expression (orbicularis oculi, orbicularis oris, buccinator)
      b. Three other muscles (stylohyoid, stapedius, and the posterior belly of the digastric)
   3. Gives rise to the following skeletal structures:
      a. Greater cornu of hyoid bone
      b. Inferior portion of the body of hyoid bone

C. Arch 3
   1. Innervated by the glossopharyngeal nerve (**CN IX**)
   2. Gives rise to the stylopharyngeus muscle
   3. Gives rise to the following skeletal structures:
      a. Greater cornu of the hyoid bone
      b. Lower portion of the body of hyoid bone

D. **Arch 4**
1. Innervated by the vagus nerve (pharyngeal and superior laryngeal branches of CN X)
2. Gives rise to the following muscles:
   a. Cricothyroid muscle
   b. All the muscles of the soft palate and pharynx except the stylopharyngeus muscle (arch 3) and tensor veli palatini (arch 1)
E. **Arch 6**
1. Innervated by the vagus nerve (recurrent laryngeal branch of CN X)
2. Gives rise to the intrinsic muscles of the larynx except the cricothyroid
F. **Arch 4 and Arch 6** fuse to give rise to the thyroid, cricoids, arytenoids, corniculate, and cuneiform cartilages.

BONE FUNCTION AND METABOLISM *(Figure 9-1)*

I. Osteoblasts
A. They synthesize type I collagen and bone matrix proteins to form an unmineralized osteoid.

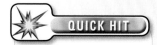
QUICK HIT

All the intrinsic muscles of the pharynx, except the cricothyroid, are innervated by the recurrent laryngeal branches of the vagus nerve. Consequently, bilateral injury to the recurrent laryngeal nerves leaves the cricothyroid unopposed, and the vocal cords become tense and adducted.

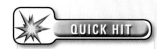
QUICK HIT

Of all the intrinsic muscles of the larynx (posterior cricoarytenoid, lateral cricoarytenoid, arytenoid, thyroarytenoid, cricothyroid, transverse arytenoid, oblique arytenoid, and vocal muscle), the posterior cricoarytenoid muscle is the only muscle that **abducts** the vocal cords.

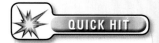
QUICK HIT

Exogenous estrogen administration (hormone replacement therapy) slows the rate of bone loss that occurs after menopause by stimulating osteoblasts via estrogen receptors.

The Musculoskeletal System

 Bone histology

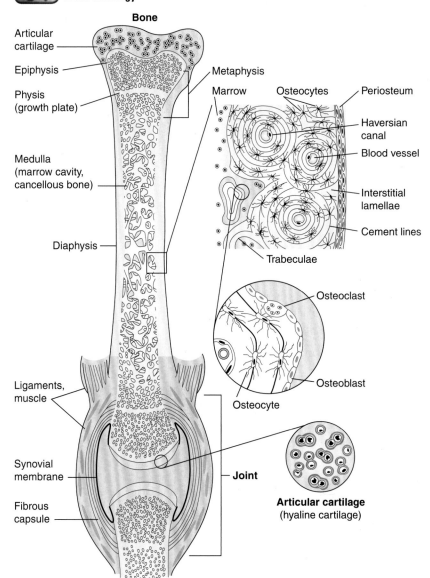

(Adapted with permission from Damjanov IM. *Histology: A Color Atlas and Textbook.* Baltimore, MD: Lippincott Williams & Wilkins; 1996.)

B. Calcium (Ca^{2+}) and phosphate (PO_4^{3-}) are deposited on the cartilaginous matrix to form mineralized bone.

C. Blood supply goes to osteoblasts via vessels within the **haversian canals**.

D. When osteoblasts become surrounded by bone matrix, they become **osteocytes**.

II. Osteocytes

A. Occupy a space called lacuna

B. Communicate with other osteocytes via cytoplasmic extensions called canaliculi

C. Are influenced by parathyroid hormone (**PTH**) to stimulate osteoclastic bone resorption

D. Resorption allows Ca^{2+} to be transferred rapidly into the blood.

E. Are not directly involved in bone resorption

III. Osteoclasts

A. Multinucleated cells formed from monocytes, which are responsible for bone resorption

B. Contain acid phosphatase

C. Resorb bone under influence of PTH

IV. Hormonal control (also see Chapter 7)

A. **PTH**
   1. Release is stimulated by hypocalcemia and hypophosphatemia
   2. Stimulates osteoclastic activity causing osteolysis and release of Ca^{2+} from bone
   3. Promotes the reabsorption of Ca^{2+} in the distal tubule of the kidney
   4. Inhibits PO_4^{3-} reabsorption in the proximal tubule of the kidney
   5. Converts vitamin D to its active form, 1,25-dihydroxycholecalciferol
   6. Raises blood Ca^{2+} and lowers blood PO_4^{3-}

B. **Calcitonin**
   1. Inhibits osteoclasts, which inhibits bone resorption
   2. Lowers blood Ca^{2+}

C. **Vitamin D**
   1. Assists PTH in the resorption of bone
   2. Increases Ca^{2+} absorption from the intestine
   3. Increases Ca^{2+} reabsorption from the kidney
   4. Increases PO_4^{3-} reabsorption from the kidney
   5. Raises blood Ca^{2+} and PO_4^{3-}
   6. Has net effect on bone growth

BONE, CARTILAGE, AND JOINT DISEASE

In the healthy adult, bone mass peaks between 20 and 25 years of age. Peak bone mass is typically higher in males and blacks. Bone diseases can adversely affect the mass and strength of the skeleton, predisposing the patient to fractures.

• **Diseases That Affect Bone Formation** (Table 9-1)

TABLE 9-1 Diseases that Affect Bone Formation

Disease	Etiology	Clinical Features
Osteitis fibrosa cystica (von Recklinghausen disease of bone)	Caused by increased levels of **PTH**; primary or secondary hyperparathyroidism	Cystic spaces in the bone that are lined with osteoclasts; often colored brown owing to hemorrhage, hence the name **"brown tumor of bone"**
Achondroplasia (dwarfism)	Caused by failure of long bones to elongate because of narrow epiphyseal plates and sealing of these plates with the metaphysis; **autosomal dominant** disease; **most common cause of dwarfism**; linked to activating mutation in gene for fibroblast growth factor-3 receptor	Short limbs; normal-size head and trunk

(continued)

TABLE 9-1 Diseases that Affect Bone Formation (Continued)

Disease	Etiology	Clinical Features
Osteogenesis imperfecta ("brittle bone disease")	Group of gene mutations that cause **defective type I collagen synthesis**; most common type of mutation is **autosomal dominant**	Multiple fractures occur with only minor trauma; **blue sclera**; deformities of teeth and skin; deafness
Osteopetrosis ("marble bone disease")	**Defective osteoclasts** cause a decrease in reabsorption leading to **increased bone density**; the most severe form is autosomal recessive	Multiple **fractures** despite increased density; narrowing of marrow spaces causes anemia; narrowing of other cavities causes blindness, deafness, and cranial nerve compression
Paget disease of bone	Increased osteoblastic and osteoclastic activity by an unknown cause; occurs most commonly in the elderly; may involve one or more bones	**Skeletal deformities**; complications include bone pain owing to fracture, multiple arteriovenous (AV) shunts in bone causing high output cardiac failure, hearing loss as a result of thickening of bony structures in ear; may lead to osteosarcoma; increased levels of serum alkaline phosphatase; three phases of disease: • Osteolytic phase—resorption owing to osteoclasts • Mixed phase—osteoclastic and osteoblastic activity leads to a **mosaic pattern** in the bone • Late phase—increase in bone density as a result of osteoblastic activity

PTH, parathyroid hormone.

Clinical Vignette 9-1

CLINICAL PRESENTATION: A 4-year-old child with the chief complaint of "belly pain" is brought to the emergency department by his mother. As you begin his physical examination, you note that the child is short for his age and that there are multiple ecchymoses on his lower extremities. The mother reports that her son bruises easily. A head, ear, eye, nose, and throat examination shows multiple dental caries and blue sclera. Physical examination shows that the abdomen is soft, nontender, and nondistended. There are normoactive bowel sounds. The patient is without organomegaly or masses. Temperature = 98.6° F; heart rate = 80 bpm; respiration rate = 18 breaths/min; blood pressure = 100/80 mm Hg.

DIFFERENTIALS: Osteogenesis imperfecta (OI), child abuse, child neglect. Short stature, multiple ecchymoses, and dental caries can be seen in each of the listed differentials. However, blue sclera is a characteristic finding of OI. Also, child abuse can be differentiated from OI based on nonskeletal manifestations such as retinal hemorrhage, intracranial bleeding, and splenic trauma.

DIAGNOSTIC WORKUP: **Radiographs** should be obtained of the skull, chest, long bones, and pelvis, looking for **type of fracture** as well as **osteopenia** (seen in OI). Diaphyseal fractures (break in the midshaft of long bone) and metaphyseal fractures (appear as corner chip of bone edge) suggest child abuse. In addition to multiple fractures, osteopenia would be seen on radiograph in OI. In child abuse, serial plain films should show healing and remineralization. In OI, fractures continue to occur in protective custody. In difficult cases, **collagen synthesis analysis** would show abnormal findings in OI.

MANAGEMENT: Medical therapy of OI is supportive, and in some cases, surgical interventions are done to improve weight bearing.

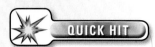

QUICK HIT

Osteoporosis versus osteopenia: Osteoporosis is a loss of bone that predisposes to fractures; osteopenia is detectable loss of bone via resorption.

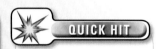

QUICK HIT

Dual-energy x-ray absorptiometry (DEXA) scan is the gold standard for diagnosis of osteoporosis.

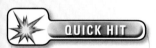

QUICK HIT

Osteochondrosis is avascular necrosis of epiphysis sites in children. Legg–Calvé–Perthes disease is avascular necrosis of the femoral head in children and often presents with limp. Osgood–Schlatter disease is an inflammation at the insertion site of the patellar tendon on the tibial apophysis.

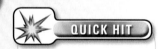

QUICK HIT

The most common cause of avascular necrosis is steroid-induced vascular compression, most commonly occurring in the femoral head.

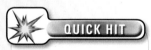

QUICK HIT

Patients with sickle cell disease contract osteomyelitis as a result of *Salmonella*, whereas intravenous drug users may be infected with *Pseudomonas*. However, *Staphylococcus aureus* continues to be the most common cause of osteomyelitis in both these groups of patients.

METABOLIC AND INFECTIOUS BONE DISEASE (Table 9-2)

TABLE 9-2 Metabolic and Infectious Bone Disease

Disease	Etiology	Clinical Features
Osteoporosis	**Primary:** **Type I:** postmenopausal, with excess loss of trabecular bone **Type II:** men and women >70 years of age, with loss of trabecular and cortical bone **Secondary:** Physical inactivity, increased parathyroid levels, hypercortisolism, hyperthyroidism, vitamin D deficiency, hypocalcemia	**Bone mineral density** is 2.5 or more standard deviations **below** normal; **decrease in bone mass** leads to fractures (especially of the weight-bearing bones of the spine); radiolucent bone seen on radiograph; DEXA scan positive
Scurvy	Lack of vitamin C intake; defective **proline and lysine hydroxylation** in collagen synthesis	Impaired bone formation and lesions result; painful subperiosteal hemorrhage; osteoporosis; bleeding gums; poor wound healing
Rickets (children); osteomalacia (adults)	Impaired calcification of bone because of deficiency of vitamin D; if caused by renal disease, termed "renal osteodystrophy"	**Children:** Skeletal malformations Craniotabes (thinned and softened bones of the skull) Late fontanelle closure Decreased height Rachitic rosary (costochondral junction thickening resembling string of beads) Pigeon breast owing to a protruding sternum **Adults:** Fractures Radiolucency on radiography
Avascular necrosis	Death of osteocytes and fat necrosis via the following mechanisms: vascular compression, vascular interruption (fracture), thrombosis (sickle cell disease, caisson disease), vessel injury	Joint pain; osteoarthritis; sites include head of the femur, shoulder, knee
Pyogenic osteomyelitis	Infection of bone most often caused by ***Staphylococcus aureus***; routes of infection include hematogenous extension from adjacent infection, open fracture, or surgery	Acute febrile illness; pain; tenderness; usually affects metaphysis of distal femur, proximal tibia, and proximal humerus; forms sequestrum and involucrum
Tuberculous osteomyelitis	Tuberculous infection spreads to bone from elsewhere in body	Seen in hips, long bones, hands, feet, and vertebrae **(Pott disease)**

DEXA, dual energy x-ray absorptiometry.

I. Bisphosphonates

The bisphosphonates, which include alendronate, risedronate, ibandronate, pamidronate, and etidronate, inhibit osteoclast-mediated bone resorption by binding to hydroxyapatite. The bisphosphonates are most commonly used to prevent or treat postmenopausal osteoporosis but can also be used for Paget disease and steroid-induced osteoporosis.

II. Tumors of bone and cartilage (*Table 9-3*)

Tumors of the bone and cartilage, although rare, occur most commonly in the lower extremities of young males. Metastases are more common than primary tumors of the bone. Tumors of the prostate, breast, and lung account for 80% of bone metastases.

TABLE 9-3 Tumors of Bone and Cartilage

Tumor	Morphology	Clinical Features
Osteochondroma	Benign bone tumor; **most common benign tumor**; originates in metaphysis of long bones; growth of mature bone (exostosis) with a cartilaginous cap	Most common in men younger than 25 years of age; usually occurs on the lower end of the femur or upper end of the tibia
Giant cell tumor	Benign bone tumor; spindle-shaped cells with multinuclear giant cells; most commonly occur in the epiphysis of the distal femur or proximal tibia	Most common in women 20–55 years of age; has **"soap bubble"** appearance on radiograph; usually occurs on the lower end of the femur or upper end of the tibia
Osteoma	Benign bone tumor; mature bone (dense tissue)	Most common in men; affects skull or facial bones; protrudes from surface; associated with Gardner syndrome
Osteoid osteoma	Benign bone tumor; **nidus** rimmed by osteoblasts and surrounded by vascular, spindled stroma; <2 cm in diameter	Most common in men 20–30 years of age; occurs near the ends of the tibia and femur; painful due to excess prostaglandin E_2 production; radiolucent **nidus** is seen on radiograph
Osteosarcoma	Malignant mesenchymal bone tumor; malignant cells produce bone matrix; origin usually in metaphyseal long bones; destructive masses with hemorrhage and necrosis; retinoblastoma, Paget disease, radiation exposure are risk factors	Bimodal distribution, most common in boys in their teenage years and in elderly; usually occurs in tibia or femur near the knee; local pain; tenderness; swelling; metastasizes to lung first; growth under bone results in the **Codman triangle and a "sunburst" appearance** on radiograph
Chondrosarcoma	Malignant cartilage tumor; lobulated translucent tumors; necrosis; calcification	Most common in men usually 40 years of age or older; central skeleton is affected such as the pelvis, ribs, shoulders, spine; radiograph shows localized area of bone destruction
Ewing sarcoma	Malignant small round cell tumors of bone and soft tissue; **t(11;22)**; sheets of small round cells producing **Homer-Wright pseudorosettes**; histologically similar to lymphoma, small cell carcinoma, rhabdomyosarcoma	Most common in boys 10–15 years of age; occurs in long bones, ribs, pelvis, scapula; early metastasis; responds to chemotherapy; painful, warm, swollen mass; "onion skin" appearance on radiograph
Fibrous dysplasia	Benign; bone replaced haphazardly by fibrous tissue	**"Chinese figures"** configuration on radiograph. Three types: Single bone involvement; Several bones involved; Several bones involved, along with precocious puberty and café au lait spots
Metastasis	Malignant; usually lytic lesions unless arising from prostate or breast	Originate from prostate, breast, kidney, lung; ectopic hormone production **(parathyroid hormone-related protein [PTHrP])**

Handwritten annotations: "not high yield"; "giant soap bubble"; "om Ån the garden"; "OO = pain!"; "aspirin"; "(Rb) + p53 Sunburst is Really Bright"

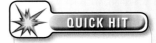

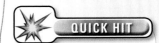

Gardner syndrome is an autosomal dominant disorder characterized by multiple colonic polyps associated with other tumors such as osteomas of the skull, fibromas, thyroid cancer, epidermoid cysts, and sebaceous cysts.

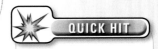

In osteosarcoma, a "sunburst" appearance on radiography is due to calcified streaks that radiate from a tumor. Codman triangle is due to periosteum lifting away from the bone due to an underlying tumor.

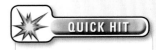

The most common bone sarcoma in children is an osteosarcoma, followed by Ewing sarcoma.

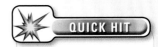

Predisposing factors for osteosarcoma include Paget disease of the bone, mutations of the p53 gene on chromosome 17 (Li–Fraumeni syndrome), familial retinoblastoma, radiation, and bone infarcts.

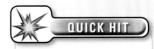

The most common malignancy of the skeleton is metastatic tumors.

The Musculoskeletal System

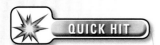
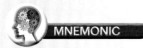
III. Arthritic joint disease (Table 9-4)

The etiology of arthritic joint diseases is not well understood. For this reason, treatment is often palliative rather than curative.

Two factors to consider in the differential diagnosis of an acutely painful joint include infection and urate deposition. These two entities may be distinguished from each other, in part, by aspiration of the joint fluid with evaluation for white blood cells (WBCs), bacteria on Gram stain, or crystals.

TABLE 9-4 Arthritic Joint Disease

Disease	Etiology	Clinical Features
Osteoarthritis (degenerative joint disease)	Degeneration of joint articular cartilage followed by growth of surrounding bone; the **most common type of arthritis**; primary type has no specific risk factor; secondary type related to trauma, metabolic disorder, or inflammatory arthropathy; knee is the most common site	Pain in joint after use, improves with rest, stiffness in the morning or after a period of immobility; **"Joint mice"** form from pieces of torn and frayed joint cartilage and broken pieces of osteophytes; erosion of cartilage results in **eburnation** (polishing) of the underlying bone; cysts visible in bone on radiograph; Heberden nodes are osteophytes at the DIP joint; Bouchard nodes are osteophytes of the PIP joints
Rheumatoid arthritis	Symmetrical, chronic inflammation of the synovium with edema and cellular infiltrate, leading to the destruction of articular cartilage of joints, most likely because of autoimmune reaction; synovial hypertrophy and hyperplasia; granulation tissue **(pannus)** over articular cartilage; **rheumatoid factor**—IgM autoantibody against the Fc receptor located on IgG; more common in women; associated with **HLA-DR4**	Ulnar deviation of MCP joints, **swan-neck**, and **boutonnière** deformity develop owing to inflammation, muscle atrophy, and contracture; **DIP joints are spared**; morning stiffness that improves throughout the day; subcutaneous rheumatoid nodules; systemic symptoms such as fever, weight loss, fatigue
Ankylosing spondylitis	Unknown cause; high association with **HLA-B27**; negative rheumatoid factor; males are more commonly affected	Bilateral sacroiliitis (inflammation of the sacroiliac joint) noted; chronic low back pain and stiffness; improves with movement; calcification of spinal ligaments and fusion of the facet joints produces a **"bamboo spine"**; may produce extraskeletal manifestations of **apical lung fibrosis, aortic insufficiency**, or **cauda equina syndrome**
Psoriatic arthritis	Unknown cause; may present similar to rheumatoid arthritis; HLA-B27 association; **no rheumatoid factor**; no male or female preponderance	**Asymmetric** involvement of **DIP joints**, PIP joints, feet, ankles, and knees; **"pencil-in-a-cup"** deformity of the proximal phalanges
Reiter syndrome	Caused by reaction to systemic illness that originated either enteropathically or urogenitally; HLA-B27 association; most common in males, usually 20–40 years of age	Classic triad of genitourinary inflammation **(urethritis)**, ocular inflammation **(conjunctivitis)**, and acute asymmetric **arthritis**

(continued)

The Musculoskeletal System

TABLE 9-4 Arthritic Joint Disease (Continued)

Disease	Etiology	Clinical Features
Gout	Inflammatory reaction in joints caused by monosodium **urate crystal** deposition; IgG opsonization of the crystals followed by phagocytosis stimulates inflammation; pathogenesis includes increased uric acid production such as Lesch–Nyhan syndrome (hypoxanthine-guanine phosphoribosyltransferase deficiency), increased activity of phosphoribosyl pyrophosphate (PRPP) synthetase, and decreased uric acid secretion such as diuretics; acidosis; often precipitated by a large, high-protein meal or by drinking excessive amounts of alcohol	First MTP joint involvement is called **podagra**; **tophi** (nodules of fibrous tissue and crystals) occur near the joints, on the ear, and on the Achilles tendon; renal damage may occur when crystals deposit in collecting tubules; urate crystals have **strong negative birefringence** under polarized light and are **needle shaped**. For treatment, see Table 9-5.

DIP, distal interphalangeal; HLA, human leukocyte antigen; Ig, immunoglobulin; MCP, metacarpophalangeal; MTP, metatarsophalangeal; PIP, proximal interphalangeal.

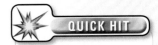

QUICK HIT

Lesch–Nyhan syndrome is an **X-linked deficiency** of **hypoxanthine-guanine phosphoribosyl transferase** (HGPRT) that results in elevated levels of uric acid and manifests as mental retardation, gout, and self-mutilation. It can be treated with allopurinol, which blocks xanthine oxidase, an important enzyme in the formation of uric acid.

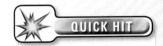

QUICK HIT

Pseudogout, caused by **calcium pyrophosphate** crystals, resembles gout in its presentation. However, calcium pyrophosphate crystals have weak **positive birefringence** under polarized light.

IV. Gout is a condition in which uric acid crystals in joints trigger intermittent inflammatory reactions. The etiologic process can be blocked at different stages (Table 9-5).
- A. Inhibition of the production of uric acid from the breakdown of DNA **purines**
- B. Increased excretion of uric acid in the urine
- C. Blunting the body's **inflammatory response** to the gout crystals (the body's reaction to gout crystals actually causes the pain and damage associated with gout)

TABLE 9-5 Drugs Used to Treat Gout

Therapeutic Agent	Mechanism of Action	Indications	Side Effects	Notes
Allopurinol	Inhibition of uric acid production—**competitive inhibitor of xanthine oxidase**, decreases conversion of **xanthine to uric acid**	Chronic gout therapy; lymphoma, leukemia (prevents tumor lysis associated urate nephropathy), uric acid stones	Rash, fever, diarrhea, occasional peripheral neuritis; enhances effect of azathioprine	Should not be used to treat acute gout
Probenecid	Increased secretion of uric acid (uricosuric)—small dose inhibits uric acid secretion; large dose inhibits uric acid reabsorption (i.e., promotes excretion)	Chronic gout therapy	**Caution: should not be used in patients with sulfa allergies**	Should not be used to treat acute gout or patients with uric acid stones
Colchicine	Anti-inflammatory—interrupts **microtubule formation**, thereby interfering with normal mitosis and inhibiting WBC migration and phagocytosis	Acute gout therapy	Diarrhea (common)	

(continued)

The Musculoskeletal System

TABLE **9-5** **Drugs Used to Treat Gout** *(Continued)*

Therapeutic Agent	Mechanism of Action	Indications	Side Effects	Notes
NSAIDs (e.g., indomethacin)	Decrease **prostaglandin** production, thereby interrupting the inflammatory process	Acute therapy	Bone marrow suppression and renal damage (indomethacin); GI distress and ulceration	
Celecoxib	Selectively inhibits cyclooxygenase-2 (COX-2)	Acute therapy	Sulfa allergy; renal damage	Less toxic to GI mucosa than NSAIDs
Glucocorticoids (prednisone)	Suppresses prostaglandin and leukotriene synthesis	Acute therapy	Osteoporosis, Cushingoid reaction, psychosis, glucose intolerance, infection, hypertension, cataracts	

GI, gastrointestinal; NSAID, nonsteroidal anti-inflammatory drug; WBC, white blood cell.

Clinical Vignette 9-2

CLINICAL PRESENTATION: A 45-year-old man presents to the emergency department with severe pain in his left **great toe** that began suddenly yesterday evening. He reports **exquisite tenderness,** saying "even the bed sheet touching my toe was intolerable." The patient also reports that yesterday afternoon, he had "gone out with the boys" and estimates drinking five to six **beers.** Patient denies both pain in other joints and having felt pain like this before. Physical examination shows swelling, erythema, rubor, and tenderness of the left great toe. His past medical history is significant for osteoarthritis of the left knee for which he takes ibuprofen. Temperature = 98.5° F; blood pressure = 135/70 mm Hg; heart rate = 85 bpm; respiration rate = 21 breaths/min.

DIFFERENTIALS: Septic arthritis, cellulitis, gout, pseudogout. Osteoarthritis and rheumatoid arthritis are ruled out in this case because they typically present as pain in multiple joints. Polyarticular pain should be thought of as inflammatory (showing signs of rubor, swelling, and erythema as in rheumatoid arthritis) and noninflammatory (as in osteoarthritis). Septic arthritis is unlikely in this case because of the location of the pain and the lack of fever. Based on the location of the pain, occurrence after a diet rich in purines, and the examination, this patient most likely is experiencing an acute gouty attack.

LABORATORY STUDIES: Appropriate workup of monoarticular pain includes **synovial fluid aspiration and analysis.** If the fluid is **inflammatory** (white blood cells >5,000), the fluid should be further evaluated by **crystal analysis** (positive in gout and pseudogout), **Gram stain,** and **culture** (showing bacteria in infectious arthritis). **Complete blood count (CBC), erythrocyte sedimentation rate (ESR),** and **blood cultures** should also be obtained to rule out septic arthritis.

MANAGEMENT: Acute gout is treated by **nonsteroidal anti-inflammatory drugs** (NSAIDs; indomethacin is traditionally used, aspirin aggravates the problem), **colchicines** (if the patient did not respond to NSAIDs), and **corticosteroids** (if patient cannot tolerate NSAIDs or colchicine). Prophylactic therapy would not be initiated in this patient because this is his first acute gouty attack. Prophylactic therapy is indicated after two gouty attacks and consists of **uricosuric drugs** or **allopurinol,** depending on the amount of uric acid excreted in urine over 24 hours. Never give allopurinol for acute gout; it makes it worse.

V. Infectious joint disease (*Table 9-6*)

TABLE **9-6** **Infectious Joint Disease**

Disease	Etiology	Clinical Features
Nongonococcal septic arthritis	Inflammation of joints; most commonly **Staphylococcus aureus** and *Streptococcus* species	Monoarticular arthritis, usually affecting the knee; chills and fever; **positive Gram stain** and cultures of synovial fluid
Gonococcal septic arthritis	Inflammation of joints and other systemic effects secondary to dissemination of sexually acquired gonococcal infection; **most common form of arthritis in sexually active adults**	Polyarticular arthritis, usually affects the knee; chills and fever; rash (including papules and pustules); Gram stain and synovial fluid cultures often negative
Lyme disease	Infection with *Borrelia burgdorferi*, which is transmitted by the tick *Ixodes dammini*; arthritis occurs late in the disease	**Erythema chronicum migrans**, a characteristic expanding bull's-eye rash; knees are most common site of arthritis; may cause myocardial, pericardial, and neurologic manifestations

SYSTEMIC LUPUS ERYTHEMATOSUS

I. Prototypical connective tissue disorder that more frequently affects women

II. Clinical features
A. Fever, lymphadenopathy, weight loss, and general malaise
B. **Immune complex deposition** in the vessels of almost all organs
C. Pulmonary fibrosis characterized by interstitial fibrosis or diffuse alveolitis
D. **Libman–Sacks endocarditis**
   1. **Mitral valve** affected
   2. Sterile verrucous lesions seen on both sides of the leaflets
E. Pericarditis and pleuritis
F. Glomerular disease
   1. May range from mild to diffuse proliferative change
   2. Subendothelial and mesangial immune complex deposits
   3. Endothelial proliferation (wire loops) and thickened basement membranes (membranous glomerulonephritis)
G. Arthralgia and arthritis
H. Vasospasm of small vessels, especially of the fingers (**Raynaud phenomenon**)
I. **Cotton-wool spot lesions in fundus of eye**
J. Skin rash
   1. Characteristic **butterfly rash** over the malar eminences of the face
   2. Rashes can also be prevalent elsewhere on the body
   3. Rashes associated with exposure to sunlight (photosensitivity)

III. Laboratory findings
A. Antinuclear antibodies (ANAs) are seen in almost all cases.
   1. ANA is a sensitive marker, but it is not specific for systemic lupus erythematosus (SLE).
   2. Presence of antibodies to **double-stranded DNA** is highly specific for SLE.
   3. Antibodies to **Smith (Sm) antigen** are also specific for SLE.

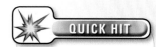

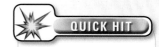

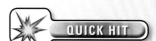

The Musculoskeletal System

QUICK HIT

SLE has a female-to-male ratio of 2:1 and is more common in African-American women.

QUICK HIT

Presence of antibodies against double-stranded DNA antibodies and Smith (Sm) antigen is practically diagnostic of SLE.

QUICK HIT

Antihistone antibodies are associated with drug-induced lupus. Common drugs that cause drug-induced lupus: hydralazine, procainamide, isoniazid, chlorpromazine, methyldopa, and quinidine.

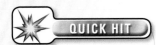

B. Decreased level of complement (C3 and C4) in the serum
C. Skin biopsies show immune complex deposition.
D. **False-positive test for syphilis**
E. **Hypercoagulable** state in vivo owing to antiphospholipid antibodies

 OTHER CONNECTIVE TISSUE DISORDERS (Table 9-7)

Inherited disorders of the bone, skin, cartilage, and blood vessels are some of the most common genetic conditions in humans. These diseases are characterized by widespread manifestations.

TABLE 9-7 Other Connective Tissue Disorders

Disease	Etiology	Clinical Features
Marfan syndrome	Abnormality of **fibrillin** (a glycoprotein in microfibrils) due to mutations in the FBN1 gene on chromosome 15; results in skeletal, visual, and cardiovascular defects; **autosomal dominant** inheritance	Abnormally long fingers (**arachnodactyly**), arms, and legs; hyperextensible joints; tall and thin body habitus; high palate; ocular lens dislocation (**ectopia lentis**); cardiovascular defects including mitral valve prolapse, proximal aorta aneurysm, aortic valve insufficiency, and **aortic dissection**
Ehlers–Danlos syndrome	Genetic defect in type I and type III **collagen and elastin** formation	Frequent hemorrhage, **hyperextensibility of joints** and skin, fragility of tissue, poor wound healing
Progressive systemic sclerosis (scleroderma)	Diffuse fibrosis and degeneration of almost every organ owing to autoimmune reaction; **anti-scl70** (ANA); anticentromere antibody present in **CREST** (**c**alcinosis cutis, **R**aynaud phenomenon, **e**sophageal dysfunction, **s**clerodactyly, and **t**elangiectasia); occurs more frequently in women	Hypertrophy of subcutaneous collagen leads to thickened skin, fixed facial expression, clawlike hand (sclerodactyly); Raynaud phenomenon; fibrosis of esophagus, GI tract, lungs, heart, and kidney
Sjögren syndrome	Autoimmune reaction; **anti-SSA (anti-Ro)** and **anti-SSB (anti-La)** antibodies; anti-SSB antibody is highly specific; occurs more often in women Enlarged parotid glands as a consequence of lymphocytic infiltration; hypergammaglobulinemia	Classic triad: • Dry eyes (xerophthalmia) • Dry mouth (**xerostomia**) • Presence of **other connective tissue or autoimmune disease** (often rheumatoid arthritis)
Polymyositis	Autoimmune inflammatory disorder; occurs more frequently in women; often **associated with malignancy**	Weakness in the proximal muscles of the extremities; high level of creatine kinase in serum; termed **dermatomyositis** when skin is involved
Mixed connective tissue disease	Autoimmune disorder; occurs more frequently in women; renal involvement is rare (as opposed to other connective tissue diseases); antinuclear ribonucleic protein (**anti-nRNP**) is a highly specific ANA	Raynaud phenomenon, arthralgia, muscle inflammation, esophageal dysmotility

ANA, antinuclear antibodies; *FBN1*, fibrillin-1; GI, gastrointestinal.

Clinical Vignette 9-3

CLINICAL PRESENTATION: A 35-year-old woman presents to her primary care physician complaining of **joint pain** in her wrist, ankle, and knee for the past several months. She also reports a **painful intermittent rash** of the same duration on her **face** that **worsens in the sun**. The patient also tells you that she has noted that her **fingers oddly become very pale, turn blue,** and then **bright red** while in the **cold outdoors.** Review of systems is positive for **fatigue and weight loss.** A head, ear, eye, nose, and throat (HEENT) examination shows an **erythematous rash over the cheeks and nasal bridge, sparing the nasolabial folds, hair thinning along the crown, and ulceration of the oral mucosa.** Examination of the forearm shows a **raised erythematous patch** with some **scaling.** Temperature = 100.2° F; blood pressure = 145/90 mm Hg; heart rate = 75 bpm; respiration rate = 20 breaths/min.

DIFFERENTIALS: SLE, drug-induced lupus, discoid lupus, mixed connective tissue disease (MCTD), scleroderma. The arthralgia, malar rash, discoid lesions on sun-exposed arms, alopecia, weight loss, oral ulcers, and mild fever all suggest SLE. **Drug-induced lupus** could be ruled out from a detailed medication history (see Quick Hit for list of drugs). Although Raynaud phenomenon is observed in SLE, it also occurs in **scleroderma.** MCTD is a disorder in which features of SLE, systemic sclerosis, dermatomyositis, polymyositis, and Sjögren syndrome can coexist and overlap. Serologic studies should be performed to differentiate these further.

LABORATORY STUDIES: When given serologic studies on the USMLE, look for the following results: A **positive antinuclear antibody (ANA)** screening test occurs in SLE, rheumatoid arthritis, scleroderma, Sjögren syndrome, MCTD, polymyositis, dermatomyositis, and drug-induced lupus. **A negative ANA** screening test suggests that the diagnosis is likely not SLE. Presence of either **anti–double-stranded DNA (dsDNA)** or **anti-Sm antibody** is diagnostic of SLE. **Antihistone antibodies** are present in 100% of cases of drug-induced lupus. If negative, drug-induced lupus can be excluded. Ribonucleoprotein (RNP) antibodies are a specific marker of MCTD. **Positive anti-scl70** indicates scleroderma, and positive **anticentromere antibody** specifically indicates CREST (calcinosis cutis, Raynaud phenomenon, esophageal motility disorder, sclerodactyly, and telangiectasia) syndrome. **Complete blood count** studies show anemia, leukopenia, lymphopenia, or thrombocytopenia in SLE. Also, **serum electrolytes** with **blood urea nitrogen (BUN)** and **creatinine** should be ordered to detect renal disease. In SLE, a **urinalysis** should also be performed, looking for **proteinuria** (evaluate further for nephrotic syndrome), **cellular casts,** and **hematuria** (evaluate further for glomerulonephritis).

MANAGEMENT: Depends on severity and type of symptoms: **mild symptoms**—NSAIDS; **acute exacerbations**—local/systemic corticosteroids; **constitutional, cutaneous, articular symptoms**—antimalarial agents (hydroxychloroquine); **active glomerulonephritis**—cytotoxic agents cyclophosphamide). Monitor for renal disease and hypertension.

The Musculoskeletal System

BRACHIAL PLEXUS (Figure 9-2)

- Lesions of the brachial plexus and its branches (Table 9-8)
- Nerve damage and regeneration (Figure 9-3)

MNEMONIC

To remember the parts of the brachial plexus: "Real Texans Drink Cold Beer" (Roots, Trunks, Divisions, Cords, Branches).

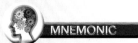

The Musculoskeletal System

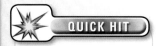

QUICK HIT

Wrist drop also occurs in lead poisoning.

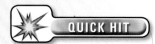

QUICK HIT

Contents of the carpal tunnel include tendons of flexor digitorum profundus, flexor digitorum superficialis, flexor pollicis longus, and the median nerve.

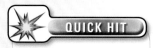

QUICK HIT

Lateral winging is caused by accessory nerve lesions leading to trapezius paralysis.

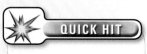

QUICK HIT

Posterior dislocations of the shoulder are common in seizure disorders and injuries caused by electrocution.

FIGURE 9-2 Brachial plexus

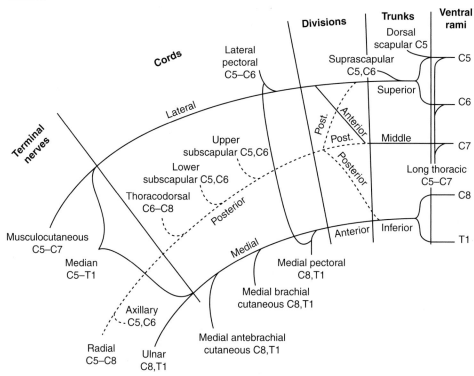

C, cervical vertebra; Post, posterior; T, thoracic vertebra.

TABLE 9-8 Lesions of the Brachial Plexus and Its Branches

Disorder	Lesion	Cause	Clinical Features
Erb–Duchenne palsy	Upper brachial plexus (C5 and C6)	**Hyperabduction** of the arm (such as trauma, shoulder dystocia during delivery)	**"Waiter's tip"** position (arm extended and adducted, forearm pronated)
Klumpke palsy	Lower brachial plexus (C8–T1)	**Hyperabduction** of the arm (shoulder dystocia during delivery)	Claw hand from ulnar nerve involvement; wrist and hand dysfunction; associated with **Horner syndrome**
Claw hand	Ulnar nerve	Occurs in children with **epiphyseal separation** of the medial epicondyle of the humerus	Weak finger adduction; medial hand numbness; dysfunction of fourth and fifth digit flexion
Radial nerve palsy	Radial nerve	**Fracture of midhumerus**	**Wrist drop**; inability to extend wrist or fingers; loss of sensation from dorsum of hand
Carpal tunnel syndrome	Median nerve	**Repetitive wrist motion** (swelling within the flexor retinaculum compresses the median nerve)	Wrist flexion elicits pain; wrist extension relieves pain; symptoms worse at night

(continued)

TABLE 9-8 Lesions of the Brachial Plexus and Its Branches *(Continued)*

Disorder	Lesion	Cause	Clinical Features
Medial winging of the scapula	Long thoracic nerve	Surgery (e.g., **mastectomy**)	Limited arm abduction and flexion; **serratus anterior paralysis**; medial scapula protrudes if patient pushes against a wall
Shoulder dislocation	Axillary nerve	**Anterior dislocation** (owing to forced abduction and extension)	Loss of innervation to deltoid; compromised shoulder flexion and extension; palpable depression under acromion
Surgical neck fracture of the humerus	Axillary nerve	A fall landing on the elbow	Loss of innervation to deltoid; compromised shoulder flexion and extension; palpable depression under acromion

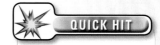

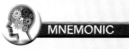

QUICK HIT

The median nerve can also be damaged in fractures of the distal third of the humerus and elbow (causing total loss of thumb opposition) or slashing of the wrist.

MNEMONIC

To remember the nerves affected by humerus fracture location, think ARM fracture from superior to inferior: **A**xillary-head of humerus; **R**adial-midshaft of humerus; **M**edian-supracondylar/distal third of humerus.

The Musculoskeletal System

FIGURE 9-3 Nerve damage and regeneration

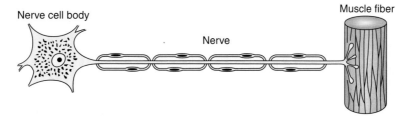

Nerve cell body

Nerve

Muscle fiber

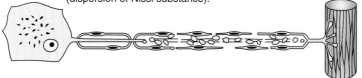

Nerve damage causes some degeneration of the distal segment. The nerve cell body undergoes chromatolysis (dispersion of Nissl substance).

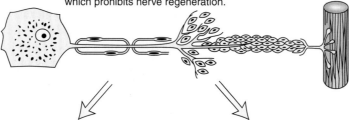

The muscle continues to atrophy for 3 weeks. In the PNS, Schwann cells proliferate and help direct the regenerating neuron. In the CNS, astrocyte proliferation forms a scar, which prohibits nerve regeneration.

If the nerve fibers do not find the degenerating segment, a neuroma is formed.

Successful nerve regeneration allows the muscle fiber to return to its original size.

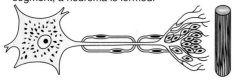

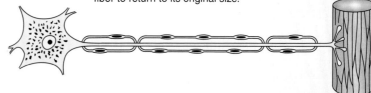

CNS, central nervous system; PNS, peripheral nervous system.

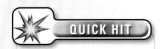

QUICK HIT

All the nerves of the sacral plexus and the pudendal nerve (S2–S4) emerge from the pelvis through the greater sciatic foramen below the piriformis muscle except the superior gluteal nerve, which passes above the piriformis.

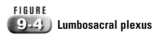

LUMBOSACRAL PLEXUS *(Figure 9-4)*

I. The lumbosacral plexus, which consists of the ventral rami of L1–S4, supplies the lower extremity.

FIGURE 9-4 Lumbosacral plexus

A. The lumbar plexus

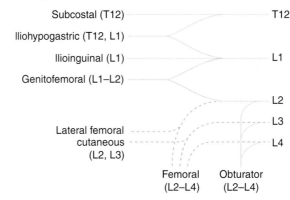

B. The sacral plexus

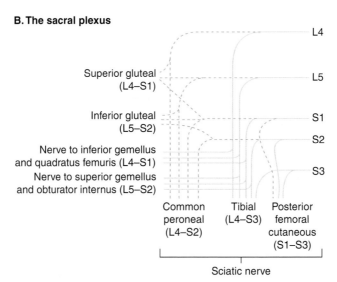

L, lumbar vertebra; S, sacral vertebra; T, thoracic vertebra.

II. Motor and sensory functions of the lumbosacral plexus

Sacral plexus lesions are commonly caused by locally invading or metastasizing carcinoma from pelvic organs (e.g., bladder, prostate, ovaries). Knowledge of the motor and sensory functions of the sacral plexus can assist in determining the deficits resulting from complications of these tumors (Tables 9-9 and 9-10).

TABLE 9-9 Segmental Nerve Functions of the Lumbosacral Plexus

Spinal Nerve	Muscle Innervation	Muscle Test	Sensory Function
L1	Cremaster	Cremasteric reflex	Inguinal region
L2	Iliopsoas	Hip flexion	Upper anteromedial thigh
L3	Medial thigh Quadriceps femoris	Hip adduction Knee extension	Lower anteromedial thigh
L4	Tibialis anterior	Ankle dorsiflexion	Anteromedial leg
L5	Extensor hallucis longus	Great toe extension	Anterolateral leg, medial dorsal foot, plantar region of great toe
S1	Gastrocnemius, soleus Posterior thigh Gluteus maximus	Ankle plantarflexion Hip extension, knee flexion Power hip extension, external rotation	Heel region, plantar foot, lateral dorsal foot
S2	Gastrocnemius, soleus Foot intrinsics	Ankle plantarflexion Abduction and adduction of toes	Posterior upper thigh and leg
S3–S4	External anal sphincter Bulbospongiosus	External anal sphincter tone Bulbospongiosus reflex	Circumanal and perineal region

TABLE 9-10 Peripheral Nerve Functions of the Sacral Plexus

Nerve	Muscle Innervation	Muscle Test	Sensory Function
Genitofemoral	Cremaster	Cremasteric reflex	Skin below middle of inguinal ligament
Lateral femoral cutaneous	None	None	Skin of lateral thigh
Femoral	Anterior thigh (quadriceps)	Knee extension	Skin of anteromedial thigh and leg
Obturator	Medial thigh	Hip adduction	Hip joint and medial skin of knee
Superior gluteal	Gluteus medius, gluteus minimus	Hip abduction and internal rotation	None
Inferior gluteal	Gluteus maximus	Power hip extension and external rotation	None
Posterior femoral cutaneous	None	None	Skin of posterior thigh and upper leg
Superficial peroneal	Lateral leg	Foot eversion	Skin of anterolateral leg and dorsum of foot
Deep peroneal	Anterior leg	Ankle dorsiflexion, foot inversion, metatarso-phalangeal joint extension	Skin of dorsum of web space between great and second toes
Tibial	Posterior thigh, gastrocnemius, soleus, deep posterior leg, planar muscles	Hip extensions, knee flexion, foot inversion, toe flexion	Skin of posterior leg and plantar foot

The Musculoskeletal System

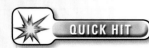

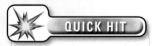

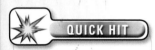

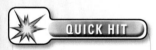

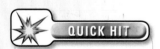

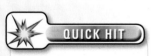

OTHER TRAUMATIC INJURIES (Table 9-11)

Musculoskeletal dysfunction can be caused by dearrangement of bone, nerve, musculature, or any combination of these elements. Insult to the body can result in problems that are acute (e.g., a torn anterior cruciate ligament) or chronic (e.g., tennis elbow).

TABLE 9-11 Other Traumatic Injuries	
Injury	**Description**
Anterior cruciate ligament (ACL) tear	Positive **anterior drawer sign** (lower leg pulled forward with knee flexed); often manifests as **"terrible triad"** (i.e., torn medial collateral ligament, lateral meniscus damage, and torn ACL), which occurs due to a force to the knee directed laterally to medially
Clavicle fracture	**Middle third** of clavicle; upward displacement of proximal fragment due to the sternocleidomastoid muscle; downward displacement of distal fragment; severe pain
Compartment syndrome	Fascial sheets separate the limbs into anterior and posterior compartments; hemorrhage into these compartments owing to crush injury or fracture, results in **compression of neurovascular structures** and further complications; emergent fasciotomy is needed
Inversion sprain of ankle	**Most common ankle injury**; results from forced inversion; stretches or tears lateral ligaments (especially the **anterior talofibular**)
Scaphoid fracture	Tenderness in the anatomical snuffbox; may lead to **avascular necrosis** if left untreated; easily missed on radiographs
Scoliosis	Complex lateral deviation and torsion of the spine; may be idiopathic or congenital or may result from a short leg, hip displacement, or polio
Shoulder separation	Downward displacement of the clavicle as a result of laxity of the acromioclavicular and coracoclavicular ligaments
Subacromial bursitis	Inflammation of the subacromial bursa
Tennis elbow (lateral epicondylitis)	Sprain of radial collateral ligament (lateral epicondyle); pain on wrist extension and forearm supination
Golfer's elbow (medial epicondylitis)	Overuse of the pronator teres, palmaris longus, and flexor carpi radialis; causes sprain of their tendinous insertion on the anterior medial epicondyle; pain on wrist flexion

(continued)

TABLE **9-11** **Other Traumatic Injuries** *(Continued)*

Injury	Description
Waddling gait	Limp caused by superior gluteal nerve injury affecting gluteus medius and gluteus minimus; inability to abduct thigh; results in **Trendelenburg sign**

 PAIN MANAGEMENT *(Figure 9-5) (Table 9-12)*

I. Musculoskeletal conditions, such as fractures and soft-tissue injuries, can result in significant disability, pain, and inflammation. Medical management of this pain and discomfort involves the use of nonnarcotic and narcotic preparations.

II. Acetaminophen

Acetaminophen (Tylenol) is a nonnarcotic analgesic with antipyretic and analgesic properties. It has little anti-inflammatory action. After acetaminophen is absorbed by the gastrointestinal (GI) tract, it is metabolized in the liver. In therapeutic doses, acetaminophen has minimal significant adverse effects. However, in large doses, depletion of liver **glutathione** levels may occur, resulting in hepatic necrosis as a result of the excess N-acetyl-p-benzoquinoneimine (NAPQI). Treatment for acetaminophen overdose is aerosolized N-**acetylcysteine, which regenerates the depleted levels of glutathione.**

III. Nonsteroidal anti-inflammatory drugs (NSAIDs)

NSAIDs are similar to acetaminophen in that they have **antipyretic** and **analgesic** properties. In addition, these agents have **anti-inflammatory** effects. NSAIDs act by inhibiting cyclooxygenase (COX) enzymes (Figure 9-5).

FIGURE
9-5 Mechanism of action of nonsteroidal anti-inflammatory drugs

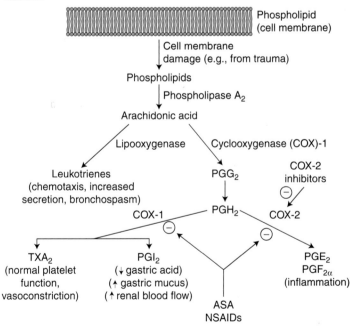
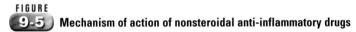

ASA, aspirin; NSAIDs, nonsteroidal anti-inflammatory drugs; PG, prostaglandin; TX, thromboxane.

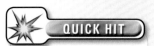
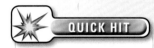
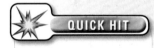
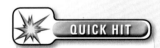
The Musculoskeletal System

A. **Aspirin**, the most common NSAID, blocks prostaglandin synthesis from arachidonic acid in the hypothalamus and in peripheral tissue, which provides its antipyretic, antiplatelet, analgesic, and anti-inflammatory benefits. Unlike other NSAIDs, its inhibitory effect on COX enzymes is irreversible.

B. A major adverse effect of aspirin and NSAIDs (e.g., ibuprofen, indomethacin, naproxen, diclofenac, ketorolac) is increased risk of **GI bleeding**. By blocking prostaglandin synthesis, NSAIDs may result in GI ulcers and hemorrhage. Prostacyclin (PGI_2) inhibits gastric acid secretion, whereas prostaglandin (PG) E_2 and $PGF_{2\alpha}$ help synthesize protective mucus in the stomach and small intestine. **COX-2 inhibitors** such as **celecoxib** may be indicated in patients who have a history of GI conditions; these NSAIDs are more specific for the inflammatory mediators (Figure 9-5).

IV. Opioids

Opioids are useful for severe pain that is uncontrolled by NSAIDs. Opioids exert their effects by interacting with protein receptors in the central nervous system (CNS) and by inhibiting G proteins and adenylyl cyclase in the peripheral nervous system. Each family of opioid receptors—μ, κ, σ, and δ—has its own set of properties and binding potency, which correlates with the amount of analgesia provided. The μ receptors primarily mediate analgesia.

The strong agonists of the various receptor families are **morphine, meperidine, methadone, fentanyl,** and **heroin**. Moderate agonists include codeine and propoxyphene. Some of these agents can produce extreme states of euphoria and become drugs of abuse because of their binding affinity and their intrinsic effects on the CNS. Methadone, which induces less euphoria and has a longer duration of action, is often used to provide controlled withdrawal from addiction to agents such as morphine and heroin.

Opioid overdose can lead to respiratory depression, depression of the cough reflex, pinpoint pupils, constipation, bronchoconstriction, diaphoresis, and urinary retention. Naloxone and naltrexone reverse the adverse effects of opioids. A rapid-acting drug, naloxone, displaces the receptor-bound opioid agents. Its effects are short-lived (approximately 2 hours). However, naltrexone works for up to 48 hours.

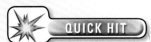

Because of the irreversible effect of aspirin on thromboxane production in platelets, it can be used as an anticoagulant. A daily low dose of aspirin has a cardio-protective effect in men.

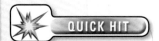

The miosis seen in opioid overdose is a result of stimulation of the Edinger–Westphal nucleus of the oculomotor nerve, which leads to enhanced parasympathetic stimulation of the eye.

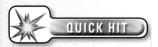

Opioids can also be used as effective medications to combat diarrhea and cough.

(sidebar, vertical) **The Musculoskeletal System**

TABLE 9-12 **Therapeutic Agents for Pain**				
Therapeutic Agent (common name, if relevant) [trade name, where appropriate]	**Class—Pharmacology and Pharmacokinetics**	**Indications**	**Side Effects or Adverse Effects**	**Contraindications or Precautions to Consider; Notes**
Acetaminophen [Tylenol]	Analgesic, antipyretic—reversibly inhibits COX centrally (inactivated peripherally); prostaglandin inhibitor, **not anti-inflammatory**	Pain, fever	Liver toxicity in high doses **(high levels deplete glutathione)**	**Overdose treated with** *N*-acetylcysteine (regenerates glutathione); unlike aspirin, **can be used in children, gout, peptic ulcer, and patients with platelet dysfunction**
Acetylsalicylic acid (aspirin)	**Anti-inflammatory, antipyretic, analgesic**—acetylates COX irreversibly	Articular, musculoskeletal pain; chronic pain; **maintenance therapy for preventing clot formation**	GI distress, **GI ulcers, inhibits platelet aggregation**; causes **hypersensitivity reactions (rash)**; reversible hepatic dysfunction	**Contraindicated for children** with the flu or chicken pox (leads to **Reye syndrome**), **patients with gout**
Ibuprofen [Advil, Motrin]	**NSAID—reversibly inhibits COX** (both COX-1 and COX-2) → decreases prostaglandin synthesis	**Inflammation, pain**	GI distress, **GI ulcers,** coagulation disorders, aplastic anemia, metabolic abnormalities, hypersensitivity, renal damage	

(continued)

TABLE 9-12 Therapeutic Agents for Pain (Continued)

Therapeutic Agent (common name, if relevant) [trade name, where appropriate]	Class—Pharmacology and Pharmacokinetics	Indications	Side Effects or Adverse Effects	Contraindications or Precautions to Consider; Notes
Naproxen [Naprosyn, Aleve]	**NSAID—reversibly inhibits COX** (both COX-1 and COX-2) → decreases prostaglandin synthesis	Inflammation, pain	GI distress, **GI ulcers**, coagulation disorders, aplastic anemia, metabolic abnormalities, hypersensitivity, renal damage	
Indomethacin [Indocin]	**NSAID—reversibly inhibits COX** (both COX-1 and COX-2) → decreases prostaglandin synthesis	Acute gout; closes patent ductus arteriosus	GI distress, **GI ulcers**, coagulation disorders, aplastic anemia, metabolic abnormalities, hypersensitivity, renal damage	
Ketorolac [Toradol]	**NSAID—reversibly inhibits COX** (both COX-1 and COX-2) → decreases prostaglandin synthesis; relieves pain and reduces swelling	**Postoperative pain**, severe pain	GI distress, **GI ulcers**, coagulation disorders, aplastic anemia, metabolic abnormalities, hypersensitivity, renal damage	
Celecoxib [Celebrex]	**NSAID—selectively inhibits COX-2**	Rheumatoid arthritis, osteoarthritis; pain, inflammation	**Increased risk of thrombosis; sulfa allergy; less toxic to GI mucosa**	COX-2 selectivity reduces inflammation while minimizing GI adverse effects (ulcers)
Morphine [MS Contin, MSIR, Roxanol]	**Opioid agonist—** converted to more potent morphine-6-glucose	Severe pain; general anesthetic; antitussive; antidiarrheal	Respiratory depression; histamine release; constipation; nausea; miosis	
Meperidine [Demerol]	**Opioid agonist**	**Pain**, acute migraine attacks	**CNS excitation at high doses**; histamine release	**Contraindicated in patients with MAOI** (results in hyperpyrexia)
Fentanyl	**Opioid agonist**	**Pain**; general anesthetic	Prolonged recovery; nausea	
Codeine	**Opioid agonist**	**Pain**; antitussive	**Constipation**	
Oxycodone [Roxicodone]	**Opioid agonist**	Severe pain; general anesthetic	Respiratory depression, constipation, nausea	
Hydromorphone [Dilaudid]	Opioid agonist	**Pain**; antitussive	Respiratory depression, constipation, nausea	
Methadone	**Opioid agonist—** synthetic	Maintenance therapy for **heroin addiction**	Respiratory depression; histamine release; constipation; nausea; miosis	
Tramadol [Ultram]	Analgesic—similar to opioid agonist	Chronic pain of **osteoarthritis**	Nausea, vomiting, constipation, drowsiness	

CNS, central nervous system; COX, cyclooxygenase; GI, gastrointestinal; MAOI, monoamine oxydase inhibitor; MSIR, morphine sulfate instant release; NSAID, nonsteroidal anti-inflammatory drug.

MUSCLE FUNCTION AND DYSFUNCTION (Figure 9-6)

FIGURE
9-6 The cross-bridge cycle of skeletal muscle

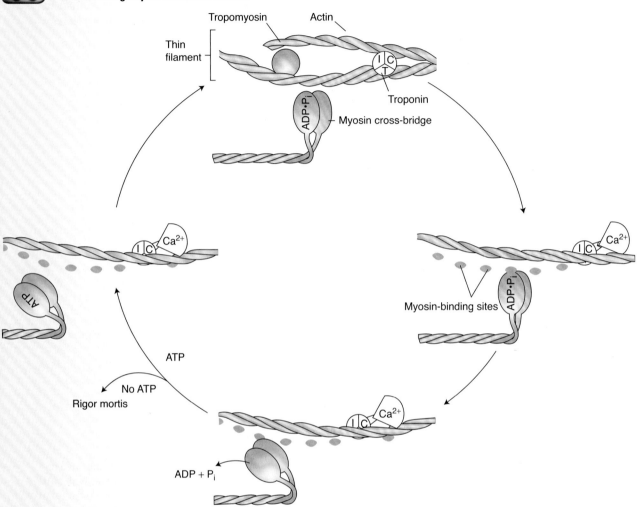

ADP, adenosine diphosphate; ATP, adenosine triphosphate; Ca^{2+}, calcium; P_i, inorganic PO_4^{3-}; T, troponin.

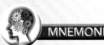

MNEMONIC

Remember the number of nuclei in muscle cells by simply noting **one** heart in the body and **one** nucleus per heart muscle cell; **many** skeletal muscles, so **many** nuclei per skeletal muscle fiber. Also, **location** of nucleus mirrors **location** in human body. The heart is in the center of the body and the nucleus is centrally located. Skeletal muscles predominate in the periphery of the body and the nuclei are at the periphery.

I. Comparison of muscle fibers (Table 9-13) (Figure 9-7)

Muscle can be divided into three subtypes with differing physiologic roles.

   A. **Smooth muscle** plays a significant role in the maintenance of the lumens of the respiratory and GI tracts and blood vessels.

   B. **Cardiac muscle** contracts the heart and propels blood through the vasculature.

TABLE **9-13** **Comparison of Muscle Fibers**

Category	Smooth Muscle Fiber	Cardiac Muscle Fiber	Skeletal Muscle Fiber
Nuclei	Centrally located single nucleus	Centrally located single nucleus	Peripherally located multiple nuclei
Banding	No distinct bands	Distinct bands	Distinct bands
Z line (convergence actin filaments)	None; dense bodies present	Present	Present

(continued)

The Musculoskeletal System

Category	Smooth Muscle Fiber	Cardiac Muscle Fiber	Skeletal Muscle Fiber
Transverse (T) tubules (membrane invaginations)	None	At Z line; diads	At A–I junction; triads
Junctional communication	Gap junctions	Intercalated discs	None
Neuromuscular junction	None	None	Present
Regeneration	High	None	Some
Calcium source	Sarcoplasmic reticulum; extracellular	Sarcoplasmic reticulum; extracellular	Sarcoplasmic reticulum
Mechanism of calcium release	IP$_3$ (inositol-1,4,5-triphosphate)	Calcium induced	Depolarization of T tubule
Calcium-binding protein	Calmodulin	Troponin	Troponin

TABLE 9-13 Comparison of Muscle Fibers *(Continued)*

FIGURE 9-7 Gross, histologic, microscopic anatomy of skeletal muscle

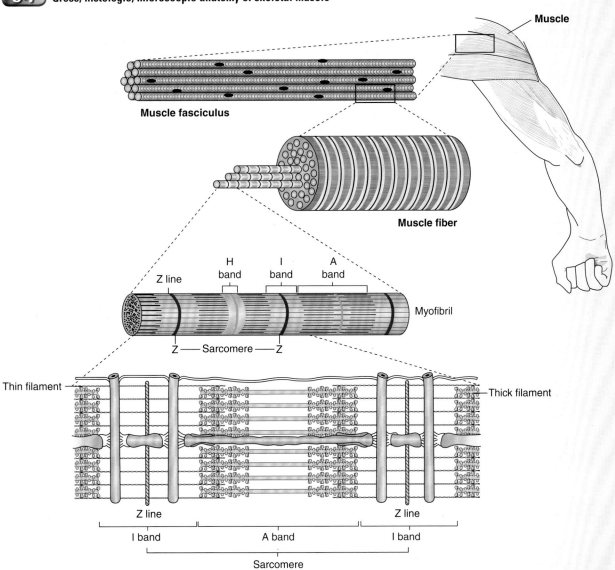

TABLE 9-14	**Types of Skeletal Muscle Fibers**	
Category	**Type 1**	**Type 2**
Action	Sustained force; weight-bearing muscles	Sudden movement; directed action
Lipid stores	Abundant	Few
Glycogen stores	Few	Abundant
Energy use	Aerobic; many mitochondria	Anaerobic; few mitochondria; easily fatigued
Twitch	Slow	Fast
Color	Red (owing to blood supply)	White

C. **Skeletal muscle maintains posture and produces movement**. There are two types of skeletal muscle fibers (Table 9-14).

II. Muscle tumors *(Table 9-15)*

Pathology of muscles can take many forms. Metabolic dyscrasias, which can be induced or inherited, are far more common than neoplasms.

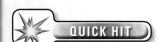

QUICK HIT

The embryonal type of rhabdomyosarcoma is related to sarcoma botryoides, resulting in a "bunch of grapes" appearance (see Chapter 8).

TABLE 9-15	**Muscle Tumors**		
	Leiomyoma	**Leiomyosarcoma**	**Rhabdomyosarcoma**
Morphology	Benign; elongated nuclei; whorled bundles of smooth muscle cells; no larger than 2 cm	Malignant; "cigar-shaped" nuclei dense bodies	Malignant; embryonal, alveolar, and pleomorphic types; rhabdomyoblast is diagnostic cell
Location	Smooth muscle, **uterus**	Smooth muscle, skin, deep soft tissues	Skeletal muscle, head and neck, genitourinary tract, retroperitoneum
Immunohistochemistry	Antibodies to actin and desmin	Antibodies to vimentin, actin, and desmin	Antibodies to vimentin, actin, desmin, and myoglobin
Prognosis	Indolent course; easily cured	Variable; prognosis worse with increased size	Aggressive; treat with surgery, radiation, chemotherapy
Notes	Afflicts women more often than men; **most common tumor in women**	Uncommon	**Most common soft tissue sarcoma of childhood** and adolescence

III. Other neuromuscular disorders *(Table 9-16)*

IV. Neuromuscular blocking agents

Neuromuscular blocking agents, which are most often encountered in the operating room, are used to produce the flaccid paralysis that is essential for many procedures, such as abdominal operations and joint replacements. These drugs affect the muscles of the body in a typical order. The small, fast-twitch muscles of the face and eyes are the first to be paralyzed, followed by the muscles of the hand, limbs, and trunk. The intercostal muscles and the diaphragm are the last to be affected. As the effects of neuromuscular blockers wear off, the muscles regain function in the reverse order.

TABLE 9-16 **Other Neuromuscular Disorders**

Disorder	Etiology	Clinical Features	Notes
Lactic acidosis	Shock, sepsis, methanol poisoning, metformin toxicity, liver failure, diabetic ketoacidosis	Increased serum lactate; **metabolic acidosis**; increased anion gap	May lead to coma or death
Myasthenia gravis	Acetylcholine receptor **autoantibodies at the neuromuscular junction**; linked to HLA-DR3; associated with thymus disorders	Muscle weakness with use; ptosis; manifests itself in facial, ocular, and limb muscles; proximal muscles affected first	Four times more common in women; diagnosis includes the edrophonium (Tensilon) test; anticholinesterase (e.g., edrophonium) improves condition
Duchenne muscular dystrophy	**X-linked recessive**; deficiency in **dystrophin** leading to lack of actin stabilization	Progressive; proximal muscle weakens, beginning with the pelvic girdle and extending to the shoulder girdle; **pseudohypertrophy** of muscles (e.g., calf); positive Gowers maneuver; leads to death via respiratory or cardiac failure	Increased serum creatine kinase and lactate dehydrogenase; clinical symptoms usually appear by age 5 years with wheelchair dependence by the end of the first decade of life and death in the 20s
Mitochondrial myopathy	Transmitted via mitochondrial DNA (mtDNA); non-Mendelian inheritance	**Ragged red fibers** seen on muscle biopsy; proximal muscle weakness	**Maternal** mode of transmission

HLA, human leukocyte antigen.

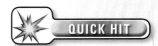

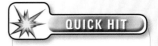

Pseudohypertrophy is initially caused by muscle hypertrophy. Then as atrophy ensues, an increase in fat and connective tissue deposition occurs.

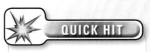

Becker muscular dystrophy is a less common and less severe variant of Duchenne muscular dystrophy that involves the same gene (Xp21) and the dystrophin protein.

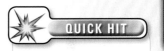

When succinylcholine is used in combination with halothane, it can cause malignant hyperthermia in certain predisposed individuals. Treatment of this condition, which is characterized by severe, prolonged muscle contractions, involves the use of dantrolene and cooling blankets.

The Musculoskeletal System

Neuromuscular blocking agents can be categorized in several ways. The most useful system divides them into central-acting and neuromuscular endplate (NMEP) blockers. The NMEP blockers can be further divided into depolarizing and nondepolarizing agents.

Centrally acting neuromuscular blocking drugs include diazepam and baclofen. **Diazepam**, a benzodiazepine, acts at γ-aminobutyric acid (GABA) receptors in the CNS. **Baclofen**, another GABA mimetic, also acts in the CNS to decrease muscle tone. Peripherally acting drugs include curare, succinylcholine, and dantrolene.

Curare acts as a nicotinic antagonist at the motor endplate to produce muscle relaxation. At low doses, this agent binds to and blocks the nicotinic receptor, a competitive blockade that can be overcome by increasing the concentration of acetylcholine. At higher doses, curare and the curare-like agents actually block ion channels at the NMEP (noncompetitive block).

Succinylcholine, the only depolarizing neuromuscular blocking agent, acts by binding to and activating the nicotinic receptor of the NMEP. In phase 1 block, a wave of fasciculations rapidly passes over the patient as the drug is administered. The drug then remains attached to the nicotinic receptor and is not broken down by acetylcholinesterase. In phase 2 block, the membrane of the NMEP repolarizes, the muscles relax, and the succinylcholine continues to block the nicotinic receptor. Plasma cholinesterase quickly breaks down the drug, and its duration of action is only a few minutes. The rapid onset and short duration of action of succinylcholine make it ideal for use during rapid-sequence endotracheal intubation and electroconvulsive therapy.

The Musculoskeletal System

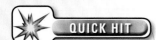

QUICK HIT

Hesselbach triangle is formed from the border of the rectus abdominis medially, inferior epigastric artery laterally, and the inguinal ligament inferiorly.

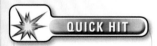

QUICK HIT

Hernias may cause small bowel obstruction. However, small bowel obstructions are most commonly caused by adhesions.

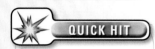

QUICK HIT

Hernia complications include small bowel entrapment (incarceration) and bowel ischemia (strangulation).

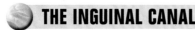

THE INGUINAL CANAL

I. The inguinal canal (*Figure 9-8*) (*Table 9-17*)

FIGURE 9-8 The inguinal canal

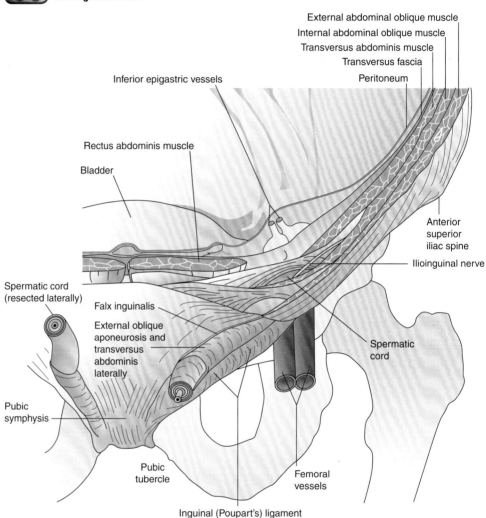

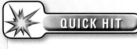

QUICK HIT

The inguinal canal contains the ilioinguinal nerve (sensory to the anterior aspect of labia or scrotum), spermatic cord in males (vas deferens, testicular artery, pampiniform plexus, genital branch of the genitofemoral nerve), and the round ligament of the uterus in females.

TABLE 9-17	The Inguinal Canal
Border	**Anatomic Composition**
Superior	Falx inguinalis: internal abdominal oblique (IAO) and transversus abdominis muscles
Inferior	Inguinal ligament
Anterior	External abdominal oblique (EAO) aponeurosis; IAO and transversus abdominis muscles laterally
Posterior	Transversalis fascia; falx inguinalis medially

II. Hernias (Table 9-18)

TABLE 9-18 Hernias

Hernia	Pathology	Clinical Features	Diagnosis
Direct inguinal hernia	Parietal peritoneum passes directly through the abdominal wall (through the **Hesselbach** triangle)	More common in older males	Medial to inferior epigastric artery; located above pubic tubercle
Indirect inguinal hernia	Parietal peritoneum passes through the internal inguinal ring and follows the inguinal canal; failure of the processus vaginalis to close properly	**Most common** type; occurs in young adult males more frequently than in females	Lateral to inferior epigastric artery; located above and medial to pubic tubercle; hernia sac may enter the scrotum in males
Femoral hernia	Parietal peritoneum passes through the femoral canal	More common in older females	Located below and lateral to pubic tubercle

DERMATOLOGY

I. Skin (Figure 9-9)

A. Stratum basale is actively mitotic and gives rise to the other four layers.

B. Epidermis forms from ectoderm and dermis forms from mesoderm.

C. Melanocytes contain melanin pigment and are derived from neural crest.

D. Skin renews every 2 to 3 weeks.

E. Function
1. Barrier to infection
2. Thermoregulation
3. Protection from desiccation

F. Two types of skin
1. Thick skin (e.g., palms and soles of feet)
   a. Stratum basale (deepest layer)
   b. Stratum spinosum
   c. Stratum granulosum
   d. Stratum lucidum
   e. Stratum corneum (most superficial layer)
2. Thin skin (e.g., face, genitalia, and back of hands): stratum lucidum is absent in thin skin (although it has all the other layers).

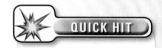

A lack of pigment, such as in albinism, predisposes one to a variety of skin disorders, including actinic keratosis, basal cell carcinoma, squamous cell carcinoma, and malignant melanoma.

The Musculoskeletal System

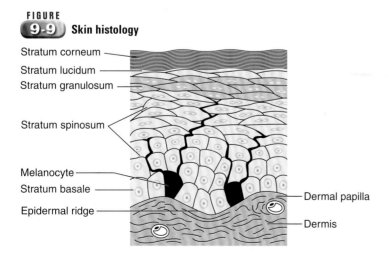

FIGURE 9-9 Skin histology

Stratum corneum

Stratum lucidum

Stratum granulosum

Stratum spinosum

Melanocyte

Stratum basale

Epidermal ridge

Dermal papilla

Dermis

II. Skin disorders (*Table 9-19*)

Skin disorders are often characterized by pruritus, inflammation, and irritability. Skin lesions that are suggestive of malignancy demonstrate asymmetry, irregular borders, variations in color, and increasing size.

- **Skin Cancers** (Table 9-20)

TABLE 9-19	Skin Disorders
Disorder	**Description**
Keloid scarring	• **Excessive scarring** that occurs after minor trauma • Results in raised, firm lesions on the skin • Occurs more frequently in Blacks • Genetic predisposition is a factor
Xanthomas	• Accumulation of foam-filled histiocytes within the dermis • Often associated with **hyperlipidemia** or lymphoproliferative disorders • Often found on the Achilles tendon, the extensor tendons of the fingers, and the eyelids
Verrucae	• "Warts" • Histology: epidermal hyperplasia, hyperkeratosis, koilocytosis
Seborrheic keratosis	• Common **benign neoplasm** in the elderly • Raised papules and plaques that appear to be "pasted on"; often dark, and can be large
Actinic keratosis	• A series of dysplastic changes that occur before the onset of **squamous cell carcinoma** • A buildup of keratin caused by excessive exposure to sunlight leads to a **"warty"** appearance • Higher incidence in lightly pigmented individuals
Albinism	• **Lack of melanin pigment** production • Ocular type limited to eyes; X linked • Oculocutaneous type involves the skin, eyes, and hair; autosomal recessive; lack of tyrosinase, which converts tyrosine to DOPA (3,4-dihydroxyphenylalanine)
Vitiligo	• Irregular areas of depigmentation due to **decreased number of melanocytes**
Melasma	• Pregnancy-associated hyperpigmentation
Acanthosis nigricans	• Velvety thickening and **hyperpigmentation** of the axilla, neck, and groin region • Associated with insulin resistance (type 2 diabetes mellitus) and sometimes with occult visceral malignancy
Hemangiomas	• Large-vessel malformation composed of masses of blood-filled channels • **Port-wine stain** birthmarks are the most common manifestation • Cavernous hemangiomas are a subset with large cavernous vascular spaces that can occur in von Hippel–Lindau disease
Psoriasis	• Plaques with **silvery scale**; plaque bleed when scraped (**Auspitz sign**) • Often affects elbows, knees, scalp, hands • Autoimmune etiology; may be associated with psoriatic arthritis • Histology: parakeratotic scaling, increased thickness of the stratum spinosum, decreased thickness of the stratum granulosum
Atopic dermatitis (eczema)	• Dry skin with pruritic inflammatory lesions that become lichenified with chronic scratching, especially in flexural areas • Commonly seen in infants and children • Associated with other atopic diseases (allergic rhinitis, asthma)

TABLE 9-20 Skin Cancers

Disorder	Description
Squamous cell carcinoma	• Malignant tumor of the skin associated with excessive exposure to sunlight (UV rays) leading to DNA damage, immunosuppresion, or xeroderma pigmentosum • Rarely metastasizes • Characterized by ulcerated, scaling nodules • Appears microscopically as islands of neoplastic cells with **whorls of keratin** ("pearls") and cells with atypical nuclei at all levels of the epidermis
Basal cell carcinoma	• **Most common skin tumor** • Appears grossly as a pearl-like papule on sun-exposed areas • Appears histologically as a dark cluster with **palisading peripheral cells** • Almost never metastasizes but can cause local invasive tissue destruction

Malignant melanoma	• Aggressive tumor that arises from melanocytes (neural crest origin)
	• Associated with excess exposure to sunlight, immunosuppression, and xeroderma pigmentosum
	• Associated with the S-100 tumor marker
	• Two growth patterns:
	  • **Benign radial manner** (growth within skin layer)
	  • **Aggressive vertical manner** (growth through deeper layers)

UV, ultraviolet.

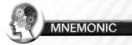

MNEMONIC

MElanoma is more likely to **ME**tastasize. Basal and squamous cell carcinoma hardly ever metastasize.

MNEMONIC

Use ABCDE to identify nevi at higher risk for melanoma: **A**symmetry, **B**order irregular, **C**olor irregular, **D**iameter greater than 0.5 cm, **E**levation irregular.

The Musculoskeletal System

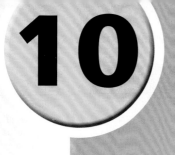

QUICK HIT

Hematopoiesis expands into fetal sites in times of hematologic stress (e.g., sickle cell anemia).

DEVELOPMENT

I. Hematopoiesis timetable

A. **Week 3: Extraembryonic visceral mesoderm** gives rise to **hemangioblasts**, which aggregate and subsequently differentiate into two cell lines:
   1. Endothelial precursor cells, which form capillaries and eventually larger vessels
   2. Primitive hematopoietic stem cells, which form primitive nucleated erythrocytes. These stem cells colonize the developing liver and then the spleen, which become the major sites of fetal hematopoiesis.

B. **Weeks 3 to 9: Yolk sac** produces primitive erythrocytes.

C. Weeks 5 to 6: Intraembryonic visceral mesoderm gives rise to another line of hematopoietic stem cells in the dorsal aorta, near the gonad/mesonephric ridge (the "AGM" region).
   1. These stem cells also migrate and colonize the liver, where they expand in number and become definitive pluripotent hematopoietic stem cells, capable of producing the myeloid and lymphoid cell lines.
   2. These definitive hematopoietic stem cells eventually migrate to the bone marrow.

D. **Weeks 6 to 34: Liver and spleen** produce red blood cells (RBCs).

E. **Week 28 through childhood: Axial** (sternum, pelvis, ribs, cranial bones, vertebrae) and **peripheral** (tibia, femur) **bone marrow** produces RBCs.

F. **Adulthood: Axial skeleton (vertebral bodies, sternum, ribs, and pelvis)** produces RBCs.

II. Hemoglobin structure

A. Normal **hemoglobin** consists of four protein ("globin") subunits and four iron-containing heme prosthetic groups.

B. **Fetal hemoglobin** (HbF) consists of hemoglobin F, which is composed of two alpha globins and two gamma globins, $\alpha_2\gamma_2$. Compared to adult hemoglobin, HbF has a lower affinity for 2,3-diphosphoglycerate (2,3-DPG) and a higher affinity for oxygen.

C. **Adult hemoglobin** mostly consists of **hemoglobin A**, which is made up of two alpha and two beta globins, $\alpha_2\beta_2$. A small quantity of hemoglobin A_2 may also be found in adult blood, consisting of two alpha and two delta globins, $\alpha_2\delta_2$.

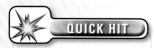

MNEMONIC

To remember the concentrations of the WBCs, think "Never Let Monkeys Eat Bananas."
Neutrophils (65%)
Lymphocytes (25%)
Monocytes (8%)
Eosinophils (3%)
Basophils (<1%)

THE CELLS (Table 10-1)

The hematopoietic lymphoreticular system is composed of a multitude of cells. Most of these cells can be found circulating in the bloodstream, although a few are found within peripheral tissues.

TABLE 10-1 The Cells of the Hematopoietic–Lymphoreticular System

Cell	Relative Amounts	Life Span	Morphology	Functions	Secretion	Notes
Neutrophils (PMNs)	40%–75% of WBCs; band form 3%–5% of WBCs	Less than 7 days	Multilobed nucleus, azurophilic granules (lysosomes)	Phagocytic; acute inflammatory response	**Myeloperoxidase**, lysozyme, lactoferrin, hydrolytic enzymes	Lysosomes contain lysozyme and myeloperoxidase, which are **bactericidal**
Basophils	<1% of WBCs	Years	Bilobate, basophilic	Allergies	Heparin, histamine, SRS-A	**Bind IgE** antibody to their membrane
Eosinophils	1%–6% of WBCs	Less than 2 weeks in connective tissues	Bilobed, azurophilic granules	Phagocytic for Ag–Ab complexes; **antiparasitic**; inactivated histamine and SRS-A	Histaminase, arylsulfatase	Large numbers found in lamina propria of GI tract
Mast cells	Found in connective tissue	9–18 months	Basophil-like, round nucleus	Bind IgE; mediate **type I hypersensitivity** reaction	ECF, histamine, leukotrienes, heparin, tryptase	**Cromolyn sodium** prevents degranulation by stabilizing membrane
Macrophages	Found **only in tissues**, not in the blood	Extended life in tissues	Ameboid	Phagocytize bacteria, RBCs, and damaged cells; APCs	IL-1, **IL-2**, TNF-α	Activated by LPS and IFN-γ
Monocytes	3%–9% of WBCs	Less than 3 days in the blood	Large, kidney-shaped nucleus	Differentiate into macrophages and osteoclasts	IL-1, IL-6	Chemotactically **attracted to sites of inflammation**
T lymphocytes	15%–18% of WBCs, 75% of lymphocytes	Years	Basophilic, large nucleus, scant cytoplasm	**Cell-mediated immune response**	IL-2, IL-3, IL-4, IL-5, IL-6, IFN-γ, TNF-α, TNF-β	Originate in bone marrow, mature in thymus
B lymphocytes	5%–7% of WBCs, 25% of lymphocytes	Months	Basophilic, large nucleus, scant cytoplasm; plasma cell has clock-faced chromatin distribution	**Humoral immune response**	IFN-α	Differentiate into plasma cells (produce large amounts of Ab specific to an Ag) and long-lived memory cells
Erythrocytes	$5 \times 10^6/\mu L$ in men, $4.55 \times 10^6/\mu L$ in women	120 days	**Anucleate, biconcave disc** (allows for large surface area to volume ratio)	Gas exchange		Anaerobic metabolism exclusively, membrane contains chloride bicarbonate antiport
Platelets	250,000–400,000/μL	7–10 days	Irregularly shaped, membrane bound, anucleate, extremely small	Prevention of bleeding by **clot formation**	Histamine, PDGF, serotonin, TXA_2, clotting factors, thrombospondin (thromboglobulin)	Disorders of number or function can result in bleeding

Ag–Ab, antigen–antibody; APC, antigen-presenting cell; ECF, eosinophilic chemotactic factor; GI, gastrointestinal; IFN, interferon; Ig, immunoglobulin; IL, interleukin; IFN, interferon; LPS, lipopolysaccharide; PDGF, platelet-derived growth factor; PMN, polymorphonuclear neutrophil; RBC, red blood cell; SRS-A, slow-reacting substance of anaphylaxis; TNF, tumor necrosis factor; TXA_2, thromboxane A_2; WBC, white blood cell.

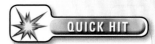

QUICK HIT

All neutrophils are hypersegmented (six to seven segments) in megaloblastic anemia.

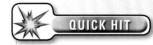

QUICK HIT

Slow-reacting substance of anaphylaxis (SRS-A) is composed of leukotriene C_4 and leukotriene D_4, which bronchoconstrict, vasoconstrict, and increase vascular permeability.

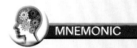

MNEMONIC

To remember the causes of eosinophilia, think DNAAACP:
Drugs
Neoplasm
Allergies/**A**sthma
Adrenal insufficiency
Acute interstitial nephritis
Collagen vascular disease
Parasites

The Hematopoietic and Lymphoreticular System

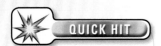

QUICK HIT

Adrenocorticotropin, steroids, estrogens, and androgens cause involution of the thymus.

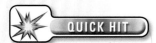

QUICK HIT

Virchow's node is a left supraclavicular node enlarged by metastasis from gastric carcinoma or other abdominal malignancy.

THE ORGANS OF THE LYMPHORETICULAR SYSTEM

I. Thymus
A. It is derived from the **third pharyngeal pouch**.
B. The cortex contains thymocytes (immature T lymphocytes).
C. The medulla contains mature T lymphocytes and **Hassall corpuscles** (whorl-like bodies that contain keratin). As T lymphocytes mature, they express T-cell receptors and cluster of differentiation (CD) receptors. T lymphocytes that are unable to recognize 'self' undergo apoptosis (positive selection). Subsequently, T lymphocytes that recognize 'self' too strongly also undergo apoptosis (negative selection). Cells that survive both positive and negative selection are released into the bloodstream.

II. Lymph nodes *(Figure 10-1)*
A. Derived from **mesenchymal cells**
B. **Outer cortex** contains B lymphocytes.
C. **Inner cortex** (also called the paracortex) contains T lymphocytes and is thymus dependent.
D. **Medulla** contains B lymphocytes, plasma cells, and macrophages.

FIGURE
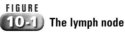 **The lymph node**

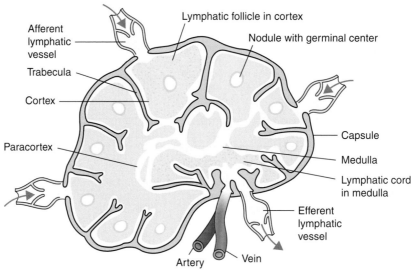

III. Lymph
A. It is the fluid that returns lipids, proteins, and water-soluble substances to the circulation via the lymphatic vessels.
B. The **left side of the head, the left thorax, the left upper limb**, and **everything below the diaphragm** drain into the **thoracic duct**. This duct terminates at the junction of the left subclavian and left internal jugular veins.
C. The **right upper quadrant of the body** (right side of the head, right upper limb, and right thorax) empties into the **right lymphatic duct**.

IV. Spleen *(Figure 10-2)*
A. It is derived from **mesenchyme** beginning in the fifth week.
B. **White pulp**: B lymphocytes surround the central artery and T lymphocytes are arranged into periarteriolar lymphatic sheaths (PALS).
C. **Marginal zone**: It is the zone where blood meets spleen parenchyma; antigen-presenting cells (APCs) and macrophages are present.
D. **Red pulp**: It contains splenic (Billroth) cords separated by sinusoids and also has plasma cells, macrophages, lymphocytes, and RBCs.

FIGURE
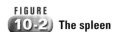
10-2 The spleen

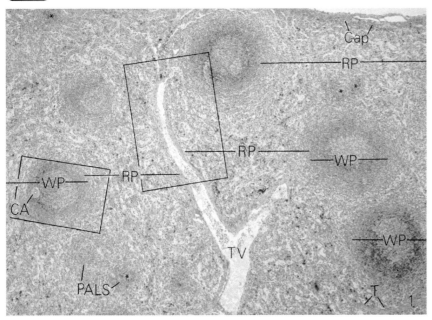

CA, central artery; Cap, capillary; PALS, periarteriolar lymphatic sheaths; RP, red pulp; T, trabeculae; TV, trabecular vein; WP, white pulp. (From Ross MH, Romrell LJ, Kaye GI. *Histology: A Text and Atlas.* 3rd ed. Baltimore, MD: Lippincott Williams & Wilkins; 1995. Used by permission of Lippincott Williams & Wilkins.)

V. Liver
A. **Endoderm** of the foregut (**hepatic diverticulum**) grows into the surrounding **mesoderm (septum transversum)**.
B. Hepatic cords from diverticulum, arranged around umbilical and vitelline veins, form **hepatic sinusoids**.
C. It produces HbF during much of fetal life.
D. It produces **clotting factors** of coagulation cascade.
E. It can function to sequester and break down RBCs if spleen is removed.

VI. Gut-associated lymphatic tissue
A. Found in **tonsils, Peyer patches** of the ileum, **appendix**, and cecum
B. **M cells**: Transcytose antigen from intestinal lumen into underlying lymphoid tissue, where it is taken up by antigen-presenting cells for presentation to lymphocytes. Also secrete IgA.

RED BLOOD CELL PHYSIOLOGY

I. Oxygen transport
A. RBCs deliver oxygen from the lungs to the tissues. Deoxyhemoglobin exists in the **tense/taut (T) state**, which has a **low affinity for oxygen**. Binding of the first oxygen molecule requires considerable energy and precipitates a conformational change from the tense state to the **relaxed (R) state**. Binding of further oxygen molecules requires less energy (**positive cooperativity**).
B. Several factors affect hemoglobin affinity for oxygen (Figure 10-3).
C. Hemoglobin binds with carbon monoxide 200 times more readily than with oxygen. The presence of carbon monoxide on one of the four heme sites causes the oxygen to bind with greater affinity. This makes it difficult for the hemoglobin to release the oxygen to the tissues and causes the hemoglobin oxygen dissociation curve to shift to the left. Therefore, increased levels of carbon monoxide can lead to severe hypoxemia while maintaining a normal P_{O_2}.

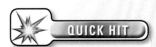

The erythrocyte relies on glucose for energy; 90% is metabolized anaerobically to lactate and 10% by the hexose monophosphate shunt.

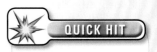

Carbon monoxide poisoning causes hypoxic injury to the basal ganglia and results in a cherry-red color of the skin and viscera. The treatment is 100% oxygen.

The Hematopoietic and Lymphoreticular System

FIGURE
10-3 Hemoglobin–oxygen dissociation curve

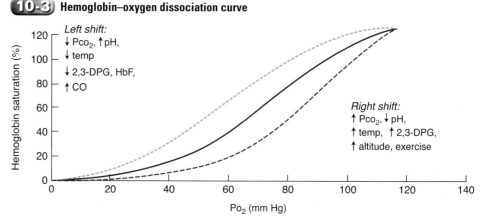

2,3-DPG, 2,3-diphosphoglycerate; CO, carbon monoxide; HbF, fetal hemoglobin; Pco_2, partial pressure of carbon dioxide; pH, hydrogen ion concentration; Po_2, partial pressure of oxygen; temp, temperature. Left shift: Hemoglobin (Hgb) molecules have more affinity for oxygen (O_2); right shift: Hgb molecules have less affinity for O_2.

II. Carbon dioxide transport (Figure 10-4)

A. RBCs carry carbon dioxide (CO_2) from the tissues to the lungs. In the tissues, CO_2 diffuses into the RBC, combines with water via **carbonic anhydrase**, and produces carbonic acid. Carbonic acid dissociates into hydrogen ions and bicarbonate. **Bicarbonate leaves** the RBC in exchange for chloride (**chloride shift**). In the lungs, this process is reversed. Thus, **bicarbonate in the plasma** is the **major route** for CO_2 transport to the lungs (90%).

B. Small amounts (5%) of CO_2 are bound to the N-terminus of globin (on hemoglobin) within the RBC. This carbaminohemoglobin favors the taut, oxygen-unloaded state.

C. A small amount (5%) of CO_2 is dissolved in the plasma.

FIGURE
10-4 Carbon dioxide transport

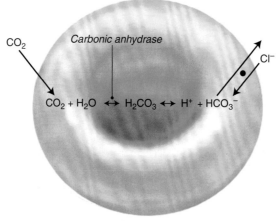

Cl^-, chloride; CO_2, carbon dioxide; H^+, hydrogen ion; HCO_3^-, bicarbonate; H_2CO_3, carbonic acid; H_2O, water.

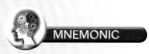

MNEMONIC

To remember which T cells interact with which MHC, think of the "=8" rule: $2 \times 4 = 8$ and $1 \times 8 = 8$; thus, MHC **II** goes with CD**4** and MHC **I** goes with CD**8**.

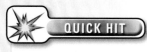

QUICK HIT

The CD4/CD8 ratio is normally 2:1. In AIDS, this ratio is **reversed**.

LYMPHOCYTE DIFFERENTIATION

T-helper (Th) lymphocytes recognize **major histocompatibility complex (MHC) class II** with **CD4 proteins** on their membranes. They participate in the cellular response to **extracellular** antigens (e.g., bacteria). Cytotoxic T lymphocytes (T-cyt) **recognize MHC class I with CD8 proteins** on their membranes. T-cyt cells are involved in the immune response to **intracellular antigens** (e.g., viruses and obligate intracellular organisms such as Chlamydiae or Rickettsiae). Natural killer (NK) cells are lymphocytes that do not pass through the thymus for maturation. As one of the body's innate defenses, NK cells kill **tumor cells** and **virus-infected cells** by secreting cytotoxins (granzymes and perforins). They do not require antibodies to kill, but their potency is increased when antibody is present (i.e., antibody-dependent cell-mediated cytotoxicity [ADCC]).

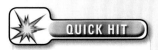

QUICK HIT

ADCC is one of the mechanisms by which type II hypersensitivity reactions can occur. Other mechanisms are complement-fixing antibodies (e.g., Goodpasture syndrome) and anti–cell surface receptor antibodies (e.g., Graves disease).

• **T-cell differentiation** (Figure 10-5)

FIGURE 10-5 T-cell differentiation and effect on other immune cells

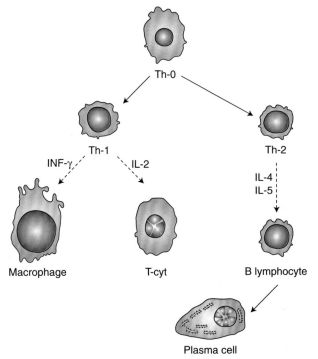

IFN-γ, interferon-γ; IL, interleukin; T-cyt, cytotoxic T lymphocytes; Th, T-helper lymphocytes.

IMMUNOGLOBULINS

I. Characteristics

    A. Structure

        1. Immunoglobulins are glycoproteins consisting of two identical **heavy (H) chains** and two identical **light (L) chains** linked by **disulfide bonds** in a "Y" shape.

        2. **Variable regions** exist on both the L and H chains.

        3. The **H chain** is composed of **Fc** and **Fab** fragment. The **L chain** is composed of **Fab** fragment only. The **Fab** is the **antigen-binding fragment**. The **Fc** fragment is <u>c</u>onstant and, in the case of immunoglobulin (Ig) M and IgG, it is <u>c</u>omplement binding. It also contains a <u>c</u>arboxy terminal and <u>c</u>arbohydrate side chains.

    B. **Antibody diversity** is created by

        1. Random recombination of the VJ (L chain) or VDJ (H chain) genes

        2. Random combination of H chains with L chains

        3. Somatic hypermutation

        4. Addition of nucleotides to DNA during recombination by terminal deoxynucleotidyl transferase

    C. **Antibody functions**

        1. **Opsonization**—in which the antibody promotes phagocytosis

        2. **Neutralization**—in which the antibody prevents pathogen adherence to cells and membranes or blocks the activity of toxins

        3. **Complement activation**—in which antibody activates complement, enhancing opsonization and lysis

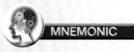

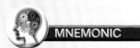

D. Allotype, isotype, and idiotype
   1. **Allotypes** are Ig epitopes that are different among the members of the same species. It is secondary to polymorphisms in the constant portion of the H chain or L chain. When trying to find appropriate transplant donors, allotypes are matched.
   2. An **isotype** is an Ig epitope that is common to a single class of immunoglobulins. For example, IgG, IgM, and IgA are different isotypes of Ig. It is determined by the constant region of the H chain.
   3. An **idiotype** is an Ig epitope that is specific for a given antigen. It is determined by the antigen-binding site contributed by the variable and hypervariable regions.

II. Types (Table 10-2)

TABLE 10-2 Immunoglobulin (Ig) Properties

	IgM	IgG	IgE	IgA	IgD
Percentage of total Ig	9%	75% (most abundant)	0.004% (least abundant)	15%	0.2%
Structure	Monomer or pentamer Pentamer held together by J chain	Monomer	Monomer	Monomer or dimer Dimer held together by J chain (secretory piece)	Monomer
Function	Fixes complement Antigen receptor on B-cell surface, **Primary response**	Fixes complement Opsonizes bacteria **Crosses the placenta** Neutralizes bacterial toxins and viruses **Secondary response**	Allergic response **(type I hypersensitivity)** Binds to basophils and mast cells (induces release of mediators) Antihelminthic (by activating eosinophils)	Found in **secretions** (including **breastmilk**) Prevents bacterial and viral attachment to mucous membranes Does not fix complement Picks up secretory component from epithelial cells before secretion	Unknown May be antigen receptor on B-cell surface

COMPLEMENT SYSTEM (Figure 10-6)

I. Function of complement
   A. Causes **direct lysis** of target cell
   B. Opsonizes target cells
   C. Promotes inflammation
   D. Promotes influx of immune cells (chemotaxis)
   E. Promotes clearane of immune complexes

II. Activation of pathways
   A. IgG and IgM activate the **classical pathway.**
      1. The activation is initiated by the binding of antibodies to antigens on a cell surface.
      2. The first step of activation involves formation of the complex by C1, C2, and C4.
   B. The **alternative pathway** is activated spontaneously.
      1. The pathway begins with hydrolysis of C3.
      2. Antigens on microbial surfaces stabilize C3b, allowing for the formation of the membrane-attack complex.
   C. Mannose chains on bacteria activate the **lectin pathway.**
      1. The activation is initiated by mannose-binding lectin (MBL) and associate protease binding to mannose residues.
      2. The first step of activation involves the MBL–mannose complex activating proteases that activate C4 and C2, which then go on to activate the rest of the classical pathway.

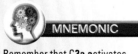

III. Properties of complement cascade components
   A. **C1**: only component not made in liver (made in gastrointestinal [GI] epithelium)
   B. C1–C4: involved in viral neutralization

C. **C3b**: involved in opsonization

D. C3a: acts as an anaphylatoxin

E. **C5a**: acts as an anaphylatoxin. Also chemotactic for neutrophils and macrophages.

F. **C5b–C9**: also known as the membrane attack complex (MAC)

G. **C1 inhibitor**: deficiency of this component leads to hereditary angioedema

H. Table 10-3 discusses alterations in the complement cascade (complement deficiencies)

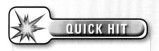

QUICK HIT

The membrane attack complex (MAC) has only one component each of C5b, C6, C7, and C8 but has numerous C9 components.

FIGURE 10-6 Complement pathway

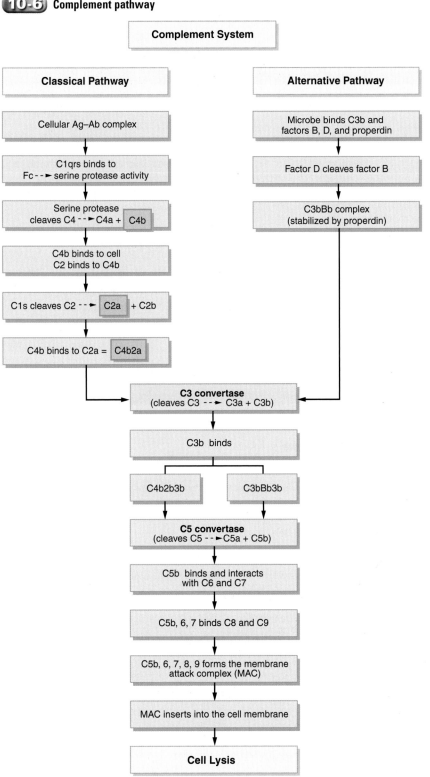

IV. Complement deficiencies

A. Deficiencies of C1, C3, C5, C6, C7, and C8 lead to increased bacterial infections.

B. C1 deficiency results in hereditary angioedema.

C. C2 deficiency is the most common complement deficiency. Manifestations of C2 and C4 deficiencies resemble autoimmune diseases such as systemic lupus erythematosus (SLE).

D. C3 deficiency causes increased susceptibility to *Staphylococcus aureus* and severe, recurrent sinus and respiratory infections.

E. C6, C7, and C8 deficiencies lead to *Neisseria gonorrhoeae* infection and meningitis.

F. Deficiency of decay accelerating factor (DAF) leads to complement-mediated lysis of erythrocytes and paroxysmal nocturnal hemoglobinuria (PNH).

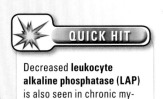

QUICK HIT

Decreased **leukocyte alkaline phosphatase (LAP)** is also seen in chronic myelogenous leukemia (CML).

TABLE 10-3 Complement Deficiencies

Disease	Defect	Significant Features
Hereditary angioedema	Decreased C1 (first component of complement) inhibitor	Increased capillary permeability; edema
PNH	Deficiency of DAF and MIRL; increased complement activation	Complement-mediated hemolysis; brown urine in the morning; **decreased LAP**

DAF, decay accelerating factor; LAP, leukocyte alkaline phosphatase; PNH, paroxysmal nocturnal hemoglobinuria; MIRL, membrane inhibitor of reactive lysis.

V. Cytokines (Table 10-4)

Cytokines are hormones that have a low molecular weight and are involved in cell-to-cell communication. Human recombinant cytokines are useful in the management of neoplasms, transplant rejection, and to stimulate the growth of various cell lines in cases of bone marrow suppression (Table 10-5).

TABLE 10-4 Cytokines

Cytokine	Secreted by	Function
IL-1	Macrophages	Endogenous **pyrogen**; stimulates T cells
IL-2	T-helper cells (Th1)	Activates T-helper and T-cytotoxic cells
IL-3	Activated T cells	Stimulates the growth and differentiation of bone marrow stem cells
IL-4	T-helper cells (Th2)	Stimulates the growth of B cells; increases IgE and IgG
IL-5	T-helper cells (Th2)	Differentiation of B cells; increases IgA
IL-10	Monocytes, T-helper cells (Th2)	Inhibits the development of Th1 cells; inhibits IFN-γ production
IL-12	Macrophages	Promotes Th1 cell development; stimulates IFN-γ production
IFN-α	Virus-infected leukocytes	Produces ribonuclease that degrades viral mRNA inhibiting viral protein synthesis
IFN-β	Virus-infected fibroblasts	Produces ribonuclease that degrades viral mRNA inhibiting viral protein synthesis
IFN-γ	T-helper cells (Th1)	Stimulates macrophages and NK cells; increases MHC expression; stimulates phagocytosis and killing
Tumor necrosis factor	Macrophages	At low concentrations, activates neutrophils and increases IL-2 receptor synthesis; at high concentrations, mediates septic shock and results in tumor necrosis
Transforming growth factor	T cells, B cells, and macrophages	Inhibits the growth and activities of T cells; enhances collagen synthesis; dampens the immune response

IFN, interferon; Ig, immunoglobulin; IL, interleukin; MHC, major histocompatibility complex; mRNA, messenger RNA; NK, natural killer.

The Hematopoietic and Lymphoreticular System

TABLE 10-5 Recombinant Cytokines				
Therapeutic Agent (common name, if relevant) [trade name, where appropriate]	Class—Pharmacology and Pharmacokinetics	Indications	Side Effects or Adverse Effects	Contraindications or Precautions to Consider; Notes
Aldesleukin [Proleukin]	Human recombinant **interleukin-2**	**Metastatic renal cell carcinoma, metastatic melanoma, AML**		
Epoetin alfa [Procrit, Epogen]	**Colony-stimulating factor**	**Anemias (especially in renal failure), AIDS**	Hypertension	
Filgrastim [Neupogen]	**Granulocyte-macrophage colony–stimulating factor**	**Recovery of bone marrow (e.g., chemotherapy-induced neutropenia)**		
Sargramostim (Leukine)	**Granulocyte-macrophage colony–stimulating factor**	**Recovery of bone marrow (e.g., bone marrow transplant failure)**	Hypertension	
Interferon α-2a [Roferon A], **α2b** [Intron A], and **α-n3** [Alferon-N]	Antiviral—decreases protein synthesis	**Genital warts, chronic hepatitis B and C, AIDS-related Kaposi sarcoma, laryngeal papillomatosis, hairy cell leukemia, malignant melanoma**	**Flulike symptoms**, headache, malaise, fever, chills, **depression**, **neutropenia**, somnolence, tachycardia	
Interferon β-1a [Avonex, Rebif]	Antiviral—decreases protein synthesis	**Multiple sclerosis**	**Flulike symptoms**, ache, fatigue, fever, pain, chills, depression	
Interferon γ-1b [Actimmune]	Antiviral—decreases protein synthesis	**Chronic granulomatous disease**	Fever, headache, chills, fatigue	
Oprelvekin [Neumega]	**Interleukin-11** stimulates multiple stages of **thrombopoiesis**, increasing the platelet production	**Thrombocytopenia**		
Thrombopoietin	Recombinant human thrombopoietin	**Thrombocytopenia**		

AML, acute myelogenous leukemia.

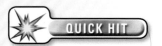

HYPERSENSITIVITY REACTIONS

MNEMONIC

Use **ACID** to help remember immunology of each hypersensitivity reaction:
Anaphylactic: Type I
Cytotoxic: Type II
Immune complex disease: Type III
Delayed hypersensitivity (cell mediated): Type IV

I.   **There are four types of hypersensitivity reactions. They vary in onset of symptoms, severity, and mechanism** (Table 10-6).

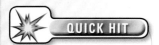
QUICK HIT

An acute allergic reaction is a type I hypersensitivity reaction.

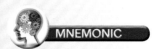
QUICK HIT

Serum sickness is more common than an Arthus reaction.

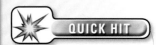
MNEMONIC

Remember poison **IV**y causes type **IV** hypersensitivity.

QUICK HIT

Graft-versus-host disease (GVHD) is caused by donor lymphocytes attacking recipient cells. It is characterized by elevated bilirubin and liver enzymes and skin lesions. It is seen commonly in bone marrow transplants.

TABLE 10-6   Hypersensitivity Reactions

Reaction Type	Description	Example
Type I (anaphylaxis)	Mediated by **IgE** antibody bound to mast cells or basophil antigens cross-link antibody Release of **histamine**, SRS-A, eosinophilic chemotactic factor, and platelet-activating factor p-tryptase, leukotrienes	Anaphylaxis Allergic rhinitis (hay fever) Asthma Wheal and flare
Type II (cytotoxic)	Antibody-dependent cellular cytotoxicity Antibody produced to specific cell-surface antigens IgM- and IgG-mediated lysis via complement Immunofluorescence, stains smooth, linear Abs staining in biopsy	Rh incompatibility Goodpasture syndrome Myasthenia gravis Hemolytic anemia Idiopathic thrombocytopenic purpura Rheumatic fever Graves disease Bullous pemphigoid
Type III (immune complex)	**Antigen–antibody complexes** induce inflammatory response Deposition of complexes in tissue	**Arthus reaction** **Serum sickness** Glomerulonephritis Rheumatoid arthritis SLE Polyarteritis nodosa
Type IV (delayed or cell mediated)	**Helper (CD4) Th1 lymphocyte mediated** Response is delayed (from hours to days) Predominantly mononuclear cell infiltration	Tuberculin (PPD) test GVHD Contact dermatitis Type 1 diabetes mellitus Multiple sclerosis Guillain–Barré syndrome Hashimoto thyroiditis

CD4, cluster of differentiation 4; GVHD, graft-versus-host disease; Ig, immunoglobulin; PPD, purified protein derivative; Rh, rhesus (factor); SLE, systemic lupus erythematosus; SRS-A, slow-reacting substance of anaphylaxis; Th, T-helper.

II. Transplant rejection timeline (Figure 10-7)

FIGURE
10-7 Transplant rejection timeline

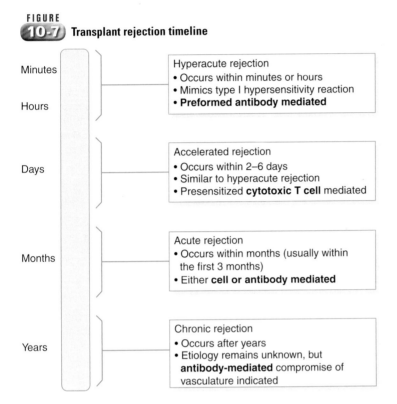

Minutes Hours	**Hyperacute rejection** • Occurs within minutes or hours • Mimics type I hypersensitivity reaction • **Preformed antibody mediated**
Days	**Accelerated rejection** • Occurs within 2–6 days • Similar to hyperacute rejection • Presensitized **cytotoxic T cell** mediated
Months	**Acute rejection** • Occurs within months (usually within the first 3 months) • Either **cell or antibody mediated**
Years	**Chronic rejection** • Occurs after years • Etiology remains unknown, but **antibody-mediated** compromise of vasculature indicated

IMMUNODEFICIENCIES

I. **Diseases affecting the immune system leave the individual prone to infection. The immune system can be affected on any level and at any time—from its development to its most distal signaling mechanisms.**

II. **Congenital B-cell deficiencies** (Table 10-7)

TABLE 10-7 Congenital B-Cell Deficiencies

Disease	Defect	Significant Features
X-linked agammaglobulinemia (of Bruton)	Lack of maturation of B cells, secondary to defective tyrosine kinase gene	Absence of plasma cells, **low levels of all immunoglobulins**; **recurrent pyogenic infections** beginning after 6 months; lymphoid tissue has **poorly defined germinal centers**
Selective IgA deficiency	Lack of maturation of B cells; failure of gene switching in H chain	**Most common congenital B-cell defect (1 in 600 newborns of European descent)**; most appear healthy; **sinus/lung infections**; possible anaphylaxis to blood product transfusions
Common variable immunodeficiency	Failure of terminal B-cell differentiation; defective Ig production	Variable: recurrent infections, autoimmune disorders, chronic lung and/or GI disease, increased risk of lymphoma

GI, gastrointestinal; Ig, immunoglobulin.

The Hematopoietic and Lymphoreticular System

III. **Congenital T-cell deficiencies** (*Table 10-8*)

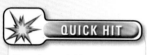

Remember the features of DiGeorge syndrome by thinking of it as the disease of Ts:
Third and fourth branchial pouch absent
Thymic aplasia
T cells absent
Twenty-**T**wo chromosome deletion
Tetany: Para**T**hyroid (decreased parathyroid hormone results in hypocalcemia).

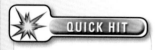

Treat hyper-IgM syndrome with pooled γ-globulin.

Measles, a paramyxovirus, results in a T-cell deficiency.

Severe combined immunodeficiency (SCID) caused by adenosine deaminase (ADA) deficiency was one of the first diseases successfully treated with gene therapy.

TABLE 10-8 Congenital T-Cell Deficiencies

Disease	Defect	Significant Features
Thymic aplasia (DiGeorge syndrome)	Deficiency of development of third and fourth branchial pouches; thymic aplasia leads to T-cell defect; commonly 22q11.2 deletion	Defective development of the thymus, parathyroid glands, ear, mandible, and aortic arch; leads to recurrent infections by **viral and fungal organisms; hypocalcemia** from low parathyroid hormone leads to tetany
Chronic mucocutaneous candidiasis	Lack of T-cell response to candidiasis	Recurrent candidal skin and mucous membrane infections; treat infections with fluconazole or ketoconazole
Hyper IgM syndrome	Mutation in CD4$^+$ Th cell interaction with CD40 on B cell prevents class switching; two main types **X linked**: deficiency of CD40 ligand on T cell **AR**: defect in CD40 on B cells	Increased IgM; decreased IgG, IgA, and IgE; normal numbers of T and B cells
IL-12 receptor deficiency	Deficiency in IL-12 receptor leads to decreased Th1 response	Patients present with disseminated mycobacterial infections

AR, autosomal recessive; CD, cluster of differentiation; Ig, immunoglobulin; IL, interleukin; Th, T-helper.

IV. **Congenital combined T- and B-cell deficiencies** (*Table 10-9*)

TABLE 10-9 Congenital Combined T- and B-Cell Deficiencies

Disease	Defect	Significant Features
Severe combined immunodeficiency (SCID)	Autosomal recessive (defect in tyrosine kinase zeta-associated protein [ZAP]-70 or adenosine deaminase deficiency); X-linked forms (interleukin [IL]-2 receptor defect)	Triad of severe **recurrent infections** (candidiasis, PCP, fatal or recurrent viral infections [RSV, VZV, HSV, measles, flu, parainfluenza]), **chronic diarrhea, failure to thrive** No thymic shadow on newborn CXR
Wiskott–Aldrich syndrome	X-linked weak IgM response to capsule polysaccharide (e.g., *Streptococcus pneumoniae*)	**Eczema, thrombocytopenia, and recurrent infections**; becomes noticeable in first year of life; low IgM, high IgA
Ataxia telangiectasia	IgA deficiency and lymphopenia (low T cells)	**Autosomal recessive**; becomes noticeable in first 2 years of life; cerebellar ataxia, poor smooth pursuit of moving target with eyes; telangiectasias of face >5 years; increased cancer risk (lymphoma and acute leukemias); radiation sensitivity (avoid x-rays); average age of death 25 years

CXR, chest x-ray; HSV, herpes simplex virus; Ig, immunoglobulin; PCP, *Pneumocystis carinii* pneumonia; RSV, respiratory syncytial virus; VZV, varicella-zoster virus.

V. Plasma cell abnormalities *(Table 10-10)*

TABLE 10-10 Plasma Cell Abnormalities

Disease	Etiology	Clinical Features	Notes
Multiple myeloma	Clonal plasma cell tumor	**"Punched-out" lytic bone lesions**, especially in the skull; hypercalcemia; back pain; anemia; hyperglobulinemia; **Bence Jones proteinuria**; renal insufficiency	Rouleaux formation ("stack of coins" appearance) of RBCs on peripheral smear
Waldenström macroglobulinemia	Excessive production of IgM by lymphoid cells	Slowly progressive course; usually in men older than 50 years of age; platelet function abnormal; hyperviscosity syndrome	No bone lesions (which differentiates this from multiple myeloma)
Benign monoclonal gammopathy	Increased production of monoclonal antibodies from an unknown origin	Asymptomatic; occurring in older individuals	Monoclonal spike without Bence Jones proteinuria (versus multiple myeloma)

Ig, immunoglobulin; RBC, red blood cell.

VI. Phagocyte deficiencies *(Table 10-11)*

TABLE 10-11 Phagocyte Deficiencies

Disease	Defect	Significant Features
Chronic granulomatous disease (CGD)	Neutrophils **lack NADPH oxidase**; no oxidative burst in macrophages	**X linked** (some AR); susceptible to organisms with catalase (e.g., *Staphylococcus aureus*, *Escherichia coli*, *Klebsiella*, *Aspergillus*, *Candida*) Diagnosis: **negative nitroblue tetrazolium (NBT) dye** (no yellow to blue-black oxidation) Treatment: prophylactic TMP-SMX, itraconazole, IFN-γ
Chédiak-Higashi syndrome	Defective LYST gene (lysosomal transport); failure of neutrophils to empty lysosomes; giant cytoplasmic granules in neutrophils	Autosomal recessive; presentation triad: **partial albinism; recurrent pyogenic infections** (e.g., *Staphylococcus*, *Streptococcus*); **neurologic disorders**
Job syndrome	T-helper lymphocytes fail to produce IFN-γ; neutrophils fail to respond to chemotactic stimuli (C5a, LTB4)	High levels of IgE and eosinophils; presentation triad: **eczema; recurrent cold *S. aureus* abscesses; coarse facial features** (broad nose, prominent forehead "frontal bossing," deep-set eyes, doughy skin); commonly have retained primary teeth (2 rows of teeth)
Leukocyte adhesion deficiency	Defect in integrins prevents phagocytes from exiting circulation	Delayed separation of umbilicus; pyogenic infections early in life

IFN-γ, interferon-γ; Ig, immunoglobulin; LTB4, leukotriene B4; NADPH, nicotinamide adenine dinucleotide phosphate; TMP-SMX, trimethoprim-sulfamethoxazole.

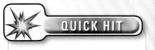

QUICK HIT

Interferon-γ (IFN-γ) is used to treat chronic granulomatous disease (CGD).

The Hematopoietic and Lymphoreticular System

VII. Acquired immunodeficiencies (Table 10-12)

TABLE 10-12	Acquired Immunodeficiencies	
Disease	**Defect**	**Significant Features**
Common variable hypogammaglobulinemia	Acquired or congenital (unknown) B-cell defects	Recurrent pyogenic bacterial infections (e.g., *S. pneumoniae*, *Haemophilus influenzae*); decreased IgG production
AIDS	**HIV virus infects CD4 cells and macrophages**	Opportunistic infections (e.g., ***Mycobacterium avium-intracellulare***, *Cryptococcus neoformans*, **Pneumocystis jirovecii**, and *Candida albicans*); increased tumors (e.g., Kaposi sarcoma)

CD4, cluster of differentiation 4; Ig, immunoglobulin.

IMMUNOSUPPRESSANTS (Table 10-13)

TABLE 10-13	Immunosuppressants			
Therapeutic Agent (common name, if relevant) [trade name, where appropriate]	**Class— Pharmacology and Pharmacokinetics**	**Indications**	**Side Effects or Adverse Effects**	**Contraindications or Precautions to Consider; Notes**
Cyclosporine [Sandimmune]	Binds **cyclophilins** → complex inhibits **calcineurin** → prevents production of **IL-2, IL-3,** and **IFN-γ** → inhibits **T-helper cell** activity	**Transplant rejection,** selected **autoimmune disorder**	**Nephrotoxic,** hepatotoxic; hypertension; **increased incidence of viral infection and lymphoma**	Nephrotoxicity preventable with mannitol diuresis
Tacrolimus (FK506) [Prograf]	Binds to **FK-binding protein** (T-cell transcription factor) → inhibits **calcineurin** → inhibits **IL-2** synthesis and T-cell signal transduction → inhibits **T-cell** activity	**Transplant rejection**	**Nephrotoxic, neurotoxic (peripheral neuropathy); hyperglycemia, hypertension, pleural effusion;** GI disturbances	Potent immunosuppressant

(continued)

TABLE 10-13 Immunosuppressants *(Continued)*

Therapeutic Agent (common name, if relevant) [trade name, where appropriate]	Class—Pharmacology and Pharmacokinetics	Indications	Side Effects or Adverse Effects	Contraindications or Precautions to Consider; Notes
Azathioprine [Imuran]	Purine antagonist; antimetabolite precursor of **6-mercaptopurine** → inhibits nucleic acid synthesis and metabolism → toxic to **proliferating lymphocytes**; blocks both CMI and humoral response	**Transplant (esp. kidney),** acute glomerulonephritis, renal component of lupus, rheumatoid arthritis, hemolytic anemia	**Bone marrow suppression,** rash, fever, nausea, vomiting, hepatotoxicity, malignancy, GI intolerance	Metabolized by xanthine oxidase; **toxic effects may be increased by allopurinol**
Muromonab (OKT3)	**Monoclonal antibody** that binds CD3 on T lymphocytes → blocks cellular interaction with CD3 protein responsible for T-cell signal transduction	Acute rejection of **renal transplants**	**Cytokine release syndrome,** hypersensitivity reaction	
Sirolimus (rapamycin)	Binds to mTOR → inhibits response to **IL-2** → inhibits **T-cell proliferation**	Immunosuppression after **kidney transplantation** (in combination with cyclosporine and corticosteroids)	**Hyperlipidemia, thrombocytopenia, and leukopenia**	
Mycophenolate mofetil [CellCept]	Inhibits de novo **guanine synthesis** → blocks **lymphocyte production**	Prevents rejection after **organ transplantation,** myasthenia gravis	Hypertension, hyperglycemia, hypercholesterolemia, leucopenia, thrombocytopenia	
Daclizumab [Zenapax]	Monoclonal antibody with high affinity for the **IL-2 receptor** on activated T cells → **prevents T-cell activation**	**Prevents rejection after kidney transplantation**		Decreased incidence of opportunistic infections when compared with other immunosuppressants

CD, cluster of differentiation; CMI, cell-mediated immunity; GI, gastrointestinal; IFN, interferon; IL, interleukin; mTOR, mammalian target of rapamycin.

The Hematopoietic and Lymphoreticular System

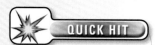

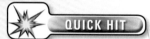

Factors II, VII, IX, and X and proteins C and S require vitamin K for their synthesis and are produced in the liver.

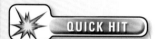

Vitamin K is administered to newborns in the United States to prevent hemorrhagic diseases.

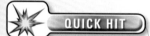

Factor VIII is the only clotting factor increased in liver disease.

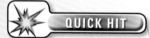

Partial thromboplastin time (**PTT**) measures the **contact activation pathway.** Therapeutic drug monitoring of heparin is measured using PTT. Heparin overdose is treated with intravenous protamine sulfate.

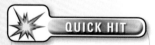

Prothrombin time (**PT**) measures the **tissue factor pathway.** Therapeutic drug monitoring of warfarin is measured using PT. Warfarin overdose is treated with the administration of vitamin K. In acute cases of hemorrhage, fresh frozen plasma may be given to quickly reverse the effects of warfarin.

The Hematopoietic and Lymphoreticular System

THROMBOSIS AND THE CLOTTING CASCADE (Figure 10-8)

The intravascular coagulation of blood involves the interaction of platelets, coagulation proteins, and endolethial cells. With intact endothelium, a balance exists between prothrombotic (platelet-derived thromboxane A₂ [TXA₂]) and antithrombotic (endothelium-derived prostaglandin 12 [PGI₂]) mediators. With damaged endothelium, exposed collagen causes adhesion of platelets through glycoprotein receptors and **von Willebrand factor (vWF)**. This adhesion triggers platelet release of adenosine diphosphate (ADP), serotonin, histamine, platelet-derived growth factor (PDGF), and TXA₂, resulting in primary plug formation and cessation of bleeding. Stabilization of the primary plug (formation of the secondary plug) is mediated by fibrin and factor XIIIa, a result of activation of the clotting cascade. Thrombosis is pathologic blood clotting that results in the obstruction of a vessel.

Factor XIa in the presence of calcium (Ca^{2+}) activates factor IX. Factor IXa requires Ca^{2+} and a phospholipid to activate factor X. Activated factor X requires Ca^{2+}, phospholipid, and factor Va to activate prothrombin to thrombin. Thrombin and Ca^{2+} activate factor XIII that promotes the cross-linking of fibrin.

- Key Players in Inhibition of Coagulation

α₁-Antitrypsin	Inhibits factor XIa
α₂-Macroglobuli	Inhibits serine proteases
Antithrombin	Inhibits factor Xa and thrombin
Inhibitor of the first component	Inhibits factor XII and kallikrein of complement (C1 INH)
Heparin cofactor II	Inhibits thrombin
Protein C	Inactivates factors Va and VIIIa
Protein S	Is a cofactor for protein C

FIGURE 10-8 Thrombosis and the clotting cascade

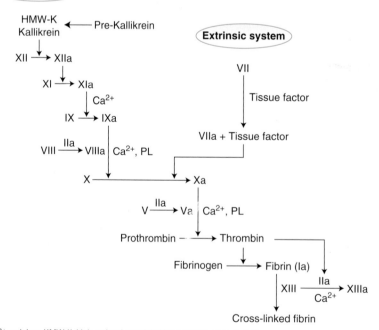

Ca^{2+}, calcium; HMW-K, high-molecular-weight kininogen; PL, phospholipid.

Clinical Vignette 10-1

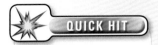

CLINICAL PRESENTATION: A 65-year-old man presents to his primary care physician complaining of **bad back pains** for the past several months aggravated by **walking or bending over.** Yesterday, he fell on his right arm while shoveling snow. Patient has no past medical or surgical history, but the patient was recently hospitalized for a **kidney stone.** Physical examination reveals tenderness to palpation over the thoracic and lumbar spine. No splenomegaly or lymphadenopathy. Plain films of the spine show several **lytic lesions in the vertebral bodies at L3–L4 levels.** Plain films of the right upper extremity show lytic lesions in the diaphysis and a **fracture line.**

DIFFERENTIALS: Fibromyalgia, herniated disk (nerve root impingement), osteoarthritis, metastatic bone lesion, and multiple myeloma. The lytic lesions, pathologic fractures, and kidney stones (evidence of hypercalcemia) suggest multiple myeloma.

LABORATORY STUDIES: In addition to the **lytic lesions on the plain film** (Figure 10-9A), **serum and urine electrophoresis** showing M-protein spike would support a diagnosis of multiple myeloma. To confirm a diagnosis of multiple myeloma, a **bone marrow biopsy** showing 10% plasma cells (Figure 10-9B) would need to be performed. A **complete blood count (CBC) showing mild anemia** and **electrolytes showing hypercalcemia and renal insufficiency** are also findings seen in multiple myeloma.

MANAGEMENT: Multiple myeloma has a poor prognosis, with median survival of few months without treatment. Treatment is reserved for patients with advanced disease and includes chemotherapy (alkylating agents), radiation therapy, and transplantation.

**FIGURE
10-9** Multiple myeloma

A. Lytic lesions

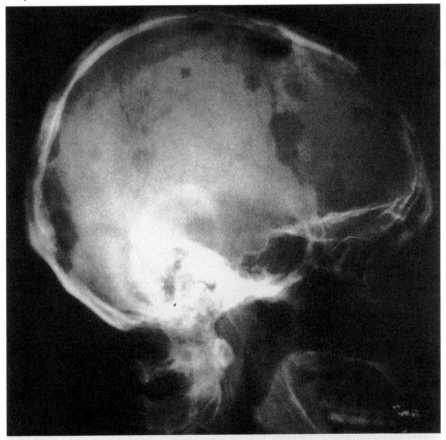

A

The Hematopoietic and Lymphoreticular System

FIGURE
10-9 Multiple myeloma *(Continued)*

B. Plasma cells

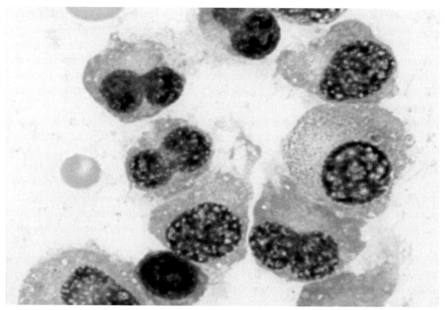

B

(Reproduced with permission from Anderson SC. *Anderson's Atlas of Hematology.* Philadelphia, PA: Wolters Kluwer Health/Lippincott Williams & Wilkins; 2003.)

ANTITHROMBOTIC THERAPEUTIC AGENTS

I. Platelet inhibitors *(Figure 10-10) (Table 10-14)*

Aspirin inhibits thromboxane-mediated platelet aggregation, ticlopidine and clopidogrel block platelet ADP receptors, and argatroban and hirudin inhibit thrombin directly.

  A. Aspirin
   1. Irreversibly acetylates **platelet cyclooxygenase (COX)**
   2. Results in disruption of TXA_2-dependent platelet aggregation
   3. Leads to less platelet hemostasis
   4. Can be used in acute myocardial infarctions (MIs) or prophylactically to reduce the likelihood of platelet-mediated vascular occlusion

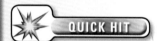

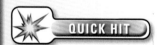

QUICK HIT

Heparin, sulfonamides, sulfonylureas, valproate, ethanol, gold, antineoplastic agents, chloramphenicol, and benzene result in drug-induced injury to the bone marrow, resulting in a decreased platelet production.

QUICK HIT

Aspirin, ticlopidine, and clopidogrel work globally to reduce the risk of thrombotic occlusion and thromboembolism regardless of the anatomic site.

FIGURE
10-10 Inhibition of platelet aggregation pathways

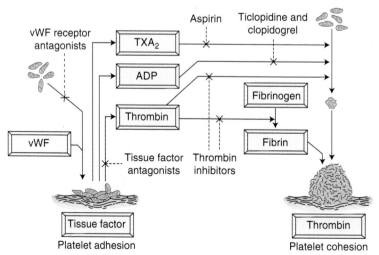

Aspirin inhibits thromboxane-mediated platelet aggregation, ticlopidine and clopidogrel block platelet ADP receptors, and argatroban and hirudin inhibit thrombin directly. ADP, adenosine diphosphate; TXA_2, thromboxane A_2; vWF, von Willebrand factor.

B. Ticlopidine and clopidogrel
   1. Irreversible **blockage of platelet ADP receptors**
   2. Can be used for the same clinical scenarios in which aspirin has failed
   3. Are at least as safe as aspirin in terms of side effects

II. Anticoagulants (*Table 10-14*)

A. Heparin
   1. Binds to antithrombin
   2. Greatly **enhances the ability of antithrombin to inhibit coagulation proteases, primarily thrombin**
   3. Is useful in a variety of situations in which anticoagulation is necessary
      a. Deep venous thrombosis (DVT) or pulmonary embolism
      b. Brain attack (thrombotic occlusion)
      c. MI
      d. Others
   4. Leads to **heparin-induced thrombocytopenia** or **thrombosis**, a notable side effect that occurs in 1% to 3% of patients. A heparin-platelet factor 4 antibody is the cause.
   5. Reversal by protamine sulfate
B. Warfarin (Coumadin)
   1. **Impairs vitamin K metabolism**
      a. Low levels of vitamin K prevent γ-carboxylation of **clotting factors II, VII, IX, and X.**
      b. Lack of γ-carboxylation leads to **hypofunctional clotting factors II, VII, IX, and X.**
   2. Is used in a variety of clinical scenarios in which oral anticoagulation is required
      a. Atrial fibrillation
      b. Prosthetic valves
      c. DVT or pulmonary embolism
      d. Postoperative anticoagulation
      e. Hypercoagulable states
   3. Use requires care because excessive anticoagulation can lead to hemorrhage.
   4. Reversal by Vitamin K and Factor VIIa

III. Thrombolytics (*Table 10-14*)

A. **Convert plasminogen to plasmin**, which disrupts vascular clot formation
B. Are useful in acute MI, acute ischemic stroke, acute arterial thromboembolic occlusion, severe DVT, and pulmonary embolism
C. Include tissue plasminogen activator (tPA), streptokinase, urokinase, and anistreplase
   1. tPA leads to the most rapid lysis of the clot and results in less systemic fibrinolysis.
   2. However, tPA is also the most expensive.
D. Require careful monitoring because of **increased risk of abnormal bleeding**

IV. Direct thrombin inhibitors (*Table 10-14*)

A. **Do not require antithrombin for activity**
B. Allow for more efficient inhibition of clot-bound fibrin
C. Include hirudin derivatives (lepirudin, bivalirudin, desirudin) and non-hirudin derivatives (argatroban and dabigatran)
D. Various drug-specific indications include prophylaxis of thrombosis in heparin-induced thrombocytopenia or nonvalvular atrial fibrillation, secondary prevention of stroke/transient ischemic attack (TIA), and postcoronary stenting.

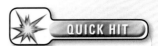

QUICK HIT

Low-molecular-weight heparins (LMWHs) such as enoxaparin and dalteparin are much more convenient than standard intravenous heparin therapy because they require no PTT monitoring and are administered subcutaneously. Uses for LMWHs include postsurgical prophylaxis against DVT and the treatment of venous thromboembolism. However, the use of LMWHs is limited in patients with renal failure.

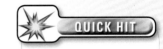

QUICK HIT

The effect of heparin is determined by measuring the activated partial thromboplastin time (aPTT). The effect of warfarin is determined by measuring the PT.

The Hematopoietic and Lymphoreticular System

The Hematopoietic and Lymphoreticular System

TABLE 10-14	**Antithrombotics**			
Therapeutic Agent (common name, if relevant) [trade name, where appropriate]	**Class—Pharmacology and Pharmacokinetics**	**Indications**	**Side Effects or Adverse Effects**	**Contraindications or Precautions to Consider; Notes**
Aspirin	**Platelet inhibitor**; anti-inflammatory, antipyretic, analgesic; **acetylates COX irreversibly** inhibiting the conversion of arachidonic acid to thromboxane A_2	Articular, musculoskeletal pain; chronic pain; acute gout; **maintenance therapy for preventing clot formation**	**Gastric ulcers, bleeding**, causes hypersensitivity reactions (rash), hyperventilation and tinnitus in overdose, **Reye syndrome**	**Contraindicated for children with the flu or chicken pox** (leads to Reye syndrome)
Clopidogrel	**Platelet inhibitor**—irreversibly blocks **ADP receptors**, inhibiting platelet aggregation; prevents **glycoprotein IIb/IIIa** expression, which inhibits fibrinogen binding	**Acute coronary syndrome, coronary stenting, prevention of thrombotic stroke**	Bleeding	
Ticlopidine	**Platelet inhibitor**—irreversibly blocks **ADP receptors**, inhibiting platelet aggregation; prevents **glycoprotein IIb/IIIa** expression, which inhibits fibrinogen binding	**Acute coronary syndrome, coronary stenting, prevention of thrombotic stroke**	Bleeding, **neutropenia**	
Abciximab	**Platelet inhibitor**—**monoclonal antibody** that binds to **glycoprotein receptor IIb/IIIa** on activated platelets → prevents platelet aggregation	**Acute coronary syndrome, PTCA**	Bleeding, thrombocytopenia	
Heparin	**Anticoagulant**—catalyzes the activation of **antithrombin**; decreases thrombin and factor Xa	**Immediate anticoagulation** for pulmonary embolism, stroke, angina, myocardial infarction, and deep vein thrombosis	**Bleeding, osteoporosis, HIT**, drug–drug interactions, overdose reversed by IV **protamine sulfate**	Fast-acting, short half-life; **laboratory monitoring with PTT; does not cross placenta**
Enoxaparin [Lovenox]	**Anticoagulant**—low-molecular-weight heparin; enhances inhibition of factor Xa and thrombin by increasing **antithrombin** activity **(preferentially increases the inhibition of factor Xa)**	**Prophylaxis of thrombosis**	**Elevated AST/ALT** (reversible), **HIT**	**Caution in recent surgery** or **active bleeding ulcers** or **internal hemorrhages; fewer bleeding complications, increased bioavailability, and longer half-life** compared to unfractionated heparin; no requirement for laboratory monitoring
Fondaparinux [Arixtra]	**Anticoagulant**—factor Xa inhibitor; binds to antithrombin to inactivate Xa	**Prophylaxis or treatment of DVT**, used off-label to treat HIT	Hemorrhage	

(continued)

TABLE 10-14 **Antithrombotics** *(Continued)*

Therapeutic Agent (common name, if relevant) [trade name, where appropriate]	Class—Pharmacology and Pharmacokinetics	Indications	Side Effects or Adverse Effects	Contraindications or Precautions to Consider; Notes
Warfarin [Coumadin]	**Anticoagulant—** inhibits potassium epoxide regeneration → **interferes with the synthesis of vitamin K–dependent clotting factors II, VII, IX, and X** and **proteins C and S**	**Chronic anticoagulation for thrombotic disorders, atrial fibrillation**	Bleeding, teratogenic, skin/tissue necrosis, drug–drug interaction	**Contraindicated in pregnancy and patients with liver, CNS, and hemostatic disease; laboratory monitoring with PT/INR**; 99% exists protein bound; metabolized by and extremely sensitive to **cytochrome P450 system**
Bivalirudin, desirudin	**Anticoagulant—direct thrombin inhibitors;** hirudin derivatives	Bivalirudin: anticoagulation in patients undergoing PTCA at risk for HIT; Desirudin: DVT prophylaxis	**Hemorrhage**	IV administration
Argatroban	**Anticoagulant—direct thrombin inhibitor**	Anticoagulation in patients with **HIT**	**Hemorrhage**	IV administration
Dabigatran [Pradaxa]	**Anticoagulant—direct thrombin inhibitor**	Prevention of thromboembolism in patients with **nonvalvular atrial fibrillation**	**Hemorrhage**	**Reduce dose in patients with moderate renal insufficiency, contraindicated in renal failure**; oral administration
tPA (alteplase)	**Thrombolytic—binds to fibrin** in a thrombus → converts entrapped plasminogen to plasmin → fibrinolysis	**Acute myocardial infarction, acute ischemic stroke, and acute pulmonary embolism**	**Hemorrhage;** contraindicated in patients with **active bleeding, history of intracranial bleeding, recent surgery, known bleeding diatheses**, or **severe hypertension**	In cases of acute **ischemic stroke,** should be given **within 3 hours of the onset of symptoms;** treat toxicity with **aminocaproic acid** that inhibits fibrinolysis
Streptokinase [Streptase], **urokinase** [Abbokinase], **anistreplase**	**Thrombolytic— plasminogen-activator converting plasminogen to plasmin →** fibrinolysis	**Lysis of clots**	**Hemorrhage;** contraindicated in patients with **active bleeding, history of intracranial bleeding, recent surgery, known bleeding diatheses,** or **severe hypertension**	**Treat toxicity with aminocaproic acid** that inhibits fibrinolysis

ADP, adenosine diphosphate; ALT, alanine transaminase; AST, aspartate transaminase; CNS, central nervous system; COX, cyclooxygenase; DVT, deep venous thrombosis; HIT, heparin-induced thrombocytopenia; IV, intravenous; PT/INR, prothrombin time/international normalized ratio; PTCA, percutaneous transluminal coronary angioplasty; PTT, partial thromboplastin time; tPA, tissue plasminogen activator.

 COAGULATION DISORDERS *(Table 10-15)*

Abnormalities of the coagulation cascade, endothelial cells, or platelets can lead to inappropriate bleeding or clot formation. These coagulopathies can be manifested as symptomatology involving skin, joints, vasculature, or internal organs.

TABLE 10-15 Coagulation Disorders

Disease	Etiology	Clinical Features	Notes
Disseminated intravascular coagulation (DIC)	Multifactorial; causes include sepsis, trauma, and neoplasms	**Thrombocytopenia, diffuse hemorrhage**, microthrombus formation, schistocytes	Activation of factors V, VIII, and protein C
Von Willebrand disease (vWD)	**Autosomal dominant** disorder	Impaired platelet adhesion, **decreased factor VIII** (vWF binds factor VIII in the blood), **increased bleeding time**	**Most common hereditary bleeding disorder**; similar deficiency diseases include Bernard–Soulier disease and Glanzmann thrombasthenia
Hemophilia A	**X-linked** factor VIII deficiency	Bleeding into muscle, subcutaneous tissues, and joints	**Most common type of hemophilia**; variable penetrance
Hemophilia B (Christmas disease)	**X-linked** factor IX deficiency	Bleeding into muscle, subcutaneous tissues, and joints	Presentation is identical to hemophilia A
Immune thrombocytopenic purpura (ITP)	**Antiplatelet antibodies**	Thrombocytopenia	Follows upper respiratory tract infection in children and is self-limiting; chronic in adults
Thrombotic thrombocytopenic purpura (TTP)	Idiopathic systemic disease	Hyaline occlusions and microangiopathic hemolytic anemia leading to schistocytes; **classic pentad**: anemia, thrombocytopenia, renal failure, neurologic changes, and fever	May cause neurologic abnormalities

vWF, von Willebrand factor.

I. von Willebrand factor deficiency versus hemophilia A (Table 10-16)

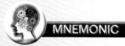

MNEMONIC

To remember the classic pentad of TTP, think **FAT RN**:
Fever
Anemia
Thrombocytopenia
Renal failure
Neurologic changes

TABLE 10-16 von Willebrand Factor (vWF) Deficiency versus Hemophilia A

	vWF Deficiency	Hemophilia A
Factor VIII: coagulant activity	↓	↓
vWF level	↓	Normal
Ristocetin[a] cofactor activity	↓	Normal
Ristocetin[a] aggregation	↓	Normal
Bleeding time	↑	Normal
Inheritance	**Autosomal dominant**	**X linked**

[a]An antibiotic not used for clinical disease; has platelet aggregation properties.

II. Clotting time algorithm (Table 10-17)

TABLE 10-17 Clotting Time Algorithm

	PT Normal	PT Prolonged
PTT normal	Factor XIII deficiency	Factor VII deficiency
PTT prolonged	Factors VIII, IX, and XI deficiencies in patients with bleeding; factor XII, prekallikrein, and HMW-K deficiencies in patients without bleeding	Common pathway deficiency: factors V, X, II, and I; severe hepatic diseases; DIC

DIC, disseminated intravascular coagulation; HMW-K, high-molecular-weight kininogen; PT, prothrombin time; PTT, partial thromboplastin time.

The Hematopoietic and Lymphoreticular System

Clinical Vignette 10-2

CLINICAL PRESENTATION: A 20-year-old woman presents to her primary care physician with the chief complaint of **frequent and prolonged nosebleeds.** Review of systems is positive for **heavy menstrual flow since menarche** and **easy bruising.** Patient **denies bleeding in joints.** Patient also recently had her wisdom teeth extracted and the oral surgeon had told her she had **bled more than expected.** Physical examination reveals **petechiae in dependent areas** and **multiple ecchymoses** on thigh and upper arms.

DIFFERENTIAL: Coagulation disorder (hemophilia A, hemophilia B, and vitamin K deficiency), platelet disorders (von Willebrand disease, aplastic anemia, Fanconi syndrome, immune thrombocytopenic purpura [ITP], thrombotic thrombocytopenic purpura [TTP], and disseminated intravascular coagulation [DIC]), and increased vascular fragility. In approaching abnormal bleeding, group the differentials according to the pathophysiology (Figure 10-11). Note that this constellation of symptoms is more consistent with a platelet disorder because of the **superficial nature of the bleeding.** On the other hand, **bleeding in joints** suggests hemophilia.

LABORATORY STUDIES: CBC should be obtained specifically to measure **platelet counts,** which, if low, define thrombocytopenia. To determine the cause of thrombocytopenia, examination of **peripheral blood smear** and **bone marrow biopsy** might be helpful. A peripheral blood smear may show schistocytes in the case of DIC or TTP (Figure 10-12). **Elevated bleeding time** indicates a *qualitative platelet dysfunction.* **Elevated partial thromboplastin time (PTT)** indicates *defect in contact activation pathway* (factors XII, XI, IX, VIII, X, V, and II). Because hemophilia A and B affect factors VIII and IX, an abnormal PTT is expected in hemophilia. **Elevated prothrombin time (PT)** indicates *defects in the tissue factor pathway* (factors VII, X, V, and II). Production of factors II, VII, IX, and X are vitamin K dependent; because these factors play a role in both contact activation and tissue factor pathways, an elevated PT and PTT is expected in vitamin K deficiency. vWF is a carrier for factor VIII and also contributes to platelet function by binding subendothelium to platelet glycoprotein Ib; thus, abnormalities in bleeding time and PTT are expected. In cases of suspected DIC, **fibrin-split products** (high), **fibrinogen** (low), and **D-dimer** (high) should also be obtained. In this case, the blood studies returned: platelet count = 300 K (normal); bleeding time = 13 seconds (high); PT = 12 seconds (normal); and PTT = 40 seconds (high). Because platelet counts are normal and bleeding time/PTT is elevated, the patient most likely has vWF, which is the most common inherited form of bleeding disorder.

MANAGEMENT: The **underlying cause** should be determined and treated. **Platelet transfusion** depends on cause and severity of thrombocytopenia. Also, **nonsteroidal anti-inflammatory drugs (NSAIDs), anticoagulants, and other antiplatelet agents should be discontinued.**

FIGURE 10-11 Causes of abnormal bleeding

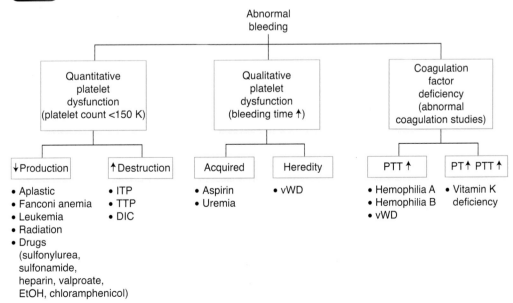

DIC, disseminated intravascular coagulation; EtOH, ethanol; ITP, immune thrombocytopenic purpura; PT, prothrombin time; PTT, partial thromboplastin time; TTP, thrombotic thrombocytopenic purpura; vWD, von Willebrand disease.

FIGURE
10-12 Schistocyte

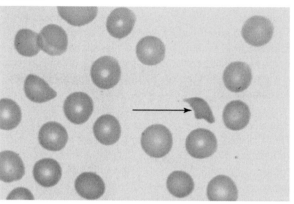

Schistocytes are seen in disseminated intravascular coagulation, thrombotic thrombocytopenic purpura, and hemolytic uremic syndrome. (Reproduced with permission from Anderson SC. *Anderson's Atlas of Hematology.* Philadelphia, PA: Wolters Kluwer Health/Lippincott Williams & Wilkins; 2003.)

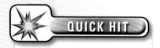

QUICK HIT

Staging of lymphoma (Ann Arbor System): (I) one node or organ affected; (II) two nodes or organs on same side of diaphragm affected; (III) both sides of diaphragm, spleen, or other organ affected; and (IV) disseminated foci.

LYMPHOMA

Tumors of the lymphoid system present as **enlarged, firm, and fixed painless nodes** and are classified as **Hodgkin** and **non-Hodgkin lymphoma** (Table 10-18).

TABLE 10-18 Hodgkin versus non-Hodgkin Lymphoma

Hodgkin Lymphoma	Non-Hodgkin Lymphoma
Number of **Reed–Sternberg cells** (binucleated giant cells) proportional to severity	Malignant neoplasm of lymphocytes (85% B cell, 15% T cell) within lymph nodes (especially periaortic)
Causes **painless cervical lymphadenopathy**, fever, **night sweats**, weight loss, hepatosplenomegaly, and pruritus	Causes painless peripheral lymphadenopathy
Usually affects **young men** (bimodal age distribution)	Usually affects White men younger than 65 years of age
Often curable	Nodular type has better prognosis than diffuse
More reactive lymphocytes signal better prognosis	Small cell type has better prognosis than large cell
Subtypes • Lymphocytic predominance (least common; best prognosis; L/H variant of RS cells; "popcorn" cells) • Mixed cellularity (most frequent, numerous RS cells) • **Nodular sclerosis** (collagen banding, lacunar cells) (most common; women = men; often found in the mediastinum) • Lymphocytic depletion (worst prognosis; rare necrosis and fibrosis of lymphocytic tissue)	**Subtypes** • Small lymphocytic cell (B cell; elderly; indolent course; CLL related) • Follicular cell (cleaved B cells); elderly • Diffuse large B cell (**most common non-Hodgkin lymphoma**; elderly and children; usually B cell; **t[14;18]**; expression of *bcl-2* oncogene) • Lymphoblastic (T cell; children; **mediastinal mass** progressing to ALL) • Burkitt lymphoma (small, noncleaved B cell, Epstein–Barr virus infection; **"starry-sky"** appearance; **t[8;14]**; expression of *c-myc* oncogene) • Cutaneous T cell (mycosis fungoides; Pautrier microabscesses; Sézary syndrome, skin lesions) • Adult T cell (associated with HTLV-1 infection; highly aggressive) • Mantle cell (B cells; poor prognosis) • Marginal cell MALToma (associated with Sjögren syndrome, Hashimoto thyroiditis, and *Helicobacter pylori*) • Intestinal T-cell lymphoma (associated with long-term celiac disease; sometimes called "enteropathy-associated T-cell lymphoma")

ALL, acute lymphocytic leukemia; CLL, chronic lymphocytic leukemia; HTLV-1, human T-lymphotropic virus type 1; MALToma, mucosa-associated lymphatic tissue lymphomas; RS, Reed–Sternberg.

LEUKEMIA *(Table 10-19)*

The symptoms of leukemia include fatigue, dyspnea on exertion, bleeding, pallor, and hepatosplenomegaly.

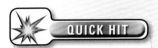

Acute lymphocytic leukemia (ALL) is the most common malignancy in children.

TABLE 10-19 Classification of Leukemia			
Acute Lymphoblastic	**Acute Myeloblastic**	**Chronic Myeloid**	**Chronic Lymphocytic**
Small lympho-blasts, decreased cytoplasm, pre-dominantly affects **children, PAS (+)**, responsive to therapy	Myeloblasts, defect in maturation beyond myeloblast or promy-elocyte stage, **Auer rods**, predominantly affects **adults, PAS (−)**, poor prognosis	t(9;22) results in **Philadelphia chromosome** (BCR-ABL), leukocytosis, **decreased leukocyte alkaline phosphatase**, splenomeg-aly, onset at **35–55** years of age, ends in blast crisis	Usually B cells, "smudge cells" in smear, warm AIHA, hypogam-maglobulinemia, lymphadenopathy, hepatosplenomegaly, more common in **men >60** years of age

AIHA, autoimmune hemolytic anemia; PAS, periodic acid-Schiff stain.

 ## ANEMIA *(Table 10-20)*

Anemia, a decrease in circulating RBC mass, is usually defined as hemoglobin <12 g/dL in female patients and <14 g/dL in male patients.

I. **Microcytic anemia**
  A. Iron deficiency
    1. **Most common anemia**
    2. **Total iron-binding capacity (TIBC) is increased. Serum iron, ferritin, and percent transferrin saturation are decreased. Bone marrow iron stores are low.**
    3. Occurs in menstruating or pregnant women, infants, and preadolescents
    4. Caused by dietary deficiency or bleeding (menorrhagia, GI bleeding, GI cancers, and inflammatory bowel disease)
    5. Pale, easy fatigability, and dyspneic; rarely associated with Plummer–Vinson syndrome (characterized by glossitis, esophageal web, and iron deficiency)
  B. Lead poisoning
    1. It inhibits heme synthesis (D-ala dehydratase and ferrochelatase).
    2. **Basophilic stippling** of RBCs is seen on peripheral smear. Examination of bone marrow may reveal ringed sideroblasts.
    3. Finger, wrist, and foot drop occur from neurotoxicity.
    4. Renal lesions, GI colic, and gingival lead lines occur.
    5. Treatment is chelation with ethylenediaminetetraacetic acid (EDTA), succimer, or dimercaprol.

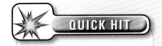

The most common chromo-somal translocations tested on the boards are t(9;22) (Philadelphia chro-mosome), associated with chronic myelogenous leuke-mia (CML) (*BCR-ABL* hybrid) t(8;14), associated with Burkitt lymphoma (activation of *c-myc*) t(14;18), associated with fol-licular lymphoma (activation of *bcl*-2) t(15;17), associated with M3 type of acute myelogenous leukemia (AML) t(11;22), associated with Ewing sarcoma t(11;14), associated with mantle cell lymphoma

TABLE 10-20 Classification of Anemia		
Microcytic (MCV <80)	**Normocytic (MCV 80–100)**	**Macrocytic (MCV >100)**
Iron deficiency	Aplastic anemia	Liver disease
Lead poisoning	Acute blood loss	Vitamin B$_{12}$ deficiency
Sickle cell	Hemolytic anemia	Folate deficiency
Chronic disease	Chronic disease	
Sideroblastic anemia		
Thalassemia		

MCV, mean cell volume.

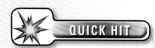

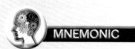

C. Sideroblastic anemia
   1. Iron stain of bone marrow reveals ringed sideroblasts.
   2. TIBC is reduced and serum iron is increased.
   3. RBC count is reduced.
D. Sickle cell disease (hemoglobin S [HbS])
   1. It is primarily seen in **Blacks**.
   2. The homozygous form is most severe. Heterozygotes are generally asymptomatic.
   3. Severe hemolytic anemia is seen.
   4. Deoxygenated HbS polymerizes within RBCs, causing the characteristic sickle shape. Sickling leads to painful crises, organ infarction (**autosplenectomy**), and strokes.
   5. Aplastic crises may occur, usually provoked by viral infection (usually parvovirus B19).
   6. Patients are especially susceptible to infection by **encapsulated bacteria** (*S. pneumoniae* and *H. influenzae*) and osteomyelitis caused by *Salmonella*.
   7. Sickle cells and Howell–Jolly bodies (due to asplenia) are seen in peripheral blood smear.
   8. Treatment is with **hydroxyurea** to increase HbF.
E. Thalassemia
   1. This is a group of genetic disorders, all in some way deficient in α- or β-globin chain synthesis.
   2. **β-Thalassemia is more common** (especially in people of Mediterranean origin)
      a. The homozygous form, called thalassemia major (also known as Mediterranean or Cooley anemia), causes splenomegaly, bone distortions, hemosiderosis, and increased HbF, and it is fatal in childhood.
      b. The heterozygous form of β-thalassemia (thalassemia minor) causes a minor anemia but has no effect on the life span.
   3. α-Thalassemia is caused by a deletion in one or more of the four α-globin genes; loss of all four genes is incompatible with life. It is seen primarily in patients of Asian or African descent.

II. Normocytic anemias

A. Anemia of chronic disease
   1. Anemia is seen in chronic disease states such as cancer and autoimmune disease due to impaired iron usage.
   2. It is the second most common anemia.
   3. Usually normocytic but can be microcytic in longstanding cases
   4. **TIBC is reduced. Ferritin is increased.** Percent transferrin saturation is generally normal.
   5. Low serum iron but high iron stores in the bone marrow are observed.
B. Aplastic anemia
   1. Dysfunctional or deficient multipotent myeloid stem cells lead to pancytopenia.
   2. It is caused by viruses, chemicals, radiation, or renal failure (via decreased erythropoietin), or may be idiopathic.
   3. Drugs causing aplastic anemia include **nonsteroidal anti-inflammatory drugs (NSAIDs)**, **benzene**, and **chloramphenicol**.
   4. Symptoms include fatigue, pallor, mucosal bleeding, and petechiae as a result of thrombocytopenia.
   5. Neutropenia occurs, leading to frequent infections.
   6. Marrow is hypocellular, with **fat infiltration**.
C. Anemia caused by acute blood loss
   1. Leads to a **transient normocytic anemia** (however, chronic bleeding can lead to iron deficiency and hence microcytic anemia)
   2. May appear macrocytic because of increased reticulocyte release from bone marrow 7 to 10 days later
D. Hemolytic anemias
   1. Increased RBC destruction leads to an increase in unconjugated bilirubin, hemoglobinemia, hemoglobinuria, and hemosiderosis and decreased serum haptoglobin.

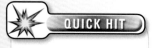

The Hematopoietic and Lymphoreticular System

2. Increase in reticulocytes occurs because of additional erythropoiesis.
3. Extracorpuscular (acquired) hemolytic anemias
   a. Warm autoimmune hemolytic immunoglobulin (AIHI) (IgG): associated with lymphoma, spherocytosis, and **positive direct Coombs test**
   b. Cold AIHI (IgM): associated with lymphoid neoplasm, mycoplasma infection, anti-I antibodies, ABO incompatibility, and **Raynaud phenomenon**. It causes hemolysis at low temperatures.
   c. Erythroblastosis fetalis (hemolytic diseases of the newborn): usually caused by Rh blood group incompatibility; can result in kernicterus and death
   d. Infections such as bartonellosis, *Clostridium*, and malaria
4. Intracorpuscular (genetic) hemolytic anemias
   a. Hereditary ovalocytosis (elliptocytosis): **autosomal dominant**
   b. Hereditary spherocytosis: **autosomal dominant**; **spectrin** deficiency
   c. PNH: deficiency of DAF and MIRL and decreased leukocyte alkaline phosphatase (LAP)
   d. Glucose-6-phosphate dehydrogenase (G6PD) deficiency: **X linked**; more common in Mediterranean and Blacks; precipitated by oxidative stress (primaquine therapy); **Heinz bodies** are seen.
   e. Pyruvate kinase deficiency: **autosomal recessive**; chronic

III. Macrocytic anemias

A. Liver disease—usually cirrhosis
   1. Excess lipid is added to RBC membrane in diseased liver.
   2. Hypersplenism occurs.
   3. Spur cells are present.
B. Vitamin B_{12} (cobalamin) deficiency
   1. **Megaloblastic anemia** characterized by **hypersegmented neutrophils** (Figure 10-13), macrocytosis, and pancytopenia
   2. Decreased DNA synthesis
   3. Most common form is **pernicious anemia**.
      a. Caused by a deficiency of intrinsic factor secondary to the destruction of parietal cells
      b. Associated with increased incidence of gastric carcinoma and achlorhydria
   4. Other etiologies for vitamin B_{12} deficiency anemia include strict vegetarian diet, distal ileum pathology, bacterial overgrowth, *Diphyllobothrium latum* infection, and type A gastritis
   5. **Neurologic symptoms** caused by demyelination of posterior and lateral columns, ataxia, and paresthesia in distal extremities

FIGURE
10-13 Hypersegmented neutrophil

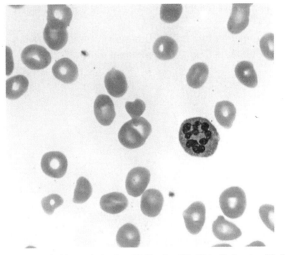

(Reproduced with permission from McClatchey KD. *Clinical Laboratory Medicine*. 2nd ed. Philadelphia, PA: Lippincott Williams & Wilkins; 2002.)

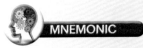

MNEMONIC

Remember the immunoglobulins associated with each type of autoimmune hemolytic anemia: Ig**G** with **warm (Georgia is warm)** and Ig**M** with **cold (Minnesota is cold)**.

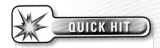

QUICK HIT

ABO transfusion reactions are almost always a result of clerical (human) error.

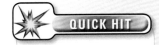

QUICK HIT

Hemolytic disease of the newborn can be prevented with **RhoGAM** (anti-D antibody), which neutralizes the mother's immunogenic response to fetal RBCs that carry the D antigen.

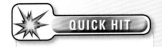

QUICK HIT

Spherocytes are characterized by osmotic fragility in hypotonic solution.

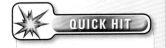

QUICK HIT

The Schilling test is used to diagnose the etiology of pernicious anemia.

The Hematopoietic and Lymphoreticular System

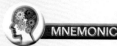

C. Folate deficiency
1. It causes megaloblastic anemia; hematologic findings are identical to vitamin B$_{12}$ deficiency.
2. **No neurologic** deficits are present.
3. Folate deficiency can mask vitamin B$_{12}$ deficiency.
4. Etiologies include dietary deficiency, tropical sprue, *Giardia lamblia* infection, oral contraceptives, **antineoplastics** (methotrexate), and pregnancy.

Clinical Vignette 10-3

CLINICAL PRESENTATION: A 28-year-old woman visits her primary care physician for her yearly physical examination. During her review of systems, she tells her physician that she has been feeling **fatigued.** She denies weight loss, diarrhea, and menorrhagia. Physical examination shows **pallor.** Blood studies show: **Hct = 32%, Hg = 11.1 g/dL,** and platelet = 300 K.

DIFFERENTIALS AND LABORATORY STUDIES: This patient is anemic. Figure 10-14 summarizes the approach to anemia. Two laboratory studies critical in working up anemia are (a) **RBC indices** and (b) **peripheral blood smear.** Tables 10-21 and 10-22 summarize the findings expected in each of these studies.

The first step in approaching blood studies for a patient with anemia is the **reticulocyte count,** which is used to determine whether the cause of the anemia is from increased destruction of RBCs (high reticulocyte count from compensatory increase in RBC production) or decreased production of RBCs (normal or low reticulocyte count). A high reticulocyte count suggests hemolysis, and the differentials would include causes intrinsic to the RBC such as hereditary spherocytosis, glucose-6-phosphate dehydrogenase (G6PD) deficiency, PNH, and sickle cell anemia. Extrinsic causes of hemolysis include thrombotic thrombocytopenic purpura (TTP), hemolytic uremic syndrome (HUS), artificial heart valve, disseminated intravascular coagulation, warm autoimmune hemolytic anemia (WAIHA), cold autoimmune hemolytic anemia (CAIHA), altered plasma components (high lipids), drugs, and infectious agents; Table 10-23 shows how these hemolytic disorders can be differentiated.

If the reticulocyte count is normal, the next step is to look at the **mean cell volume (MCV)** that categorizes the anemia as hypochromic microcytic (MCV <80), normochromic (MCV 80 to 100), and hyperchromic macrocytic (MCV >100). If MCV values suggest microcytic anemia, the differentials are iron (Fe) deficiency, anemia of chronic disease, thalassemia, sideroblastic anemia, and lead poisoning. These can be differentiated based on **serum Fe, serum ferritin,** and **TIBC** (Table 10-24). Also, **lead levels** will be high in lead poisoning. Note that hemolytic anemias can also produce an MCV <80. If macrocytic anemia is observed, the differentials include vitamin B$_{12}$ deficiency, folate deficiency, and liver disease. To differentiate, **check vitamin B$_{12}$** and **folate levels** and **liver function tests.** If normocytic anemia is observed, the causes could be primary involvement of bone marrow, such as aplastic anemia, or secondary to other underlying disease. **Bone marrow examination** can also be done but is not needed in all patients with anemia.

MANAGEMENT: In acute cases, **transfusion** may be necessary. Otherwise, treat underlying cause of anemia. For iron, vitamin B$_{12}$, or folate deficiency, **supplement diet** with appropriate nutrient.

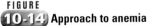

FIGURE 10-14 Approach to anemia

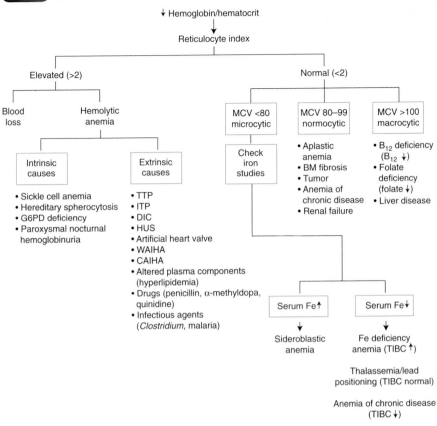

BM, bone marrow; CAIHA, cold autoimmune hemolytic anemia; DIC, disseminated intravascular coagulation; Fe, iron; G6PD, glucose-6-phosphate dehydrogenase; HUS, hemolytic uremic syndrome; ITP, immune thrombocytopenic purpura; MCV, mean cell volume; TIBC, total iron-binding capacity; TTP, thrombotic thrombocytopenic purpura; WAIHA, warm autoimmune hemolytic anemia.

TABLE 10-21 Approach to Laboratory Blood Studies

Blood Lab Study	Definition	Notes
Hemoglobin (Hgb)	Concentration of Hgb in 100 mL of blood	**Increased**: severe dehydration, erythrocytosis, polycythemia, severe burn, shock, COPD, CHF, high altitudes, drugs (gentamicin, methyldopa) **Decreased**: hyperthyroidism, leukemia, liver disease, hemolytic reaction, over-hydration, pregnancy, drugs (acetaminophen, antineoplastic agents, chloramphenicol, hydralazine, MAOI, nitrites, penicillin, tetracycline, sulfonamide)
Hematocrit	Percentage of RBCs in a volume of whole blood; not reliable indicator of anemia immediately after blood loss or blood transfusion	**Increased**: severe dehydration, erythrocytosis, polycythemia, severe burns, shock, high altitudes **Decreased** (defined as anemia): hyperthyroidism, leukemia, liver disease, hemolytic reactions, pregnancy, and causes of macrocytic, normocytic, and microcytic anemia (see below)
MCV	Represents volume of single RBC; indicator of cell size	**Increased** (>100) (defined as macrocytic anemia): vitamin B_{12} deficiency, folate deficiency, liver disease, alcoholism **Decreased** (<80) (defined as microcytic anemia): iron deficiency, thalassemia, lead poisoning, sideroblastic anemia; some hemolytic anemias, possibly anemia of chronic disease
MCHC	Represents average concentration of Hgb in RBC	**Increased**: spherocytosis
MCH	Represents average weight of Hgb in RBCs; confirms accuracy of MCV value	**Increased**: macrocytic anemia (see above) **Decreased**: microcytic anemia (see above)
Reticulocyte count	Reticulocyte is nonnucleated immature RBC formed in bone marrow; increased values indicate accelerated erythropoiesis	**Increased**: hemolytic anemias, sickle cell disease, pregnancy, splenectomy, hemorrhage **Decreased**: aplastic anemia, chronic infection, radiation therapy

CHF, congestive heart failure; COPD, chronic obstructive pulmonary disease; MAOI, monoamine oxidase inhibitor; MCH, mean corpuscular hemoglobin; MCHC, mean corpuscular hemoglobin concentration; MCV, mean cell volume; RBC, red blood cell.

The Hematopoietic and Lymphoreticular System

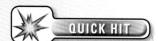

TABLE 10-22 Peripheral Blood Smear Findings

Peripheral Blood Smear	Conditions Associated
Hypersegmented neutrophils (Figure 10-13)	Folate/B_{12} deficiency
Basophilic stippling of RBCs	Lead poisoning
Echinocytes (Burr cells)	Uremia
Spherocytes	Spherocytosis
Microspherocytes	Coombs hemolysis
Schistocytes (fragmented cells, helmet cells) (Figure 10-12)	Disseminated intravascular coagulation, TTP, HUS
Poikilocytes (irregularly shaped cells)	Thalassemia
Target cells	Liver disease, thalassemia
Acanthocytes (spur cells)	Liver disease, abetalipoproteinemia
Sickle cells	Sickle cell anemia
Howell–Jolly bodies	Asplenia
Heinz bodies	Glucose-6-phosphate dehydrogenase deficiency
Teardrop cells	Myeloid metaplasia with myelofibrosis

HUS, hemolytic uremic syndrome; RBC, red blood cell; TTP, thrombotic thrombocytopenic purpura.

TABLE 10-23 Differential for Platelet Destruction

Lab Study	DIC	HUS	TTP	ITP
Blood smear	Schistocytes	Schistocytes	Schistocytes	Normal
PT/PTT	Markedly increased	Normal or mildly increased	Normal or mildly increased	Normal
Fibrin-split products	Increased	Normal	Normal	Normal
Fibrinogen	Decreased	Normal	Normal	Normal
Notes	Platelets trapped in fibrin mesh deposited in blood vessels	*E. coli* often implicated in pathogenesis; usually occurs in **children**	Idiopathic	Autoimmune: autoantibody-mediated platelet destruction; follows URI in children
	Risk factors: sepsis, trauma, obstetric complications, malignancy, transfusions	Symptoms: anemia, thrombocytopenia, acute renal failure, **bloody diarrhea, abdominal pain, seizures**	**Classic pentad**: anemia, thrombocytopenia, renal failure, **neurologic changes, fever**	

DIC, disseminated intravascular coagulation; HUS, hemolytic uremic syndrome; ITP, immune thrombocytopenic purpura; PT/PTT, prothrombin time/partial thromboplastin time; TTP, thrombotic thrombocytopenic purpura; URI, upper respiratory infection.

TABLE 10-24 **Differential for Microcytic Anemia**

Lab Study	Iron Deficiency Anemia	Beta Thalassemia	Anemia of Chronic Disease	Sideroblastic Anemia
Serum iron	Low	Normal/high	Low	**High**
Serum ferritin	Low	Normal	Normal/high	High
TIBC	High	Normal	Low	Normal/low
% Transferrin saturation	Low (<12%)	Normal/high	Normal (>18%)	High

TIBC, total iron-binding capacity.

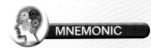

MNEMONIC

To remember the findings of TIBC in iron deficiency and chronic disease, use **TIBC**: **T**op = **I**ron, **B**ottom = **C**hronic disease. TIBC levels are high (**top**) in iron deficiency anemia and low (**bottom**) in chronic disease.

MYELOPROLIFERATIVE DISORDERS

The myeloproliferative disorders include four diseases, all of which have features of hepatosplenomegaly, increased risk of converting into a blastic leukemia, or a spent phase of marrow fibrosis: (1) polycythemia vera, (2) myelofibrosis, (3) essential thrombocythemia, and (4) chronic myelogenous leukemia (CML).

I. Polycythemia vera
A. Chronic increase in the number of red cells caused by bone marrow hyperplasia of unknown etiology
B. Clinical manifestations
   1. Presents in middle age
   2. Symptoms include vision disturbances, erythromelalgia (burning pains in the hands/feet, associated with erythema, pallor, or cyanosis), pruritus, facial plethora, hepatosplenomegaly, and thrombosis.
C. Differential diagnosis
   1. Absolute polycythemia vera
      a. Primary polycythemia—**appropriately low erythropoietin levels**
      b. **Secondary polycythemia**—elevated erythropoietin levels
         • Appropriate: response to hypoxia
         • Inappropriate: secondary to inappropriate secretion of erythropoietin (renal cell carcinoma, pheochromocytoma, hepatocellular carcinoma, hemangioblastoma)
   2. Relative polycythemia vera (e.g., dehydration) often caused by a decrease in extracorpuscular volume, thus causing a relative increase in the hematocrit level
D. Diagnosis
   1. Major diagnostic criteria
      a. Increased RBC mass (hematocrit)
      b. Normal arterial oxygen saturation (≥92%)
      c. Splenomegaly
   2. Minor diagnostic criteria
      a. Thrombocytosis
      b. Leukocytosis
      c. Elevated LAP
      d. Elevated serum vitamin B_{12}
   3. Diagnosis requires either all three major criteria *or* increased RBC mass plus normal arterial oxygen saturation plus at least two minor criteria including leukocytosis and thrombocytosis.

II. Myelofibrosis
A. Generalized fibrosis of bone marrow characterized by pancytopenia in the face of increased megakaryocytes in the marrow

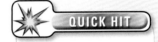

QUICK HIT

Myelodysplastic syndromes also exist: refractory anemia, refractory anemia with ringed sideroblasts, refractory anemia with excess blasts, refractory anemia with excess blasts in transformation, and chronic myelomonocytic leukemia.

The Hematopoietic and Lymphoreticular System

B. Clinical manifestations
1. Presents in patients in their late 50s
2. **Teardrop deformity** of RBCs occurring along with splenomegaly and extra-medullary hematopoiesis
3. "Dry tap" seen on bone biopsy
C. Differential diagnosis
1. Primary myelofibrosis
   a. Marrow fibrosis
   b. Extramedullary hematopoiesis
2. Secondary myelofibrosis
   a. Infections: tuberculosis, osteomyelitis
   b. Metastatic carcinoma
   c. Paget disease

III. Essential thrombocythemia
A. A primary disorder of unknown etiology resulting in increased platelets
B. Clinical manifestations
1. Thrombocytosis
2. Megakaryocytic hyperplasia
3. Splenomegaly
4. Hemorrhage and thrombosis
5. Increased bone marrow reticulin and absence of *BCR-ABL* gene

IV. Chronic myelogenous leukemia
A. The t(9,22) translocation of the *ABL* proto-oncogene to *BCR*, creating a *BCR-ABL* fusion gene (Philadelphia chromosome)
B. Clinical manifestations
1. Hepatosplenomegaly and lymphadenopathy
2. Normocytic to macrocytic anemia
3. Platelet derangement (either a thrombocytosis during active phase or thrombocytopenia in spent phase can occur)
4. Bone marrow hypercellular
5. Blast crisis in late stages

 CHEMOTHERAPEUTICS (*Table 10-25*)

The chemotherapeutics can be classified based on where they act in the cell cycle (mitotic phase, DNA synthesis phase, etc.) and **chemical structure** (e.g., alkylating agent, etoposide, and nitrosoureas).

TABLE 10-25 Chemotherapeutics

Therapeutic Agent (common name, if relevant) [trade name, where appropriate]	Class—Pharmacology and Pharmacokinetics	Indications	Side Effects or Adverse Effects	Contraindications or Precautions to Consider; Notes
Methotrexate [Rheumatrex]	S phase specific antimetabolite—folic acid analog (dihydrofolate reductase inhibitor) → decreases dTMP → decreases DNA and protein synthesis; **immunosuppressant**	**Acute lymphocytic and myelogenous leukemia, lymphoma**, choriocarcinoma, sarcoma, bone marrow transplant, **abortion, ectopic pregnancy, rheumatoid arthritis, psoriasis**	Oral and GI ulceration, **myelosuppression**, thrombocytopenia, leukopenia, hepatotoxicity, **fibrotic lung disease**, mucositis	**Leucovorin is given as an adjuvant after treatment (reverses myelosuppression)**

(continued)

TABLE 10-25 **Chemotherapeutics** *(Continued)*

Therapeutic Agent (common name, if relevant) [trade name, where appropriate]	Class—Pharmacology and Pharmacokinetics	Indications	Side Effects or Adverse Effects	Contraindications or Precautions to Consider; Notes
5-Fluorouracil	**S phase specific antimetabolite—pyrimidine analog** → bioactivated to 5F-dUMP → binds folic acid → complex inhibits thymidylate synthase → decreases dTMP and DNA synthesis	**Colon cancer, solid tumors, basal cell carcinoma, and actinic keratosis (topical)**	**Myelosuppression, photosensitivity**	Acts **synergistically with methotrexate**; myelosuppression is not reversible with leucovorin but with **thymidine**
6-Mercaptopurine [Purinethol]	**S phase specific antimetabolite—purine analog** → inhibits purine synthesis → disrupts DNA and RNA synthesis	**Acute lymphoblastic leukemia**, Crohn disease, ulcerative colitis	**Myelosuppression, liver toxicity** (intrahepatic cholestasis and focal centrilobular necrosis)	Metabolized by **xanthine oxidase**, therefore increased toxicity with **allopurinol**
Cytarabine	**S phase specific antimetabolite—pyrimidine analog**; inhibits DNA polymerase	**AML**	Leukopenia, thrombocytopenia, megaloblastic anemia	
Cyclophosphamide [Cytoxan]	**Cell cycle nonspecific agent—alkylating agent** → cross-links DNA strands → decreases DNA synthesis and prevents cell division → destroys proliferating lymphoid cells; alkylates the resting cells; potent immunosuppressant	**Transplant rejection, rheumatic arthritis, non-Hodgkin lymphoma, breast and ovarian carcinoma**	**GI and bone marrow toxicity, hemorrhagic cystitis** (can be partially prevented by mesna)	Requires bioactivation by liver
Ifosfamide	**Cell cycle nonspecific agent—alkylating agent** → cross-links DNA strands → decreases protein and DNA synthesis → prevents cell division	**Testicular cancer**	**GI and bone marrow toxicity, hemorrhagic cystitis** (can be partially prevented by mesna)	Requires bioactivation by liver
Carmustine, lomustine, semustine, streptozocin	**Cell cycle nonspecific agent (nitrosoureas)—alkylating agent** → cross-links DNA and RNA strands	**Brain tumors** (including glioblastoma multiforme)	**CNS toxicity** (dizziness, ataxia)	**Crosses blood–brain barrier to CNS;** requires bioactivation
Cisplatin, carboplatin, oxaliplatin	**Cell cycle nonspecific agent—alkylating agent** → cross-links DNA and RNA strands	**Bladder, testicular, ovarian, and lung carcinomas**	**Nephrotoxicity, acoustic nerve damage**	
Busulfan	**Cell cycle nonspecific agent—alkylating agent** → cross-links DNA and RNA strands	**Chronic myelogenous leukemia**	**Pulmonary fibrosis, hyperpigmentation**	
Doxorubicin [Adriamycin]	**Cell cycle nonspecific agent—generates free radicals; also intercalates into DNA** → breaks DNA; affects plasma membrane	**Hodgkin lymphoma; myeloma**; sarcoma; solid tumors of breast, ovary, and lung	Cardiac changes resulting in cumulative **cardiotoxicity**, myelosuppression, alopecia, and toxic extravasation	Part of the ABVD combination regimen for Hodgkin lymphoma

(continued)

TABLE 10-25 **Chemotherapeutics** (Continued)

Therapeutic Agent (common name, if relevant) [trade name, where appropriate]	Class—Pharmacology and Pharmacokinetics	Indications	Side Effects or Adverse Effects	Contraindications or Precautions to Consider; Notes
Daunorubicin [DaunoXome, Cerubidine]	**Cell cycle nonspecific agent—oxidizes free radicals; also intercalates into DNA** → breaks DNA; affects plasma membrane	**Hodgkin lymphoma; myeloma**; sarcoma; solid tumors of breast, ovary, and lung	Cardiac changes resulting in cumulative **cardiotoxicity**, myelosuppression, alopecia, and toxic extravasation	Part of the ABVD combination regimen for Hodgkin lymphoma
Dactinomycin [Cosmegen]	**Cell cycle nonspecific agent—intercalates into DNA**	**Wilms tumor, Ewing sarcoma, rhabdomyosarcoma**	**Skin eruptions, hyperkeratosis, myelosuppression**	
Bleomycin [Blenoxane]	**G2 phase–specific agent—generates free radicals** that bind, intercalate, and cut DNA	**Testicular cancer, Hodgkin disease**	**Pulmonary fibrosis**, fever, **blistering, stomatitis**, hypersensitivity reactions (anaphylaxis)	**Minimal myelosuppression**; part of the ABVD regimen for Hodgkin lymphoma
Hydroxyurea [Hydrea]	**S phase–specific agent—binds ribonucleotide reductase** → inhibits formation of DNA	**Melanoma, CML, sickle cell disease**	**Nausea, vomiting, bone marrow suppression**	
Etoposide	**G2 phase specific— inhibits topoisomerase II → increases DNA degradation**	**Small cell lung cancer**, prostate and testicular carcinoma	**Myelosuppression**, nausea, vomiting, **alopecia**	
Prednisone	**Glucocorticoid— inhibits protein synthesis**; reduces lymph node and spleen size; **inhibits cell cycle activity of lymphoid cells; lyses T cells; suppresses antibody, prostaglandin, and leukotriene synthesis; blocks monocyte production of IL-1**	**CLL, Hodgkin lymphoma**, rheumatic arthritis; **autoimmune disorders; allergic reaction; asthma; organ transplantation (esp. during rejection crisis)**	**Osteoporosis, Cushingoid reaction, psychosis, hyperglycemia, immunosuppression, infection, hypertension, cataracts, acne, peptic ulcers**	Part of the MOPP regimen for Hodgkin lymphoma
Tamoxifen [Nolvadex]	**Selective estrogen receptor modulator— competitively binds estrogen receptors; breast (estrogen antagonist)**: prevents proliferation of estrogen receptor positive tumor cells; **endometrium (partial agonist)**; bone (agonist): decreases bone turnover and increases bone density	**Treats estrogen-dependent breast cancer in postmenopausal women**; reduces contralateral breast cancer; osteoporosis prevention	**May increase the risk of endometrial cancer; hot flashes;** flushing	

(continued)

TABLE **10-25** **Chemotherapeutics** *(Continued)*

Therapeutic Agent (common name, if relevant) [trade name, where appropriate]	Class—Pharmacology and Pharmacokinetics	Indications	Side Effects or Adverse Effects	Contraindications or Precautions to Consider; Notes
Raloxifene [Evista]	**Selective estrogen receptor modulator— breast (estrogen antagonist); endometrium (estrogen antagonist)**: prevents proliferation of endometrium; **bone (estrogen agonist)**: decreases bone turnover and increases bone density; **cardiovascular (estrogen agonist)**: decreases LDL	**Osteoporosis, breast cancer**	**Hot flashes**, sinusitis, weight gain, muscle pain, leg cramps, **increased risk of blood clots**	Unlike estrogen, raloxifene **does not decrease HDL**
Trastuzumab [Herceptin]	**Monoclonal antibody against HER2**; binds to tumor cells overexpressing HER2 → mediates antibody-dependent cytotoxicity → destruction of tumor cells	**Metastatic breast cancer**	**Cardiotoxicity**	
Imatinib [Gleevec]	**Tyrosine kinase inhibitor—inhibits BCR-ABL tyrosine kinase** (abnormal product of **Philadelphia chromosome** in CML) blocks proliferation → induces apoptosis in BCR-ABL positive cell lines and fresh leukemic cells	**CML**, GI stromal tumors	**Fluid retention**	
Vincristine [Oncovin]	**M phase specific (vinca alkaloid)— blocks polymerization of microtubules** → mitotic spindle cannot form	**Hodgkin lymphoma, Wilms tumor, choriocarcinoma, acute leukemia**	**Peripheral neuritis, areflexia**, paralytic ileus	Part of the MOPP regimen for Hodgkin lymphoma
Vinblastine [Velban]	**M phase specific (vinca alkaloid)— blocks polymerization of microtubules** → mitotic spindle cannot form	**Hodgkin lymphoma, Wilms tumor, choriocarcinoma**	**Myelosuppression**	
Paclitaxel [Taxol]	**M phase specific (Taxol)—stabilizes polymerization of microtubules** → mitotic spindle cannot break down → anaphase cannot occur	**Ovarian and breast cancer**	**Myelosuppression, hypersensitivity**	

ABVD, Adriamycin, bleomycin, vinblastine, and dacarbazine; AML, acute myelogenous leukemia; CLL, chronic lymphoblastic leukemia; CML, chronic myelogenous leukemia; CNS, central nervous system; dTMP, deoxythymidine monophosphate; dUMP, deoxyuridine monophosphate; G2 phase, synthesis of components needed for mitosis; GI, gastrointestinal; HDL, high-density lipoprotein; HER2, human epidermal growth factor receptor 2 protein; IL, interleukin; LDL, low-density lipoprotein; MOPP, Mustargen, Oncovin, procarbazine, prednisone; M phase, mitotic phase; S phase, DNA synthesis phase.

The Hematopoietic and Lymphoreticular System

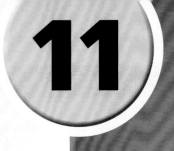

Biochemistry and Genetics

GENETICS

Nucleic Acids

A. **Purine Synthesis**

1. <u>Overall reaction</u>: Ribose-5-phosphate → adenosine monophosphate (AMP) or guanosine monophosphate (GMP). This requires the amino acids glycine, aspartate, and glutamine. It also requires tetrahydrofolate.

2. <u>Rate-limiting step</u>: phosphoribosyl pyrophosphate (PRPP) → β-5-phosphoribosylamine (β-5PRA) by **glutamine PRPP amidotransferase**. This step requires glutamine.

3. Initially, ribose-5-phosphate is converted to PRPP, which is then converted to β-5-PRA.

4. After several more steps, β-5-PRA is converted to inosine monophosphate (IMP).

5. IMP can then be converted to either GMP or AMP.
   a. The conversion of IMP to GMP is catalyzed by inosine monophosphate dehydrogenase.
   b. This enzyme is inhibited by the drug mycophenolate.

B. **Purine Catabolism** (*Figure 11-1*)

1. <u>Overall reaction</u>: AMP, IMP, GMP → uric acid.

2. GMP is converted to guanosine, which is then converted to guanine, followed by xanthine.

3. IMP is converted to inosine, which is then converted to hypoxanthine, followed by xanthine.

4. AMP is converted to adenosine. Adenosine is then converted to inosine by adenosine deaminase. Inosine is then converted to hypoxanthine, followed by xanthine.

5. Xanthine is converted to uric acid by xanthine oxidase. This enzyme is inhibited by the drug allopurinol.

C. **Purine Salvage**

1. <u>Overall reaction</u>: Adenine → AMP requires adenosine phosphoribosyl transferase (APRT). Hypoxanthine → IMP and guanine → GMP require hypoxanthine guanine phosphoribosyl transferase (HGPRT).

2. **Lesch-Nyhan syndrome**: X-linked recessive deficiency of HGPRT. The lack of purine salvage causes accumulation of uric acid. This causes mental retardation, self-mutilation, choreoathetosis, and gout. It is treated with allopurinol.

D. **Pyrimidine Synthesis**

1. <u>Overall reaction</u>: Glutamine + bicarbonate → uridine diphosphate (UDP), then UDP → uridine triphosphate (UTP) → cytosine triphosphate (CTP) (which requires glutamine) or UDP → deoxyuridine monophosphate (dUMP) → thymidine monophosphate (TMP) (which requires tetrahydrofolate). Both require aspartate, and bicarbonate.

2. <u>Rate-limiting step</u>: Glutamine + bicarbonate → carbamoyl phosphate by carbamoyl phosphate synthase II.

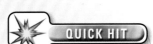

Tetrahydrofolate is regenerated by **dihydrofolate reductase**, which is inhibited by methotrexate in eukaryotes and by trimethoprim in prokaryotes.

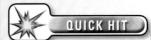

Adenosine deaminase deficiency is the most common cause of **severe combined immunodeficiency** (SCID).

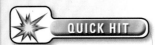

Allopurinol increases the toxicity of **azathioprine** and **6-mercaptopurine,** since both are metabolized by xanthine oxidase.

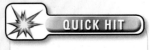

Carbamoyl phosphate synthase I is an enzyme in the urea cycle.

FIGURE 11-1 Purine catabolism

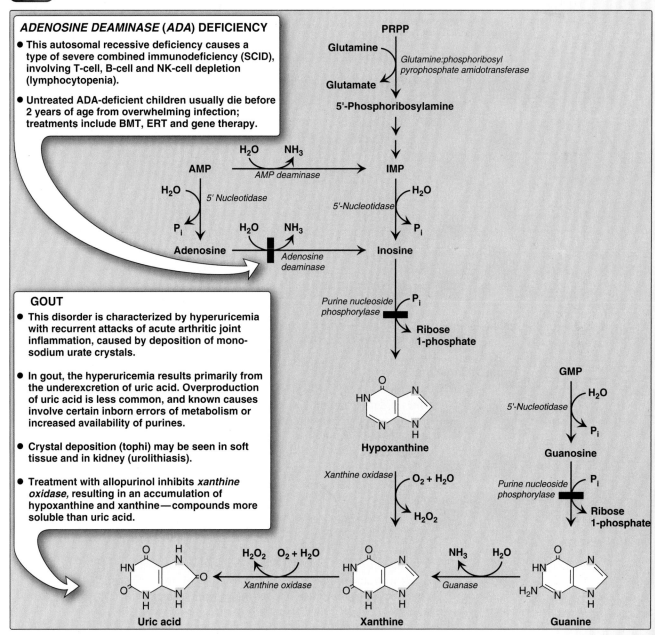

ADENOSINE DEAMINASE (ADA) DEFICIENCY
- This autosomal recessive deficiency causes a type of severe combined immunodeficiency (SCID), involving T-cell, B-cell and NK-cell depletion (lymphocytopenia).
- Untreated ADA-deficient children usually die before 2 years of age from overwhelming infection; treatments include BMT, ERT and gene therapy.

GOUT
- This disorder is characterized by hyperuricemia with recurrent attacks of acute arthritic joint inflammation, caused by deposition of mono-sodium urate crystals.
- In gout, the hyperuricemia results primarily from the underexcretion of uric acid. Overproduction of uric acid is less common, and known causes involve certain inborn errors of metabolism or increased availability of purines.
- Crystal deposition (tophi) may be seen in soft tissue and in kidney (urolithiasis).
- Treatment with allopurinol inhibits *xanthine oxidase*, resulting in an accumulation of hypoxanthine and xanthine—compounds more soluble than uric acid.

The degradation of purine nucleotides to uric acid, illustrating some of the genetic diseases associated with this pathway. (Adapted with permission from Harvey RA, Ferrier DR. *Lippincott's Illustrated Reviews: Biochemistry.* 5th ed. Baltimore, MD: Lippincott Williams & Wilkins; 2011.)

3. Carbamoyl phosphate is converted to orotic acid.
4. Orotic acid is converted to UMP in a reaction that requires PRPP.
5. UMP is phosphorylated to UDP, which is then converted to CTP. Alternatively, UDP is converted to deoxyuridine diphosphate (dUDP), then dUMP, and finally deoxythymidine monophosphate (dTMP).
   a. The conversion of UDP to dUDP is catalyzed by ribonucleotide reductase.
   b. Ribonucleotide reductase is inhibited by **hydroxyurea**.
6. **Orotic aciduria:** Deficiency of UMP, due to an autosomal recessive defect in UMP synthase. This results in elevated orotic acid in the urine, and megaloblastic anemia that is nonresponsive to B_{12} or folate supplementation. Uridine supplementation is indicated instead.

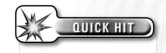

QUICK HIT

Orotic acid in urine is also seen in ornithine trans-carboxylase deficiency, where it is accompanied by hyperammonemia.

FIGURE
11-2 Nucleosomes

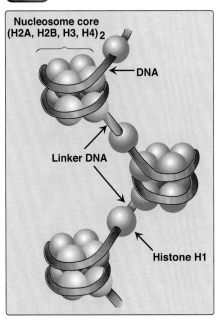

Nucleosome core
(H2A, H2B, H3, H4)₂

DNA

Linker DNA

Histone H1

Organization of human DNA, illustrating the structure of nucleosomes. (Adapted with permission from Harvey RA, Ferrier DR. *Lippincott's Illustrated Reviews: Biochemistry.* 5th ed. Baltimore, MD: Lippincott Williams & Wilkins; 2011.)

DNA Structure

A. DNA Strand
1. Purines: Adenine, guanine
2. Pyrimidines: Thymine, cytosine, uracil
3. Adenine binds thymine (or uracil) through two hydrogen bonds.
4. Cytosine binds guanine through three hydrogen bonds.
5. Adjacent nucleotide pairings are linked by a phosphodiester backbone, which is what gives DNA its negative charge.

B. Chromosomes
1. DNA wraps twice around a core of histone proteins to form **nucleosomes** (*Figure 11-2*). Negatively charged DNA binds easily to the positively charged lysine and arginine residues in histone proteins.
2. The histone core is composed of four proteins: two each of H2A, H2B, H3, and H4.
   a. Prior to transcription, histones are acetylated, relaxing the DNA coiling.
   b. After transcription, histones are methylated, causing the DNA to coil more tightly.
3. H1 is the only histone protein that is not found in the histone core. It holds the DNA in place around the core, and also interacts with linker DNA.
4. This combination of DNA and proteins is known as **chromatin**.
   a. **Heterochromatin** is condensed and transcriptionally inactive.
   b. **Euchromatin** is less condensed and transcriptionally active.
5. Supercoiling and packing of chromatin forms **chromosomes**.

DNA Replication and Repair

A. DNA Replication (*Figure 11-3*)
1. Replication is started at the origin of replication by the pre-replication complex.
2. DNA helicase unwinds the DNA at the replication fork.
3. Topoisomerase relieves supercoiling at the other end of the DNA strand.
4. Single-strand binding proteins prevent the two strands from reannealing.
5. Each DNA strand is synthesized from the 5′ end to the 3′ end.
6. An RNA primer must be added to the DNA strand to allow replication by DNA polymerases.
   a. In eukaryotes, this function is carried out by DNA polymerase α.
   b. In prokaryotes, this function is carried out by primase.

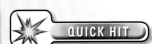

QUICK HIT

Because CG pairs have more bonds than AT pairs, a higher CG content increases the melting temperature of DNA.

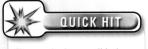

QUICK HIT

Fluoroquinolone antibiotics inhibit prokaryotic topoisomerase. Etoposide inhibits eukaryotic topoisomerase.

Biochemistry and Genetics

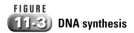

FIGURE
11-3 **DNA synthesis**

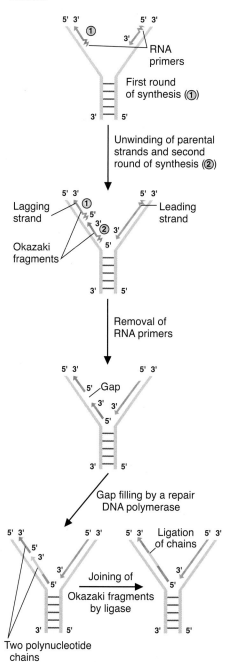

(Reprinted with permission from Lieberman M, Marks AD. *Marks' Basic Medical Biochemistry: A Clinical Approach.* 4th ed. Philadelphia, PA: Lippincott Williams & Wilkins; 2013.)

7. Eukaryotic DNA replication
    a. DNA polymerase α synthesizes the initial RNA primer on the leading and lagging strands.
    b. DNA polymerase δ replicates the leading strand in a continuous fashion.
    c. DNA polymerase α replicates the lagging strand in short, discontinuous segments called Okazaki fragments, which are later joined together by DNA ligase.
    d. DNA polymerase γ replicates mitochondrial DNA.
8. Prokaryotic DNA replication
    a. Primase synthesizes the initial RNA primers.
    b. DNA polymerase III replicates the leading strand in a continuous fashion and also synthesizes the Okazaki fragments on the lagging strand.

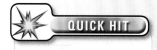

Diffuse scleroderma is caused by autoantibodies against topoisomerase.

Biochemistry and Genetics

c. DNA polymerase I degrades the RNA primers and fills in gaps in the DNA.

d. DNA ligase joins the Okazaki fragments together.

9. **Telomerase** adds nucleotides to the 3′ ends of chromosomes to compensate for the loss of nucleotides during replication.

a. In eukaryotes, DNA is linear, so the polymerase cannot reach the end of the strand. As a result, chromosomes get shorter with each replication.

b. Germ cells express telomerase, which allows them to grow and divide for many generations.

c. Somatic cells do not normally express telomerase. As they lose nucleotides from the ends of their chromosomes, they eventually reach a point where DNA replication is impaired and cells can no longer grow and divide.

d. Somatic cancer cells often express telomerase, which is thought to be a major factor in their continued growth and division.

B. **DNA Mutations**

1. **Silent mutation:** A mutation in the third position of a codon that does not change the resulting amino acid. This is due to transfer RNA (tRNA) wobble, which allows for tolerance of some of these mutations.

2. **Missense mutation:** A mutation that results in an amino acid substitution. This can cause a change in the folding and/or function of the resulting protein.

3. **Nonsense mutation:** A mutation that creates an early stop codon, resulting in termination of transcription and a shortened protein.

4. **Frameshift mutation:** Addition or deletion of a nucleotide shifts the reading frame, resulting in a completely different set of codons.

5. **Pyrimidine dimer:** Inappropriate binding of thymine to a neighboring thymine on the same DNA strand (or cytosine to cytosine, which is less common). This mutation is often caused by ultraviolet (UV) radiation.

C. **DNA Repair**

1. **Nucleotide excision repair:** A segment of single-stranded DNA containing bulky, helix-distorting damage is removed by an endonuclease. The section is then filled in by DNA polymerases, and DNA ligase joins the ends. This is most commonly used to repair pyrimidine dimers.

2. **Base excision repair:** The damaged base is removed by a glycosylase, and the apurinic/apyrimidinic site is removed by an endonuclease. The gap is filled by a polymerase and sealed by ligase. This is most commonly used to remove uracil, hypoxanthine, or 3-methyladenine from DNA.

a. Spontaneous deamination of cytosine forms uracil.

b. Spontaneous deamination of adenine forms hypoxanthine.

c. Methylation of adenine creates 3-methyladenine.

3. **Mismatch repair:** Mismatched nucleotides are removed by an endonuclease. This occurs immediately after the synthesis of the strand, just upstream of the DNA polymerase. The gap is filled by another polymerase and sealed by a ligase.

4. **Nonhomologous end joining:** Repair of double-stranded breaks by joining overhanging ends of DNA by a ligase. The gaps are filled in by polymerase and sealed by another ligase.

D. **DNA Repair Defects**

1. **Xeroderma pigmentosum:** Autosomal recessive deficiency in nucleotide excision repair. This causes extreme sensitivity to UV light, along with multiple skin malignancies. Patients must avoid all sunlight.

2. **Ataxia telangiectasia:** Autosomal recessive defect of the ATM protein, resulting in the inability to repair double-stranded DNA breaks. This causes many problems, including gait ataxia, immunodeficiency, telangiectasia, and an increased risk of cancer.

3. **Bloom syndrome:** Autosomal recessive defect of the BLM protein, which is a helicase that is important in both DNA repair and DNA replication. This causes hypersensitivity to UV light, short stature, immunodeficiency, and an increased risk of leukemia or lymphoma.

4. **Hereditary nonpolyposis colorectal cancer (HNPCC):** Autosomal dominant defect in mismatch repair. This greatly increases the risk of colorectal cancer, as well as other cancers (especially endometrial cancer).

5. **BRCA1/BRCA2 mutation:** A defect in the proteins BRCA1 or BRCA2, which are involved in the repair of double-stranded DNA breaks. This greatly increases the risk of breast cancer, as well as other cancers (especially ovarian cancer).

RNA Transcription

A. Important Terms

1. **Operon:** A region of DNA containing transcribed genes under the control of a single promoter region, as well as structural DNA and operator sequences. Operons are generally found in prokaryotes, although they do occur less commonly in eukaryotes.

2. **Promoter:** The region of DNA to which RNA polymerase binds prior to the initiation of transcription.

3. **Operator:** A specialized region of DNA within the promoter of an inducible (*lac* operon) or repressible operon. This region binds inducer proteins or repressor proteins that either promote or prevent binding of RNA polymerase.

4. **Repressor:** A protein that binds to the operator region of a promoter and prevents transcription by RNA polymerase.

5. **Corepressor:** A substance that facilitates the binding of a repressor protein to an operator sequence.

6. **Inducer:** A substance that prevents the binding of a repressor protein to an operator sequence.

7. **Transcription factor:** Any protein that binds to DNA and regulates transcription.

8. **Response element:** Any region of DNA that is bound by a transcription factor.

9. **General transcription factor:** A protein that binds in or near the promoter region and facilitates the binding of RNA polymerase. General transcription factors are required for initiation of transcription. They bind to conserved sequences such as the TATA box (TATAAA, or a variation), or the CAAT box (GGCCAATCT), which are located approximately 25 base pairs and 40 base pairs respectively upstream of the start site.

10. **Enhancer:** A regulatory region of DNA that allows control of transcription through folding of the DNA. Enhancer regions are far more common in eukaryotes than in prokaryotes. They may be located near the promoter but are often thousands of base pairs upstream or downstream. Enhancer-bound proteins do not initiate or prevent transcription. They only affect the rate at which it occurs.

11. **Activator/Repressor:** A protein that binds to an enhancer region and either stimulates or inhibits transcription, either through direct interactions with RNA polymerase or indirectly through interactions with transcription factors, other activators, or other repressors. Enhancer-bound repressors merely slow transcription, whereas operator-bound repressors prevent transcription.

B. Transcription Factors

1. **Helix-loop-helix:** Characterized by two α helices connected by an amino acid loop. These generally form dimers when binding DNA. An example of a helix-loop-helix transcription factor is Myc, the mutated form of which is associated with Burkitt lymphoma.

2. **Helix-turn-helix:** Characterized by two α helices connected by a short strand of amino acids. Helix-turn-helix transcription factors bind DNA as monomers. The *lac* repressor contains a helix-turn-helix motif.

3. **Zinc finger:** These transcription factors have a DNA-binding domain containing an atom of zinc. GATA-3, a transcription factor that regulates type 2 immune responses, has a zinc-finger binding domain.

4. **Leucine zipper:** Transcription factors that bind DNA through two α helices that are held together by leucine residues. CREB, a transcription factor that regulates many of the effects of cyclic adenosine monophosphate (cAMP) signaling, has a leucine zipper domain.

C. RNA Polymerases

1. Eukaryotic RNA polymerases
   a. RNA Pol I: Transcribes ribosomal RNA (rRNA) in the nucleolus.
   b. RNA Pol II: Transcribes messenger RNA (mRNA) in the nucleoplasm.
   c. RNA Pol III: Transcribes tRNA in the nucleoplasm.

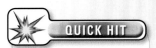

QUICK HIT

Prokaryotic RNA polymerase can bind directly to the DNA unassisted, although transcription factors can still increase its affinity.

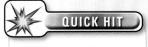

QUICK HIT

RNA polymerase II is inhibited by α-amanitin, a toxin found in certain mushrooms.

Biochemistry and Genetics

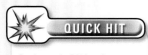

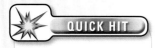

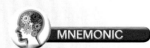

2. Prokaryotic RNA polymerase
   a. Prokaryotes only have one RNA polymerase, and it transcribes rRNA, mRNA, and tRNA.

D. *lac* Operon
   1. Inducible operon that responds to an increase in levels of lactose by transcribing RNA that will then be translated to β-galactosidase.
   2. Allolactose, a lactose derivative, binds the *lac* repressor that is bound to the operator region of the promoter, causing it to dissociate.
   3. Catabolite activator complex (CAP), an activator that is required by RNA polymerase, only binds in the absence of glucose.
   4. Thus, β-galactosidase will only be synthesized in the presence of lactose and the absence of glucose.

E. Termination of Prokaryotic Transcription
   1. Rho factor uses its adenosine triphosphatase (ATPase) activity to dissociate RNA polymerase from the DNA strand.
   2. In intrinsic termination, the RNA polymerase encounters an RNA stem loop that forms in a region rich in guanine and cytosine. This stem loop is followed by a sequence of adenine-uracil base pairs between the nascent RNA strand and the template DNA. This promotes the release of RNA polymerase (the mechanism is unclear).

RNA Translation

A. Codons
   1. Sequences of mRNA, each three bases in length, that code for specific amino acids.
   2. The start codon, AUG, codes for methionine in eukaryotes and N-formyl-methionine in prokaryotes.
   3. The sequences UGA, UAA, and UAG are stop codons, each signaling the termination of translation.

B. mRNA
   1. RNA within the nucleus is known as heterogeneous nuclear RNA (hnRNA).
   2. Precursor mRNA (pre-mRNA) is the term for transcribed RNA that has not yet undergone processing into mRNA.
      a. hnRNA and pre-mRNA are not synonymous. Pre-mRNA only makes up a small portion of hnRNA.
      b. Most hnRNA is composed of RNA transcripts that remain in the nucleus and regulate gene expression.
   3. Pre-mRNA is processed in the nucleus.
      a. Pre-mRNA is capped at the 5′ end with 7-methylguanosine. This requires S-adenosyl-methionine.
      b. The 3′ end is capped with a string of adenine residues known as the poly(A) tail. The site of this is determined by a polyadenylation signal sequence (5′-AAUAAA-3′).
      c. Introns are removed in a process known as RNA splicing.
   4. The processed mRNA then leaves the nucleus to enter translation.

C. tRNA
   1. Transports amino acids to the ribosome, where they can be attached to the growing amino acid chain.
   2. The characteristic cloverleaf structure has an anticodon loop that attaches to the mRNA and a nucleic acid sequence of CCA at the 3′ end.
   3. The amino acid is attached to the 3′ end of the tRNA by an aminoacyl tRNA synthetase. This process is known as tRNA charging.

D. Protein Synthesis (*Figure 11-4*)
   1. Ribosomal subunits are synthesized in the nucleus and then transported into the cytosol.
      a. Eukaryotes have an 80s ribosome, composed of a 40s and a 60s subunit.
      b. Prokaryotes have a 70s ribosome, composed of a 30s and a 50s subunit.
   2. In initiation, Initiation Factors (IF) facilitate the attachment of the smaller ribosomal subunit (30s or 40s) to the mRNA strand just upstream of the start codon (AUG). This positions the ribosomal subunit so that the P site can accept the aminoacyl tRNA containing methionine.

Continued at top of next page

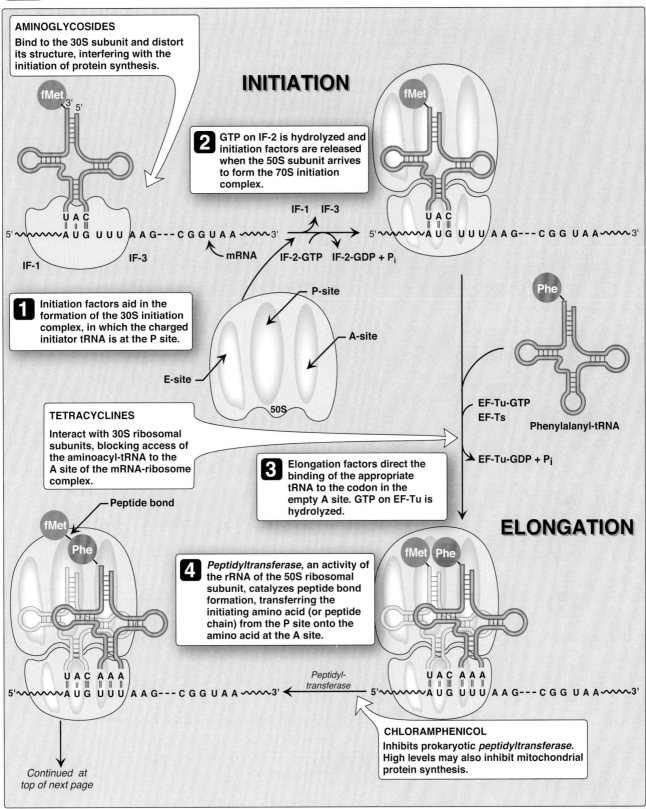

FIGURE 11-4 Protein synthesis

A, adenine; Arg, arginine; C, cytosine; EF, elongation factor; fMET, formyl methionine; G, guanine; GDP, guanosine diphosphate; GTP, guanosine triphosphate; IF, initiation factor; Phe, phenylalanine; Pᵢ, inorganic phosphate; RF, release factor; T, thymine; tRNA, transfer RNA; U, uracil. (Adapted with permission from Harvey RA, Ferrier DR. *Lippincott's Illustrated Reviews: Biochemistry.* 5th ed. Baltimore, MD: Lippincott Williams & Wilkins; 2011.)

FIGURE 11-4 *(Continued)*

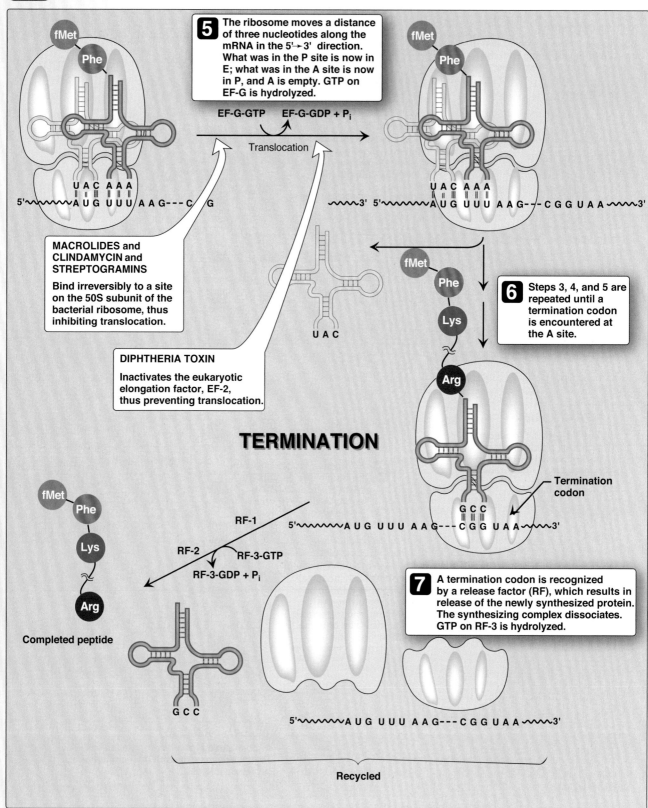

5 The ribosome moves a distance of three nucleotides along the mRNA in the 5'→3' direction. What was in the P site is now in E; what was in the A site is now in P, and A is empty. GTP on EF-G is hydrolyzed.

EF-G-GTP → EF-G-GDP + P$_i$

Translocation

MACROLIDES and CLINDAMYCIN and STREPTOGRAMINS

Bind irreversibly to a site on the 50S subunit of the bacterial ribosome, thus inhibiting translocation.

DIPHTHERIA TOXIN

Inactivates the eukaryotic elongation factor, EF-2, thus preventing translocation.

6 Steps 3, 4, and 5 are repeated until a termination codon is encountered at the A site.

Termination codon

TERMINATION

RF-1

RF-2   RF-3-GTP

RF-3-GDP + P$_i$

7 A termination codon is recognized by a release factor (RF), which results in release of the newly synthesized protein. The synthesizing complex dissociates. GTP on RF-3 is hydrolyzed.

Completed peptide

Recycled

3. The aminoacyl tRNA binds, and the larger ribosomal subunit (50s or 60s) binds to the smaller ribosomal subunit. At the same time, the IFs are released from the complex through hydrolysis of guanosine triphosphate (GTP).

4. As <u>elongation</u> occurs, the incoming aminoacyl tRNAs bind to the A site of the ribosome.

5. A peptidyltransferase then attaches the amino acid from the aminoacyl tRNA at the P site to the amino acid at the A site.
    a. In prokaryotes, the peptidyltransferase is found in a 23s subunit that is part of the larger 50s subunit.

6. In <u>translocation</u>, the ribosome complex hydrolyzes GTP and moves 3 nucleotides down the mRNA strand. This requires elongation factor G (EF-G) in prokaryotes and elongation factor 2 (EF-2) in eukaryotes.

7. The newly uncharged tRNA moves to the E site, while the tRNA attached to the amino acid chain moves to the P site. As the incoming aminoacyl tRNA binds to the A site, the empty tRNA is ejected from the E site.

8. This process repeats until the stop codon is reached. Release factors then facilitate the release of the amino acid strand.

9. The amino acid must undergo posttranslational modifications prior to becoming a functional protein. This may include removal of N-terminal or C-terminal polypeptides, phosphorylation, glycosylation, hydroxylation, and many others.

E. **Drugs that Inhibit Translation**
1. **Aminoglycosides** bind the 30s ribosomal subunit in prokaryotes and inhibit initiation.
2. **Linezolid** binds the 50s subunit and prevents formation of the initiation complex.
3. **Tetracycline** antibiotics bind to the A site of the 30s ribosome subunit and prevent the attachment of aminoacyl tRNAs.
4. **Chloramphenicol** binds the 50s subunit and prevents the action of peptidyltransferase.
5. **Macrolides**, lincosamides (including **clindamycin** and lincomycin), and **streptogramins** bind the 50s subunit and inhibit translocation of the ribosome complex.

Inheritance

A. **Modes of Inheritance**
1. **Autosomal dominant:** Phenotype requires only one allele. Structural gene defects are often inherited in this pattern. Offspring with heterozygous parents have a 75% chance of expressing the associated phenotype.
2. **Autosomal recessive:** Phenotype requires two alleles. Enzyme defects are often inherited in this pattern. Offspring have a 75% chance of inheriting at least one allele from heterozygous parents, but only a 25% chance of expressing the associated phenotype.
3. **X-linked dominant:** Phenotype requires only one X-linked allele. Offspring from a heterozygous mother have a 50% chance of expressing the associated phenotype. If the father carries the allele, female offspring have a 100% chance of expressing the associated phenotype.
4. **X-linked recessive:** Phenotype requires two X-linked alleles in women, but only one X-linked allele in men. Offspring with a heterozygous mother have a 50% chance of inheriting the allele. Male offspring will then express the associated phenotype, while female offspring will only be carriers.
5. **Mitochondrial:** Phenotype always manifests, and a mother will always pass mitochondria to both male and female offspring.

B. **Important Terms**
1. **Codominance:** Both alleles are expressed at the same time (e.g., ABO blood groupings).

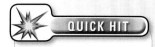

Because men only have one X chromosome, X-linked recessive diseases affect men far more often than women.

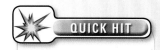

Mitochondrial diseases always affect both male and female offspring but are only inherited through the mother.

Biochemistry and Genetics

2. **Variable expression:** The effect of the genes varies from one individual to another (e.g., neurofibromatosis, tuberous sclerosis).
3. **Pleiotropy:** A single gene has more than one effect on phenotype (e.g., phenylketonuria).
4. **Locus heterogeneity:** Several different genes can cause the same phenotype (e.g., genes related to Marfan syndrome and homocystinuria can both cause Marfanoid habitus).
5. **Mosaicism:** A condition when cells within the same individual differ in genetic makeup. This may result from mutations during development or genetic re-combination during mitosis.
6. **Loss of heterozygosity:** Deletion or interruption of an allele, leaving only one functional allele. Loss of heterozygosity often has no effect because one functioning allele remains. However, in some cases (notably oncogenes), deletion of one allele is sufficient to cause a phenotypic change.
7. **Anticipation:** Phenotypes manifest earlier in the offspring than in the parents. This can continue through multiple generations. In the case of a disease, this may also manifest as an increase in severity in successive generations (e.g., Huntington disease).
8. **Incomplete penetrance:** Alleles do not always express the associated phenotype (e.g., BRCA1and BRCA2 mutations do not always cause breast cancer).
9. **Imprinting:** Phenotypes resulting from the same alleles differ depending on whether the allele came from the mother or the father (e.g., Prader–Willi syndrome, Angelman syndrome).
   a. **Prader–Willi syndrome:** Deletion of a paternal allele on chromosome 15 and inactivation of the corresponding maternal allele. It presents in infancy with hypotonia, poor feeding, and characteristic facial features. Later in life, it causes childhood osteoporosis, polyphagia and obesity, short stature, mental retardation, behavioral disorders, and incomplete sexual development.
   b. **Angelman syndrome:** Deletion of a maternal allele on chromosome 15 and inactivation of the corresponding paternal allele. It presents with mental retardation, seizures, ataxia, and inappropriate laughter.
10. **Dominant negative mutation:** A recessive allele in a heterozygous individual that interferes with the function of the normal, dominant allele. Transcription factors with a mutation that renders them nonfunctional may still bind DNA, preventing the binding of nonmutated transcription factors.
11. **Linkage disequilibrium:** The tendency for alleles at two or more loci to occur together more or less often than expected by random chance.
12. **Heteroplasmy:** The occurrence of both normal and mutated mitochondrial DNA. This causes variable expression of mitochondrial-associated diseases.
13. **Uniparental disomy:** The inheritance of two copies of a chromosome from one parent and no copies from the other parent, rather than one copy from each parent.

C. **Hardy–Weinberg Population Genetics**
1. Assumptions
   a. p and q are the frequencies of two separate alleles in a population.
   b. Allelic frequencies are equally distributed among the sexes.
   c. The population is infinitely large.
   d. Everyone produces the same number of offspring.
   e. There are no mutations at the locus.
   f. There is no selective pressure for any of the genotypes.
   g. Mating is completely random.
   h. There is no net migration of alleles into or out of the population, i.e., the population is closed.
2. Hardy–Weinberg equilibrium
   a. $p + q = 1$
   b. $p^2 + 2pq + q^2 = 1$
   c. $p^2 =$ frequency of individuals homozygous for the first allele
   d. $q^2 =$ frequency of individuals homozygous for the second allele
   e. $2pq =$ frequency of heterozygous individuals

MNEMONIC

To remember Prader–Willi syndrome and Angelman syndrome, use the phrase, "**MAMA** and **POP**":
Maternal gene deletion
Angelman syndrome
Mood (happy, laughter)
Ataxia
and
Prader–Willi syndrome
Overeating/Obesity
Paternal gene deletion

Biochemistry and Genetics

f. For X-linked recessive alleles, the frequency of phenotypic expression is q for males and q^2 for females.

g. Evolution does not occur in Hardy–Weinberg equilibrium, and allelic frequencies do not change from generation to generation. Obviously, in reality, this never occurs.

Genetics Laboratory Methods

A. Polymerase Chain Reaction (PCR)

1. Used to create many copies of a segment of DNA.

2. DNA is mixed with DNA primers, heat-stable DNA polymerase, and deoxyribonucleotides.

3. First, DNA is denatured by heating the solution to a high temperature. This separates the strands.

4. Second, the solution is rapidly cooled to a relatively low temperature, allowing the primers to anneal to the DNA strands. The primers are designed so that they bind sequences that flank the DNA segment of interest.

5. Third, the solution is heated to an intermediate temperature, which allows the polymerase to synthesize DNA using the primers as a starting point.

   a. PCR-denaturing Ztemperatures will also denature most DNA polymerases. Therefore, PCR systems use Taq polymerase, a heat-stable DNA polymerase isolated from bacteria that live in hydrothermal vents.

6. After the initial cycle, the primers will also bind the newly synthesized DNA. These three steps are repeated many times (typically 30 to 40 cycles) resulting in many copies of the region of interest.

B. Gel Electrophoresis

1. Used to separate segments of DNA (or RNA) according to size.

2. Samples are mixed with a fluorescent stain and loaded into wells at one end of a gel.

3. The gel is covered with a buffer solution and a current is passed through it.

4. Negatively charged DNA or RNA will migrate toward the positive pole.

5. Migration will occur at different rates because smaller segments of DNA or RNA can move more quickly through the gel matrix.

6. Samples are usually run alongside a control sample with segments of known size.

7. This technique can reveal the size of a segment (may reveal insertions or deletions in genes) or allow for isolation of the DNA or RNA segment (can be cut out of the gel and analyzed further).

8. Gel electrophoresis can also be used to separate proteins. Because proteins may be positive or negative, they are placed in wells in the middle of the gel, and they may migrate toward either end.

C. Blots

1. Used to analyze DNA, RNA, or proteins through the use of labeled probes.

2. Samples are hybridized to a membrane or filter and treated with a labeled probe that is specific for a nucleotide sequence or an amino acid sequence.

3. The probe is then detected by color change, fluorescence, or radioactivity.

4. **Southern blot:** DNA is denatured in an alkaline solution and treated with a labeled DNA (or RNA) probe that is complementary to the sequence of interest.

5. **Northern blot:** RNA is treated with a labeled RNA (or DNA) probe that is complementary to the sequence of interest. Normally, no denaturing solution is required because RNA is single stranded (except in the case of certain viruses).

6. **Western blot:** Protein samples are treated with a labeled antibody that recognizes the protein of interest.

7. **Southwestern blot:** Protein is treated with labeled oligonucleotides. This identifies proteins that bind specific DNA sequences, i.e., transcription factors.

8. Blots are almost always paired with gel electrophoresis. DNA, RNA, or proteins that have been separated are transferred directly from the gel to the membrane or filter.

9. Microarrays utilize these same techniques to analyze samples with thousands of probes at once. Special cartridges called chips contain tiny spots with very small amounts of probe material. The sample is added to the chip and analyzed using special equipment.

D. **Enzyme-Linked Immunosorbent Assay (ELISA)**
  1. Uses antigen–antibody interactions to detect antigens or antigen-specific antibodies in a sample.
  2. **Traditional ELISA (Indirect):** Used to detect protein-specific antibodies in a serum sample. Serum is added to a well or vial coated with a protein of interest. Serum antibodies that recognize the protein will then bind. Unbound antibodies are washed away, and an enzyme-linked secondary antibody is added to bind the serum antibody.
  3. **Sandwich ELISA (Direct):** Used to detect specific proteins in a serum sample. Serum is added to a well or vial coated with an antibody that recognizes the protein of interest. Surface-bound antibodies bind the proteins, and unbound proteins are washed away. An enzyme-linked antibody specific for the protein is then added.
  4. In both assays, a substrate for the enzyme is then added, resulting in a color change. The magnitude of the color change reflects either the concentration of protein or protein-specific antibodies in a sample.

E. **Fluorescence In Situ Hybridization (FISH)**
  1. Used to detect specific nucleic acid sequences within chromosomes or within cells.
  2. Fluorescently labeled DNA or RNA probes are added to isolated chromosomes, where they will bind complementary sequences, revealing the location of the segment of interest.
  3. Probes can also be added to fixed cells or tissue sections to study gene expression. Because probes cannot access coiled DNA, they only bind segments that are being actively transcribed. In this way, they can reveal which cells or tissues are expressing certain genes. Alternatively, probes can be designed to bind mRNA.

F. **Cloning**
  1. Used to study DNA sequences for specific genes by using bacterial systems to make copies.
  2. Reverse transcriptase is used to make complementary DNA (cDNA) from mRNA.
  3. The cDNA is then inserted into a bacterial plasmid, which is then taken up by bacterial cells.
  4. As the bacteria grow and divide, the plasmids are replicated. This creates many copies of the cDNA, which can then be isolated.
  5. cDNA is different from normal DNA because it lacks introns. This means that it contains only the coding sequences of the gene, and it can be studied without having to distinguish between the exons and introns.
  6. This system can also be used to manufacture bacterial proteins for study.

G. **Modifications of Gene Expression**
  1. Knockout: Deletion or disruption of a gene. The function of many genes can be determined by analyzing the effect of the loss of those genes. This technique is often used in bacteria and in mice, although it can theoretically be used in any animal model.
  2. Knock-in: The targeted insertion of a gene. Homologous recombination is used to replace one allele with another, ensuring that it is found in the same place and will be expressed as it normally would.
  3. Transgenic animal: A gene is inserted into the genome of an animal, but its insertion is random. Because the gene contains the promoter and many of the necessary response elements, it will often be transcribed normally. However, this method risks disruption of other genes if the gene of interest is inserted into another reading frame. In addition, multiple copies may insert at different sites, resulting in overexpression of the gene. This method is quicker and easier than knocking in, but it is less accurate.
  4. Small interfering RNA (siRNA): Short RNA strands that are complementary to mRNA from genes of interest are either inserted into cells or inserted into the genome so that they will be directly transcribed by the cells. These RNA molecules may bind to mRNA and prevent its translation or activate an RNA-induced silencing complex that targets the mRNA for degradation. The result is a knockdown of the protein.

5. Cre-Lox system: A system used for conditional deletions of specific DNA segments. Special recognition sequences, known as LoxP sequences, can be inserted into the genome flanking the DNA segment to be deleted. Cre recombinase, an enzyme that recognizes LoxP sites, can be inserted downstream from a specific promoter. Once Cre recombinase is synthesized, it will excise the portion of DNA between the LoxP sites. This allows for specific genes to be deleted only after the activation of another gene within the same cell.

6. Karyotyping: Metaphase chromosomes are stained, paired, and ordered according to size, banding pattern, and morphology. This is useful in diagnosing chromosomal imbalances.

 # PROTEIN

Amino Acids

A. Classifications

1. Essential amino acids: **Phe, Val, Thr, Trp, Ile, Met, His, Arg, Leu, Lys**.
2. Acidic amino acids: **Aspartic acid (Asp), Glutamic acid (Glu)**. These carry a negative charge at normal body pH.
3. Basic amino acids: **Lys, Arg, His**. Lys and Arg carry a positive charge at normal body pH. His is neutral.

B. Important Amino Acid Derivatives

1. Phenylalanine: Can be converted to tyrosine.
2. Tyrosine: Dopa, dopamine, norepinephrine, epinephrine, melanin.
3. Arginine: Urea, and nitric oxide. Arginine is also required for creatine synthesis.
4. Tryptophan: Niacin, nicotinamide adenine dinucleotide (NAD), nicotinamide adenine dinucleotide phosphate (NADP), serotonin, melatonin.
5. Histidine: Histamine.
6. Glycine: Porphyrin (part of heme synthesis).
7. Glutamate: γ-aminobutyric acid (GABA), glutathione.
8. Methionine: S-adenosylmethionine (SAM; transfers methyl units in the synthesis of both epinephrine and creatine).

C. Amino Acid Disorders

1. Phenylketonuria
   a. Autosomal recessive deficiency of **phenylalanine hydroxylase** or **tetrahydrobiopterin** (less common).
   b. Phenylalanine cannot be converted to tyrosine. Phenylalanine then accumulates and is converted to phenylketones (i.e., phenylacetate, phenylpyruvate, phenyl-lactate).
   c. **Presentation:** Fair skin and hair, eczema, intellectual disability, musty or mousy odor, seizures, microcephaly.
   d. **Labs:** ↑ Phenylalanine, cranial demyelination (in untreated, older patients).
   e. **Treatment:** Decreased dietary phenylalanine and/or increased dietary tyrosine. Tetrahydrobiopterin supplementation may also be indicated.
      i. Restriction of phenylalanine within the first few weeks of life prevents developmental abnormalities.
      ii. Patients remain largely asymptomatic as long as the diet is strictly followed.
   f. **Maternal phenylketonuria:** Phenylalanine intake in phenylketonuric mothers during pregnancy may result in fetal defects such as microcephaly, mental retardation, growth retardation, and congenital heart defects.

2. Alkaptonuria
   a. Autosomal recessive deficiency of homogentisic acid oxidase, an enzyme involved in tyrosine catabolism.
   b. Alkaptonuria is a relatively benign condition, but it may manifest with moderate to severe arthralgia.
   c. **Presentation:** Grayish-brown sclera, ochronosis (darkened tissues), dark urine, decreased joint mobility (due to deposition of homogentisic acid in joints), calcifications in affected areas.
   d. **Labs:** ↑ Homogentisic acid in urine, spinal disk degeneration and calcification.

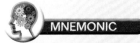 **MNEMONIC**

Remember the essential amino acids with **"PVT. TIM HALL"** (Private Tim Hall):
Phenylalanine (Phe)
Valine (Val)
Threonine (Thr)
Tryptophan (Trp)
Isoleucine (Ile)
Methionine (Met)
Histidine (His)
Arginine (Arg)
Leucine (Leu)
Lysine (Lys)

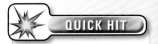 **QUICK HIT**

Arginine is normally only essential in children because they are unable to synthesize enough to meet growth demands. Adults can generally synthesize an adequate amount.

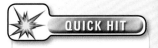 **QUICK HIT**

Newborns are not screened for phenylketonuria until 2–3 days after birth. Prior to this, phenylketone levels may appear normal, giving a false negative result.

e. **Treatment:** Decreased dietary phenylalanine and tyrosine, vitamin C supplementation. Nitisinone may also be indicated (inhibits homogentisic acid synthesis).

3. Albinism
   a. Autosomal recessive deficiency of tyrosinase or a defect of tyrosine transport into cells. Albinism may also result from a defect or deficiency of melanocytes (less common).
   b. This results in the inability to synthesize melanin, which increases the risk of skin cancer.
   c. **Presentation:** Hypopigmentation of the skin and hair, iris depigmentation, visual impairment, photosensitivity,
   d. **Labs:** ↓ Tyrosinase activity (in some cases). Genetic tests provide the most definitive diagnosis.
   e. **Treatment:** Treatment is normally not indicated.

4. Homocystinuria
   a. Autosomal recessive deficiency of cystathionine synthase, an enzyme involved in the synthesis of cysteine from homocysteine.
   b. Homocystinuria may also be due to a deficiency of cofactors in the synthesis of methionine from homocysteine.
   c. The result is the accumulation of homocysteine.
   d. **Presentation:** Mental retardation, subluxation of the lenses of the eyes, **Marfanoid habitus** (tall stature, long limbs, joint hypermobility, and long fingers [arachnodactyly]).
   e. **Labs:** ↑ Homocysteine, ↑ methionine (only in cystathionine synthase deficiency), osteoporosis, kyphosis, atherosclerosis.
   f. **Treatment:** Supplementation with vitamins B_6, B_{12}, and folic acid; increased dietary cysteine; decreased dietary methionine.

5. Cystinuria
   a. Autosomal recessive defect of the renal tubular transporter of COLA (cysteine, ornithine, lysine, arginine).
   b. Cysteine reabsorption is impaired.
   c. **Presentation:** Recurrent urinary tract infections.
   d. **Labs:** The presence of hexagonal crystals in urine is considered pathognomonic for cystinuria. Bilateral renal calculi and renal colic are also common.
   e. **Treatment:** Hydration, potassium citrate (alkalinizes urine), penicillamine or α-mercaptopropionylglycine (bind cystine and increase its solubility).

6. Maple syrup urine disease
   a. Autosomal recessive deficiency of branched-chain α-ketoacid dehydrogenase, an enzyme that breaks down branched-chain amino acids (i.e., Ile, Leu, Val).
   b. This causes accumulation of branched-chain amino acids and their corresponding α-ketoacids.
   c. **Presentation:** Urine that smells like maple syrup (Ile excretion), mental retardation, CNS defects (Leu accumulation).
   d. **Labs:** Serum alloisoleucine, ↑ urine organic acids.
   e. **Treatment:** Decreased dietary branched-chain amino acids, dialysis (severe cases).

7. Hartnup disease
   a. Autosomal recessive defect of neutral amino acid transporters in the kidneys and intestines.
   b. Causes malabsorption of tryptophan and lack of niacin synthesis.
   c. Hartnup disease is generally asymptomatic except in cases of poor diet.
   d. **Presentation:** Niacin deficiency causes dementia, dermatitis, and diarrhea (pellagra). Photosensitivity is also common.
   e. **Labs:** ↑ Neutral amino acids in urine.
   f. **Treatment:** High dietary protein, decreased exposure to sunlight, nicotinic acid or nicotinamide supplementation.

Collagen

A. **Classification**
  1. Collagen is the most abundant protein in the body. It provides structure and substance to extracellular space.
  2. **Type I:** Found in skin, bones, dentin, and scar tissue. This is the most common type of collagen.
  3. **Type II:** Found in cartilage, vitreous body of the eye, and nucleus pulposus.
  4. **Type III:** Found in blood vessels, skin, uterus, fetal tissue, and granulation tissue.
  5. **Type IV:** Found in basement membrane.

B. **Synthesis and Structure** (*Figure 11-5*)
  1. Collagen is composed of very long chains with a regular structure of Gly-Pro-X, or Gly-X-hydroxyproline.
  2. Collagen synthesis begins inside fibroblasts, then finishes outside of the cells.
      a. Alpha chains (**preprocollagen**) are synthesized in the rough endoplasmic reticulum (RER) of fibroblasts.
      b. Lysine and proline residues are then hydroxylated in a reaction that requires **vitamin C.**
      c. Hydroxylated lysine residues are then glycosylated, and hydrogen and sulfide bonds are formed as alpha chains are linked into a triple helix (**procollagen**).
      d. Procollagen is exocytosed, and the terminal regions are cleaved (**tropocollagen**).
      e. Finally, tropocollagen chains are cross-linked through covalent bonds between lysine and hydroxylysine residues to form large collagen fibrils (**collagen**).

C. **Osteogenesis Imperfecta (OI)**
  1. Most commonly an autosomal dominant deficiency of collagen synthesis involving type I collagen.
  2. OI causes weak bones, hence its alternate name, "brittle bone disease."
  3. Subtypes:
      a. **Type I:** Mildest and most common subtype. Type I collagen is normal but is synthesized at a low level. Alternatively, type I collagen may be abnormal, although this is less frequent.
      b. **Type II:** Collagen is deficient in both quantity and quality. This is a very severe condition that causes intrauterine death or early postnatal death.
      c. There are many other subtypes of OI with varying severity.
  4. **Presentation:** Blue sclerae (the choroid is visible through the thin collagen mesh), skin and teeth deformities, hearing loss, scoliosis, limb deformities, frequent fractures from minimal trauma.
  5. **Radiology:** Fractures on X-ray, excessive callus formation, thoracic cage deformity, skull changes, low bone density.
  6. **Treatment:** Surgical correction, pamidronate (inhibits osteoclasts), increased dietary intake of calcium, phosphorus, and vitamin D.

D. **Ehlers–Danlos Syndrome**
  1. May be either autosomal dominant or recessive. Ehlers–Danlos may be caused by varying defects in different types of collagen, but it affects connective tissue rather than bone.
  2. Causes weakness of blood vessels, joint cartilage, and skin.
  3. **Presentation:** Muscle weakness, easy bruising, hemorrhages, hyperelastic skin, joint hypermobility. Aneurysms are also common.
  4. **Radiology:** Opaque nodules on X-ray, disorderly dermal collagen fibers.
  5. **Treatment:** There is no treatment for Ehlers–Danlos syndrome. Only the symptoms can be managed.

E. **Alport Syndrome**
  1. Most commonly an X-linked dominant defect in type IV collagen, although it may also be autosomal dominant or recessive.
  2. This causes weakness of the basement membrane, which is most evident in the kidneys.
  3. **Presentation:** Hypertension, hearing loss, lenticonus, dot-and-fleck retinopathy.
      a. Lenticonus is a thinning of the capsule around the lens of the eye.

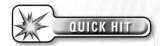

QUICK HIT

Vitamin C deficiency impairs collagen synthesis and causes **scurvy.**

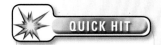

QUICK HIT

A scar with excess collagen is called a **keloid**. It can be treated by glucocorticoid injection, which inhibits collagen synthesis.

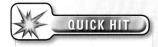

QUICK HIT

Osteogenesis imperfecta types VII and VIII are rare and are caused by mutations in proteins other than type I collagen. They are the only types of OI known to have an autosomal recessive pattern of inheritance.

Biochemistry and Genetics

Biochemistry and Genetics

FIGURE
11-5 Collagen synthesis

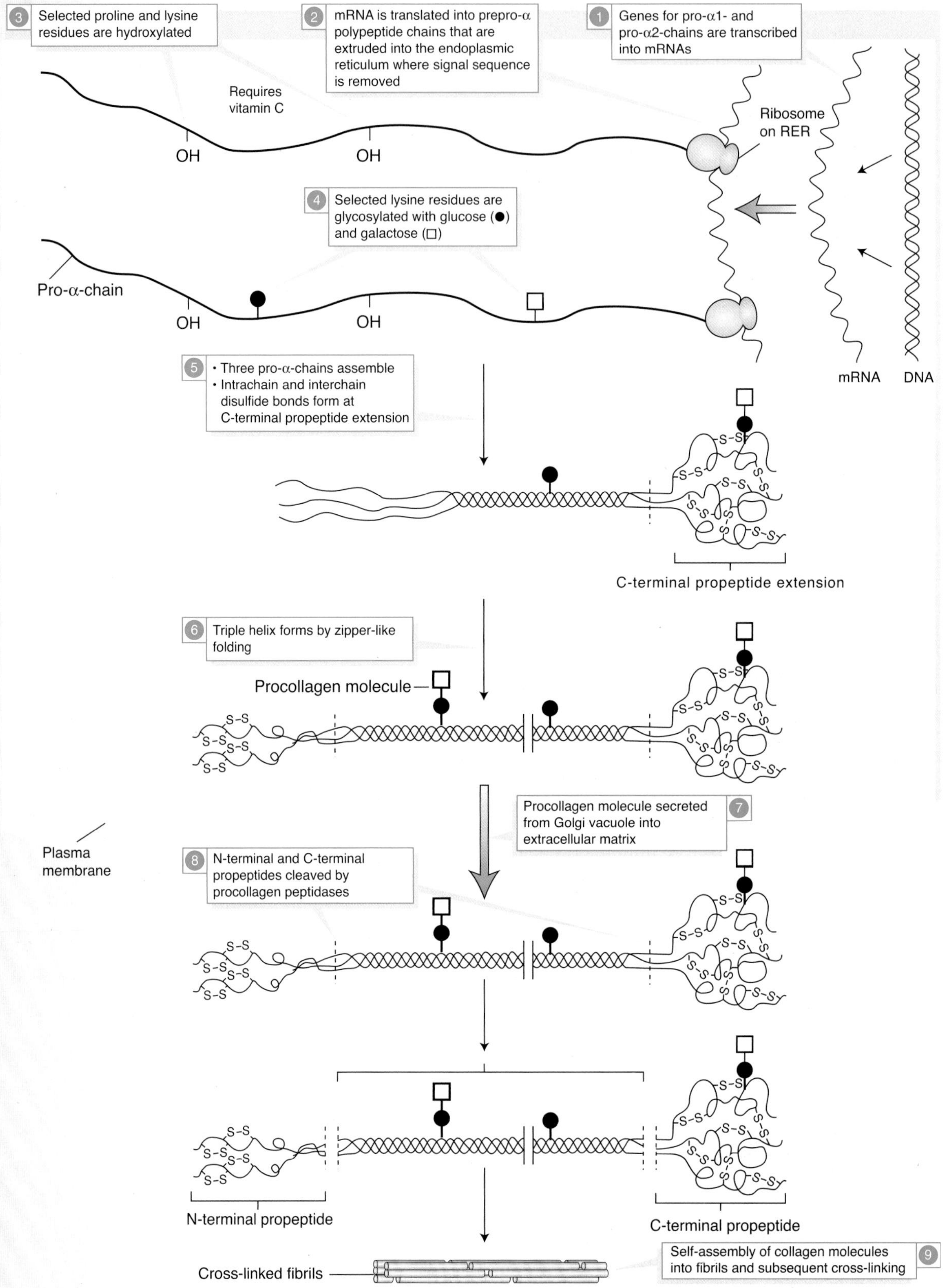

3 Selected proline and lysine residues are hydroxylated

2 mRNA is translated into prepro-α polypeptide chains that are extruded into the endoplasmic reticulum where signal sequence is removed

1 Genes for pro-α1- and pro-α2-chains are transcribed into mRNAs

Requires vitamin C

OH   OH

Ribosome on RER

4 Selected lysine residues are glycosylated with glucose (●) and galactose (□)

Pro-α-chain

OH   OH

mRNA   DNA

5 • Three pro-α-chains assemble
• Intrachain and interchain disulfide bonds form at C-terminal propeptide extension

C-terminal propeptide extension

6 Triple helix forms by zipper-like folding

Procollagen molecule

7 Procollagen molecule secreted from Golgi vacuole into extracellular matrix

Plasma membrane

8 N-terminal and C-terminal propeptides cleaved by procollagen peptidases

N-terminal propeptide

C-terminal propeptide

9 Self-assembly of collagen molecules into fibrils and subsequent cross-linking

Cross-linked fibrils

mRNA, messenger RNA; RER, rough endoplasmic reticulum. (Adapted with permission from Champe PC, Harvey RA, Ferrier DR. *Lippincott's Illustrated Reviews: Biochemistry.* 2nd ed. Philadelphia, PA: Lippincott-Raven, 1994:41.)

4. **Labs:** Hematuria, proteinuria, nephritis, red blood cell (RBC) casts.

5. **Treatment:** There is no definite treatment for Alport syndrome. Kidney transplantation is indicated for end-stage renal disease.

Elastin

A. **Structure**

1. Elastin is an extracellular matrix protein. It is not as strong as collagen, but it stretches more.

2. Found in blood vessels (especially arteries) and alveoli of lungs, larynx, and ligamenta flava of the spine.

3. Contains high amounts of proline and glycine. In contrast to collagen, these residues are nonhydroxylated.

4. Tropoelastins are held together by a matrix of fibrillin.

B. **Marfan Syndrome** *(Figure 11-6)*

1. Autosomal dominant defect of fibrillin.

2. This causes weakness of blood vessels, skeletal deformities, cardiovascular abnormalities (e.g., aortic dissection), and pulmonary difficulties.

FIGURE 11-6 Marfan syndrome

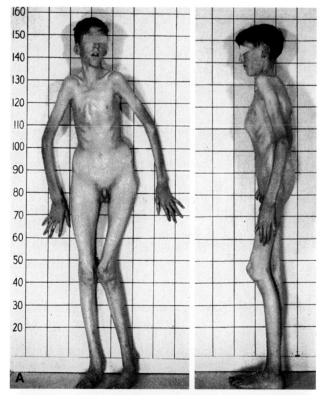

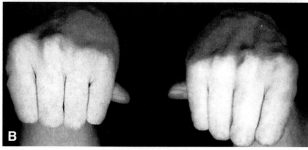

A. Marfan syndrome in a 14-year-old boy. Note arachnodactyly, relatively long limbs (dolichostenomelia), pectus carinatum, sparse subcutaneous fat, unilateral genu valgum, and pes planus. The patient also had scoliosis. This patient died of aortic rupture at age 15 years. **B.** A positive Steinberg thumb sign consists of protrusion of the distal phalanx of the thumb beyond the ulnar border of the clenched fist, and reflects both longitudinal laxity of the hand and a long thumb. (Reproduced with permission from Koopman WJ, Moreland LW. *Arthritis and Allied Conditions A Textbook of Rheumatology.* 15th ed. Philadelphia, PA: Lippincott Williams & Wilkins; 2005.)

3. **Presentation:** Pectus carinatum, pectus excavatum, genu valgum, subluxation of the lens of the eye, tall stature, long limbs, long fingers (arachnodactyly), joint hypermobility, positive **Steinberg sign** (Figure 11-6B), scoliosis.
4. **Labs:** There are no specific lab tests for Marfan syndrome other than screening for genetic markers.
5. **Treatment:** β-blockers for heart conditions, surgical intervention.

C. **α₁-Antitrypsin Deficiency**

1. Autosomal recessive deficiency of α_1-antitrypsin, which inhibits elastase.
2. The lack of elastase inhibition leads to the systemic breakdown of elastin.
3. Defective α_1-antitrypsin proteins may also accumulate and polymerize in hepatocytes.
4. **Presentation: Panacinar emphysema** and associated dyspnea (most common), cirrhosis, hepatitis.
    a. Panacinar emphysema affects the entire alveolus at once. In contrast, centri-acinar emphysema affects the bronchioles and spreads to the alveoli, whereas paraseptal emphysema affects only the distal alveolar ducts and sacs.
5. **Labs:** ↓ Serum α_1-antitrypsin, ↑ AST, ↑ ALT, ↓ pulmonary function.
6. **Treatment:** Prolastin (plasma proteins will replace missing enzymes), liver or lung transplantation.

Nitrogen Metabolism

A. **Urea Cycle** (*Figure 11-7*)

1. <u>Overall reaction</u>: $NH_3 \rightarrow$ urea. This requires three adenosine triphosphate (ATP) and aspartate.
2. <u>Rate-limiting step</u>: Ammonia + bicarbonate → carbamoyl phosphate via carbamoyl phosphate synthase I.
3. This pathway excretes excess nitrogen from amino acid metabolism in the form of urea.

B. **Alanine Cycle** (*Figure 11-8*)

1. Pathway for the movement of nitrogen to the liver for conversion to uric acid.
2. Pyruvate and glutamate are converted to alanine and α-ketoglutarate in the cells via **alanine aminotransferase** (ALT). This requires vitamin B_6 (in the form of pyridoxal phosphate).
3. Alanine is released into the blood, where it travels to the liver.
4. Alanine and α-ketoglutarate are converted back to pyruvate and glutamate in the liver, also via ALT and vitamin B_6.
5. Glutamate then undergoes deamination, donating its amino group to the urea cycle and regenerating α-ketoglutarate.
6. **Transamination:** The exchange of an amine group for a keto group between two molecules. In this case, an amino acid (glutamate, alanine) exchanges an amine group for a keto group from an α-ketoacid (pyruvate, α-ketoglutarate).

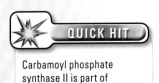

QUICK HIT

Carbamoyl phosphate synthase II is part of pyrimidine synthesis.

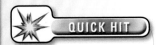

QUICK HIT

ALT is commonly measured as part of a liver function panel.

Biochemistry and Genetics

FIGURE
11-7 Urea cycle

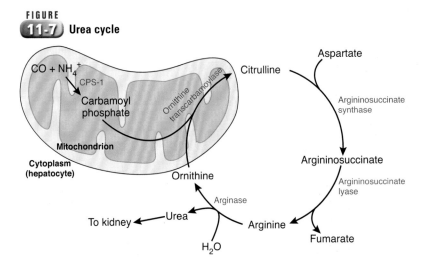

CPS-1, Carbamoyl phosphate synthase I.

FIGURE
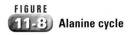 **Alanine cycle**

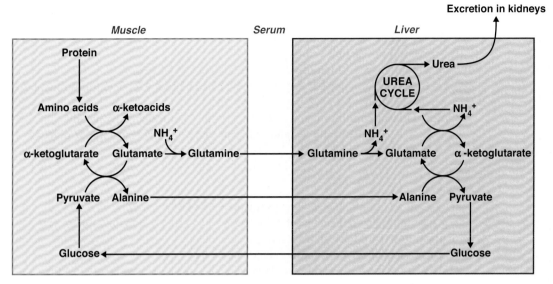

C. Ornithine Transcarbamoylase Deficiency
1. X-linked recessive. This is the most common disorder of the urea cycle.
2. Ornithine transcarbamylase (OTC) deficiency results in an inability to synthesize citrulline from carbamoyl phosphate and ornithine. This causes the urea cycle to stall. Ammonia then accumulates, causing hyperammonemia.
3. **Presentation:** Slurred speech, somnolence, vomiting, blurred vision.
4. **Labs:** Hematuria, orotic acid in the blood and urine, cerebral edema, decreased blood urea nitrogen (BUN) (due to decreased production of urea).
5. **Treatment:** Phenylbutyrate, which binds glutamine and facilitates its excretion.

D. Hyperammonemia
1. Various causes. It may be hereditary or acquired.
2. Excess ammonia depletes α-ketoglutarate, which impairs the tricarboxylic acid (TCA) cycle.
3. **Presentation:** Similar to OTC deficiency. Additional symptoms are associated with the underlying cause.
4. **Labs:** Alkalosis of blood, ↑ serum glutamine, ↑ serum alanine.
5. **Treatment:** Treated with lactulose, a sugar that cannot be absorbed by enterocytes. It then travels to the intestines, where it is broken down by bacteria, creating an acidic environment. Ammonia in the blood diffuses through intestinal enterocytes, where it is protonated by hydrogen ions, becoming ammonium. Ammonium cannot reenter the blood, and is excreted in the stool.

CARBOHYDRATE METABOLISM

Glucose Uptake and Processing
A. Glucose Transporters
1. Glucose enters the body through enterocytes in the gut. Once in circulation, it enters cells through glucose transporters (GLUT).
2. **GLUT-1:** Found on RBCs and the endothelium of the blood–brain barrier, as well as many other tissues. Mediates basal (low-level) uptake of glucose.
3. **GLUT-2:** Found on cells that regulate glucose (e.g., hepatocytes, pancreatic beta cells), although there is some evidence that beta cell GLUT-1 may be more important for stimulating insulin release.
4. **GLUT-3:** Found mainly on neurons and the placenta.
5. **GLUT-4:** Found on skeletal muscle and adipose tissue. This is the insulin-dependent glucose transporter.

B. Hexokinase and Glucokinase

1. Enzymes that phosphorylate glucose to **glucose-6-phosphate**, which confers a negative charge. It can no longer cross the membrane and thus remains inside the cell.
2. **Glucokinase:** Found in hepatocytes and pancreatic beta cells. Induced by insulin.
   a. Very high K_m (low affinity for glucose; high concentration to reach half of maximum reaction velocity).
   b. Very high V_{max} (high capacity to phosphorylate glucose).
   c. Glucokinase activity is very low except when glucose concentration increases substantially.
3. **Hexokinase:** Found in many cells of the body. Not induced by insulin.
   a. Low K_m (high affinity for glucose), but low V_{max} (low capacity for glucose phosphorylation).

Glycolysis *(Figure 11-9)*

A. Overview

1. <u>Overall reaction</u>: Glucose → 2 pyruvate + 2 ATP.
2. <u>Rate-limiting step</u>: Fructose-6-phosphate → **fructose-1,6-bisphosphate** via **phosphofructokinase-1** (PFK-1).
3. This process does not require oxygen.
4. All cells of the body can break down glucose, but it occurs mainly in RBCs (other cells obtain most of their energy through aerobic respiration).

B. Important Steps

1. Glucose → glucose-6-phosphate via hexokinase or glucokinase
2. Fructose-6-phosphate → fructose-1,6-bisphosphate via PFK-1
   a. Promoted by AMP and **fructose-2,6-bisphosphate**
   b. Inhibited by ATP and citrate (feedback inhibition from TCA cycle)
3. Fructose-1,6-bisphosphate → **glyceraldehyde-3-phosphate** and dihydroxyacetone phosphate (DHAP)
4. DHAP → glyceraldehyde3-phosphate

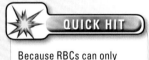

QUICK HIT

Because RBCs can only perform glycolysis, glycolytic enzyme deficiencies cause hemolytic anemia. **Pyruvate kinase** deficiency is the most common cause.

FIGURE
11-9 Glycolysis and Gluconeogenesis

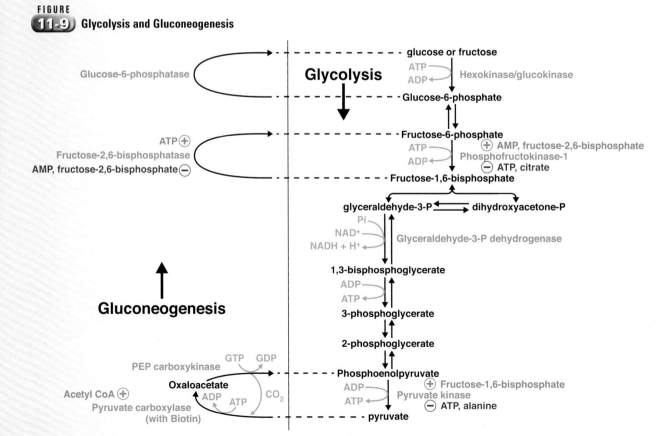

Enzymes are in blue; enzyme stimulators are in green; enzyme inhibitors are in red.

5. Glyceraldehyde-3-phosphate → 1,3-bisphosphoglycerate via **glyceraldehyde-3-phosphate dehydrogenase** (GAPDH)
6. Phosphoenolpyruvate (PEP) → pyruvate via **pyruvate kinase**
   a. Promoted by fructose-1,6-bisphosphate
   b. Inhibited by ATP and alanine
7. **Phosphofructokinase-2/fructose bisphosphatase-2** (PFK-2/FBP-2) can promote either glycolysis or gluconeogenesis.
   a. Fed state: PFK-2 promotes glycolysis by converting glucose-6-phosphate to fructose-2,6-bisphosphate, which allosterically activates PFK-1.
   b. Fasting state: Glucagon binds cellular receptors, stimulating adenylyl cyclase to convert ATP to cAMP. cAMP activates protein kinase A, which phosphorylates PFK-2, inactivating it, and activating FBP-2. FBP-2 then converts fructose-1,6-bisphosphate to fructose-6-phosphate, which can then enter gluconeogenesis.

Gluconeogenesis (*Figure 11-9*)

A. Overview
1. Overall reaction: 2 pyruvate→ glucose. This requires four ATP, two GTP, and two nicotinamide adenine dinucleotide (NADH).
2. Rate-limiting step: Fructose-1,6-bisphosphate → fructose-6-phosphate via fructose-1,6-bisphosphatase.
3. The steps of gluconeogenesis are essentially the steps of glycolysis reversed, with a few exceptions (Table 11-1).
4. Whereas all cells can perform glycolysis, most cannot perform gluconeogenesis. This occurs mainly in the liver, as well as the kidneys and small intestine under fasting conditions.
5. Nongluconeogenic cells lack **glucose-6-phosphatase**. These cells cannot convert glucose-6-phosphate (G6P) to glucose in the final step of gluconeogenesis. G6P is then shunted into the glycogenesis pathway.
6. Pyruvate may come from a number of sources, including TCA cycle intermediates and amino acids.

B. Important Steps
1. Pyruvate → **oxaloacetate** via pyruvate carboxylase. This requires biotin and ATP.
   a. Promoted by acetyl-CoA.
2. Oxaloacetate → malate, which requires NADH. Malate is then transported out of the mitochondrion into the cytosol. Malate → oxaloacetate, which requires NAD^+.
   a. Gluconeogenesis mainly occurs in the cytosol, but oxaloacetate cannot cross the mitochondrial membrane. It must first be converted to malate, which can move across via transporter proteins. Once in the cytosol, malate is converted back into oxaloacetate.
3. Oxaloacetate → PEP via PEP carboxykinase. This requires GTP.
4. 3-phosphoglycerate → 1,3-bisphosphoglycerate. This requires ATP.
5. Fructose-1,6-bisphosphate → fructose-6-phosphate via fructose-1,6-bisphosphatase.
   a. Promoted by ATP
   b. Inhibited by AMP and fructose-2,6-bisphosphate
6. Glucose-6-phosphate → glucose via glucose-6-phosphatase. Glucose can now exit the cell.

C. Cori Cycle (*Figure 11-10*)
1. Overall reaction: Pyruvate → lactate → pyruvate.
2. This is also known as the lactic acid cycle.
3. Pyruvate is converted to lactate via lactate dehydrogenase in cells.
4. Lactic acid is then released into the blood where it travels to the liver.
5. Lactate is converted to pyruvate in the liver, also via lactate dehydrogenase.
6. Pyruvate then enters gluconeogenesis, and is converted to glucose.

Glycogenesis

A. Overview
1. Overall reaction: Glucose → glycogen, requiring one ATP per glucose molecule.
2. Rate-limiting step: UDP-glucose attachment to glycogen molecule via **glycogen synthase**.

TABLE **11-1** Glycolysis vs. Gluconeogenesis			
Glycolysis Enzymes	**Intermediates**	**Gluconeogenesis Enzymes**	**Reversible?**
	Glucose		
Hexokinase/Glucokinase	↓ ↑	**Glucose-6-phosphatase**	**No**
	Glucose-6-phosphate		
Phosphoglucose isomerase	↓↑	Phosphoglucose isomerase	Yes
	Fructose-6-phosphate		
PFK-1/FBP-2	↓ ↑	PFK-1/**FBP-2**	**No**
	Fructose-1,6-bisphosphate		
Aldolase	↓↑	Aldolase	Yes
	Glyceraldehyde-3-P + DHAP		
Glyceraldehyde-3-phosphate dehydrogenase	↓↑	Glyceraldehyde-3-phosphate dehydrogenase	Yes
	1,3-bisphosphoglycerate		
Phosphoglycerate kinase	↓↑	Phosphoglycerate kinase	Yes
	3-phosphoglycerate		
Phosphoglycerate mutase	↓↑	Phosphoglycerate mutase	Yes
	2-phosphoglycerate		
Enolase	↓↑	Enolase	Yes
	Phosphoenolpyruvate		
Pyruvate kinase	↑	**PEP carboxykinase**	
↓	**Oxaloacetate**		**No**
	↑	**Pyruvate carboxylase**	
	Pyruvate		

PFK-2/FBP-2, Phosphofructokinase-2/Fructose-1,6-bisphosphatase-2.

FIGURE
11-10 Cori cycle

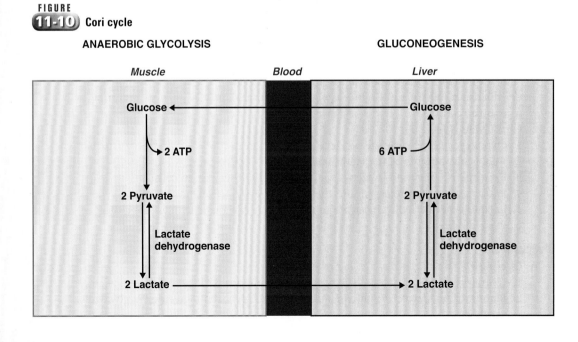

3. Glucose is converted into chains and attached to existing glycogen molecules.

4. Glucose conversion to glucose-6-phosphate requires one ATP, but glycogenesis mainly begins with glucose-6-phosphate from gluconeogenesis.

5. Occurs in skeletal muscles and hepatocytes.

B. Important Steps

1. Glucose → glucose-6-phosphate via glucokinase or hexokinase. This requires ATP.

2. Glucose-6-phosphate → glucose-1-phosphate via phosphoglucomutase.

3. Glucose-1-phosphate → UDP-glucose via UDP-glucose phosphorylase. This requires UTP.

4. UDP-glucose is attached to a glucose chain on the glycogen molecule through an α-1,4 linkage via glycogen synthase.

5. Glucose chains are attached to other glucose chains midstrand through α-1,6 linkages. This is catalyzed by **branching enzyme**.

Glycogenolysis (Figure 11-11)

A. Overview

1. <u>Overall reaction</u>: Glycogen → glucose. This does not consume ATP.

2. <u>Rate-limiting step</u>: Breakdown of α-1,4 linkages by **glycogen phosphorylase**.

3. Glucose monomers are sequentially removed from glycogen, and processed into glucose.

4. Requires the breakdown of both the α-1,4 and the α-1,6 linkages.

B. Important Steps

1. α-1,4 linkages are broken down by glycogen phosphorylase to yield glucose-1-phosphate.
   a. Promoted by epinephrine and glucagon
   b. Inhibited by insulin

2. Glucose-1-phosphate → glucose-6-phosphate via phosphoglucomutase.

3. Glucose-6-phosphate → glucose via glucose-6-phosphatase.
   c. Because most cells cannot perform this step, glucose-6-phosphate is then used to generate ATP through glycolysis.

4. α-1,6 linkages are broken down by α-1,6 glucosidase. This reaction produces glucose directly.

Glycogen Storage Diseases (Figure 11-11)

A. McArdle Disease

1. Autosomal recessive deficiency of **myophosphorylase** (muscle isoform of glycogen phosphorylase). This is also known as type V glycogen storage disease.

2. Muscle cells are unable to break down the α-1,4 linkages of glycogen.

3. Muscle cells then swell due to increased glycogen as well as osmotic influx of water.

4. Lysis of muscle cells releases myoglobin, which can interfere with kidney function (**rhabdomyolysis**).

5. **Presentation:** Muscle cramps, muscle weakness, fatigue, burgundy-colored urine.

6. **Labs:** ↑ Creatine kinase, myoglobinuria.

7. **Treatment:** Restriction of intense physical activity.

B. Von Gierke Disease

1. Autosomal recessive deficiency of glucose-6-phosphatase. It is also known as type I glycogen storage disease.

2. The inability to synthesize glucose (either from gluconeogenesis or glycogenolysis) affects hepatocytes, kidney cells, and small intestine cells.

3. Glucose-6-phosphate is shunted into glycogenesis, resulting in excess glycogen.

4. **Presentation:** Seizures (due to severe hypoglycemia), hepatomegaly, hypertension, xanthomas.

5. **Labs:** ↑ Serum lactate, hyperlipidemia, nephropathy, gout.

6. **Treatment:** Diet containing high protein and cornstarch (cornstarch takes longer to break down, resulting in a slow, steady release of glucose that can prevent hypoglycemia in glycogen storage diseases). Liver transplantation may be necessary in severe cases.

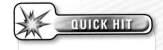

QUICK HIT

Cornstarch is ineffective in the treatment of McArdle disease, where liver glycogen storage is normal.

Biochemistry and Genetics

FIGURE
11-11 Glycogenolysis and glycogen storage disorders

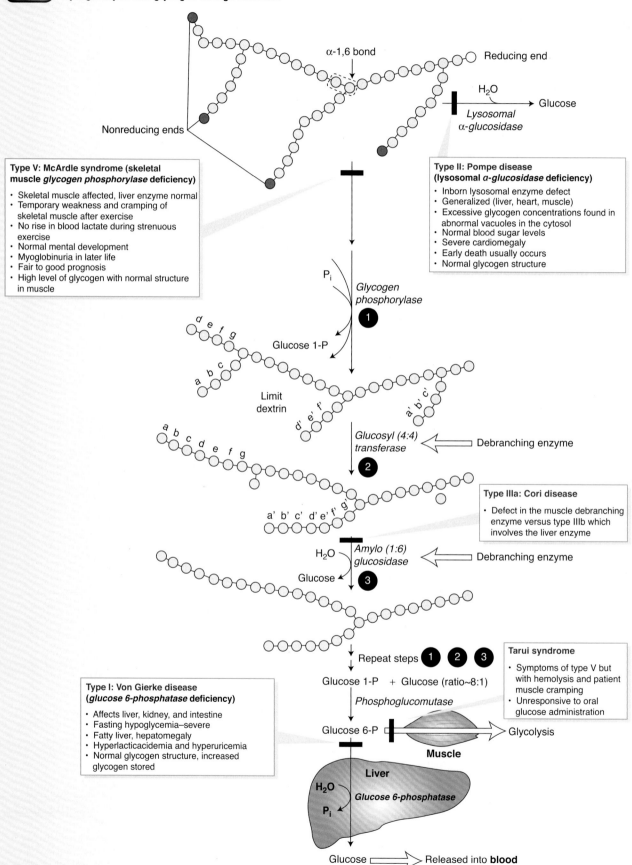

Type V: McArdle syndrome (skeletal muscle _glycogen phosphorylase_ deficiency)

- Skeletal muscle affected, liver enzyme normal
- Temporary weakness and cramping of skeletal muscle after exercise
- No rise in blood lactate during strenuous exercise
- Normal mental development
- Myoglobinuria in later life
- Fair to good prognosis
- High level of glycogen with normal structure in muscle

Type II: Pompe disease (lysosomal _a-glucosidase_ deficiency)

- Inborn lysosomal enzyme defect
- Generalized (liver, heart, muscle)
- Excessive glycogen concentrations found in abnormal vacuoles in the cytosol
- Normal blood sugar levels
- Severe cardiomegaly
- Early death usually occurs
- Normal glycogen structure

Type IIIa: Cori disease

- Defect in the muscle debranching enzyme versus type IIIb which involves the liver enzyme

Tarui syndrome

- Symptoms of type V but with hemolysis and patient muscle cramping
- Unresponsive to oral glucose administration

Type I: Von Gierke disease (_glucose 6-phosphatase_ deficiency)

- Affects liver, kidney, and intestine
- Fasting hypoglycemia–severe
- Fatty liver, hepatomegaly
- Hyperlacticacidemia and hyperuricemia
- Normal glycogen structure, increased glycogen stored

(Adapted with permission from Champe PC, Harvey RA, Ferrier DR. _Lippincott's Illustrated Reviews: Biochemistry._ 2nd ed. Philadelphia, PA: Lippincott-Raven; 1994:41.)

C. Cori Disease
   1. Autosomal recessive deficiency of debranching enzyme. It is also known as type III glycogen storage disease.
   2. Cells are unable to break down the α-1,6 linkages of glycogen (α-1,4 linkages can still be broken down by glycogen phosphorylase).
   3. This is generally mild compared to McArdle disease.
   4. **Presentation:** Seizures, hepatomegaly, splenomegaly, growth retardation.
   5. **Labs:** Hypoglycemia, myoglobinuria, hyperlipidemia, ↑ serum lactate (in some cases).
   6. **Treatment:** Treatment is unnecessary in many cases. A diet containing high protein and cornstarch may be helpful.
D. Pompe Disease
   1. Autosomal recessive deficiency of **lysosomal α-1,4 glucosidase** (part of glycogenolysis in lysosomes).
   2. Glycogen accumulates in lysosomes, disrupting many cellular functions.
      a. Incidental lysosomal uptake of glycogen from the cytosol is normal, and a small percentage of glycogen can be found in the lysosomes of most cells.
      b. The enzymes in lysosomal glycogenolysis must function at a lower pH, and thus differ from enzymes in cytosolic glycogenolysis.
   3. **Presentation:** Breathing difficulty, muscle weakness, macroglossia, hepatomegaly, depressed reflexes.
   4. **Labs:** Aneurysms, cardiomegaly, vacuolar myopathy.
   5. **Treatment:** Alglucosidase alfa (infants only), pulmonary hygiene, high protein diet.

Other Carbohydrates
A. Fructose Metabolism
   1. **Essential fructosuria:** Autosomal recessive deficiency of fructokinase, which converts fructose to fructose-1-phosphate. Fructose appears in the blood and urine and causes mild diuresis. This is a relatively benign condition.
      a. Essential fructosuria does not cause osmotic damage because unphosphorylated fructose simply diffuses back out of the cells.
   2. **Aldolase B deficiency:** Autosomal recessive disease in which fructose metabolism stalls, resulting in the accumulation of fructose-1-phosphate. This trapping of phosphate impairs glycolysis and gluconeogenesis, and causes hypoglycemia, vomiting, jaundice, and cirrhosis. The treatment is decreased fructose/sucrose intake.
B. Galactose Metabolism
   1. **Galactokinase deficiency:** An autosomal recessive disease that causes the accumulation of galactitol. This causes cataracts because the lens of the eye is particularly sensitive to sugar accumulation.
      a. Galactose is reduced to galactitol by intracellular aldose reductase, an enzyme that is normally involved in the synthesis of fructose from glucose.
   2. **Galactosemia:** An autosomal recessive deficiency of galactose-1-phosphate uridylyltransferase. This causes accumulation of galactose-1-phosphate, which causes more severe cataracts than in galactokinase deficiency. It also causes hepatomegaly, jaundice, failure to thrive, and mental retardation. The treatment is galactose and lactose restriction.
C. Lactose Metabolism
   1. **Lactase deficiency:** An autosomal recessive disease that causes lactose intolerance. Lactose is a dimer, so it does not get absorbed by enterocytes. It then moves into the intestine, where it is processed by bacteria. This causes gas, bloating, and osmotic diarrhea. This can be treated with lactase supplementation or dairy restriction.
      a. Temporary lactase deficiency can result from infections that erode microvilli, the main source of lactase.
D. Ethanol Metabolism
   1. Ethanol can be converted to acetaldehyde via **alcohol dehydrogenase**. This generates NADH.
      a. Alcohol dehydrogenase follows zero-order kinetics. This means that its rate is independent of the concentration of ethanol.

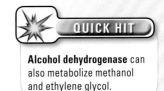

Alcohol dehydrogenase can also metabolize methanol and ethylene glycol.

Biochemistry and Genetics

2. Acetaldehyde is further converted to acetate via **acetaldehyde dehydrogenase**. This also generates NADH.
   a. NADH made in this manner does not usually enter the electron transport chain because ethanol metabolism takes place in the liver.
   b. NADH builds up and must be reoxidized to NAD^+. The liver accomplishes this by converting pyruvate to lactate and oxaloacetate to malate. This impairs the TCA cycle and gluconeogenesis and causes hypoglycemia.
3. Acetate can then be converted to acetyl-CoA, resulting in more NADH and $FADH_2$.
4. **Fomepizole:** Inhibits alcohol dehydrogenase. It is used as an antidote for methanol and ethylene glycol poisoning.
5. **Disulfiram:** Inhibits acetaldehyde dehydrogenase. Buildup of acetaldehyde causes vomiting, and flushing. Thus, disulfiram is prescribed to recovering alcoholics to deter drinking.

OXIDATIVE PROCESSES

Aerobic Respiration (Oxidative Phosphorylation)

A. **Electron Transport Chain** (*Figure 11-12*)
1. Occurs in the mitochondria. Electrons are transferred from NADH or $FADH_2$ to membrane-bound protein complexes.
2. Electrons move down chain through a series of redox reactions. This provides energy for each complex to pump protons from the mitochondrial matrix to the intermembranous space.
3. This creates an electrochemical gradient. Protons then flow down the gradient through **ATP synthase**, which uses the energy to synthesize ATP.

FIGURE
 Electron transport chain

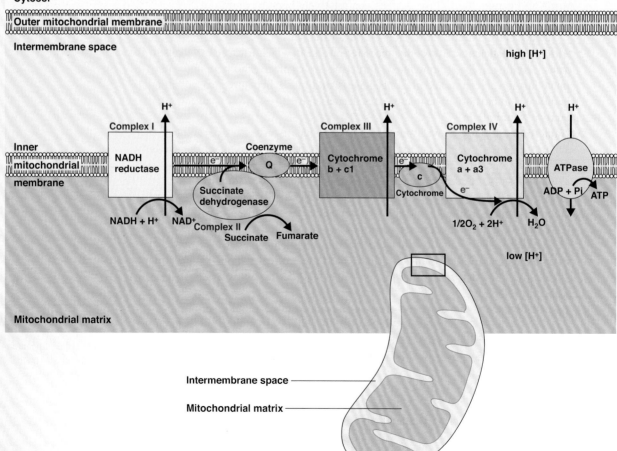

NAD, nicotinamide adenine dinucleotide; e⁻, electron.

B. Important Steps

1. **Complex I:** Also known as NADH dehydrogenase. It converts NADH to NAD^+.
2. **Complex II:** Also known as succinate dehydrogenase. It converts $FADH_2$ to FAD. This requires **coenzyme Q**.
   a. The transfer of electrons from $FADH_2$ to complex II occurs at a lower energy level than at complex I. This is why $FADH_2$ provides fewer ATP molecules than NADH.
3. **Complex III:** Contains cytochromes B and C1. This transfers electrons to **cytochrome C**.
4. **Complex IV:** Cytochromes A and A3. It accepts electrons from cytochrome C. Electrons join oxygen and hydrogen to form water.
5. **Complex V:** ATP synthase. Protons travel through this complex from the inter-membranous space to the mitochondrial matrix. This powers the synthesis of ATP from ADP and P_i.

C. Inhibitors of the Electron Transport Chain

1. **Complex I:** Inhibited by amobarbital (barbiturate), rotenone, and methyl-phenyl-pyridinium (MPP).
   a. MPP comes from the in vivo processing of 1-methl-4-phenyl-1,2,3,6-tetrahydropyridine (MPTP), a neurotoxin that destroys dopaminergic neurons. MPTP is an impurity that can form during the attempted synthesis of 1-methyl-4-phenyl-4-propionoxypiperidine (MPPP), an opioid and meperidine analog.
2. **Complex III:** Inhibited by antimycin A.
3. **Complex IV:** Inhibited by cyanide, sodium azide, carbon monoxide, hydrogen sulfide.
4. **Uncoupling agents:** Allow protons to bypass ATP synthase when crossing the membrane. This wastes energy, generating heat.
   a. **Thermogenin:** Natural substance found in brown fat. It generates heat in cold temperatures.
   b. **2,4-Dinitrophenol:** Found in wood preserving agents.
   c. **Aspirin:** Uncoupling action causes hyperthermia in aspirin overdose.

Other Oxidative Processes

A. Tricarboxylic Acid Cycle (Figure 11-13)

1. <u>Overall reaction</u>: Pyruvate → Oxaloacetate + 3 NADH + 1 $FADH_2$ + 1 GTP.
2. <u>Rate-limiting step</u>: Isocitrate → α-ketoglutarate via isocitrate dehydrogenase.
3. Replenishes reducing agents and provides precursors and intermediates for a number of reactions.
4. Pyruvate is converted to acetyl-CoA via the **pyruvate dehydrogenase complex**. This reaction requires thiamine pyrophosphate (TPP), lipoic acid, coenzyme A (CoA), flavin adenine dinucleotide (FAD), and nicotinamide adenine dinucleotide (NAD^+).
   a. **Pyruvate dehydrogenase deficiency:** Pyruvate is shunted into other pathways. Excess conversion of pyruvate to lactate causes lactic acidosis. Neurologic defects are common. Diets high in fat can provide other substrates for acetyl-CoA synthesis. Ketogenic amino acids (Lys, Leu) are also helpful.
   b. The most common form displays an X-linked dominant pattern of inheritance. Other forms are autosomal recessive.
   c. This may be an acquired deficiency, often due to **arsenic poisoning** or lack of thiamine (common in alcoholics).
5. Acetyl-CoA is converted to citrate via citrate synthase.
6. Isocitrate is converted to α-ketoglutarate via isocitrate dehydrogenase. This step produces NADH, and requires the exact same cofactors as pyruvate dehydrogenase.
7. α-Ketoglutarate is then converted to succinyl-CoA via α-ketoglutarate dehydrogenase. This step produces NADH.

B. Hexose Monophosphate (HMP) Shunt (Pentose Phosphate Pathway)

1. <u>Overall reaction</u>: Glucose-6-phosphate → nicotinamide adenine dinucleotide phosphate (NADPH) and **ribulose-5-phosphate**.
2. NADPH is required for fatty acid synthesis, cholesterol synthesis, oxygen free radical generation, protection from oxidative damage, and cytochrome p450 activities.
3. Ribulose-5-phosphate is used to generate PRPP, which is required for nucleotide synthesis.

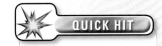

QUICK HIT

Coenzyme Q supplementation may optimize this process. Heart attack patients receive coenzyme Q to maximize the capacity of cardiac myocytes to generate ATP.

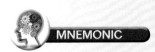

MNEMONIC

Remember the cofactors for **pyruvate dehydrogenase** by the phrase, "Tender Loving Care For Nobody":
TPP
Lipoic acid
CoA
FAD
NAD$^+$

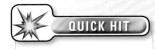

QUICK HIT

Arsenic inhibits lipoic acid. Arsenic poisoning presents with garlic breath, rice water stool, and vomiting.

Biochemistry and Genetics

FIGURE
11-13 Tricarboxylic acid cycle

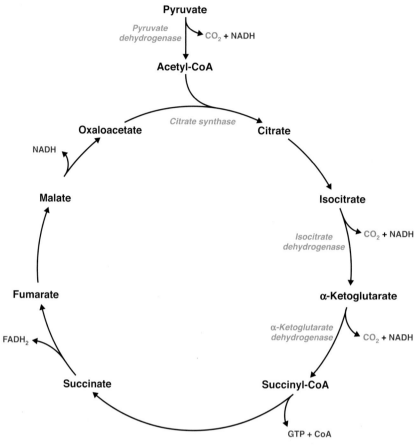

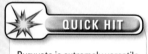

TABLE 11-2 Paths of Pyruvate

Reaction	Enzyme	Subsequent Pathway
Pyruvate → Oxaloacetate	Pyruvate carboxylase	Gluconeogenesis
Pyruvate → Lactate	Lactate dehydrogenase	Cori cycle
Pyruvate → Alanine	Alanine transaminase	Alanine cycle
Pyruvate → Acetyl-CoA	Pyruvate dehydrogenase	TCA cycle

C. Antioxidant Functions
   1. Protects cells against oxidative damage.
   2. RBCs convert H_2O_2 to H_2O via glutathione peroxidase. This requires glutathione
      and NADPH.
   3. **Glucose-6-phosphate dehydrogenase deficiency:** X-linked recessive disease, re-
      sulting in the inability to synthesize NADPH. RBCs are vulnerable to oxidative
      damage, resulting in hemolytic anemia. Heinz bodies and bite cells are seen on
      blood smear. Patients must avoid substances that cause oxidative damage, such
      as fava beans, sulfonamides, and antimalarial drugs.
D. Oxidative Burst
   1. There are two different reactive oxygen species that are used in the oxidative
      burst: superoxide and hydrogen peroxide. In addition, hydrogen peroxide can
      be used to create hypochlorous acid.
   2. O_2 + NADPH → $NADP^+$ + H^+ + O_2^- (superoxide) via **NADPH oxidase**.
   3. O_2^- + H^+ → O_2 + H_2O_2 (hydrogen peroxide) via superoxide dismutase.

4. $H_2O_2 + Cl^- \rightarrow H_2O + HOCl$ (hypochlorous acid) via myeloperoxidase.

5. Superoxide, hydrogen peroxide, and hypochlorous acid are all important in antibacterial immune functions.

6. **Chronic granulomatous disease:** X-linked recessive or autosomal recessive deficiency of NADPH oxidase. Macrophages cannot synthesize reactive oxygen species, although they can still utilize exogenous hydrogen peroxide. However, this is ineffective against catalase-positive organisms (e.g., *Staphylococcus aureus*, *Aspergillus*), making patients vulnerable to these infections.

 ## LIPID METABOLISM

Lipoproteins (*Table 11-3*)

A. **Transport**

1. Triglycerides are broken down in the small intestine by pancreatic lipase.

2. **Chylomicrons:** Created from dietary fat by enterocytes and released into the lymph via ApoB48. Chylomicrons enter the blood, where peripheral cells pull triglycerides from them as they circulate. The remnants travel to the liver and are taken up by lipoprotein-related receptor protein (LRP).

   a. Peripheral cells take triglycerides from lipoproteins using the enzyme lipoprotein lipase.

3. **VLDL:** Very low-density lipoprotein (VLDL) is created from chylomicron remnants, and is released into the blood via ApoB100.

4. **IDL:** Once VLDL has lost a significant amount of triglycerides, it is known as intermediate density lipoprotein (IDL).

5. **LDL:** When IDL has lost most of its remaining triglycerides, it is known as low-density lipoprotein (LDL). It can serve as a cholesterol source for other cells (especially hepatocytes) via clathrin-mediated endocytosis or LRP.

6. **HDL:** High-density lipoprotein (HDL) is synthesized in the liver and can accept excess cholesterol from cells via lecithin cholesterol acyltransferase (LCAT). It may then donate cholesterol to VLDL or to LDL via cholesterol ester transfer protein (CETP) or to hepatocytes via scavenger receptor B1 (SRB1). For this reason, the cholesterol content of HDL varies widely.

7. **Abetalipoproteinemia:** Autosomal recessive mutation in microsomal triglyceride transfer protein (MTTP) that prevents synthesis of ApoB48 and ApoB100. Enterocytes cannot release chylomicrons into lymph. This causes steatorrhea in infancy, and failure to thrive. Swollen enterocytes are seen on biopsy. Acanthocytes, night blindness, and ataxia are also common. This can be treated with vitamin E.

B. **Apolipoproteins**

1. ApoB48: Mediates secretion of chylomicrons from intestine

2. ApoB100: Found on VLDL, IDL, and LDL

3. ApoE: Mediates extra remnant uptake

4. ApoA1: Activates LCAT. Found on HDL

5. ApoC2: Cofactor for lipoprotein lipase

TABLE 11-3 **Lipoprotein Composition**		
Lipoprotein	**% Triacylglycerols**	**% Cholesterol**
Chylomicrons	84–86	5
VLDL	55	19–25
IDL	31	29–30
LDL	6–10	50
HDL	4–6	16–50 (highly variable)

Biochemistry and Genetics

FIGURE
11-14 Signs of hyperlipidemia

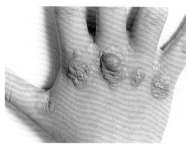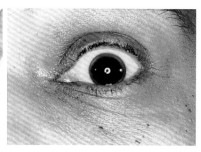

A. Xanthomas in the skin and tendons. **B**. Corneal arcus lipoides represents the deposition of lipids in the peripheral cornea. (Reprinted with permission from Rubin E, Farber JL. *Pathology*. 3rd ed. Philadelphia, PA: Lippincott-Raven; 1999.)

C. Dyslipidemia
   1. An abnormal amount of lipids in the blood. Most cases of dyslipidemia are classified as hyperlipidemia.
   2. **Type I hyperlipidemia:** Autosomal recessive mutation of lipoprotein lipase or ApoC2 (activates lipoprotein lipase). This causes hyperchylomicronemia, which leads to acute pancreatitis, hepatosplenomegaly, and eruptive xanthomas.
   3. **Type IIa hyperlipidemia:** Autosomal dominant mutation that causes a decrease or absence of LDL receptors. This leads to increased LDL causing familial hypercholesterolemia. The result is accelerated atherosclerosis, tendon xanthomas (especially the Achilles tendon), xanthomas around the eyelids, and corneal arcus (grayish-blue ring around the cornea) (*Figure 11-14*).
      a. Homozygosity in type IIa hyperlipidemia causes earlier onset of symptoms.
   4. **Type IV hyperlipidemia:** Autosomal dominant defect in VLDL production in the liver. This leads to familial hypertriglyceridemia, which causes acute pancreatitis.

Cholesterol and Fatty Acids
   A. Cholesterol Synthesis
      1. <u>Overall reaction</u>: Acetyl-CoA + acetoacetyl-CoA → cholesterol
      2. <u>Rate-limiting step</u>: 3-Hydroxy-3-methylglutaryl coenzyme A (HMG-CoA) → mevalonate via **HMG-CoA reductase**
      3. Inhibited by statins
   B. Fatty Acid Synthesis
      1. <u>Overall reaction</u>: Acetyl-CoA → fatty acids.
      2. <u>Rate-limiting step</u>: Acetyl-CoA → malonyl-CoA via acetyl-CoA carboxylase.
      3. Occurs in the cytoplasm of hepatocytes.
      4. Citrate is transferred out of the mitochondria to the cytoplasm.
      5. Citrate and CoA are then converted to oxaloacetate and acetyl-CoA.
      6. Acetyl-CoA is then converted to malonyl-CoA, or to Acetyl-ACP.
         a. Acyl carrier protein (ACP) is a specialized protein that binds acyl groups from acyl-CoA.
      7. Malonyl-CoA is then converted to malonyl-ACP.
      8. Malonyl-CoA and acetyl-CoA are converted to butyryl-ACP.
      9. The reaction is repeated to elongate the chain into palmitoyl-ACP (a 16-carbon chain), which is then hydrolyzed to palmitate.
   C. Fatty Acid Oxidation
      1. <u>Overall reaction</u>: Fatty acid → acetyl-CoA.
      2. <u>Rate-limiting step</u>: Acyl-CoA + carnitine → acyl carnitine by carnitine acyltransferase I. After the fatty acid chain is bound to a molecule of CoA, it is then bound to carnitine for transfer from the cytoplasm through the mitochondrial membrane.
      3. In the mitochondria, beta oxidation breaks down fatty acids into molecules of acetyl-CoA.
      4. **Carnitine acyltransferase deficiency:** Accumulation of fatty acids in the cytoplasm causes weakness, hypotonia, and hypoketotic hypoglycemia.

D. Omega-3 Fatty Acids

1. Essential fatty acids (meaning they cannot be synthesized in the body). They are found in fish oils and flaxseed oil.
2. Omega-3 fatty acids are named for the position of the unsaturated bond at the third carbon.
3. Three forms: eicosapentanoic acid (EPA), docosahexanoic acid (DHA), and alpha linolenic acid (ALA).
4. Omega-3 fatty acids are supplemented in hypertriglyceridemia to lower serum triglyceride levels. They can reduce arrhythmias and may augment nerve and eye development in utero. Additionally, they also reduce inflammation in rheumatoid arthritis.

MALNUTRITION

A. Ketogenesis

1. <u>Overall reaction</u>: 2 acetyl-CoA → acetoacetate.
2. <u>Rate-limiting step</u>: Acetoacetyl-CoA → HMG-CoA via HMG-CoA synthase.
3. Synthesized in the liver. Fatty acids and amino acids are metabolized to **acetoacetate**.
4. Acetoacetate and NADH can then be converted to β-**hydroxybutyrate**. Acetoacetate and β-hydroxybutyrate are two of the three ketone bodies (the third is **acetone**).
5. Ketone bodies can be used by many cells but most importantly, muscle and brain cells.
6. Ketogenesis occurs when the oxidative capacity of the TCA cycle is exceeded due to excess acetyl-CoA from fatty acid breakdown or when oxaloacetate is depleted due to increased gluconeogenesis, as in starvation.
7. Ketone bodies are metabolized into 2 acetyl-CoA upon reaching other sites.
8. Acetoacetate can spontaneously lose a carbon dioxide (CO_2) to become acetone. This causes fruity-smelling breath, a hallmark of ketosis and diabetic ketoacidosis.

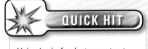

QUICK HIT

Urinalysis for ketones tests for acetoacetate but not β-hydroxybutyrate.

B. Fasting State

1. Postabsorptive period:
   a. Glucose is produced in the liver through glycogenolysis and gluconeogenesis.
   b. Fatty acids are produced from adipocytes beginning 4 to 6 hours after the last meal.
   c. Glycogen stores are depleted 10 to 18 hours after the last meal.
2. Starvation mode:
   a. Glycogenolysis is low because glycogen stores have been depleted.
   b. Gluconeogenesis is occurring at a high rate.
   c. Fatty acids are being released and broken down.
   d. The brain predominantly uses glucose at this point, whereas the muscles and other tissues mainly use fatty acids.
   e. Ketogenesis begins in intermediate starvation.

C. Malnutrition States

1. **Kwashiorkor:** Caused by protein malnutrition. The inability to maintain skin regeneration causes lesions. Patients develop fatty liver. Low serum protein creates an osmotic imbalance and causes edema.
   a. Fatty liver is due to an inability to synthesize ApoB100, which normally allows lipoproteins to leave the liver.
2. **Marasmus:** A condition resulting from total caloric malnutrition. This is characterized by tissue and muscle wasting, loss of subcutaneous fat, and variable edema.
3. **Refeeding syndrome:** The result of sudden food intake after prolonged starvation. During fasting, the body adapts by releasing osmotically active substances (e.g., potassium, phosphates) into the blood to maintain osmotic balance. A sudden increase in caloric intake causes all cells to shift from fasting to fed state at once, resulting in uptake of many nutrients in blood. This depletion of magnesium, phosphate, potassium, etc. from the blood can cause arrhythmias and neurologic problems.

ENZYMATIC CATALYSTS

Minerals

A. Iron

  1. Found in hemoglobin and myoglobin. Iron is stored in the liver, spleen, and bone marrow.

  2. **Ferritin:** Binds iron and stores it within cells. Ferritin is found in high concentration in hepatocytes. It is also an acute-phase reactant (the liver releases ferritin to bind up free iron, in order to sequester it from pathogens).

  3. **Transferrin:** Binds free ferric molecules and transports them through the plasma. Transferrin is increased in cases of iron deficiency.

  4. **Iron poisoning:** Causes peroxidation of lipid membranes and free radical generation. Iron poisoning initially results in gastric bleeding and hypovolemic shock. Metabolic acidosis follows, and gastrointestinal (GI) scarring can create obstructions weeks later.

B. Zinc

  1. Common cofactor for many enzymatic reactions.

  2. Zinc is required for zinc-finger DNA transcription factors, as well as lactate dehydrogenase, and carbonic anhydrase. Zinc is also required for optimal immune responses.

  3. Zinc is supplemented in patients healing from wounds because these patients have a higher zinc requirement due to increased DNA transcription.

  4. **Zinc deficiency:** Causes delayed wound healing, decreased immune response, acrodermatitis enteropathica (rash around eyes, mouth, nose, and anus), anorexia, diarrhea, growth retardation, depressed mental function, poor night vision, infertility.

C. Calcium

  1. Parathyroid hormone (PTH) regulates calcium metabolism. Excess PTH causes hypercalcemia and "stones, bones, groans, and psychiatric overtones."

  2. Hypocalcemia presents with Trousseau sign (carpal muscle spasm upon tightening of blood pressure cuff), and Chvostek sign (facial muscle spasm upon tapping the cheek).

  3. Calcium is required for muscle contraction, neurotransmitter release, platelet function, coagulation cascades, and various intracellular processes including the utilization of ATP and glucose.

D. Lead

  1. **Lead poisoning:** Decreased IQ, hearing problems, growth impairment, peripheral neuropathy, wrist drop, foot drop, lead lines in bone *(Figure 11-15)* and gingivae, anemia, nephropathy, encephalopathy.

  2. Children living in homes that were painted before 1978 are at greater risk of lead poisoning (lead paint was common before 1978).

  3. The treatment is removal of exposure and chelation (succimer, EDTA, dimercaprol in severe cases).

E. Mercury

  1. **Mercury poisoning:** Mercury accumulates in the kidneys and brain. This causes neurologic problems (e.g., tremor), neuropsychiatric problems (e.g., excitability, insomnia), acrodynia, and abdominal pain.

  2. Poisoning can come from eating too much of certain fish. Mercury is also found in old thermometers and batteries.

Fat-Soluble Vitamins

A. Vitamin A

  1. Forms

    a. **Retinol** is the form in which vitamin A is stored in the liver.

    b. **Retinal** is created from retinol and NAD^+, and it is the active form of vitamin A.

    c. Beta carotene is cleaved in the intestine to yield two molecules of retinal.

    d. **Retinoic acid** is the irreversibly oxidized form of retinol.

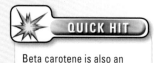

QUICK HIT

Beta carotene is also an antioxidant.

Biochemistry and Genetics

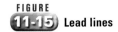

FIGURE
11-15 Lead lines

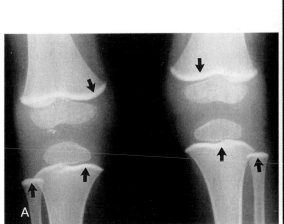
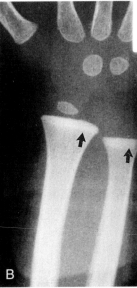

A. AP bilateral knees. **B.** PA wrist. Note the radiodense metaphyseal bands (arrows). (Reprinted with permission from Yochum TR, Rowe LJ. *Yochum and Rowe's Essentials of Skeletal Radiology*. 3rd ed. Philadelphia, PA: Lippincott Williams & Wilkins; 2004.)

2. Function
   a. Retinol and retinal are both required for vision as well as reproduction.
   b. Retinoic acid is required for various functions including maintenance of skin and epithelium (especially mucus-secreting cells) as well as growth.
3. Vitamin A deficiency
   a. Causes night blindness, xerophthalmia (failure to produce tears), and keratomalacia (wrinkling and clouding of the cornea).
   b. Vitamin A deficiency also presents with Bitot spots (dry, silver-gray plaques on the bulbar conjunctiva).
4. Vitamin A toxicity
   a. Results in headache, nausea, vomiting, stupor, dry skin, pruritus, and pseudotumor cerebri (increased intracranial pressure).
   b. Hepatomegaly and cirrhosis may also be seen along with bone and joint pain.
   c. Excess vitamin A can inhibit neural crest cell migration and is contraindicated in pregnant women.
5. Medical uses
   a. Topical retinoic acid is used to treat psoriasis and acne as well as to reduce wrinkles.
   b. Isotretinoin is an oral retinoic acid derivate used to treat acne. It is better known as Accutane.
   c. Vitamin A is also useful in the treatment of measles and acute myelogenous leukemia.

B. Vitamin D
1. Forms
   a. Vitamin D_2, ergocalciferol
   b. Vitamin D_3, cholecalciferol
   c. 1,25-dihydroxy-vitamin D, **calcitriol** (active form of vitamin D)
2. Function
   a. Affects gene expression through interactions with DNA.
   b. Vitamin D also increases calcium and phosphate uptake in the intestines and the distal tubules.
3. Synthesis of active form
   a. Initially, vitamin D_2 is absorbed in the intestine.
   b. Alternatively, vitamin D_3 is synthesized from 7-dehydrocholesterol in the skin in a reaction that is stimulated by UV light.

c. D_2 or D_3 binds to α_1-globulin and is then transported to the liver.
d. In the liver, vitamin D is converted to 25-hydroxy-vitamin D by 25-hydroxylase. This can also happen in macrophages.
e. 25-hydroxy-vitamin D leaves the liver and travels to the kidney, where it is converted to 1,25-dihydroxy-vitamin D by α_1-hydroxylase. This is the active form.

4. Vitamin D deficiency
   a. Known as osteomalacia in adults and rickets in children.
   b. Deficiency of vitamin D causes hypocalcemia, which increases PTH. PTH then promotes bone resorption and decreases renal calcium excretion. PTH also promotes excretion of phosphate, leading to inhibition of bone mineralization because bone is mostly calcium phosphate.
   c. Symptoms include lumbar lordosis, pectus carinatum, bow-legged appearance, and rachitic rosary (overgrowth of the cartilage or osteoid tissue at the costochondral junctions).
   d. Dark-skinned individuals may be deficient in vitamin D. Increased melanin in the skin absorbs UV light that might otherwise be used for vitamin D production.

5. Vitamin D toxicity
   a. Excess vitamin D can cause hypercalcemia.
   b. Sarcoidosis can lead to excess vitamin D. Macrophages in granulomas may overproduce 25-hydroxy-vitamin D.

C. Vitamin E
1. Forms
   a. The most common form is also known as **gamma-tocopherol**.
   b. α-**Tocopherol** is the second most common and it is the most biologically active form.
2. Function
   a. Important in the regulation of enzymatic reactions, gene expression, and platelet aggregation. Vitamin is also important for neurologic function.
   b. Vitamin E is an important antioxidant, and it is incorporated into cell membranes to protect cells from oxidative damage.
3. Vitamin E deficiency
   a. Results in peripheral neuropathy and muscle weakness.
   b. Vitamin E deficiency also causes spinocerebellar degeneration, resulting in ataxia.

D. Vitamin K
1. Forms
   a. Vitamin K_1, also known as phylloquinone, is found in green, leafy vegetables.
   b. Vitamin K_2 is the main form in animals.
2. Function
   a. Involved in the synthesis of clotting factors as well as proteins C and S.
3. Vitamin K deficiency
   a. Results in hemorrhagic disease.
   b. Newborns are particularly prone to this. They lack the commensal gut bacteria that synthesize vitamin K, and breast milk is very low in vitamin K.
   c. Warfarin, certain anticonvulsants, and antibiotics that kill off gut bacteria can all cause vitamin K deficiency.

Water-Soluble Vitamins
A. Vitamin C
1. Forms
   a. Also known as **ascorbic acid**. There is only one form of vitamin C.
2. Function
   a. Catalyzes the hydroxylation of proline and lysine residues during collagen synthesis.
   b. Vitamin C is also required for the synthesis of norepinephrine from dopamine, and it serves as a circulating antioxidant in the blood.
   c. The absorption of iron is facilitated by vitamin C, which maintains iron in the reduced state.

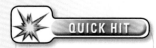

QUICK HIT

Bone resorption is the result of the body's attempt to maintain a minimum level of serum calcium because calcium is involved in muscle contraction, platelet function and coagulation, and neurotransmitter release.

Biochemistry and Genetics

3. Vitamin C deficiency
   a. Also known as scurvy.
   b. Lack of vitamin C causes sore and spongy gums, loose teeth, hemorrhages due to fragile blood vessels, swollen joints, hemarthrosis, impaired wound healing, and anemia.

B. Vitamin B$_{12}$ and Folic Acid
   1. Forms
      a. Vitamin B$_{12}$ is also known as **cobalamin**, named for the cobalt element at its center.
      b. **Tetrahydrofolate** is the biologically active form of folic acid.
      c. N-methyl folate is the intracellular storage form of folic acid.
   2. Function
      a. Required for purine and pyrimidine synthesis.
      b. B$_{12}$ is required for the regeneration of tetrahydrofolate and also for the synthesis of methionine.
      c. B$_{12}$ is also required for the conversion of methylmalonyl-CoA to succinyl-CoA, which can then enter the TCA cycle.
   3. Biosynthesis
      a. Neither plants nor animals can synthesize vitamin B$_{12}$. Bacteria synthesize it effectively though, and this is where all B$_{12}$ ultimately originates. Animals require B$_{12}$, which is why animal products in the diet are the main source of B$_{12}$. Plants do not require B$_{12}$, and thus are very poor sources.
      b. Animals cannot synthesize folate either, but plants can. Plants are thus an important dietary source of folate.
   4. Vitamin B$_{12}$ and folic acid deficiencies
      a. Results in megaloblastic anemia.
      b. B$_{12}$ and folic acid deficiencies can also cause neural tube defects *in utero* and growth failure in children.
      c. B$_{12}$ deficiency can cause a folic acid deficiency.
      d. B$_{12}$ deficiency can also cause homocystinuria, methyl-malonic acid in urine, and myelin degeneration resulting in neurologic symptoms (B$_{12}$ neuropathy is also known as **subacute combined degeneration**).
      e. **Pernicious anemia** is the most common cause of B$_{12}$ deficiency.
      f. **Crohn disease** and **celiac disease** can also cause B$_{12}$ deficiency because both affect the distal ileum where B$_{12}$ is absorbed.

C. Vitamin B$_6$
   1. Forms
      a. There are three natural forms: pyridoxamine, pyridoxine, and pyridoxal.
      b. **Pyridoxal phosphate** is the active form of B$_6$.
   2. Function
      a. Cofactor for amino acid metabolism.
      b. B$_6$, or rather pyridoxal phosphate, is also required for the synthesis of heme, niacin, histamine, GABA, dopamine, epinephrine, and norepinephrine.
   3. Vitamin B$_6$ deficiency
      a. Causes angular cheilitis (*Figure 11-16*), glossitis, hyperirritability, and peripheral neuropathy.
      b. B$_6$ deficiency also causes convulsions due to the lack of the inhibitory neurotransmitter GABA.
      c. Isoniazid can cause B$_6$ deficiency.

D. Thiamine
   1. Forms
      a. Also known as vitamin B$_1$.
      b. **Thiamine pyrophosphate** is the active form of thiamine.
   2. Function
      a. TPP is required for the conversion of pyruvate to acetyl-CoA and the conversion of α-ketoglutarate to succinyl-CoA.
      b. TPP is also needed to convert ribose-5-phosphate to glyceraldehyde-3-phosphate.

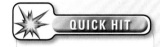

QUICK HIT

The minimum RDA for folic acid in pregnant women is 0.4 mg.

Biochemistry and Genetics

FIGURE
11-16 Angular cheilitis

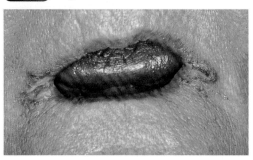

(Reproduced with permission from Neville B, et al. *Color Atlas of Clinical Oral Pathology.* Philadelphia, PA: Lea & Febiger; 1991.

3. Thiamine deficiency
   a. Thiamine deficiency causes **beriberi**. Dry beriberi affects the peripheral nervous system and presents with muscle weakness and peripheral neuropathy. Wet beriberi affects the cardiovascular system, leading to peripheral edema and heart failure.
   b. Thiamine deficiency also causes **Wernicke–Korsakoff syndrome**. This affects the CNS and presents with ocular disturbances, nystagmus, gait ataxia, and **Korsakoff syndrome**, which is characterized by retrograde recall problems, inability to acquire new information, and confabulations.
E. **Riboflavin**
   1. Forms
      a. Also known as vitamin B_2.
      b. The biological forms are **flavin mononucleotide** (FMN) and **flavin adenine dinucleotide** (FAD).
   2. Function
      a. FMN and FAD are cofactors for redox reactions.
   3. Riboflavin Deficiency
      a. Causes dermatitis, angular cheilitis, and glossitis.
F. **Niacin**
   1. Forms
      a. Also known as vitamin B_3.
      b. The biologic forms of niacin are NAD and NADP.
   2. Function
      a. NAD and NADP are important in both DNA repair and steroid hormone synthesis.
   3. Niacin deficiency
      a. Also known as **pellagra**. This presents with dermatitis, diarrhea, and dementia (the three D's of pellagra).
   4. Medical uses
      a. Niacin is used to treat type IIb hyperlipoproteinemia (hypercholesterolemia). It inhibits lipolysis in adipose tissue, leading to decreased fatty acids. This decreases synthesis of VLDL and thus LDL.
      b. Niacin is normally administered with aspirin to avoid a flushing reaction.
G. **Pantothenic Acid**
   1. Forms
      a. Also known as vitamin B_5.
   2. Function
      a. Pantothenic acid is a component of coenzyme A, and is required for the creation of acetyl-CoA.
      b. Pantothenic acid is needed for the TCA cycle, and for the synthesis and oxidation of fatty acids.

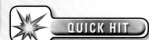

QUICK HIT

Pellagra is common in populations that subsist on corn, which has almost no tryptophan.

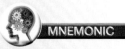

MNEMONIC

Remember the **3 Ds** *of* **pellagra**:
Dementia
Dermatitis
Diarrhea

H. Biotin
  1. Forms
     a. Biotin is also known as vitamin B_7.
  2. Function
     a. Biotin is a cofactor for carboxylation reactions.
  3. Biotin deficiency
     a. Avidin, a glycoprotein found in raw egg whites, can impair absorption of biotin.
     b. Certain antibiotics can also cause biotin deficiency.

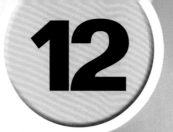

Microbiology

 BACTERIA

I. Bacterial Basics

A. Structure

1. **Gram-positive bacteria** possess a phospholipid membrane surrounded by a thick cell wall (*Figure 12-1, Figure 12-2A*).

2. **Gram-negative bacteria** possess an inner phospholipid membrane surrounded by a thin cell well, which is further surrounded by an outer phospholipid membrane (*Figure 12-1, Figure 12-2B*).

3. **Peptidoglycan:** The main component of bacterial cell walls. It is a rigid sugar backbone with cross-linked side chains.

4. **Teichoic acid:** Provides rigidity to the cell walls of gram-positive bacteria. Teichoic acid also induces secretion of tumor necrosis factor alpha (TNF-α) and interleukin-1 by immune cells.

5. **Periplasm:** Also known as the periplasmic space, this is the area between the inner and outer membranes in gram-negative bacteria, and contains the peptidoglycan cell wall layer. This is the location of β-lactamases.

   a. The space between the gram-positive membrane and the cell wall is also sometimes referred to as the periplasmic space.

6. **Lipopolysaccharide (LPS):** A type of endotoxin, LPS is typically found in the outer membrane of gram-negative bacteria, and induces the secretion of

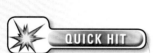

Some bacteria, such as *Mycoplasma*, lack cell walls. Others, such as *Chlamydia*, have atypical cell walls and are not typically classified as gram positive or negative.

 FIGURE 12-1 Gram-negative and gram-positive cell walls

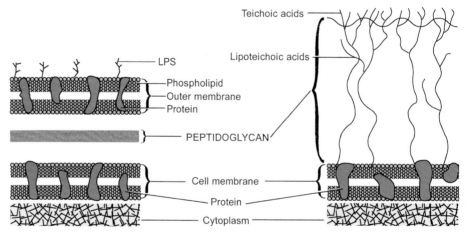

Gram Negative Cell Wall

Gram Positive Cell Wall

(Reprinted with permission from Engelkirk PG, Burton GRW. *Burton's Microbiology for the Health Sciences.* 8th ed. Philadelphia, PA: Lippincott Williams & Wilkins; 2007.)

Microbiology

TNF-α and interleukin-1 by immune cells. Specifically, the immune system responds to a component of LPS called Lipid A.

7. **Glycocalyx:** A polysaccharide layer that surrounds bacteria. When it is highly organized, it is referred to as the bacterial capsule. If it is diffuse and loosely attached, it is simply called a slime layer. It can protect cells from phagocytosis and mediate attachment to foreign surfaces (e.g., catheters, implanted devices).
   a. A capsule can be detected by the addition of anticapsular sera to a bacterial culture, which causes the cells to swell. This is called the **quellung reaction**.

8. **Pili and fimbriae:** Rigid structures extending from the surface of bacteria that mediate attachment to other bacteria or to host cells and tissues. Pili are present in low numbers and are generally used for bacterial conjugation (exchange of genetic material). Fimbriae are present in higher numbers and are used more commonly in biofilm formation.

9. **Flagella:** Long, filamentous structures that provide motility to bacteria.

10. **Plasmids:** Circular DNA found in bacterial cytoplasm. Plasmids are separate from chromosomal DNA and tend to contain genes that code for toxins, antibiotic resistance, and certain enzymes. Plasmids are exchanged between bacteria during conjugation.

B. **Morphology**
1. **Bacilli:** Rod-shaped bacteria. Most genera of bacteria fall into this category, including *Clostridium*, *Salmonella*, *Pseudomonas*, *Bacillus*, *Yersinia*, *Legionella*, *Mycobacteria*, *Listeria*, *Shigella*, *Klebsiella*, *Enterobacter*, *Proteus*, and *Escherichia*. (*Figure 12-2B*)
   a. A "bacillus" is any rod-shaped bacterium, whereas *Bacillus* is a specific genus of bacteria. To further complicate the matter, *Bacilli* is a taxonomic class that contains many non–rod-shaped bacteria, including *Streptococcus*.

2. **Cocci:** Spherical bacteria. Examples include *Streptococcus*, *Staphylococcus*, and *Neisseria* (*Figure 12-2A*).

3. **Coccobacilli:** A bacterial shape between defined rods and defined spheres. Examples include *Gardnerella*, *Coxiella*, *Haemophilus*, and *Bordetella*.

4. **Spirilla:** Spiral-shaped bacteria. Examples include *Borrelia*, *Treponema*, *Leptospira*, and *Spirillum* (rat-bite fever).

5. **Branching filament:** Some bacteria, such as *Nocardia* and *Actinomyces*, grow in a pattern similar to that of fungi. These are called branching filamentous bacteria.

6. **Endospores:** Certain bacteria form endospores under stressful conditions (e.g., low nutrients, low moisture, temperature extremes). These are tough structures encompassing the bacterial DNA and part of the cytoplasm. Examples of endospore-forming bacteria include *Bacillus* and *Clostridium* species.

C. **Aerobes vs. Anaerobes**
1. **Obligate aerobes:** Require oxygen for growth. Obligate aerobic bacteria do not have fermentation mechanisms for energy production. Examples include *Pseudomonas*, *Nocardia*, *Mycobacterium tuberculosis*, and some strains of *Bacillus*.
   a. Certain strains of *Pseudomonas* can use nitrogen compounds instead of oxygen in the electron transport chain and are thus considered to be facultative anaerobes (see following).

2. **Obligate anaerobes:** Incapable of growth in the presence of oxygen. Obligate anaerobic bacteria often lack the enzymes catalase and superoxide dismutase, which would otherwise prevent damage from reactive oxygen species. They obtain energy through fermentation or through the use of alternate electron acceptors. Examples include *Clostridium*, *Bacteroides*, *Actinomyces*, and *Treponema*.
   a. Some obligate anaerobes express both catalase and superoxide dismutase, yet still cannot grow in the presence of oxygen. The reason for this is still under investigation.

3. **Facultative anaerobes:** Bacteria that can obtain energy through aerobic respiration or fermentation, depending on the environment. Examples include *Staphylococcus*, *Escherichia coli*, *Listeria*, *Vibrio*, *Salmonella*, *Shigella*, *Klebsiella*, and some strains of *Haemophilus influenzae*.

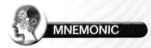

To remember the common encapsulated bacteria, use the sentence, "**E**ven **S**ome **P**retty **N**asty **K**illers **H**ave **S**hiny **B**odies":
- **E**scherichia coli
- **S**treptococcus pneumoniae
- **P**seudomonas aeruginosa
- **N**eisseria meningitides
- **K**lebsiella pneumoniae
- **H**aemophilus influenzae type B
- **S**almonella typhi
- Group **B** Strep

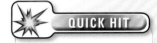

Vibrio species are "comma-shaped" organisms. Depending on the source of information, they may be classified as a form of bacilli, as a form of spirilla, or as neither.

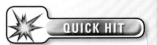

Aminoglycoside antibiotics must be taken up by bacteria through oxygen-dependent transport mechanisms and are thus ineffective against obligate anaerobes. Clindamycin and metronidazole are generally used instead.

Microbiology

4. **Microaerophile:** A specific type of obligate aerobe that requires oxygen but at a lower concentration than is found in the atmosphere. If the oxygen concentration is too high or too low, they will either die or cease to thrive. Examples include *Streptococcus pyogenes*, *Helicobacter pylori*, *Borrelia burgdorferi*, and *Campylobacter*.

5. **Aerotolerance:** Anaerobic bacteria that can thrive in the presence of oxygen, although they cannot use it for energy production. These bacteria are rare, and aerotolerance is generally strain-specific.

D. **Bacterial Genetics**

1. **Conjugation:** Bacteria connect with each other through pili interaction. Plasmids can then be copied and transferred to other bacteria. Chromosomal bacteria can also be transferred through this process, but this is less common.

2. **Transposition:** "Jumping genes" can move from chromosomal DNA to plasmid DNA and vice versa. When coupled with conjugation, this is another method that chromosomal DNA can be transferred between bacteria.

3. **Transduction:** A bacteriophage (a virus that infects bacterial cells) may inadvertently package bacterial DNA into virions and then transfer them into other bacterial cells during subsequent infections.

E. **Bacterial Staining Techniques**

1. **Gram stain:** A staining method for identifying bacteria based on the characteristics of their cell walls (*Figure 12-2*).

a. Bacteria are treated with crystal violet stain, which enters the cells.

b. Iodine is added, forming a large complex with intracellular crystal violet.

c. Cells are treated with alcohol or acetone. Gram-positive bacteria become dehydrated, and the thick peptidoglycan layer shrinks, closing the pores and trapping the crystal violet complexes inside. Gram-negative bacteria lose their outer membrane, and the thin peptidoglycan layer allows the stain to leak out of the cell.

d. Cells are treated with a different stain to allow visualization of the gram-negative bacteria.

e. **Poorly staining bacteria:** *Treponema* (too thin to be visualized), *Mycobacteria* (high lipid content in cell wall interferes with stain), *Mycoplasma* (lack a cell wall), *Legionella pneumophila* (high LPS content interferes with stain), *Chlamydia* (atypical cell wall, intracellular), and *Rickettsia* (primarily intracellular).

2. **Giemsa stain:** Binds phosphate groups of DNA. Used to identify intracellular parasites and bacteria (e.g., *Plasmodium*, *Trypanosoma*, *Histoplasma*, *Chlamydia*).

FIGURE
12-2 Gram stain

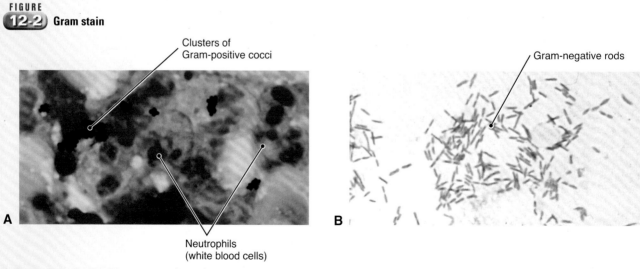

A. Gram-positive cocci (*Staphylococcus aureus*) in pus (large, dark-red globules are white cell nuclei). B. Gram-negative bacilli (*Escherichia coli*), from a culture plate. (Reprinted with permission from McConnell TH. *The Nature of Disease Pathology for the Health Professions.* Philadelphia, PA: Lippincott Williams & Wilkins; 2007.)

Microbiology

3. **Periodic acid-Schiff (PAS) stain:** Detects glycogen, glycoproteins, and proteoglycans. Used commonly to stain macrophages infected with *Tropheryma whipplei* (Whipple disease) because these bacteria have a high amount of glycoprotein in their cell membranes.

4. **Ziehl-Neelsen stain:** Allows differentiation between acid-fast and non–acid-fast organisms. Used to identify bacteria such as *Mycobacterium* and *Nocardia*. (It can also be used to identify *Cryptosporidium*.) Acid-fast organisms have cell walls that contain mycolic acid, which interferes with crystal violet uptake during Gram staining. In the Ziehl-Neelsen method, they are stained instead with carbol fuchsin, which has a high affinity for mycolic acid. When treated with acid or alcohol, they will retain the stain (hence the term "acid-fast"), while non–acid-fast organisms will not.

5. **India ink:** Used in negative staining, where encapsulated organisms are visualized by the empty spaces they form in the dark ink background. This is normally used to stain for *Cryptococcus neoformans*.

6. **Silver stain:** Used to identify fungi, as well as *Legionella*, which stains poorly with Gram stain. Treatment with chromic acid oxidizes polysaccharides in the organisms' cell walls. Further treatment with a silver compound produces a deep black color.

F. **Culture and Identification**

1. **Growth curve:** Used to determine the speed at which a bacterial strain reproduces (*Figure 12-3*).

   a. **Lag phase:** Metabolic activity in preparation for cell division.

   b. **Exponential phase:** Rapid cell division at which point the replication speed reaches its maximum. Also known as the "log phase."

   c. **Stationary phase:** As nutrients in the growth medium are depleted, replication slows to the point that it matches the rate of cell death.

   d. **Death phase:** Nutrient depletion reaches a point where the medium can no longer sustain the bacteria, and they begin to die and break down.

2. **Special growth requirements:** Although most bacteria can grow effectively on standard media (i.e., LB broth/agar, tryptic soy broth/agar, MH broth/agar), others have specific requirements.

   a. *Haemophilus influenzae*: Chocolate agar (MH agar with lysed red blood cells) fortified with V factor (NAD^+) and X factor (hematin)

   b. *Bordetella pertussis*: Bordet-Gengou agar (LB agar containing potato solids and blood)

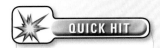

QUICK HIT

PAS stains may also be used in the diagnosis of a number of noninfective conditions, such as glycogen storage diseases, certain adenocarcinomas, and α_1-antitrypsin deficiency.

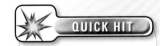

QUICK HIT

India ink is also used in pathology to visualize tumor margins.

Microbiology

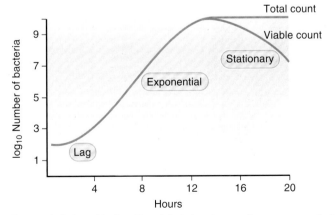

FIGURE 12-3 **Bacterial growth curve**

The growth of a bacterial culture. Bacteria in the inoculum sometimes resume growth slowly (lag phase, hours 0 to 5). They then enter the exponential phase of growth (hours 5 to 10). When foodstuff is exhausted or toxic material accumulates, they enter the stationary phase (hours 10 onward). During the stationary phase, bacterial cultures may lose their viability, as reflected in the viable count, often without losing cell integrity (maintaining a constant total count). (Reprinted with permission from Engleberg NC, Dermody T, DiRita V. *Schaecter's Mechanisms of Microbial Disease.* 4th ed. Baltimore, MD: Lippincott Williams & Wilkins; 2007.)

c. *Corynebacterium diphtheriae*: Grown on Loeffler serum medium (contains animal protein and dextrose) followed by growth on Hoyle agar (contains tellurite and beef extract)

d. *Mycobacterium tuberculosis*: Lowenstein-Jensen agar (Bordet-Gengou agar with asparagine, penicillin, and nalidixic acid)

e. *Mycoplasma pneumoniae*: Eaton agar (LB agar with animal protein, yeast extract, penicillin, and animal serum)

f. *Legionella species*: Buffered charcoal yeast extract agar (charcoal, yeast extract, α-ketoglutarate, cysteine, and iron)

3. **Oxidase test:** The oxidase test determines if a bacterial strain possesses cytochrome c oxidase (complex IV of the electron transport chain).

   a. Oxidase-negative bacteria do not necessarily perform anaerobic respiration. They may simply use a different cytochrome other than cytochrome c for aerobic respiration.

4. **Catalase test:** Catalase degrades hydrogen peroxide into oxygen and water. Bacterial production of catalase is an adaptation that prevents hydrogen peroxide from being converted to reactive oxygen species by host myeloperoxidase. The catalase test simply involves mixing hydrogen peroxide with a sample of bacteria; frothing or bubbling indicates the degradation of the hydrogen peroxide.

5. **Coagulase test:** Coagulase converts fibrinogen to fibrin. The test involves mixing a sample of bacteria with plasma. If coagulase is present, clumping will be observed. This test is classically used to differentiate coagulase-positive *Staphylococcus aureus* from other staphylococci, which are coagulase-negative.

6. **Hemolysis test:** The hemolytic capability of bacteria can be tested by plating samples onto agar containing blood (traditionally sheep or rabbit blood) (*Figure 12-4*).

   a. **α-Hemolysis**, sometimes referred to as partial hemolysis, is seen as a dark green area around the colonies. This is due to oxidation of the hemoglobin in the blood. The term is a misnomer, as no cell lysis actually takes place.

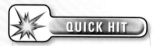

QUICK HIT

A third type of hemolysis, known as γ-hemolysis, actually refers to the total absence of hemolytic activity.

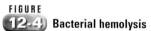

FIGURE 12-4 Bacterial hemolysis

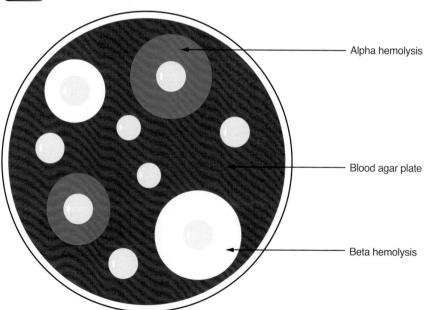

Diagram illustrating the three types of hemolysis that can be observed on a blood agar plate: α-hemolysis (a green zone around the bacterial colony), β-hemolysis (a clear zone around the bacterial colony), and γ-hemolysis (neither a green nor a clear zone around the bacterial colony). Gamma-hemolytic bacteria (also referred to as nonhemolytic bacteria) produce neither of these enzymes and, therefore, cause no change in the red blood cells. (Reprinted with permission from Engelkirk PG, Burton GRW. *Burton's Microbiology for the Health Sciences.* 8th ed. Philadelphia, PA: Lippincott Williams & Wilkins; 2007.)

In clinical microbiology, the classic α-hemolytic bacteria is *Streptococcus pneumoniae*, although Viridans strep are also α-hemolytic.

b. **β-Hemolysis** is complete lysis of the red blood cells and appears on the agar as a cleared area around the colonies. Group A strep are commonly associated with β-hemolysis, although some group B strep, as well as *Listeria* and *Clostridium*, may also display β-hemolysis.

7. **Carbohydrate fermentation test:** Tests the ability of bacteria to ferment various carbohydrates by detecting gas bubbles and acidification of media. Most carbohydrates, such as lactose, maltose, glucose, etc., can be tested. This is generally used to differentiate gram-negative bacteria.

a. MacConkey agar is a lactose-supplemented growth medium that can be used to differentiate gram-negative bacteria based on lactose fermentation. Lactose fermenters appear pink, whereas non-fermenters appear white.

II. Bacterial Toxins

A. Endotoxins

1. Endotoxin is a general term for any toxin found within a cell or attached to a cell membrane/wall.

2. The only endotoxin relevant to human disease is **LPS**, and the two terms are often used interchangeably.

a. Gram-negative bacteria are the only organisms that express LPS.

b. LPS stimulates the secretion of the cytokines interleukin-1, interleukin-6, and TNF-α by immune cells, especially macrophages. This results in inflammation.

c. LPS stimulates the secretion of nitric oxide by macrophages, which causes vasodilation. This is the chief mechanism behind septic shock in endotoxemia.

d. LPS activates the complement pathway, which also causes inflammation as well as histamine release, further contributing to hypotension.

e. Finally, LPS activates factor XII in the coagulation cascade, which can cause disseminated intravascular coagulation (DIC).

3. Several other examples of endotoxins can be found in bacteria that infect plants and insects.

B. Exotoxin Basics

1. Toxins that are secreted are called exotoxins. Unlike endotoxins, there are many different types of exotoxins.

2. Exotoxins are generally polypeptides and, as such, tend to be more antigenic than endotoxin (generate an antibody response).

a. Antibodies are readily generated against protein antigens.

b. Carbohydrate antigens (such as LPS) preferentially stimulate a T cell–independent antigen response, which produces lower affinity IgM rather than IgG. This, combined with the variability of the structure of LPS, makes LPS a relatively poor antigen.

3. Unlike endotoxin, exotoxins can be directly damaging to cells and tissue. They may be encoded by chromosomal DNA, plasmid DNA, or even bacteriophage DNA or RNA. (In contrast, LPS is only encoded by chromosomal DNA.)

4. **Superantigen:** A specialized exotoxin that binds T-cell receptors and major histocompatibility complex (MHC) class II cell surface molecules. This causes generalized, nonspecific T-cell activation, which can result in dangerous systemic inflammation.

a. Normally, the interaction of a T-cell receptor with MHC class II on an antigen-presenting cell is transient. However, when the T-cell receptor recognizes the antigen, the interaction is stabilized long enough for T-cell activation to occur.

b. Superantigens bind both the T-cell receptor and MHC class II outside of the binding groove, artificially stabilizing the interaction, resulting in T-cell activation in the absence of antigen recognition.

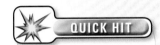

Some texts may report that *Listeria monocytogenes* is unique in that it is the only gram-positive bacterium that expresses LPS. However, this is based on outdated research and has since been disproven.

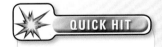

Normal antigens activate 0.0001%–0.001% of T cells. Superantigens have been observed activating up to 20% of all T cells.

Microbiology

C. Common Exotoxins

1. *Staphylococcus aureus*: Different Staph strains secrete various toxins that can cause a range of different symptoms through varying mechanisms of action:
   a. **α-Toxin:** Pore-forming toxin that breaks down red blood cells as well as endothelial and epithelial cells.
   b. **β-Toxin:** A two-component sphingomyelinase that may be important for iron scavenging. Its role in human disease is not clear.
   c. **γ-Toxin:** A two-component exotoxin that is formed from the combination of several different proteins. γ-Toxin preferentially lyses leukocytes, although its importance to pathogenesis is unclear.
   d. **Panton-Valentine leukocidin:** A two-component exotoxin common in methicillin-resistant *Staphylococcus aureus* (MRSA), which lyses a variety of cell types. This is the chief cause of necrotizing pneumonia in MRSA infections.
   e. **Enterotoxins:** A family of specialized exotoxins that disrupt the gut. These are the main cause of food poisoning symptoms.
   f. **Toxic shock syndrome toxin (TSST):** TSST is a superantigen that causes toxic shock syndrome. Staph strains expressing TSST often infect mucosal sites.
   g. **Exfoliating toxins:** Disrupt cell-to-cell interactions by breaking down desmoglein. This is the cause of scalded skin syndrome.

2. *Streptococcus pyogenes*: Also known as group A Strep, this is the organism that causes scarlet fever. It produces several toxins:
   a. **Streptolysin O:** One of the main exotoxins of *S. pyogenes*, responsible for red blood cell lysis. Antibodies against streptolysin O are used to detect the infection in lab tests.
   b. **Streptolysin S:** A hemolytic cardiotoxin that is not immunogenic (no antibodies are produced against it).
   c. **Pyogenic exotoxins:** Streptococcal pyogenic exotoxins A, B, and C (also known as erythrogenic toxins) are superantigens that are responsible for the symptoms of scarlet fever.
      i. Pyogenic exotoxins are also responsible for the symptoms of streptococcal toxic shock syndrome.

3. *Shigella* species: Produce Shiga toxin, which cleaves 60s ribosomal RNA, thus inhibiting protein synthesis (this is the same mechanism as ricin). Shiga toxin also activates complement and induces signaling cascades that lead to cytokine release. This is the mechanism behind the symptoms of TTP-HUS.
   a. *E. coli* O157:H7 produces Shiga-like toxins, which are VERY similar to Shiga toxin. It is believed that the strain acquired Shiga toxin through genetic transfer at some point in the past.

4. *Escherichia coli*: In addition to Shiga-like toxin (which is rare), *E. coli* produces two other exotoxins of note, both of which cause the symptoms of traveler's diarrhea:
   a. **Heat-labile enterotoxin:** Activates adenylate cyclase through ribosylation of G_s protein-coupled receptors. This raises intracellular cyclic adenosine monophosphate (cAMP) levels, leading to the secretion of chloride ions and water into the gut lumen, causing diarrhea.
   b. **Heat-stable enterotoxin:** Activates guanylate cyclase, which raises intracellular cyclic guanosine monophosphate (cGMP) levels, leading to ion secretion and diarrhea.

5. *Yersinia enterocolitica*: Produces Yersinia stable toxin, which activates guanylate cyclase. This raises intracellular cGMP levels, causing ion secretion and diarrhea (blood in the stool is from bacterial invasion of the intestinal wall).

6. *Bacillus anthracis*: The etiologic agent behind anthrax secretes an exotoxin called edema factor. It acts as an adenylate cyclase, which increases intracellular cAMP. This leads to ion release and edema.

7. *Vibrio cholerae*: Secretes cholera toxin, which stimulates G_s protein-coupled receptors. This activates adenylate cyclase, which increases intracellular cAMP.

This causes ion and water release into the gut lumen, leading to rice-water diarrhea.

8. *Bordetella pertussis*: Pertussis toxin inhibits G_i protein-coupled receptors (inhibitory G protein-coupled receptors), which leads to increased activation of adenylate cyclase. This raises intracellular cAMP, which leads to increased insulin release and hypoglycemia. This same mechanism is thought to be responsible for the characteristic whooping cough.

9. *Corynebacterium diphtheriae*: Diphtheria toxin catalyzes the transfer of NAD^+ to eukaryotic elongation factor 2 (eEF2), which inactivates eEF2, inhibiting protein synthesis. This causes pseudomembranous pharyngitis and can damage nerves and cardiac cells.

10. *Pseudomonas aeruginosa*: Secretes exotoxin A, which adenosine diphosphate (ADP) ribosylates eEF2. This inactivates eEF2 and inhibits protein synthesis, resulting in cell death.

11. *Clostridium tetani*: Secretes tetanospasmin, which is a metalloproteinase. It binds to nerves and travels to the central nervous system (CNS), where it binds gangliosides. It then inhibits γ-aminobutyric acid (GABA) and glycine, which causes the characteristic muscle rigidity and spasms.

12. *Clostridium botulinum*: Botulinum toxin cleaves proteins required for the fusion of intracellular vesicles with membranes. This inhibits the release of acetylcholine from cholinergic neurons, leading to flaccid paralysis, urinary retention, and constipation.

13. *Clostridium perfringens*: Secretes an alpha toxin that hydrolyzes phospholipids and produces diacylglycerol. This activates a variety of signaling cascades leading to the production of inflammatory mediators. This also generates gaseous byproducts, causing gas gangrene.

III. Gram-Positive Bacteria

A. *Staphylococcus* species

1. *Staphylococcus aureus*
   a. Coagulase-positive, catalase-positive cocci
   b. Normally found as a commensal organism in the nasal cavity and on the skin
   c. May cause infections involving skin, wounds, organs, respiratory tract, urinary tract, heart, meninges, joints, digestive tract, and bones
   d. *S. aureus* also causes scalded skin syndrome, toxic shock syndrome, and bacteremia, as well as necrotizing fasciitis.
   e. These infections can be much more difficult to treat if the infection involves MRSA.
   f. Produce Protein A, which inhibits opsonin-mediated phagocytosis
   g. Certain strains also secrete TSST, alpha toxin, beta toxin, delta toxin, and Panton-Valentine leukocidin.
   h. Some strains produce staphyloxanthin, a golden pigment that acts as an antioxidant.

2. *Staphylococcus epidermidis*
   a. Coagulase-negative, catalase-positive cocci
   b. Normally found as a commensal organism on the skin
   c. Commonly forms biofilms on catheters on implanted devices

3. *Staphylococcus saprophyticus*
   a. Coagulase-negative, catalase-positive cocci
   b. Adheres readily to urogenital mucosa
   c. Responsible for 10%–20% of all urinary tract infections in females

B. *Streptococcus* species

1. *Streptococcus pneumoniae*
   a. Catalase-negative, α-hemolytic, encapsulated cocci
   b. Most common cause of meningitis, otitis media, pneumonia, and sinusitis
   c. May also cause conjunctivitis, bacteremia, septic arthritis, osteomyelitis, various soft tissue infections, endocarditis, and pericarditis

      d. Secretes IgA protease, which allows it to more efficiently colonize mucosal surfaces

      e. Asplenic patients are at higher risk for *S. pneumoniae* infection.

  2. Viridans group strep

      a. Catalase-negative, α-hemolytic cocci

      b. Viridans group strep can be differentiated from *S. pneumoniae* through an optochin test. Viridans group strep are resistant to optochin, which is toxic to *S. pneumoniae*.

      c. Viridans group strep lack a polysaccharide capsule, and can also be differentiated from *S. pneumoniae* through a quellung test.

      d. Commonly cause dental caries (especially *S. mutans*) and subacute bacterial endocarditis (especially *S. sanguinis*)

      e. *S. mutans* and *S. sanguinis* are both found in dental plaques and may enter the bloodstream during dental procedures. It may then cause endocarditis in patients with existing endothelial damage.

  3. Group A streptococci

      a. Catalase-negative, β-hemolytic cocci. *Streptococcus pyogenes* is the most important member of this group.

      b. May cause pharyngitis, necrotizing fasciitis, or toxic shock syndrome

      c. Group A strep may also cause some of the same conditions as *Staphylococcus* species, such as folliculitis, cellulitis, or impetigo.

      d. Group A strep infections can also lead to autoimmune disorders, such as acute glomerulonephritis and rheumatic fever.

  4. Group B streptococci

      a. Catalase-negative, β-hemolytic, encapsulated cocci

      b. *Streptococcus agalactiae* is the only member of this group.

      c. Generally found as commensal vaginal flora

      d. Commonly causes pneumonia, sepsis, and meningitis in children, especially infants

  5. Group D streptococci

      a. Catalase-negative, γ-hemolytic (rarely α-hemolytic) cocci

      b. Non-enterococcal group D strep still includes *Streptococcus bovis* and *Streptococcus equinus*.

      c. *S. bovis* can cause bacteremia and subacute bacterial endocarditis. It is also strongly associated with colon cancer (found in 15% of patients).

      d. *S. equinus* is extremely rare in humans, although it has been reported to cause endocarditis and peritonitis.

C. *Enterococcus* Species

  1. Catalase-negative, nonhemolytic (γ-hemolytic) spherical bacteria. Certain strains are encapsulated.

  2. Normal gut flora that only cause disease when they invade a different environment.

  3. Previously considered group D strep, but now classified as a unique genus.

  4. May cause urinary tract infections, bacterial endocarditis, and biliary tract infections.

  5. Vancomycin-resistant *Enterococci* (VRE) are an emerging problem.

D. *Corynebacterium diphtheriae* Infection (Diphtheria)

  1. Gram-positive bacilli

  2. Cause diphtheria and secrete an exotoxin that inactivates eEF2

  3. Progression of disease may lead to myocarditis and cranial nerve deficits.

  4. Generally affects children younger than 12 years

  5. Diphtheria is rare in the United States today due to the widespread use of immunizations (DTaP and DPT). It is still a problem in developing countries.

  6. **Presentation:** Pseudomembranous pharyngitis, cervical lymphadenopathy, malaise, fever, headache, sore throat, dysphagia, cough

  7. **Labs:** Positive throat and/or sinus cultures, positive Elek test (diphtheria toxin), leukocytosis, proteinuria

  8. **Treatment:** Antibiotics, diphtheria antitoxin, supportive care

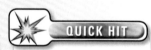

QUICK HIT

Group C streptococci are found mostly in animals, although one member of this group, *Streptococcus dysgalactiae*, can rarely cause group A strep–like infections in humans.

E. *Clostridium tetani* Infection (Tetanus, "Lockjaw")
  1. Gram-positive, spore-forming bacilli that cause tetanus
  2. Secretes tetanospasmin (tetanus toxin), which enters motor neurons and travels to the spinal cord. It then inhibits the release of glycine and GABA from central inhibitor neurons. This causes muscle rigidity and lockjaw.
      a. This is an irreversible process. Antitoxin can only neutralize unbound tetanospasmin. Recovery requires new nerve terminals and formation of new synapses.
  3. Commonly acquired through minor wounds
  4. Primarily affects older, unvaccinated adults. Neonatal tetanus is a major cause of infant mortality in underdeveloped countries.
  5. **Presentation:** Sore throat, dysphagia, local muscle rigidity, general muscle rigidity, lockjaw, stiffness, reflex spasms, positive spatula test
  6. **Labs:** No specific laboratory tests exist for diagnosing tetanus, although they may be necessary to rule out strychnine poisoning
  7. **Treatment:** Tetanus immune globulin, wound debridement, anticonvulsants. Antibiotics have questionable efficacy.

F. *Clostridium botulinum* Infection (Botulism)
  1. Gram-positive, spore-forming bacilli
  2. Commonly acquired from improperly canned food. Most cases of botulism involve infants, typically after ingestion of honey.
  3. Botulinum toxin binds irreversibly to nerves, blocking acetylcholine release. Respiratory muscle weakness may progress to respiratory failure. Low mortality, but high morbidity.
  4. **Presentation:** Nausea, vomiting, dysphagia, diplopia, fixed and/or dilated pupils, dry mouth unrelieved by drinking fluids, descending paralysis
  5. **Labs:** Laboratory tests are generally not helpful. Mouse neutralization bioassay can confirm the presence of botulinum toxin.
  6. **Treatment:** Heptavalent botulism antitoxin, supportive care

G. *Clostridium perfringens* Infection (Gas Gangrene)
  1. Gram-positive, spore-forming bacilli
  2. Most common cause of clostridial gas gangrene. Mortality is 20%–30% with treatment (100% without treatment).
  3. **Presentation:** Acute pain, edema bullae, erythema with purplish-black discoloration, crepitant tissue
  4. **Diagnostics:** Fine gas bubbles within soft tissues, sialidase in serum and wound discharge, gram-positive rods in wound discharge, possible hepatic dysfunction, possible azotemia, possible renal failure, possible metabolic acidosis
      a. Blood and wound discharge cultures can confirm the presence of *Clostridium* but require a minimum of 48 hours. Thus, they are rarely used for diagnosis because this delay will almost always result in the patient's death.
  5. **Treatment:** Supportive care, hyperbaric oxygen therapy, tissue debridement, amputation, antibiotics

H. *Clostridium difficile* Infection (Pseudomembranous Colitis)
  1. Gram-positive, oxidase-negative, spore-forming bacilli
  2. Secretes Toxin B, a cytotoxin that kills enterocytes, causing pseudomembranous colitis
  3. *C. difficile* infection has low mortality but high morbidity.
  4. Associated with antibiotics. Generally occurs in hospitalized patients.
      a. *C. difficile* is ubiquitous in nature and colonizes the intestines of a small percentage of humans. It only causes disease when the normal balance of intestinal flora is disturbed, as with a course of broad-spectrum antibiotics.
  5. **Presentation:** Watery diarrhea, abdominal pain, fever
  6. **Diagnostics:** Leukocytosis (which can be very pronounced), hypoalbuminemia, leukocytes and erythrocytes in stool, positive stool culture, positive glutamate dehydrogenase assay, positive stool cytotoxin test, positive *C. difficile* PCR on stool sample, pseudomembranes on colonoscopy
  7. **Treatment:** Supportive care, cessation of the causative antibiotic, metronidazole, vancomycin, or fidaxomicin

I. *Bacillus anthracis* Infection (Anthrax)
   1. Gram-positive, encapsulated bacilli that cause anthrax
   2. Anthrax is generally a mild cutaneous infection, although it can be serious if it progresses to bacteremia.
      a. Inhalation anthrax is rare, but the mortality is extremely high. It is normally contracted from farm animals.
      b. *B. anthracis* secretes edema toxin, which increases intracellular cAMP, causing fluid to accumulate in tissues.
      c. *B. anthracis* also secretes lethal toxin, which causes cell death through a poorly understood mechanism.
   3. **Presentation:** Black skin lesions, black eschar, necrosis surrounded by an edematous ring, flu-like symptoms (inhalation anthrax), fever (inhalation anthrax), chest pain (inhalation anthrax), myalgias (inhalation anthrax), cyanosis (inhalation anthrax)
   4. **Diagnostics:** Widening of the mediastinum, lung crackles, positive exudate/ pleural fluid culture, pleural effusion, positive blood culture, hemorrhagic cerebrospinal fluid (CSF)
   5. **Treatment:** Antibiotics, raxibacumab, supportive care
J. *Listeria monocytogenes* Infection
   1. Gram-positive bacilli that cause listeriosis
   2. Contracted through ingestion of contaminated food, especially dairy products and deli meats
   3. Generally affects infants and elderly patients, as well as immunocompromised individuals
   4. Maternal listeriosis can lead to chorioamnionitis, premature labor, spontaneous abortion, and stillbirth. It can also be transmitted to the infant during childbirth.
   5. Mortality is relatively low, except in the case of early-onset neonatal listeriosis
   6. **Presentation:** Flu-like symptoms, headache, fever, diarrhea, cyanosis (neonatal listeriosis), tachypnea
   7. **Diagnostics:** Positive culture of CSF or affected tissues, abscesses in brain
   8. **Treatment:** Antibiotics, supportive care
K. *Actinomyces* Infection
   1. Gram-positive, filamentous bacilli that cause actinomycosis. Most species are facultative anaerobes, growing best in an an anaerobic environment.
   2. Cervicofacial actinomycosis is the most common form. It generally follows oral surgery and results in oral and facial abscesses that spread. These form sinuses that exude sulfurous fluid.
   3. **Presentation:** Oral/facial nodules, sulfurous exudates, lockjaw (if the mastication muscles are affected)
   4. **Labs:** Anemia, leukocytosis (mild), elevated C-reactive protein (CRP) and sedimentation rate, positive exudate culture
   5. **Treatment:** Antibiotics, surgical excision of sinus tracts and fibrotic lesions, drainage of abscesses
L. *Nocardia* Infection
   1. Gram-positive, filamentous bacilli that are partially acid-fast that cause nocardiosis
   2. Causes pulmonary symptoms in immunocompromised hosts
   3. **Presentation:** Fever, productive cough
   4. **Diagnostics:** Endobronchial masses, pulmonary abscesses, localized or diffuse pneumonia, cavitation, pleural effusion
   5. **Treatment:** Antibiotics, surgical abscess removal

IV. Gram-Negative Bacteria
A. *Shigella* Infection (Shigellosis)
   1. Common cause of bloody diarrhea, due to secretion of Shiga toxin. Major public health problem in developing countries. Has a very low minimum infective dose (as few as 10 organisms).
   2. Shigellosis is generally self-limiting in the United States, although it has a 20% mortality rate in underdeveloped countries.

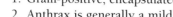

QUICK HIT

Bloody diarrhea often results from invasion and destruction of the intestinal wall by pathogens such as:
- *E. coli* O157:H7
- *Shigella*
- *Campylobacter*
- *Salmonella*

Microbiology

3. Spread through fecal–oral transmission, often in contaminated water or food. It is less commonly transmitted through sexual contact.
4. **Presentation:** Fever; dehydration; abdominal tenderness; emesis; large-volume, watery diarrhea
5. **Labs:** Stool with fecal blood, leukocytes, and *Shigella* organisms. Blood tests are normally inconclusive, although a left shift in the leukocyte count may be seen.
6. **Treatment:** Treatment is only indicated in severe cases. Penicillins, cephalosporins, fluoroquinolones, macrolides, sulfonamides, or tetracyclines may all be used. Antidiarrheals are contraindicated because they may exacerbate the infection. Zinc supplementation may also decrease the duration and severity of the disease in children.

B. *Salmonella* **Infection**
  1. Common cause of bloody diarrhea
  2. Common foodborne pathogen found in beef, poultry, and eggs. It may also be found in contaminated fruits, vegetables, dairy products, and shellfish.
     a. *Salmonella* may also be contracted through contact with pet reptiles (turtles) and amphibians.
  3. Generally a self-limited disease, although mortality is relatively high if the infection progresses to bacteremia (rare).
  4. **Presentation:** Diarrhea (occasionally large volume), fever, abdominal cramping, headache, myalgias, rose spots on chest and abdomen (typhoid fever only)
  5. **Labs:** Positive stool culture (except typhoid fever), positive bone marrow aspirate culture (more sensitive than blood culture in typhoid fever), positive urine culture (typhoid fever only), leukopenia, neutropenia, anemia
  6. **Treatment:** Supportive care is normally indicated. Antibiotics are not recommended unless the patient is at risk for invasive disease because they do not shorten illness.

C. *Escherichia coli* **(*E. coli*)**
  1. Enterotoxigenic *E. coli* (ETEC) infection
     a. ETEC generally affects the small intestine and is a common cause of traveler's diarrhea (a self-limited infection).
     b. ETEC produces a heat-labile enterotoxin and a heat-stable enterotoxin.
     c. **Presentation:** Watery diarrhea, dehydration, abdominal cramps
        i. Because ETEC does not invade the intestinal wall, there is no fever and no blood in the stool.
     d. **Labs:** Not generally done. Diagnosis is made based on symptoms.
     e. **Treatment:** Antibiotics (fluoroquinolones or azithromycin) for moderate to severe disease, along with supportive care.
  2. Enterohemorrhagic *E. coli* (EHEC) infection
     a. Generally affects the large intestine, causing hemorrhagic colitis
     b. E. coli O157:H7 serotype can cause hemolytic uremic syndrome (HUS).
     c. EHEC secretes a Shiga toxin.
     d. Presentation: Bloody diarrhea, fever, dehydration, hemolysis, uremia, HUS symptoms (thrombocytopenia, anemia, acute renal failure)
     e. Labs: Stool cultures may test positive for 0157:H7 (other serotypes are not generally tested).
     f. Treatment: Supportive care only (antibiotics are not known to be beneficial and may worsen the clinical course)
  3. Enteropathogenic *E. coli* (EPEC) infection
     a. A common cause of diarrhea in children, especially in developing countries or nurseries
     b. EPEC generally affects the small intestine, where it adheres to intestinal wall and flattens the villi, prevents absorption.
     c. **Presentation:** Watery diarrhea (lower volume than ETEC infection), dehydration
     d. **Labs:** EPEC may be detected through adherence assays, serotyping, and DNA probes, although these tests are rarely performed.
     e. **Treatment:** Supportive care, antibiotic therapy in more severe cases
  4. Enteroinvasive *E. coli* (EIEC) infection
     a. EIEC affects the large intestine and causes a *Shigella*-like dysentery, although infections are rare.

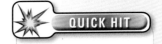

QUICK HIT

Salmonella typhi, which causes typhoid fever, is unique among *Salmonella* species in that it does not cause diarrhea.

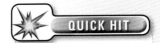

QUICK HIT

Salmonella infection may cause osteomyelitis in patients with sickle cell disease.

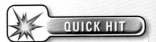

QUICK HIT

E. coli strains may be classified by their antigens:
• Somatic O antigen is associated with lipopolysaccharide in the outer membrane.
• H antigen is found in the flagella.
• K antigen is part of the polysaccharide capsule and may contribute to virulence.

Microbiology

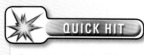

Campylobacter jejuni infection is often associated with Guillain-Barré syndrome and reactive arthritis.

    b. **Presentation:** Bloody diarrhea, fever, dehydration, abdominal cramps, tenesmus

    c. **Labs:** Not normally done, but DNA probe and animal pathogenicity tests may be performed.

    d. **Treatment:** Fluoroquinolones, along with supportive care. Antimotility agents are contraindicated.

D. *Campylobacter jejuni* **Infection**

  1. Gram-negative, oxidase-positive bacilli from the family *Campylobacteriaceae*

  2. Common cause of foodborne diarrhea in the United States. Common cause of diarrhea (sometimes bloody) in children. Self-limited disease generally lasting 1–2 weeks.

  3. Fecal–oral transmission, or from contaminated poultry, meat, and unpasteurized milk

  4. **Presentation:** Fever, headache, myalgias, abdominal pain, diarrhea (sometimes bloody), vomiting, tenesmus

  5. **Labs:** Positive stool culture, fecal leukocytes and erythrocytes, peripheral blood leukocytosis

  6. **Treatment:** Supportive care. Antibiotics only for those who have severe disease or at risk for severe disease. Antimotility agents are contraindicated because they may prolong disease.

E. *Yersinia enterocolitica* **Infection**

  1. Common cause of diarrhea in developing countries. May also cause enterocolitis, terminal ileitis, mesenteric lymphadenitis, and pseudoappendicitis.

  2. Most often affects children. Self-limited and generally responsive to therapy. Mortality is high if disease progresses to bacteremia.

  3. Commonly contracted from contaminated pork, milk, water, and tofu. Also rarely associated with household pets.

  4. **Presentation:** Diarrhea (sometimes bloody), fever, abdominal pain, emesis, erythema nodosum

  5. **Labs:** Leukocytosis, positive stool culture, positive blood culture

  6. **Treatment:** Supportive care, antibiotics may be used in severe cases

F. *Vibrio cholerae* **Infection**

  1. Gram-negative, oxidase-positive bacilli in the family *Vibrionaceae*

  2. Secretes cholera toxin, which causes rice-water diarrhea. High mortality in developing countries.

  3. Usually transmitted through contaminated food and water (classically shellfish/oysters)

  4. Increased free iron (as seen in hemolytic anemia or hemochromatosis) also increases the risk of disseminated infections, although more commonly associated with *Vibrio vulnificus* than *Vibrio cholerae*.

  5. **Presentation:** Diarrhea, abdominal pain, nausea, vomiting, fever, headache, myalgias

  6. **Labs:** Fecal leukocytes and erythrocytes, gram-negative bacteria in stool

  7. **Treatment:** Supportive care, including urgent rehydration, and antibiotics

G. *Proteus* **Infection**

  1. Most human *Proteus* infections are caused by *Proteus mirabilis*. *Proteus vulgaris* and *Proteus penneri* can also cause disease.

  2. Common cause of **urinary tract infections.** Proteus species are capable of producing urease, which converts urea into ammonia and CO_2. This results in the formation of struvite (magnesium-ammonium-phosphate). Struvite stones can enlarge to create **staghorn calculi** in the renal pelvis and calyces.

  3. **Presentation:** Dysuria, increased frequency of urination, back pain, suprapubic pain, fever

  4. **Labs:** Positive urine culture, alkaline urine, pyuria, hematuria, renal calculi. *Proteus* species demonstrate swarming motility, and it is difficult to isolate single colonies from culture plates.

  5. **Treatment:** Antibiotics, surgical removal of renal calculi

H. *Klebsiella pneumoniae* **Infection**

  1. Common cause of lobar community-acquired pneumonia in patients with alcoholism or diabetes, as well as health care–associated pneumonia and UTI.

  2. *Klebsiella* pneumonia, especially when complicated by bacteremia, has a high mortality rate.

    3. Generally affects debilitated middle-aged men and older men with alcoholism. Nosocomial infections may also affect children or immunocompromised adults.

    4. **Presentation:** Red "currant jelly" sputum, fever, chills, flu-like symptoms, productive cough

    5. **Diagnostics:** Leukocytosis, gram-negative bacteria in sputum, bulging fissure in affected lung lobes, cavitation, pleural effusion

    6. **Treatment:** Antibiotics, surgical care for drainage or debridement as necessary

I. *Neisseria gonorrhoeae* Infection

    1. Gram-negative cocci that cause gonorrhea. Most commonly acquired through sexual contact.

    2. Also a common cause of septic arthritis in young, sexually active individuals

    3. May also cause neonatal conjunctivitis (contracted from the mother during birth), pelvic inflammatory disease, and Fitz-Hugh-Curtis syndrome

       a. Fitz-Hugh-Curtis syndrome is a rare complication of pelvic inflammatory disease. It occurs when the spread of the infection results in inflammation of the liver capsule.

    4. Infections may become bloodborne and cause osteomyelitis, meningitis, endocarditis, acute respiratory distress syndrome (ARDS), or septic shock.

    5. **Presentation:** Arthralgias (septic arthritis), rash (disseminated gonococcal infection), pharyngitis and cervical lymphadenopathy (oral–genital transmission), right upper quadrant pain (perihepatitis), purulent conjunctivitis (autoinoculation). Other symptoms differ between men and women, as well as between adults and neonates.

       a. Women: Vaginal discharge, dysuria, intermenstrual bleeding, dyspareunia, abdominal pain, tenesmus

       b. Men: Urethritis, serous or purulent penile discharge, acute epididymitis, abnormal urine stream, tenesmus

       c. Neonates: Purulent conjunctivitis, eye pain, redness

    6. **Labs:** Positive PCR on genital swab or urine, positive culture (specific to infected site), mildly elevated sed rate

    7. **Treatment:** Antibiotics, drainage of infected joints

J. *Neisseria meningitidis* Infection

    1. Gram-negative, encapsulated cocci that cause meningococcal meningitis. It is naturally found on mucosal surfaces of the nasopharynx and, less commonly, the urogenital and anal mucosa.

    2. Infections are likely the result of colonization with a new strain, in which the bacteria spread prior to the development of protective antibodies.

    3. Risk factors include smoking, concurrent respiratory infection, and crowded living conditions.

    4. Ten percent to 20% of infections progress to bacteremia, which can then progress to meningitis. Mortality is relatively high in underdeveloped countries.

    5. Children may develop Waterhouse–Friderichsen syndrome, which occurs when a bacterial infection causes hemorrhage into the adrenal glands, resulting in adrenal insufficiency. This can lead to shock, DIC, and sepsis.

    6. **Presentation:** Headache, fever, nausea, vomiting, photophobia, stiff neck, lethargy, petechial rash, seizures (mainly in children)

    7. **Diagnostics:** Increased nuchal rigidity, increased CSF proteins, decreased CSF glucose, increased polymorphonuclear leukocytes in CSF, positive CSF culture, meningeal lesions, cerebral edema, cerebral ischemia

    8. **Treatment:** Antibiotics, anti-inflammatories, surgical intervention for complications

K. *Haemophilus influenzae* Infections

    1. Gram-negative coccobacilli that cause a variety of infections

       a. *H. influenzae* most commonly causes epiglottitis, especially in children.

       b. May also cause bacteremia, meningitis, otitis media, sinusitis, pneumonia, and empyema

       c. Mortality is very low, with the exception of *H. influenzae* meningitis in underdeveloped countries.

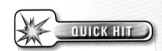
QUICK HIT

H. influenzae was originally believed to be the cause of influenza, hence its name. However, it is now known that influenza is actually caused by influenza viruses.

Microbiology

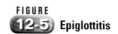

FIGURE 12-5 Epiglottitis

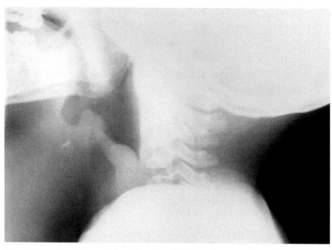

Thumb sign on inspiratory soft-tissue lateral neck radiograph, suggesting epiglottitis. (Reprinted with permission from Harwood-Nuss A, Wolfson AB, et al. *The Clinical Practice of Emergency Medicine*. 3rd ed. Philadelphia, PA: Lippincott Williams & Wilkins; 2001.)

2. Certain strains are encapsulated.
3. Transmitted through direct contact or inhalation of respiratory droplets
4. **Epiglottitis presentation:** Fever, sore throat, dysphagia, drooling, "sniffing dog position," progressive respiratory difficulty
   a. The "sniffing dog position" is seen when a patient lifts his or her head and extends his or her neck in an effort to open the airway as he or she attempts to breathe.
5. **Diagnostics:** Thumb sign on x-ray (dilation of the hypopharynx in epiglottitis) (*Figure 12-5*), straightened cervical spine, positive culture of fluid from infected site, positive blood culture
6. **Treatment:** Antibiotics, intubation as necessary, supportive care

L. *Legionella pneumophila* **Infection**
1. Gram-negative bacilli that cause two notable clinical illnesses:
   a. Legionnaires disease (pneumonia with alveolitis and bronchiolitis).
   b. Pontiac fever (a self-limited, flu-like illness that presents without pneumonia)
2. Transmitted through aerosolized, contaminated water
3. Mortality rate is dependent on factors such as age, underlying conditions, and delay in treatment but may be anywhere between 5% and 80%.
4. **Presentation:** Fever, weakness, fatigue, malaise, myalgias, nonproductive cough progressing to productive cough, chest pain, headache, confusion, cerebellar ataxia
5. **Diagnostics:** Hypotension, proteinuria, hematuria, elevated sed rate, elevated CRP, hyponatremia, hypophosphatemia, elevated creatine kinase, positive sputum culture, positive urinary antigen, lung infiltrates on chest x-ray (CXR)
6. **Treatment:** Antibiotics, supportive care

M.*Pseudomonas aeruginosa* **Infection**
1. Gram-negative bacilli that have many toxins and virulence factors, including exotoxin A, which inactivates eEF2
2. It is one of the most common causes of health care–associated pneumonia.
   a. May cause otitis externa, urinary tract infections, surgical site infections, and osteomyelitis. Progression to bacteremia is common.
   b. *P. aeruginosa* also commonly causes hot tub folliculitis.
3. *P. aeruginosa* rarely affects healthy individuals. Most patients are immunocompromised or have a disruption in physical barriers (e.g., burns, intravenous [IV] lines, catheters). Because of this, *Pseudomonas* infections have a high mortality rate.
4. **Diagnostics:** azotemia, leukocytosis, elevated erythrocyte sedimentation rate (ESR) and CRP, rapid progression of CXR findings

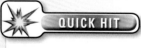

QUICK HIT

Pseudomonas infections are especially common in cystic fibrosis and burn patients.

5. **Treatment:** Fluoroquinolones, cefepime, aztreonam, piperacillin-tazobactam, meropenem. Surgical drainage of abscesses and additional treatment based on specific site of infection may also be indicated.

N. *Helicobacter pylori* **Infection**

1. Gram-negative, spiral-shaped bacteria that causes gastritis
2. Found in the gastrointestinal (GI) tract of more than 50% of the world population. Most common cause of duodenal ulcers (~90%). Increases the risk of gastric adenocarcinoma and lymphoma.
3. **Presentation:** Generally asymptomatic. Symptoms may include nausea, vomiting, abdominal pain, diarrhea, heartburn, and halitosis.
4. **Labs:** Positive fecal antigen test, positive carbon-13 urea breath test
5. **Treatment:** Antibiotics combined with a proton pump inhibitor

V. Nonstaining Bacteria

A. *Mycobacterium tuberculosis* **Infection**

1. *M. tuberculosis* is considered to be gram-positive, although they do not stain properly due to a waxy outer layer and their intracellular life cycle.
2. Transmitted in airborne particles.
3. Tuberculosis (TB) is a common cause of death worldwide. This is due to a combination of factors, including drug resistance, lack of public health infrastructure, and HIV co-infection.
   a. **Primary tuberculosis:** Infection in an individual who has not been previously exposed. Often asymptomatic. The patient recovers, often without any indications of the infection. However, the mycobacteria is not always cleared, and instead enters a dormant (latent) state.
   b. **Secondary tuberculosis:** Latent TB can reactivate and cause severe respiratory symptoms. This may also lead to extrapulmonary tuberculosis, which can cause CNS lesions and meningitis.
      i. TB in the vertebral bodies is known as Pott disease.
      ii. **Miliary tuberculosis** is caused by hematogenous spread of TB that causes many tiny lesions (1–5 mm) throughout the lung.
4. **Presentation:** Cough, rales, weight loss, fever, night sweats, hemoptysis, chest pain, fatigue, lymphadenopathy
5. **Diagnostics:** Positive tuberculin skin test, positive interferon gamma release assay, positive acid-fast bacilli (AFB) smear on sputum, cavitary lesions on CXR, hilar lymphadenopathy and Ghon focus on CXR (collectively called the Ghon complex) (Figure 12-6). Diagnostic culture of *M. tuberculosis* takes 2–6 weeks to grow on agar.

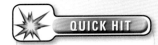

HIV-infected patients can develop a life-threatening primary TB infection.

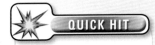

Patients who have been previously exposed to TB (or who have received the BCG vaccine) may have a positive tuberculin skin test, although they may not actually have the disease.

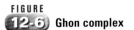

FIGURE
12-6 Ghon complex

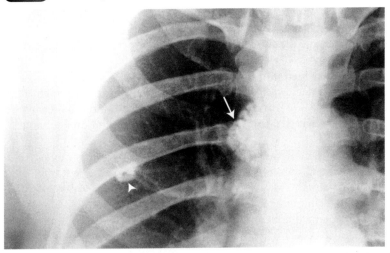

A Ghon focus (*arrowhead*) is a peripheral calcified pulmonary granuloma. A Ghon complex is a Ghon focus plus hilar lymphadenopathy. The *white arrow* indicates a calcified hilar lymph node. (Reprinted with permission from Yochum TR, Rowe LJ. *Yochum And Rowe's Essentials of Skeletal Radiology.* 3rd ed. Philadelphia, PA: Lippincott Williams & Wilkins; 2004.)

Microbiology

6. **Treatment:** Rifampin, isoniazid, pyrazinamide, and ethambutol. Other antibiotics may be needed for multidrug resistant strains. Surgical resection of infected lung tissue may be indicated in refractory cases.

B. *Mycobacterium leprae* Infection
1. Causes Hansen disease (leprosy). There are two forms: lepromatous and tuberculoid.
   a. **Lepromatous leprosy** occurs when infected individuals mount a minimal cellular immune response. Manifests with extensive skin lesions and symmetric peripheral nerve involvement.
   b. **Tuberculoid leprosy** occurs when infected individuals mount a strong cellular immune response. Manifests with limited skin lesions and asymmetric peripheral nerve involvement.
2. Route of transmission may be through respiratory droplets. Also associated with direct contact with infected armadillos.
3. Although leprosy can be a debilitating disease due to nerve damage, it has low mortality and low infectivity. Most exposed individuals never develop the disease.
4. **Presentation:** Nodules and thick plaques on fingers, peripheral neuropathy, muscle weakness, clawed hands, foot drop, leonine facies (advanced leprosy)
5. **Labs:** Positive nasal smear or skin biopsy, positive anti-phenolic glycolipid-1 antibody test (less specific for tuberculoid leprosy), positive or negative lymphocyte migration inhibition test (tuberculoid or lepromatous leprosy respectively)
6. **Treatment:** Dapsone, clofazimine, and rifampin

C. *Leptospira interrogans* Infection (leptospirosis)
1. *Leptospira interrogans* is a motile spirochete. It is one of the most common zoonotic organisms in the world, although it is most commonly seen in tropical climates.
2. Found in water contaminated with animal urine
3. It produces a range of clinical presentations:
   a. Subclinical infection without noticeable symptoms
   b. Self-limited, mild disease presenting with flu-like symptoms
   c. Severe disease causing kidney and liver failure
   d. Can also present as pulmonary disease, with hemorrhage, acute respiratory distress syndrome, and multiorgan failure
4. Morbidity from leptospirosis can be high, although mortality is low. When death does occur, it is commonly due to pulmonary involvement.
5. **Presentation:** Flu-like symptoms (fever, myalgias), headache, abdominal pain, jaundice, photophobia, conjunctivitis, tachycardia, hypotension, oliguria
6. **Diagnostics:** Elevated creatinine and blood urea nitrogen (BUN), pulmonary edema and/or myocarditis on CXR, alveolar lung disease, positive cultures, positive serology
7. **Treatment:** Antibiotics, supportive care in severe cases

D. *Borrelia burgdorferi* Infection (Lyme disease)
1. *B. burgdorferi* is a motile spirochete that causes Lyme disease.
2. Most common tick-borne disease in the United States (specifically transmitted by ticks from the genus *Ixodes*)
3. Lyme disease can be divided into three stages:
   a. Stage 1: Localized infection. Nonspecific, flu-like symptoms, accompanied by erythema migrans around the tick bite, occurring about 1 month after tick bite. Many patients will clear the infection during this stage, some without any symptoms.
   b. Stage 2: Disseminated infection. Occurs several weeks to several months after initial infection. Manifests with neurologic and cardiac symptoms.
   c. Stage 3: Chronic disease. May occur several months to several years after the initial infection. Debilitating arthritis and encephalitis are seen.
4. Diagnosis is problematic due to a number of factors:
   a. Early lyme disease occurs when the erythema migrans first appears. IgM and IgG may be negative at this early stage. If the patient has been in an endemic area recently and erythema migrans is present, the patient should be treated empirically.

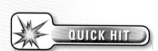

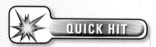

Microbiology

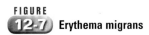

FIGURE 12-7 Erythema migrans

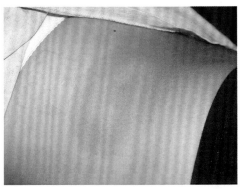

Acute Lyme disease (erythema migrans). Note the target-like concentric rings with no scale. (Reprinted with permission from Goodheart HP. *Goodheart's Photoguide of Common Skin Disorders.* 2nd ed. Philadelphia, PA: Lippincott Williams & Wilkins; 2003.)

b. When the patient has early disseminated disease, he or she may have multiple erythema migrans lesions on exam, as well as possible meningitis, carditis, and facial palsy. Serology (IgM and IgG) should be positive at this point.

c. Lyme disease is difficult to diagnose if the erythema migrans lesion is not present or if it is hidden under hair.

5. Prognosis is favorable with timely treatment, but chronic musculoskeletal symptoms, neurologic impairment, and chronic fatigue may be seen if treatment is delayed for an extended period of time. Lyme disease is very rarely fatal.

6. **Presentation:** Varies depending on disease stage:

a. Stage 1: Erythema migrans (Figure 12-7), fever, myalgias, fatigue, flu-like symptoms

b. Stage 2: Additional skin lesions, musculoskeletal and neurologic symptoms, inflammatory arthritis, Bell palsy

c. Stage 3: Myalgias, hemiparesis, ataxia, seizures, cognitive impairment, acrodermatitis chronic atrophicans

7. **Diagnostics:** Varies depending on disease stage. Positive antibody titer, mononuclear cells in CSF; electrocardiogram (ECG) may reveal atrioventricular block or other cardiac abnormalities

8. **Treatment:** Doxycycline, amoxicillin, cefuroxime

E. *Treponema pallidum* Infection (Syphilis)

1. *Treponema pallidum* is a spirochete that causes syphilis. It is commonly transmitted through sexual contact with infected individuals. Also transmitted vertically from mother to fetus.

2. Syphilis is divided into four stages: primary, secondary, latent, and tertiary.

a. **Primary syphilis:** Normally presents with a single, painless chancre 3–6 weeks after initial exposure. Few patients will seek treatment for this.

b. **Secondary syphilis:** Develops 4–10 weeks after the appearance of the initial lesion. This coincides with the dissemination of *Treponema* throughout the body.

c. **Latent syphilis:** During this period, patients are often asymptomatic, although they still carry the bacteria. This period can last for a very long period of time (25 years in some cases).

d. **Tertiary syphilis:** Relatively rare manifestation that may occur years after initial exposure. Three presentations include:

i. Gummatous syphilis: Characterized by the appearance of gummas (granulomatous lesions). These are found on skin, in bones, and even in internal organs.

ii. Cardiovascular syphilis: Commonly causes aortitis and predisposes to aneurysms of the ascending aorta, aortic dissection, and possibly aortic valve pathology.

iii. Neurosyphilis: May cause meningitis, hearing loss, tabes dorsalis, Argyll Robertson pupil, and various neurologic abnormalities.

Microbiology

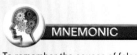

  e. **Congenital syphilis:** Vertical transmission from mother to fetus can cause the child to develop abnormalities such as saber shins, saddle nose, Hutchinson teeth, mulberry molars, and frontal bossing.
  3. **Presentation:** Varies according to stage:
    a. Primary syphilis: Painless chancre
    b. Secondary syphilis: Fever, malaise, chills, maculopapular rash that classically involves palms/soles, alopecia areata, condylomata lata
    c. Latent syphilis: Generally asymptomatic
    d. Tertiary syphilis: Gummas, positive Romberg sign, sensory ataxia, Argyll Robertson pupil, deafness, dementia, altered mental status
  4. **Labs:** Positive rapid plasma reagin (RPR) or Venereal Disease Research Laboratory (VDRL) test, positive fluorescent treponemal antibody absorption (FTA-ABS) test. The FTA-ABS test is necessary to confirm the result of a positive RPR or VDRL, which can produce false positives.
  5. **Treatment:** Penicillin is the antibiotic of choice. Doxycycline can be used in the case of penicillin allergy.
F. *Gardnerella vaginalis* Infection
  1. *Gardnerella vaginalis* is a poorly staining, nonmotile coccobacillus that is associated with bacterial vaginosis (BV).
    a. BV is not considered a sexually transmitted disease. It is often spread through sexual contact but can also be acquired in other ways.
    b. Antibiotics, IUDs, douching, and low estrogen can also predispose to BV.
    c. Untreated infections may cause endometritis, salpingitis, pelvic inflammatory disease, and pregnancy/labor complications.
    d. BV also increases the chances of contracting HIV through sexual contact.
  2. Although *Gardnerella* is usually involved in cases of BV, evidence indicates that the disease is the result of synergism between *Gardnerella* and one or more additional bacteria.
  3. **Presentation:** Gray vaginal discharge, vaginal odor, vulvar irritation
  4. **Labs:** Clue cells in discharge, discharge pH >4.5, positive whiff test. Cultures are not useful due to the polymicrobial nature of the infection.
  5. **Treatment:** Metronidazole or clindamycin
G. *Rickettsia* Infection
  1. *Rickettsia* are obligate intracellular bacteria that stain poorly with Gram stain, although they do have gram-negative cell walls.
    a. *Rickettsia rickettsii* causes Rocky Mountain spotted fever.
    b. *Rickettsia typhi* causes endemic typhus, transmitted by rat fleas.
    c. *Rickettsia prowazekii* cause epidemic typhus, transmitted by lice.
      i. Infections with *Rickettsia prowazekii* have a high mortality rate in untreated, elderly patients.
  2. **Presentation:** Headache, fever, and rash (rickettsial triad); abdominal pain; diarrhea; conjunctivitis; mental confusion; delirium; rales
  3. **Labs:** No rapid tests are available for early diagnosis of rickettsial infections. Thrombocytopenia, elevated LFTs. Positive Weil-Felix agglutination test, positive anti-rickettsial antibodies on indirect fluorescent antibody (IFA) test.
  4. **Treatment:** Doxycycline is the treatment of choice. Chloramphenicol may be used as an alternative.
H. *Coxiella burnetii* Infection (Q fever)
  1. *Coxiella burnetii* is an obligate intracellular bacterium that was originally classified as *Rickettsia*. It stains poorly with Gram stain, although it does have gram-negative cell walls.
  2. Transmitted in aerosolized form from urine, feces, milk, and birth products of animal hosts. *Coxiella* is extremely infective, requiring fewer than 10 organisms in some cases.
  3. Causes Q fever, which is generally a self-limited disease with an excellent prognosis, although it may progress to atypical pneumonia or hepatitis.
  4. **Presentation:** Fever, headache, myalgias, chills, fatigue, sweating, crackles on chest auscultation, nonproductive cough

5. **Diagnostics:** Elevated liver enzymes, mild thrombocytopenia, elevated sed rate, negative Weil-Felix agglutination test, atypical pneumonia on CXR, hepatomegaly. Serologic tests are not useful in determining treatment because they require 3–4 weeks.

6. **Treatment:** Doxycycline or other antibiotics

I. *Chlamydophila psittaci* Infection (Psittacosis)

1. *Chlamydophila psittaci* is an intracellular bacterium that causes psittacosis. Infection normally manifests as pneumonia but may progress to a systemic disease that causes gastrointestinal, neurologic, and dermatologic sequelae.

2. Transmitted to humans through aerosolized bird secretions or feces, especially those of exotic birds.

3. With antibiotic therapy, fatalities are extremely rare.

4. **Presentation:** Fever, chills, malaise, nonproductive cough, dyspnea, pharyngitis, epistaxis, Horder spots (which resemble the rose spots of typhoid fever, but are found on the face), splenomegaly

5. **Labs:** Mildly elevated liver enzymes, mild proteinuria, anti-*Chlamydophila* antibodies

6. **Treatment:** Antibiotics, supportive care as needed

J. *Chlamydophila pneumoniae* Infection

1. *Chlamydophila pneumoniae* is an intracellular bacterium that causes pneumonia.

2. *Chlamydophila pneumoniae* is responsible for 10%–20% of all cases of community-acquired pneumonia. It causes mild disease in adolescents and young adults but may cause more severe disease in older adults.

3. **Presentation:** Nonproductive cough, malaise, fever, sinus percussion tenderness, pharyngeal erythema, rhonchi, rales

4. **Diagnostics:** Atypical pneumonia, anti-*Chlamydophila* antibodies, pleural effusion. White blood cell count is not typically elevated.

5. **Treatment:** Tetracyclines, macrolides

K. **Chlamydia trachomatis** Infection

1. Intracellular bacteria that cause a variety of diseases depending on the serotype.

2. **Trachoma:** Caused by serotypes A, B, Ba, and C.
   a. The leading infectious cause of blindness
   b. Transmitted chiefly between children and caregivers
   c. Repeated reinfection can lead to conjunctival scarring.
   d. Untreated infections can cause blindness.

3. **Chlamydial genitourinary infection:** Caused by serotypes D–K.
   a. The most commonly reported sexually transmitted disease in the United States.
   b. Common cause of infertility and ectopic pregnancies in women. Also causes pelvic inflammatory disease and Fitz-Hugh-Curtis syndrome.
   c. May also cause neonatal conjunctivitis and neonatal pneumonia due to exposure during passage through the birth canal
   d. Many infections can be subclinical, especially in women. Because these women do not seek treatment, this increases the risk of transmission as well as pregnancy complications.

4. **Lymphogranuloma venereum:** Caused by serotypes L1, L2, and L3
   a. Rare infection that causes acute lymphadenitis and primary ulcers
   b. May cause rectal disease that is commonly mistaken for inflammatory bowel disease
   c. If left untreated, disfiguring ulcerations and genital enlargement can occur.
   d. Generally presents with self-limited ulcers or papules, followed by lymphadenopathy after 2–6 weeks. Proctocolitis may occur years later.
   e. Mortality is very low with proper treatment.

5. **Presentation:** Varies by disease
   a. **Trachoma:** Self-epilation of eyelashes, blepharospasm, mucopurulent keratoconjunctivitis, corneal follicles, trichiasis, corneal opacity

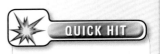

QUICK HIT

Fitz-Hugh-Curtis syndrome was initially described as a complication of *Neisseria gonorrheae*, but it is probably more commonly associated with *Chlamydia trachomatis* infection.

Microbiology

  b. **Chlamydial genitourinary infection:** Urethritis, cervicitis, salpingitis, epididymitis, proctitis, conjunctivitis, urethral or vaginal discharge, dysuria, dyspareunia

  c. **Lymphogranuloma venereum:** Inguinal and/or femoral lymphadenopathy, genital ulcers, genital papules, rectal ulcerations, proctocolitis, fever, chills, malaise, myalgias, tenesmus

  6. **Labs:** Positive polymerase chain reaction (PCR) test, peripheral eosinophilia, positive urine culture, positive anti-chlamydial antibodies

  7. **Treatment:** Antibiotics

L. *Mycoplasma pneumoniae* Infection

  1. Non–gram-staining bacteria that lack a cell wall

  2. A common cause of community-acquired pneumonia ("walking pneumonia"). Generally seen in patients under age 40 years and in military barracks and prisons. Only 5%–10% of infected patients actually develop pneumonia.

  3. **Presentation:** Headache, nonproductive cough, fever, malaise, nontoxic appearance, rhonchi, rales

  4. **Labs:** Atypical pneumonia on CXR, positive cold agglutinin test. Sputum cultures are not helpful due to the slow growth rate of *M. pneumoniae*.

  5. **Treatment:** Antibiotics

ANTIBIOTICS

I. Cell Wall Inhibitors

A. Penicillins

1. Inhibit the formation of bacterial cell walls by interfering with the enzyme transpeptidase, which normally catalyzes the cross-linking of peptidoglycan strands

2. Contain a β-lactam ring structure

3. Most penicillins are considered bactericidal.

4. Generally used in gram-positive infections (e.g., *Streptococcus*, *actinomyces*, *Staphylococcus*) as well as certain spirochete infections (e.g., syphilis).

5. There are four different categories of penicillins:

  a. **Natural penicillins:** Include **penicillin G** (intravenous) and **penicillin V** (oral).

  b. **β-lactamase-resistant penicillins:** Include **nafcillin, oxacillin,** and **dicloxacillin.** Less susceptible to inactivation by penicillinase (β-lactamase). Sometimes referred to as anti-staphylococcal penicillins, due to their efficacy in Staph infections.

  c. **Aminopenicillins:** Include **amoxicillin** and **ampicillin.** Have a wider spectrum than other categories of penicillins. Commonly used for urinary tract infections.

  d. **Extended-spectrum penicillins:** Include **ticarcillin, carbenicillin,** and **piperacillin.** Also known as antipseudomonal antibiotics, these are used for *Pseudomonas* infections. They are also effective against a number of gram-negative rods.

6. To protect against β-lactamase inactivation, some of these are administered along with β-lactamase inhibitors (i.e., clavulanic acid, tazobactam, sulbactam).

7. Commonly cause hypersensitivity reactions. Ampicillin and amoxicillin may also cause a full body rash when administered to mononucleosis patients.

B. Cephalosporins

1. Inhibit the formation of bacterial cell walls by interfering with the enzyme transpeptidase, which normally catalyzes the cross-linking of peptidoglycan strands

2. Contain a β-lactam ring structure

3. Most cephalosporins are bactericidal.

4. Generally less susceptible to penicillinases compared to penicillins

5. More effective against gram-negative bacteria compared to penicillins

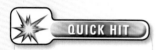

QUICK HIT

The chief mechanism of β-lactam resistance is production of β-lactamase.

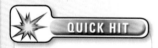

QUICK HIT

Methicillin resistance in *Staphylococcus* is determined in a laboratory setting. Methicillin is not used in humans.

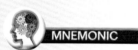

MNEMONIC

To remember the gram-negative bacteria that are susceptible to aminopenicillins, use
HELPSS:
Haemophilus influenzae
Escherichia coli
Listeria monocytogenes
Proteus mirabilis
Salmonella
Shigella

6. Cephalosporins are divided into four generations. Each generation is more effective against gram-negative bacteria than the previous generation but generally less effective against gram-positive bacteria.
   a. **First generation:** Includes **cefazolin**, **cefadroxil**, and **cephalexin**. Effective against the gram-negatives *Proteus mirabilis*, *E. coli*, and *Klebsiella*, as well as many gram-positive bacteria. Commonly used to treat urinary tract infections.
   b. **Second generation:** Includes **cefoxitin**, **cefaclor**, **cefuroxime**, **cefotetan**, and **cefprozil**. Effective against the same gram-negative bacteria as first generation cephalosporins, with the addition of *H. influenzae*, *Enterobacter*, *Neisseria*, and *Serratia*.
   c. **Third generation:** Includes **ceftriaxone**, **cefotaxime**, **ceftazidime**, **cefditoren**, **cefixime**, **cefpodoxime**, and **cefdinir**. Used against serious gram-negative infections and pneumococcal meningitis. Ceftazidime in particular is effective against *Pseudomonas*.
   d. **Fourth generation:** Includes **cefepime** and **ceftaroline**. Broad-spectrum antibiotics that are effective against a wide range of gram-negative bacteria, as well as many gram-positive bacteria.
7. Cephalosporins are generally ineffective against *Listeria*, MRSA, *Enterococcus*, *Mycoplasma*, and *Chlamydia*.
8. Fewer than 10% of individuals with type I, IgE-mediated penicillin allergies or hypersensitivities also react to cephalosporins.
9. Cephalosporins increase the risk of nephrotoxicity when combined with aminoglycoside antibiotics.

C. **Aztreonam**
1. Aztreonam is the only monobactam (monocyclic β-lactam) antibiotic that is used in humans.
2. It inhibits cell wall synthesis by binding the transpeptidase enzyme, although at a different site than penicillins and cephalosporins.
3. It works synergistically with aminoglycoside antibiotics to increase killing ability. Aztreonam has no cross-reactivity with penicillins and is safe to use in patients with penicillin allergies.
4. Effective against gram-negative rods. Ineffective against gram-positive bacteria and anaerobic bacteria.

D. **Carbapenems**
1. **Imipenem/cilastatin, meropenem, ertapenem, doripenem**
   a. Imipenem is always administered with cilastatin, which inhibits renal-dehydropeptidase. This prevents enzymatic inactivation of imipenem.
2. Powerful, broad-spectrum antibiotics that are β-lactamase-resistant
3. Effective against both gram-positive and gram-negative bacteria, including anaerobic bacteria and *Pseudomonas*
   a. Carbapenems are not effective against MRSA.
4. Generally used to treat life-threatening infections
5. Carbapenems have a number of potential side effects, including rash, GI distress, and CNS toxicity.

E. **Vancomycin**
1. A glycopeptide antibiotic that inhibits cell wall formation by binding the peptidoglycan strands themselves, rather than the transpeptidase enzyme
2. Vancomycin is effective against many gram-positive bacteria, including several drug-resistant species. These include MRSA, *Clostridium difficile*, and various enterococci.
3. Although vancomycin does have oral formulations, it has very poor oral bioavailability and is generally administered intravenously. Oral vancomycin is only indicated for the treatment of *C. difficile* colitis.
4. Generally used only in serious or refractory cases
5. Side effects include nephrotoxicity, ototoxicity, thrombophlebitis, and red man syndrome (a diffuse flushing of the entire body due to mast cell degranulation). Red man syndrome is a relatively common side effect of vancomycin and can often be prevented by slowing the infusion and pretreatment with an antihistamine.

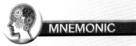

MNEMONIC

To remember the gram-negative bacteria affected by first-generation cephalosporins, use **PEcK**:
Proteus mirabilis
Escherichia coli
Klebsiella

To remember the gram-negative bacteria affected by second-generation cephalosporins, use **HENPEcKS**:
Haemophilus influenzae
Enterobacter
Neisseria
Proteus mirabilis
Escherichia coli
Klebsiella
Serratia

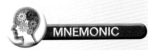

MNEMONIC

To remember the bacteria that are resistant to cephalosporins, use **LAME**:
Listeria
Atypical bacteria (*Mycoplasma*, *Chlamydia*)
MRSA
Enterococcus

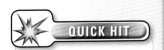

QUICK HIT

The glycopeptide class also includes the less commonly used telavancin and teicoplanin antibiotics as well as the antineoplastic drug bleomycin.

Microbiology

Microbiology

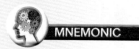

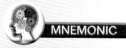

II. Protein Synthesis Inhibitors

A. Aminoglycosides
1. **Gentamicin, neomycin, amikacin, tobramycin, kanamycin, streptomycin**
2. Bind the 30S ribosome, interfering with protein synthesis
3. Aminoglycosides are generally bactericidal, but they require oxygen for uptake. This means they are ineffective against anaerobic bacteria.
4. Used to treat severe gram-negative infections. Also work synergistically with β-lactam antibiotics for some infections.
5. Side effects include nephrotoxicity and ototoxicity.
6. Aminoglycosides are contraindicated in pregnancy.

B. Linezolid
1. Binds the 50S ribosome, interfering with protein synthesis
2. Linezolid may be either bactericidal or bacteriostatic depending on the infection.
3. Mainly used to treat MRSA infections and VRE infections
4. Good oral bioavailability allows for the treatment of these infections on an outpatient basis.
5. Linezolid is not approved for the treatment of gram-negative bacterial infections.
6. In patients who are taking antidepressants, linezolid increases the risk of serotonin syndrome (excess serotonin causes restlessness and agitation, diarrhea, tachycardia, hypertension, cognitive impairment, and loss of coordination).

C. Tetracyclines
1. **Tetracycline, doxycycline, demeclocycline, minocycline, tigecycline**
2. Bind the 30S ribosome, interfering with protein synthesis
3. Tetracyclines are usually bacteriostatic.
4. Due to the fact that they are chiefly excreted in the feces, tetracyclines are suitable for use in patients with renal failure.
5. Used to treat *Vibrio cholerae*, *Chlamydia*, *Ureaplasma urealyticum*, *Mycoplasma pneumoniae*, *H. pylori*, *B. burgdorferi*, *Rickettsia*, and tularemia, as well as acne
6. Tetracyclines should not be taken with milk, antacids, or iron-containing preparations. Calcium, iron, and magnesium will inhibit the absorption.
7. Side effects include GI distress, discoloration of teeth and inhibition of bone growth in children, and photosensitivity. Minocycline in particular can cause patients to develop bluish-gray skin pigmentation with prolonged use.
8. Tetracyclines are contraindicated in pregnancy.

D. Macrolides
1. **Erythromycin, azithromycin, clarithromycin**
2. Bind the 50S ribosome, interfering with protein synthesis
3. Macrolides are usually bacteriostatic antibiotics.
4. Used to treat atypical pneumonias (i.e., *Mycoplasma*, *Chlamydia*, *Legionella*), respiratory tract infections (sinusitis, bronchitis), and sexually transmitted diseases
5. Side effects included prolonged QT interval (especially with erythromycin), GI distress, eosinophilia, and rashes.
6. Macrolides inhibit the activity of hepatic enzymes and can thus increase the serum concentration of drugs such as theophylline and warfarin.

E. Chloramphenicol
1. Inhibits the 50S ribosome, interfering with protein synthesis
2. Chloramphenicol is bacteriostatic.
3. Rarely used. Only indicated when a serious infection is refractory to other treatment.
4. Effective against *H. influenzae*, *N. meningitidis*, and *Streptococcus pneumoniae*
5. Side effects include dose-dependent anemia, aplastic anemia, and gray baby syndrome when administered to neonates

F. Clindamycin
1. Inhibits the 50S ribosome, interfering with protein synthesis
   a. Clindamycin belongs to a class of antibiotics called lincosamides.
   b. Lincomycin is the only other lincosamide approved for humans, and it is rarely used.

2. Clindamycin is bacteriostatic.
3. One of a small number of medications used to treat anaerobic infections
4. Also effective against *C. perfringens* and MRSA
5. Side effects include GI symptoms, pseudomembranous colitis, and Stevens-Johnson syndrome.

G. **Streptogramins**
1. **Quinupristin, dalfopristin**
2. Alone, each of the streptogramins is bacteriostatic. However, used together (which they always are), they can be bactericidal.
3. Dalfopristin binds the 50S ribosome, causing a conformational change that enhances the binding of quinupristin. Together they inhibit peptide transfer and protein chain elongation.
4. Used against gram-positive organisms. Notable for their effectiveness against MRSA, and vancomycin-resistant enterococci.
5. Side effects include arthralgias and myalgias, which significantly limit their use. Also cause cytochrome p450 inhibition.

III. Antimycobacterial Antibiotics

A. **Isoniazid**
1. Inhibits the synthesis of mycolic acid, which is a component of the mycobacterial cell wall
2. Isoniazid is generally bactericidal.
3. The only drug that is used for solo prophylaxis against tuberculosis
4. Commonly used together with rifampin, pyrazinamide, and ethambutol to treat active tuberculosis
5. Side effects include drug-induced lupus, hepatotoxicity, and neurotoxicity (which can be prevented with concomitant administration of pyridoxine).

B. **Rifampin**
1. Binds DNA-dependent RNA polymerase, preventing RNA transcription
2. Rifampin is bactericidal.
3. Rifampin is used to treat tuberculosis, usually in combination with isoniazid, pyrazinamide, and ethambutol.
   a. Rifampin should not be used as monotherapy because resistance can develop rapidly.
   b. May also be used in combination with dapsone and clofazimine to treat leprosy
4. Sometimes used for prophylaxis against meningitis from *N. meningitidis* and *H. influenzae*
5. Side effects include reddish-orange body fluids. Also promotes the upregulation of cytochrome P450.

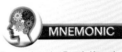

MNEMONIC

Remember the **R**s of rifampin:
RNA polymerase inhibitor
Revs up cytochrome P450
Rapid resistance if used alone
Reddish-orange body fluids

C. **Pyrazinamide**
1. Inhibits the synthesis of mycolic acid
2. Generally bacteriocidal for intracellular organisms
3. Used exclusively to treat tuberculosis and almost always in combination with rifampin, isoniazid, and ethambutol
4. Side effects include hyperuricemia and hepatotoxicity.

D. **Ethambutol**
1. Inhibits arabinosyltransferase, preventing the attachment of mycolic acids to peptidoglycans in the cell wall
2. Ethambutol is bacteriostatic.
3. Used in combination with rifampin, pyrazinamide, and isoniazid to treat tuberculosis
4. Side effects include optic neuropathy leading to reversible red-green color blindness.

E. **Dapsone**
1. Inhibits the synthesis of folic acid by mycobacteria.
2. Used in combination with rifampin and clofazimine to treat leprosy. Also used to treat dermatitis herpetiformis and acne vulgaris and as prophylaxis against *Pneumocystis* pneumonia.

3. May be either bactericidal or bacteriostatic depending on the bacterial strain
4. Side effects include hemolysis and methemoglobinemia.

F. Clofazimine
1. Binds bacterial DNA, inhibiting replication and transcription
2. Clofazimine is bactericidal.
3. Generally used in combination with dapsone and rifampin to treat leprosy
4. Clofazimine has many side effects, including skin discoloration and ichthyosis.

IV. Other Antibiotics

A. Fluoroquinolones
1. **Ciprofloxacin, levofloxacin, moxifloxacin, gemifloxacin, norfloxacin, ofloxacin**
2. Inhibits topoisomerase and DNA gyrase, interfering with DNA replication
3. Used mainly to treat gram-negative infections, although some gram-positive bacteria are also susceptible. Commonly used for respiratory tract and urinary tract infections.
4. Fluoroquinolones should not be taken with antacids or supplements that include calcium, iron, or magnesium because these can inhibit their absorption
5. Side effects include GI distress and tendonitis.
   a. Fluoroquinolones are not absolutely contraindicated in pregnant women and children but are strongly recommended against due to the possibility of arthropathies related to developmental abnormalities and damage to articular cartilage.
   b. Fluoroquinolones are recommended for use in children with cystic fibrosis, although they require monitoring of the joints.

B. Sulfonamides
1. **Sulfamethoxazole, sulfisoxazole, sulfadiazine**
2. Inhibit dihydropteroate synthetase, interfering with folic acid synthesis
   a. Effective against some gram-negative and some gram-positive bacteria, although it is mainly used to treat urinary tract infections, *Pneumocystis* pneumonia, and sometimes MRSA infections
   b. Also effective in shigellosis and salmonellosis
3. Generally bacteriostatic when used alone. However, sulfonamides antibiotics are most commonly administered in with trimethoprim. This combination is bactericidal.
4. The most common side effect is hypersensitivity reactions because sulfa allergies are common.
   a. Symptoms include fever, pruritic rash, hemolytic anemia, thrombocytopenia, agranulocytosis, and urticaria.
   b. Reactions to sulfa drugs can be life threatening.
5. Other side effects include nephrotoxicity, photosensitivity, hemolysis, kernicterus in infants, and Stevens-Johnson syndrome.

C. Trimethoprim
1. Inhibits dihydrofolate reductase, interfering with folic acid synthesis
2. Almost always used in conjunction with a sulfonamide antibiotic. The combination of the two is bactericidal.
3. Side effects are generally related to folic acid deficiency, such as megaloblastic anemia, leukopenia, and granulocytopenia. Folic acid supplementation reverses these.

D. Nitrofurantoin
1. Undergoes reduction inside bacterial cells, producing reactive products that can inactivate ribosomes and other proteins, as well as damage DNA
2. Nitrofurantoin is bactericidal.
3. Used almost exclusively to treat urinary tract infections
4. Not used to treat pyelonephritis because its poor tissue availability makes it largely ineffective
   a. Nitrofurantoin is generally taken with food to improve its absorption.
5. Side effects include nausea, headaches, and diarrhea.

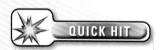

QUICK HIT

Early-generation quinolones (e.g., ofloxacin, ciprofloxacin) are less effective against gram-positive bacteria, but later-generation drugs (e.g., levofloxacin, moxifloxacin) have improved gram-positive coverage.

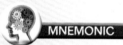

MNEMONIC

To remember the antibiotics that are contraindicated during pregnancy, remember, "**C**ountless **SAF**e **M**oms **T**ake **R**eally **G**ood **C**are":
Clarithromycin
Sulfonamides
Aminoglycosides
Fluoroquinolones
Metronidazole
Tetracyclines
Ribavirin
Griseofulvin
Chloramphenicol

Microbiology

E. Metronidazole
1. Selectively absorbed by anaerobic bacteria and certain protozoa, metronidazole is reduced intracellularly. The metabolites then inactivate enzymes and degrade DNA.
2. Uses:
   a. Used against anaerobic bacteria and *Gardnerella vaginalis*
   b. Also indicated for *Giardia*, *Entamoeba*, and *Trichomonas* infections
   c. Also used in conjunction with tetracycline and bismuth subsalicylate in *H. pylori* infection (triple therapy)
3. Side effects include a disulfiram-like reaction when alcohol is consumed.
F. Polymyxins
1. **Polymyxin B, colistin (polymyxin E)**
2. May be either bactericidal or bacteriostatic, depending on the infection
3. Act as detergents, altering bacterial membranes and destabilizing them. Also bind and inactivate endotoxins.
4. Used to treat gram-negative infections
5. Side effects include acute renal tubular necrosis and neurotoxicity. Polymyxins are almost always used as topical treatments.

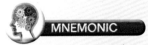

To remember the infections that are commonly treated with metronidazole, remember "**GET GAP** on the **Metro**":
Giardia
Entamoeba
Trichomonas
Gardnerella vaginalis
Anaerobic bacteria
Pylori (*H. pylori*)

 VIRUSES

I. Viral Basics
A. Viral Structure
1. Wide range of genome sizes, roughly 3 kb to 300 kb
2. Repeating elements (e.g., capsid structure) simplify the genetic requirement because fewer genes are needed.
3. Nucleocapsid contains either DNA or RNA.
4. Surface proteins facilitate attachment to host cells.
5. Some viruses are surrounded by a lipid envelope, usually acquired from a host cell. Viral envelopes may be derived from the cell membrane, the nuclear membrane, or even the endoplasmic reticulum (see Table 12-1).
   a. Enveloped viruses are more sensitive to desiccation and, thus, are generally transmitted through droplets, sexual contact, or parenteral invasion.
   b. Nonenveloped viruses can withstand much harsher conditions and are more likely to spread via the fecal–oral route.
B. Viral Genetics
1. **Reassortment:** When two or more viruses infect the same cell, genetic material from one virion may be mistakenly packaged into a different virion. This can lead to the creation of viruses with properties that they would otherwise not possess.
   a. This only occurs when viruses have segmented genomes.
   b. In humans, reassortment only occurs with RNA viruses.
2. **Recombination:** When two or more viruses infect the same cell, crossover between homologous regions of DNA (similar to homologous recombination in humans) can produce new viral progeny with different properties.
   a. This almost always involves DNA viruses, or retroviruses, due to their DNA phase.
3. **Complementation:** When a virus has a mutation that prevents it from effectively replicating, it may be able to replicate by infecting a cell at the same time as a fully functional virus. Proteins from the functional virus may be able to participate in the replication of the mutated virus, thus temporarily overcoming the mutation.
   a. This is only effective for one generation because the virus will encounter the same problems upon infection of subsequent cells.
4. **Phenotypic mixing:** When two viruses infect the same cell, progeny may be packaged with the proper genetic material, but with coat components from both parents. This can alter the tissue specificity of the virion, allowing to temporarily infect different cells.

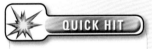

All viruses are haploid (only one copy of DNA or RNA) with the exception of retroviruses, which are diploid.

TABLE 12-1 Viral Taxonomy

Genome		Family (**enveloped viruses)	Clinically Important Virus
DNA	dsDNA	Herpesviridae**	Herpes simplex virus 1 (HSV-1) Herpes simplex virus 2 (HSV-2) Varicella zoster virus (VZV) Epstein–Barr virus (EBV) Cytomegalovirus (CMV) Human herpes virus 6 (HHV-6) Human herpes virus 8 (HHV-8)
		Papillomaviridae	Human papillomavirus (HPV)
		Adenoviridae	Adenoviruses
		Poxviridae**	Variola virus (small pox) Cowpox virus Molluscum contagiosum virus
		Polyomaviridae	JC virus
	dsDNA-RT	Hepadnaviridae**	Hepatitis B virus
	ssDNA	Parvoviridae	Parvovirus B19
RNA	dsRNA	Reoviridae	Rotavirus *Genus: Coltivirus* Colorado tick fever virus

	(+)ssRNA	Picornaviridae	Hepatitis A virus
			Genus: Enterovirus
			  • Echovirus
			  • Poliovirus
			  • Rhinovirus
			  • Coxsackievirus

		Caliciviridae	Norwalk virus
		Flaviviridae**	Yellow fever virus Dengue virus West Nile virus St. Louis encephalitis virus
		Togaviridae**	Rubella virus
		Coronaviridae**	Coronaviruses
	(−)ssRNA	Orthomyxoviridae**	Influenza virus
		Paramyxoviridae**	Human parainfluenza virus Rubeola virus Mumps virus Respiratory syncytial virus (RSV)
		Rhabdoviridae**	Rabies virus
		Bunyaviridae**	Hantavirus
	dsRNA-RT	Retroviridae**	HIV Human T-cell leukemia virus (HTLV)

DNA, deoxyribonucleic acid; dsDNA, double-stranded DNA; dsRNA, double-stranded RNA; RNA, ribonucleic acid; RT, reverse transcriptase; ssDNA, single-stranded DNA; (+)ssRNA, positive-sense single-stranded RNA; (−)ssRNA, negative-sense single-stranded RNA.

Microbiology

5. **Naked viral genome infectivity:** Not all viruses require a capsid or an envelope to infect cells. The genetic material from viruses that only use host enzymes is often infectious on its own. Naked double-stranded viral DNA is infectious on its own (except poxvirus and hepatitis B), as is positive, single-stranded RNA.

   a. Negative single-stranded RNA and double-stranded RNA are not infectious.

C. **DNA vs. RNA Viruses** (*Table 12-1*)

   1. DNA viruses

      a. Most DNA viruses contain double-stranded DNA. (Exception: Parvovirus is the only single-stranded DNA virus that infects humans.)

      b. DNA genomes are normally linear. (Exceptions: Papillomavirus and polyomavirus have circular genomes.)

      c. Replication of DNA viruses generally occurs in the nucleus because they must use host enzymes for translation. (Exception: Poxvirus possesses its own RNA polymerase, which allows it to replicate in the cytoplasm.)

   2. RNA viruses

      a. Most RNA viruses contain single-stranded RNA. (Exception: Reoviruses and retroviruses contain double-stranded RNA.)

      b. Positive-sense RNA, which can be immediately translated into proteins, is more common (see *Table 12-1*).

      c. Replication of RNA viruses generally occurs in the cytoplasm because they do not require the host nuclear RNA polymerase. (Exceptions: Influenza virus uses an exonuclease to cleave the 5′ end of methylated host RNA, which then acts as a primer for the synthesis of viral RNA. Retroviruses must enter the nucleus so that the DNA that is transcribed from viral RNA can then be inserted into the host genome.)

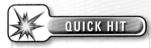

QUICK HIT

The Hepadnaviruses, which include hepatitis B, have a unique, partially double-stranded, partially circular genome. The two strands are different lengths, and only the longer strand forms a closed loop.

II. DNA Viruses

A. Herpesviruses

   1. **Herpes simplex virus 1 (HSV-1)** (human herpesvirus 1)

      a. Causes oral herpes labialis (cold sores). Also causes gingivostomatitis, keratoconjunctivitis, and temporal lobe encephalitis. May less commonly cause genital herpes.

      b. It can be transmitted through any mucosal surface or through abraded skin.

      c. The virus lies dormant in the trigeminal ganglia, occasionally causing disease and then resolving again.

   2. **Herpes simplex virus 2 (HSV-2)** (human herpesvirus 2)

      a. Most common cause of genital herpes (*Figure 12-8*)

      b. The virus lies dormant in the sacral nerve root ganglia, occasionally causing disease and then resolving again.

FIGURE
12-8 Herpes simplex virus

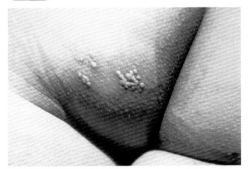

This herpes simplex outbreak on the buttock demonstrates the classic herpetic lesions: grouped vesicles on an erythematous base. (Reprinted with permission from Goodheart HP. *Goodheart's Photoguide of Common Skin Disorders*. 2nd ed. Philadelphia, PA: Lippincott Williams & Wilkins; 2003.)

Microbiology

c. Normally transmitted through sexual contact, although it can be transmitted through any mucosal surface or through abraded skin
   i. Infants born to HSV-positive mothers often contract HSV as they pass through the birth canal, provided the mother is actively shedding the virus.
   ii. If the mother has a primary infection (as opposed to a reactivation), transmission may occur *in utero*.

3. **Varicella zoster virus** (VZV) (human herpesvirus 3)
   a. Primary VZV infection causes chicken pox. Reactivation is known as herpes zoster (shingles).
   b. May cause encephalitis and pneumonia. This is rare in children but more common in adults (especially immunocompromised patients).
   c. VZV lies dormant in the dorsal ganglia. Reactivation causes vesicle formation only on the affected dermatome.
   d. Transmission of primary VZV may be through skin contact or through the respiratory route. In contrast, transmission of reactivated VZV requires direct contact with active lesions.
   e. Disseminated herpes zoster, which is almost entirely restricted to immunocompromised patients, can be transmitted through the respiratory route as well.

4. **Epstein–Barr virus** (EBV) (human herpesvirus 4)
   a. Causative agent in infectious mononucleosis
   b. Generally spread through oral secretions of infected individuals
   c. Infects B cells, which prompts a strong T-cell response. This results in the atypical lymphocytosis that is characteristic of EBV infection.
      i. These atypical lymphocytes (**Downey cells**) are large, basophilic cells with abundant cytoplasm.
   d. Infectious mononucleosis presents with malaise, fever, sore throat, and posterior cervical lymphadenopathy. Splenomegaly is common, and requires restriction of physical activity.
   e. Diagnosis often uses a monospot test that detects heterophile antibodies.
      i. Heterophile antibodies are not specific for EBV. Rather, they are the result of nonspecific B cell activation by EBV and may bind antigens to which the body has never been exposed.
      ii. In the case of the monospot test, antibody-mediated agglutination of equine, ovine, or bovine red blood cells indicates a positive result.
   f. EBV is also associated with Hodgkin lymphoma, Burkitt lymphoma, nasopharyngeal carcinoma, diffuse large cell lymphoma, oral hairy leukoplakia, and various other lymphoproliferative disorders.

5. **Cytomegalovirus** (CMV) (human herpesvirus 5)
   a. Causes mononucleosis-like symptoms with a negative result on monospot
   b. Common perinatal infection. Also may be spread through infected bodily fluids, including saliva and breast milk.
   c. Infections can be severe in immunosuppressed (e.g., transplant recipients) or immunocompromised patients (e.g., AIDS).
      i. CMV may cause acute retinitis in AIDS patients that can blind them permanently in a matter of days.
      ii. CMV may also cause GI ulcerations in AIDS patients that is initially mistaken for *Candida* infection.
   d. CMV-infected cells can be identified by their characteristic "owl eye" appearance of inclusion bodies (*Figure 12-9*).

6. **Human herpesvirus 6** (HHV-6)
   a. Causes **roseola** in children (also known as exanthem subitum, and "sixth disease")
   b. Most children are infected with HHV-6 by age 2 years.
   c. Roseola manifests with 3–5 days of high fever (>102°) without accompanying symptoms. This is followed by a maculopapular rash as the fever breaks. Roseola may also cause febrile seizures.
   d. Like all herpesviruses, HHV-6 causes a lifelong latent infection. However, there are few long-term consequences because reactivations are generally asymptomatic.

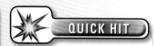

QUICK HIT

Because mononucleosis resembles streptococcal pharyngitis, patients are often mistakenly prescribed penicillin antibiotics. This may cause a pruritic, maculopapular rash, which may be further misdiagnosed as a penicillin allergy.

QUICK HIT

Mononucleosis-like symptoms in a patient with a negative monospot test is usually the result of CMV infection. It may also be the result of HIV.

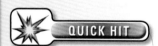

QUICK HIT

The term "owl eye" is commonly used to describe both CMV-infected cells and the Reed-Sternberg cells seen in Hodgkin lymphoma.

FIGURE
12-9 Cell infected with cytomegalovirus

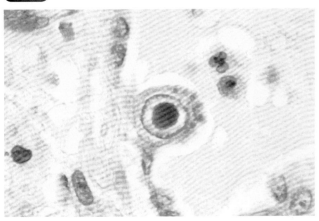

Lung tissue with characteristic "owl eye" nuclear inclusion. Cytoplasmic inclusions are also present. (Reprinted with permission from McClatchey KD. *Clinical Laboratory Medicine.* 2nd ed. Philadelphia, PA: Lippincott Williams & Wilkins; 2002.)

7. **Human herpesvirus 7** (HHV-7)
   a. Almost all humans have been infected with HHV-7 by age 5 years.
   b. It may cause roseola-like symptoms, but this often occurs in older children as compared to HHV-6.
   c. HHV-7 may also reactivate later in life, although it is generally asymptomatic.
8. **Kaposi sarcoma–associated herpesvirus** (KSHV) (human herpesvirus 8)
   a. Only 5% of the U.S. population is infected with KSHV.
   b. It infects spindle cells from vascular and lymphatic endothelium. This results in the formation of vascular tumors (Kaposi sarcoma).
   c. KSHV generally causes symptoms only in HIV and AIDS patients or in some immunosuppressed patients.
   d. Kaposi sarcoma may also affect immunocompetent individuals, although this form produces slow-growing, benign tumors.

B. **Human Papillomavirus (HPV)**
   1. There are more than 120 types of HPV.
   2. Types 1 and 2 are associated with common warts and plantar warts.
   3. Types 6 and 11 cause about 90% of all genital warts.
   4. Types 16 and 18 are responsible for 70% of all cases of invasive cervical cancer. They may also cause cancers of the vulva, vagina, anus, and penis.

C. **Adenovirus**
   1. Family of viruses that generally cause an upper respiratory infection followed by conjunctivitis. This is commonly accompanied by diarrhea.
   2. Various serotypes of adenovirus can also cause febrile pharyngitis, acute hemorrhagic cystitis, and pneumonia.

D. **Poxvirus**
   1. Smallpox is caused by an enveloped version of poxvirus called variola virus. It has been eradicated, although it remains of concern due to its potential as a bioterrorism agent.
   2. Cowpox is caused by a poxvirus called Vaccinia. It can cause "milkmaid's blisters" in people who make contact with infected cow udders.
   3. Molluscum contagiosum is a type of poxvirus that causes flesh-colored dome lesions with a central dimple or umbilication (*Figure 12-10*). It is generally benign and usually resolves on its own in immunocompetent patients. In immunocompromised individuals, it can cause chronic skin lesions.

E. **Polyomavirus**
   1. The most common polyomavirus in humans is JC virus.
   2. JC virus causes progressive multifocal leukoencephalopathy (PML) in HIV patients.

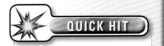

QUICK HIT

Vaccinia is the live virus that was successfully used to confer protection against smallpox. It is the origin of the term "vaccine."

Microbiology

FIGURE
12-10 Molluscum contagiosum

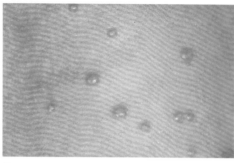

Characteristic dome-shaped, shiny, flesh-colored papules have a central dimple or umbilication. (Reprinted with permission from Goodheart HP. *Goodheart's Photoguide of Common Skin Disorders*. 2nd ed. Philadelphia, PA: Lippincott Williams & Wilkins; 2003.)

F. Hepadnavirus
1. The most important hepadnavirus in humans is hepatitis B virus (see Chapter 5).
2. Transmitted sexually, parenterally, or perinatally
3. Most patients are asymptomatic, although 10% will progress to chronic hepatitis (80%–90% of immunocompromised individuals).
4. Infants are vaccinated for hepatitis B shortly after birth.

G. Parvovirus B19
1. The smallest DNA virus in humans. It is also the only single-stranded DNA virus that infects humans.
2. Disease presentations
   a. Causes "fifth disease" in children, which manifests with a classic "slapped cheek" rash on the face.
   b. Infection in adults rarely results in a cheek rash but may cause acute inflammatory arthritis.
   c. Parvovirus can cause a transient aplastic crisis in sickle cell patients.
   d. In pregnancy, parvovirus can cause miscarriage or hydrops fetalis.

III. RNA Viruses

A. Rotavirus
1. A virus of the *Reoviridae* family that is the primary cause of fatal diarrhea in children worldwide
2. Severe diarrhea and vomiting cause dehydration and electrolyte abnormalities.
3. Outbreaks are less severe in the United States and generally occur in small children in day care centers or playgrounds.

B. Coltivirus
1. A virus of the *Reoviridae* family that causes Colorado tick fever
2. Spread by wood ticks, which are found in mountainous regions of the western United States and Canada
3. Causes an acute, self-limited, flu-like illness

C. Picornavirus
1. *Picornaviridae* is a family of small ("pico") RNA viruses including hepatitis A virus and the genus *Enterovirus*.
   a. They are primarily spread through the fecal–oral route, although enteroviruses can also be transmitted in respiratory secretions.
   b. Human enteroviruses are further divided into *Echovirus*, *Poliovirus*, *Rhinovirus*, and *Coxsackievirus*.
2. **Hepatitis A**
   a. A virus of the family *Picornaviridae* that is transmitted through the fecal–oral route, most commonly in contaminated food or water
   b. Presents with fatigue, abdominal pain, nausea, and jaundice
   c. Unlike hepatitis B, hepatitis A does not cause a latent infection and produces no chronic disease. Patients generally recover completely (see Chapter 5).

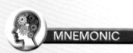

MNEMONIC

Remember that **fifth** disease causes a rash on the cheeks, which are innervated by cranial nerve **V** (5).

Microbiology

3. **Echovirus**
   a. An enterovirus that causes aseptic meningitis, myocarditis, and upper respiratory tract infections
   b. Echovirus-associated meningitis is less severe than bacterial meningitis and may not require hospital care
4. **Poliovirus**
   a. An enterovirus that infects the gray matter of the anterior horn of the spinal cord and the motor neurons of the pons and medulla
   b. Causes paralysis and eventual death
   c. Polio vaccines have made cases rare in the United States, but they are common in other parts of the world.
5. **Rhinovirus**
   a. Rhinovirus is one of the top two causes of the common cold (along with coronavirus). There are more than 100 types of rhinovirus.
   b. Rhinovirus was once classified as its own genus, but has recently been reclassified and is now considered to be part of the *Enterovirus* genus.
6. **Coxsackievirus**
   a. An enterovirus that also causes aseptic meningitis and myocarditis, along with pericarditis, herpangina, and hand, foot, and mouth disease
   b. Coxsackievirus is the most common cause of viral myocarditis in the United States.
   c. Hand, foot, and mouth disease presents with vesicular or papular lesions on posterior oropharynx as well as the palms and soles of the feet (*Figure 12-11*).

FIGURE 12-11 Coxsackie hand, foot, and mouth disease

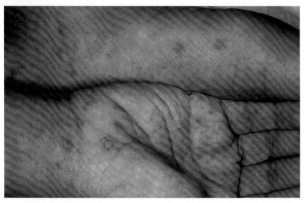

A hand and a foot of this child show isolated vesicles (in contrast to the grouped vesicles seen in patients with herpetic infections). The child also had palatal lesions. (Reprinted with permission from Fleisher GR, Ludwig W, Baskin MN. *Atlas of Pediatric Emergency Medicine*. Philadelphia, PA: Lippincott Williams & Wilkins; 2004.)

D. **Norwalk Virus**
   1. A virus of the family *Caliciviridae* that causes gastroenteritis. This results in vomiting and diarrhea.
   2. Spread through fecal–oral route, although vomitus can also spread it
   3. Often seen in point-source outbreaks (e.g., cruise ships, nursing homes)
E. **Yellow Fever Virus**
   1. A virus in the family *Flaviviridae* that causes yellow fever
   2. It is an arbovirus that is transmitted by mosquitoes. Commonly seen in sub-Saharan Africa and South America. Fatal in up to 50% of cases.
   3. Presents with high fever, hemorrhagic disease, jaundice, and "coffee ground" emesis (due to the presence of dark brown, partially digested blood in the vomitus)
F. **Dengue Virus**
   1. A virus of the family *Flaviviridae*, that causes dengue fever. Classified as an arbovirus, although it can also be transmitted by nonhuman primates.

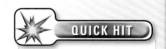

QUICK HIT

"Arbovirus" is not a taxonomic classification but rather a designation for viruses transmitted by arthropods (e.g., ticks, mosquitoes).
• Yellow fever virus
• Dengue virus
• West Nile virus
• St. Louis encephalitis virus

Microbiology

2. Dengue fever is possibly the most common mosquito-borne illness in the world, more than 50 million cases per year.
    a. Presents with severe headache (especially retro-orbital headache), myalgias, arthralgias, and rarely hemorrhagic fever (due to thrombocytopenia).
    b. Dengue fever is also known as "breakbone fever," due to the severe musculo-skeletal pain it causes.

G. **West Nile Virus (WNV)**
    1. A virus of the family *Flaviviridae*. Also classified as an arbovirus, although birds are the natural host (mosquitoes only transfer it from birds to humans).
    2. May cause symptoms in incidental human hosts but cannot be transmitted from one person to another.
    3. WNV infections generally present with flu-like symptoms, including fever, headache, malaise, back pain, myalgias, and anorexia. Approximately 1 in 150 patients experiences severe neurologic problems, including meningitis, encephalitis, muscle weakness, and flaccid paralysis.
    4. Diagnosis is usually made by identifying anti-WNV IgM antibodies in the CSF. (IgM indicates acute disease. IgG against WNV is not diagnostic because it is likely that many people have been exposed to WNV at some point.)
    5. Treatment is supportive only. There are currently no antivirals that are effective against WNV.

H. **St. Louis Encephalitis Virus (SLEV)**
    1. A virus in the family *Flaviviridae*. Also classified as an arbovirus.
    2. SLEV infection generally presents with flu-like symptoms, along with confusion, disorientation, and tremors. In severe cases, meningitis, encephalitis, and convulsions are seen, along with cranial nerve palsies and coma.
    3. SLEV-specific IgM in the CSF is used to diagnose the infection.
    4. Supportive care is indicated because there are no antivirals that are effective.

I. **Rubella Virus**
    1. A virus in the family *Togaviridae* that causes rubella, also known as German measles
    2. Presents with fever, lymphadenopathy, arthralgias, and rash
    3. Causes congenital defects *in utero*, including patent ductus arteriosus and pulmonic stenosis

J. **Coronavirus**
    1. *Coronaviridae* is a family of viruses that cause the common cold (along with rhinovirus).
    2. Also the causative agent behind severe acute respiratory syndrome (SARS)

K. **Influenza Virus**
    1. An enveloped virus in the family *Orthomyxoviridae*
    2. Contains **hemagglutinin** (promotes viral attachment) and **neuraminidase** (releases progeny virions from host cell)
    3. Rapid genetic changes occur due to mutations (**genetic drift**) and reassortment (**genetic shift**).
    4. Flu vaccines contain three different influenza viruses that are determined to be the most likely to cause infection based on data from flu cases in the previous year.
    5. **Presentation:** Sudden onset of headache, fever, myalgias (especially back and body aches), malaise, and nonspecific upper respiratory symptoms (nasal discharge, sore throat, cough). Despite popular perception, gastrointestinal complaints are relatively uncommon.
        a. Influenza virus can cause severe complications, such as viral pneumonia.
        b. Influenza infection can also increase the risk of secondary bacterial infection, which is the most common cause of mortality.
    6. **H5N1 influenza:** Also known as avian influenza ("bird flu"). It has a 60% mortality rate in humans but is currently only transmitted directly from birds to humans (no human-to-human transmission has been observed). Treatment is oseltamivir.
    7. **H1N1 influenza:** Sometimes commonly called as "swine flu." Derived from swine, avian, and human flu viruses. Presents with typical influenza symptoms, along with diarrhea and vomiting. Treatment is oseltamivir or zanamivir.

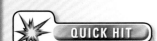

QUICK HIT

Influenza virus strains are distinguished by the types of hemagglutinin and neuraminidase they express. This is how they are named (e.g., H1N1, H5N1).

Microbiology

FIGURE 12-12 Steeple sign

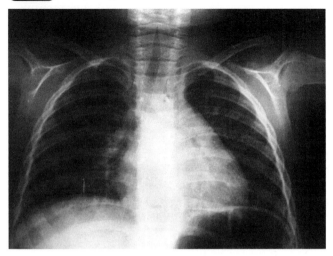

Croup. Steeple sign on a soft-tissue neck radiograph. (Reprinted with permission from Harwood-Nuss A, Wolfson AB, et al. *The Clinical Practice of Emergency Medicine*. 3rd ed. Philadelphia, PA: Lippincott Williams & Wilkins; 2001.)

L. **Parainfluenza Virus**
1. An enveloped virus in the family *Paramyxoviridae* that causes croup (laryngotracheobronchitis).
2. Presents with a barking seal cough, hoarseness, and stridor. Respiratory distress can occur.
3. CXR may reveal the steeple sign (narrowing of the trachea proximal to the larynx) (*Figure 12-12*).
4. Treatment involves cool mist, steam, or cool air. In severe cases, racemic epinephrine, steroids, and oxygen can be used.

M. **Respiratory Syncytial Virus (RSV)**
1. RSV is an enveloped virus in the family *Paramyxoviridae* that causes bronchiolitis and pneumonia. Common in young children in winter months.
2. RSV has a transmembrane protein called F protein that allows infected cells to fuse with uninfected cells (forming syncytia).
3. Presents with fever, nasal congestion, cough, wheezing, and respiratory distress in severe cases
4. Supportive care is the preferred treatment. Antivirals, bronchodilators, and corticosteroids are not recommended.

N. **Rubeola Virus (Measles)**
1. An enveloped virus in the family *Paramyxoviridae* that causes measles
2. Presents with coryza (runny nose), cough, and conjunctivitis, along with Koplik spots (bluish-gray specks on the buccal mucosa) (*Figure 12-13*) followed by generalized rash.

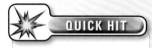

QUICK HIT

Palivizumab is a monoclonal antibody that can be administered to infants during the winter months to protect against RSV. This is generally only used in at-risk cases, such as premature infants or infants with lung conditions.

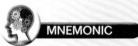

MNEMONIC

Remember the three **C**'s of measles:
Coryza
Cough
Conjunctivitis

FIGURE 12-13 Koplik spots

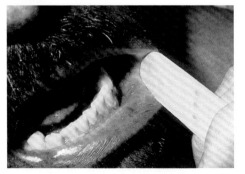

Koplik spots are an early sign of measles. This patient has the pathognomonic exanthem opposite his premolar teeth. (Reprinted with permission from Goodheart HP. *Goodheart's Photoguide of Common Skin Disorders*. 2nd ed. Philadelphia, PA: Lippincott Williams & Wilkins; 2003.)

Microbiology

3. Rubeola virus can also cause acute and chronic encephalitis as well as fetal loss and premature birth in pregnant women.
   a. The chronic form is known as subacute sclerosing panencephalitis (SSPE) and may manifest years after the patient has seemingly recovered.
4. In immunocompromised patients, rubeola virus can cause giant cell pneumonia.

O. **Mumps Virus**
   1. An enveloped virus in the family *Paramyxoviridae* that causes inflammation of the parotid glands (parotitis), or, less commonly, viral meningitis
   2. Mumps virus can also cause orchitis (inflammation of the testes) that may result in sterility

P. **Rabies Virus**
   1. An enveloped virus with a bullet-shaped capsid in the family *Rhabdoviridae*
   2. Mainly infects animals, although it can infect humans after contact with infected animals
   3. Rabies virus travels along the peripheral nerves and infects the CNS. Infected tissues contain Negri bodies, which are eosinophilic cytoplasmic inclusions that contain the capsids (*Figure 12-14*).

FIGURE
12-14 Negri body

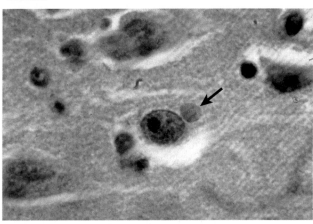

A Negri body in a neuron of a rabid dog. (Reprinted with permission from Rubin E, Farber JL. *Pathology.* 3rd ed. Philadelphia, PA: Lippincott Williams & Wilkins; 1999.)

   4. **Presentation:** Symptoms may present up to a year after infection and include fever, malaise, nausea, vomiting, and neurologic abnormalities, particularly hydrophobia. This eventually progresses to coma and death.

Q. **Hantavirus**
   1. An enveloped virus in the family *Bunyaviridae*
   2. Hantavirus infection manifests as either hemorrhagic fever or pulmonary syndrome, presenting with pulmonary edema and respiratory failure.
   3. Spread through aerosolized mouse urine, specifically from the deer mouse in the United States

R. **Retrovirus**
   1. A unique family of RNA viruses that contains double-stranded RNA
   2. HIV is the most well known retrovirus. Human T-cell leukemia virus (HTLV) is another prominent retrovirus.

IV. HIV

A. **Structure** (*Figure 12-15*)
   1. Diploid genome (2 RNA strands)
   2. Conical capsid around RNA, composed of viral protein **p24** (encoded by the *gag* gene)
   3. Capsid surrounded by spherical viral envelope, a lipid bilayer into which are embedded glycoproteins **gp120** and **gp41**. (The *env* gene codes for the protein gp160. Cleavage of this protein yields gp120 and gp41.)

FIGURE 12-15 Cross section of HIV

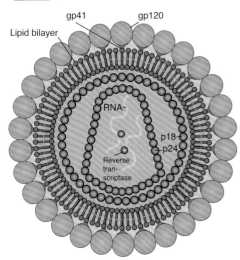

4. Contains the enzymes **reverse transcriptase** and **integrase** (both encoded by the *pol* gene) as well as **protease**

B. **Replication**

1. gp120 recognizes and binds CD4 on the surface of T cells, macrophages, or dendritic cells.

2. gp120 then undergoes a conformational change, allowing it to bind a coreceptor molecule on the cell (either CXCR4 or CCR5).

   a. **Tropism** is the tendency for a virus to preferentially infect cells that express a specific receptor.

   b. HIV strains are differentiated based on whether they bind CXCR4 (called X4 strains) or CCR5 (called R5 strains).

3. Binding of the coreceptors allows gp41 to insert itself into the cell membrane. The virus then fuses with the host cell, and the viral capsid is internalized.

   a. Initial infections mostly involve macrophages and dendritic cells because these are found at mucosal surfaces. This requires viral recognition of CCR5.

   b. As the infection progresses, viruses that recognize CXCR4 begin to predominate, permitting infection of T cells. This is known as a **tropism switch**.

4. Reverse transcriptase synthesizes DNA from the RNA genome. When cells begin to divide, this DNA integrates into the cell's genome.

   a. Once integrated into the host DNA, the provirus can remain latent for years.

   b. In quiescent cells, the viral DNA may remain in the cytoplasm for an extended period of time until cell division occurs.

5. Viral DNA is then translated by the host cell polymerases into viral proteins.

6. Cells are killed through a combination of viral actions and immune responses (the chief mechanism of cell death in HIV infections is still uncertain).

C. **Disease Progression** (*Figure 12-16*)

1. Patients are generally asymptomatic for at least the first month after exposure. These patients may also test negative for HIV during this time.

2. One to 2 months after exposure, patients may experience flu-like or mononucleosis-like symptoms (acute retroviral syndrome). These symptoms resolve on their own after several weeks.

3. The patient then enters an asymptomatic period that corresponds with low-level viral reproduction (clinical latency). This phase may last for years.

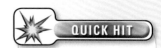

QUICK HIT

Certain strains of HIV can effectively bind both CXCR4 and CCR5. This is known as **dual tropism**.

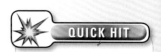

QUICK HIT

HIV displays **clinical latency**, which is the absence of symptoms despite continuous low-level viral reproduction. This is different from **viral latency**, which refers to a dormant period prior to the eventual onset of viral reproduction (e.g., herpesvirus).

Microbiology

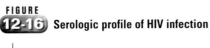

Serologic profile of HIV infection

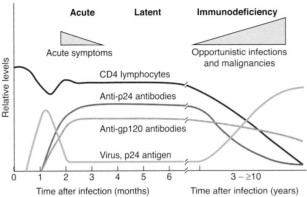

4. As T cell levels decrease, the patient begins to experience opportunistic infections.

D. **Diagnosis**

1. Diagnosis of HIV

   a. Initial screening is conducted using an enzyme-linked immunosorbent assay (ELISA) test. This will detect anti-HIV antibodies in the patient's serum. This test is highly sensitive but has some false positive results.

   b. Positive results on the HIV ELISA screen are confirmed using a Western blot, which also detects anti-HIV antibodies. This test has a very high specificity.

   c. PCR tests are used to determine the **viral load**, and this may be used to confirm the diagnosis if the patient's antibody titer is not high enough to yield positive results on the ELISA and/or Western blot screens (i.e., the initial 1–2 months postinfection). Viral load can also be used to monitor the effectiveness of drug therapy.

2. Diagnosis of AIDS

   a. A CD4 T-cell count <200 cells/μL is sufficient for a diagnosis of AIDS. (Healthy patients generally have CD4 counts between 500 and 1,500 cells/μL.)

   b. Alternatively, an AIDS diagnosis can be confirmed if the amount of CD4 T cells as a percentage of total lymphocytes drops below 14%. (A normal CD4 percentage is about 40%.)

   c. The presence of certain opportunistic infections that are seen almost exclusively in AIDS patients (e.g., *Pneumocystis jirovecii*) can also be considered diagnostic of AIDS.

E. **Opportunistic infections and associated conditions**

1. *Pneumocystis jirovecii*: Fungus that causes interstitial pneumonia

2. *Mycobacterium tuberculosis*: Generally occurs very early in the course of AIDS. May involve only the lungs or may spread to other organs, depending on the degree of immunodeficiency.

3. *Mycobacterium avium* **complex (MAC)**: Also known as *Mycobacterium avium intracellulare* (MAI). Generally occurs after the CD4 count falls below 50 cells/μL.

4. *Histoplasma capsulatum*: Causes a systemic disease characterized by hepato-splenomegaly, fever, and cough, especially with CD4 counts <100 cells/μL.

5. *Cryptococcus neoformans*: Eighty percent to 90% of cryptococcosis cases occur in patients with AIDS, often manifesting as meningitis.

6. *Cytomegalovirus*: CMV retinitis most commonly occurs when CD4 cell counts fall below 50 cells/μL. It may also cause esophagitis and/or colitis, although CMV can manifest as disseminated disease in rare cases.

7. *Toxoplasma gondii*: Toxoplasmosis is the cause of 50% of all CNS lesions in AIDS patients. These tend to manifest as ring-enhancing lesions.

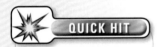

PCR tests are also useful for diagnosing HIV infections in newborns from HIV-positive mothers.

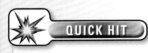

Pneumocystis pneumonia is commonly referred to as "PCP."

Microbiology

8. **JC virus:** PML is the result of reactivation of latent JC virus.
9. *Cryptosporidium:* Causes chronic diarrhea that can lead to significant wasting in AIDS patients. (The disease is self-limited in immunocompetent individuals.)
10. *Candida albicans:* Candidiasis is the most common fungal infection in AIDS patients. It generally affects the oral cavity and often occurs in asymptomatic individuals. Its appearance generally heralds the transition to AIDS. In individuals with CD4 counts <100 cells/μL, it can also affect the esophagus and the vagina.
11. **Herpes simplex virus:** HSV causes ulcers in most infected individuals, but AIDS patients have longer, more severe outbreaks.
12. **Epstein–Barr virus (EBV):** Often causes oral hairy leukoplakia in AIDS patients.
13. **Non-Hodgkin lymphoma:** AIDS patients are particularly susceptible to primary CNS lymphoma and large B-cell lymphoma, both of which are associated with EBV infection.
14. **Human papillomavirus:** May cause squamous cell carcinomas of the cervix or anus.
15. **Kaposi sarcoma:** Common neoplasm in AIDS patients. Vascular tumors cause the appearance of cutaneous purple lesions (Figure 12-17). These lesions may also appear on mucous membranes or internal organs. This condition is associated with HHV-8.

FIGURE
12-17 Kaposi sarcoma

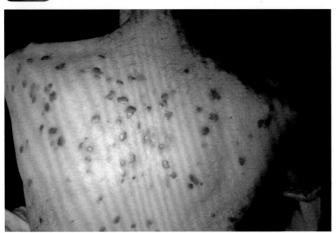

Lesions of AIDS-related Kaposi sarcoma. Whereas some patients may have lesions that remain flat, others experience extensively disseminated, raised lesions with edema. (Reprinted with permission from DeVita VT, Hellaman S, Rosenberg S. *AIDS: Etiology, diagnosis, treatment, and prevention.* 4th ed. Philadelphia, PA: Lippincott-Raven; 1997.)

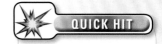

QUICK HIT

Bacillary angiomatosis due to *Bartonella henselae* causes the formation of highly vascular cutaneous lesions, which may be mistaken for Kaposi sarcoma.

F. **Treatment**
1. Antiretroviral therapy (*Table 12-2*)
   a. The standard regimen is called highly active antiretroviral therapy (HAART), a combination of three different drugs designed to inhibit viral replication as well as to avoid the development of resistance.
   b. HAART generally involves two different nucleoside reverse transcriptase inhibitors (NRTI), known as the "NRTI backbone," combined with a third drug from a different class.
   c. Indicated for all patients with CD4 counts <350 cells/μL or a diagnosis of AIDS, although it is recommended for all HIV-positive patients.
2. Prophylaxis for opportunistic infections
   a. **CD4 <200 cells/μL:** Begin PCP prophylaxis with TMP-SMX, with or without aerosolized pentamidine. In sulfa-allergic patients, the drug of choice is dapsone, although patients must be evaluated for glucose-6-phosphate dehydrogenase (G6PD) deficiency.

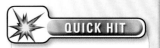

QUICK HIT

NRTIs must be activated (phosphorylated) by thymidine kinase before becoming functional.

Microbiology

TABLE 12-2 Therapeutic Agents in HIV

Therapeutic Agent (common name, if relevant)	Class—Pharmacology and Pharmacokinetics	Indications	Side or Adverse Effects	Contraindications or Precautions to Consider; Notes
Zidovudine (ZDV, formerly AZT)	**NRTI—guanosine analog** → inhibits viral reverse transcriptase → prevents integration of DNA copy of viral genome into host DNA	**HAART; HIV pregnant women** to reduce fetal transmission	**Bone marrow suppression (neutropenia, anemia)**, peripheral neuropathy, pancreatitis, lactic acidosis	**Effects of bone marrow suppression can be reduced by the addition of GM-CSF**
Didanosine (ddI)	**NRTI—guanosine analog;** (similar to Zidovudine)	HAART	Bone marrow suppression, **peripheral neuropathy, pancreatitis,** lactic acidosis, **hepatic steatosis**	
Abacavir (ABC)	**NRTI—guanosine analog** (similar to Zidovudine)	HAART	Bone marrow suppression, peripheral neuropathy, pancreatitis, lactic acidosis, **hypersensitivity reaction (can be fatal)**	Check HLA-B*5701 test prior to starting ABC to avoid giving to patients at risk for hypersensitivity reactions
Lamivudine (3TC)	**NRTI—cytidine analog** → inhibits viral reverse transcriptase → prevents integration of DNA copy of the viral genome into the host DNA	HAART	Bone marrow suppression, peripheral neuropathy, pancreatitis, and lactic acidosis	
Emtricitabine (FTC)	**NRTI—cytidine analog** (similar to Lamivudine)	HAART	Bone marrow suppression, peripheral neuropathy, pancreatitis, lactic acidosis	
Tenofovir (TDF)	**Nucleotide reverse transcriptase inhibitor— adenosine analog** → inhibits viral reverse transcriptase	HAART	Nausea, vomiting, headache, renal dysfunction	Although it is often classified with the NRTIs, it is actually a **nucleotide** reverse transcriptase inhibitor.
Nevirapine, delavirdine, efavirenz, etravirine, rilpivirine	**NNRTI—noncompetitively** bind viral reverse transcriptase and inhibits the movement of protein domains → terminates viral DNA synthesis → prevents integration of viral genome into the host DNA	HAART	**Rash,** bone marrow suppression, peripheral neuropathy; **Efavirenz causes neuropsychiatric problems (nightmares, depression),** and dizziness and is **teratogenic**	
Saquinavir (SQV), ritonavir (RTV), indinavir (IDV), nelfinavir, fosamprenavir, lopinavir, tipranavir, atazanavir, darunavir	**Protease inhibitors—HIV-1** protease is responsible for the final step of viral proliferation; inhibits protease in progeny virions → assembly of nonfunctional viruses	**HAART**	**GI intolerance (nausea, diarrhea), hyperglycemia, hyperlipidemia, lipodystrophy,**	All protease inhibitors end in -navir; **metabolized cytochrome P450** (many potential drug interactions)
Enfuvirtide	**Fusion inhibitor—binds** viral gp41 subunit → inhibits conformation change (required for fusion with CD4 cell) → blocks viral entry and replication	**Patients with persistent viral replication on antiretroviral therapy**	**Hypersensitivity reactions and injection site reactions;** increased risk of bacterial pneumonia	Used in combination with other antiretroviral drugs

TABLE 12-2 Therapeutic Agents in HIV *(Continued)*

Therapeutic Agent (common name, if relevant)	Class—Pharmacology and Pharmacokinetics	Indications	Side or Adverse Effects	Contraindications or Precautions to Consider; Notes
Raltegravir, elvitegravir	**Integrase inhibitors**— inhibit the final step in integration of viral DNA into host DNA	HAART	**Hyperglycemia, hyperlipidemia**, pancreatitis, hepatotoxicity	
Maraviroc	**CCR5 antagonist**—inhibits viral CCR5 coreceptor → blocks viral entry to host cell	HAART	Fever, cough, upper respiratory infections, peripheral neuropathy, dizziness	

CCR5, C-C chemokine receptor type 5; CD4, cluster of differentiation 4; GI, gastrointestinal; GM-CSF, granulocyte-macrophage colony-stimulating factor; HAART, highly active antiretroviral therapy; NRTI, nucleoside reverse transcriptase inhibitor; NNRTI, non-nucleoside reverse transcriptase inhibitor.

    b. **CD4 <100 cells/μL:** Begin prophylaxis against reactivation of toxoplasmosis with TMP-SMX. In sulfa-allergic patients, a combination of dapsone, pyrimethamine, and leucovorin is used.

    c. **CD4 <50 cells/μL:** Begin MAC prophylaxis with azithromycin.

 FUNGI

I. Yeast Infections

  A. *Candida albicans* Infection (Candidiasis)

    1. Skin-resident yeast that causes candidiasis. *Candida albicans* is also found in the GI tract and in the female genital tract.

    2. Diseases

      a. Severe infections only affect immunocompromised patients, although *C. albicans* can cause superficial infections in immunocompetent individuals.

      b. Vaginal candidiasis is not uncommon in immunocompetent women, although the risk is increased in diabetics and women who have recently undergone treatment with antibiotics.

      c. Diaper rash in infants

      d. Intertrigo is a candidal rash in the skin folds of obese patients or underneath the breasts.

      e. *Candida* can enter the bloodstream of IV drug users or patients with central lines. It can then cause multiple organ conditions, including endocarditis, hepatosplenic candidiasis, or endophthalmitis. Disseminated candidiasis has a mortality rate of 30%–40%.

    3. **Presentation:** Oral thrush, esophagitis, painful swallowing, dysphagia, substernal chest pain, vulvovaginitis, vaginal itch, vaginal discharge, rash with satellite lesions, intertrigo

    4. **Labs:** Positive blood culture, positive urine culture, positive β-glucan detection assay

    5. **Treatment:** Nystatin, clotrimazole, fluconazole, amphotericin B, caspofungin, micafungin, anidulafungin

  B. *Cryptococcus neoformans* Infection

    1. Encapsulated yeast that causes cryptococcosis and cryptococcal meningitis

    2. Cryptococcus is found in soil and pigeon droppings and primarily transmitted via the respiratory route. Generally only affects immunocompromised individuals, particularly cryptococcal meningitis, which is often fatal.

    3. **Presentation:** Cough, pleuritic chest pain, fever, dyspnea, lymphadenopathy, altered mental status (cryptococcal meningitis)

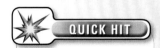

QUICK HIT

Oral thrush from *Candida* can be scraped off and will leave bleeding mucosa. It should not be confused with EBV-induced oral hairy leukoplakia, which cannot be scraped off.

4. **Diagnostics:** "Soap-bubble" brain lesion, positive blood culture, cryptococci in CSF, nodules and hilar lymphadenopathy on CXR, granulomas on biopsy
5. **Treatment:** Amphotericin B, flucytosine, fluconazole

C. *Pneumocystis jirovecii* Infection

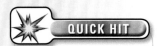

1. Yeast that causes *Pneumocystis* pneumonia (PCP). Generally only affects immunocompromised patients. It is the most common opportunistic infection in HIV-positive patients and has a mortality rate of 10%–20%.
2. *Pneumocystis jirovecii* is commonly found in the respiratory tract and is believed to be transmitted in an airborne manner.
3. **Presentation:** Dyspnea, nonproductive cough, fever, crackles on auscultation, tachypnea, tachycardia
4. **Diagnostics:** Atypical pneumonia on CXR, *Pneumocystis* in bronchial lavage, ground glass appearance of interstitial infiltrates on CXR, elevated LDH, positive β-glucan assay
5. **Treatment:** Trimethoprim/sulfamethoxazole, corticosteroids (only in severe cases)

D. *Malassezia furfur* Infection (Tinea Versicolor)
1. *Malassezia furfur* is a yeast that causes tinea versicolor, a condition named for the hypopigmented and hyperpigmented skin patches that result from the infection.
2. Immunocompromised individuals and individuals on corticosteroid therapy have a mildly increased risk for tinea versicolor.
3. **Presentation:** Round, scaly, nonpruritic macules on the trunk and proximal limbs; papules; patches of hyperpigmentation or hypopigmentation (*Figure 12-18*)
4. **Labs:** "Spaghetti and meatball" appearance on KOH test. Cultures are rarely performed.
5. **Treatment:** Topical antifungals, high rate of recurrence

FIGURE 12-18 Tinea versicolor

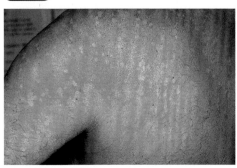

(Reprinted from Goodheart HP. *Goodheart's Photoguide of Common Skin Disorders.* 2nd ed. Philadelphia, PA: Lippincott Williams & Wilkins; 2003.)

II. Mold Infections

A. *Aspergillus* Infection
1. Multiple species of *Aspergillus* cause human disease and are found ubiquitously in nature.
2. *Aspergillus fumigates* and *Aspergillus flavus* are the most common causes in humans, although there are more than 200 different species of *Aspergillus*.
3. May cause allergic bronchopulmonary aspergillosis (ABPA) or necrotizing pneumonia or may form aspergillomas in the lungs
4. Immunocompromised patients are susceptible to disseminated aspergillosis, which has a very high mortality rate.
5. Rarely affects immunocompetent individuals
6. **Presentation:** Fever, productive cough, hemoptysis, dyspnea, pleuritic chest pain
7. **Diagnostics:** Acute-angled hyphae on plate culture, neutropenia, eosinophilia (ABPA), positive *Aspergillus* antigen skin test (ABPA), *Aspergillus*-specific serum antibodies, pulmonary infiltrates on CXR, positive sputum culture (invasive aspergillosis)

P. jirovecii was formerly called *P. carinii*. Thus, "PCP" stood for "*Pneumocystis carinii* pneumonia" but now stands for "*Pneumocystis* pneumonia."

8. **Treatment:** Voriconazole, posaconazole, amphotericin B lipid formulation, corticosteroids (not recommended in immunocompromised patients), surgical care for refractory cases of necrotizing pneumonia

B. **Mucormycosis**
1. *Rhizopus* and *Mucor* molds are the most common causes. Both are ubiquitous in the environment.
2. Mucormycosis is a rare disease that generally occurs in immunocompromised individuals, especially patients with diabetic ketoacidosis.
3. The most common form is rhinocerebral mucormycosis, although it may also be pulmonary, cutaneous, gastrointestinal, or disseminated.
   a. The rhinocerebral form has a mortality rate of 50%–70%.
   b. The disseminated form has a mortality rate of nearly 100%.
   c. Cutaneous mucormycosis has the lowest mortality rate at 15%.
4. **Presentation:** Headache, facial pain, numbness, fever, hyposmia, black nasal discharge, diplopia, vision loss, black eschars in the palate or the nose, orbital swelling, facial cellulitis
5. **Diagnostics:** Right-angled hyphae on plate culture, *Mucoraceae* in tissue biopsy, mucosal thickening, bony erosions, sinusitis. Blood cultures are generally negative.
6. **Treatment:** Amphotericin B lipid formulation, posaconazole. Surgical debridement of necrotic tissue is mandatory.

C. **Dermatophytosis**
1. Caused by a group of molds known as dermatophytes. This includes *Trichophyton*, *Microsporum*, and *Epidermophyton*. These molds may be resident in human skin, soil, or animals, depending on the species.
2. Dermatophytes cause a wide variety of superficial skin conditions.
   a. **Tinea pedis:** Affects the soles of the feet. Also known as athlete's foot. Most common presentation of dermatophytosis. *Trichophyton rubrum* is the most common cause.
   b. **Tinea cruris:** Affects the groin. Also known as jock itch. Second most common presentation of dermatophytosis. *Trichophyton rubrum* and *Epidermophyton floccosum* are the most common causes.
   c. **Tinea corporis:** Affects the glabrous (hairless) skin. Most commonly caused by *Trichophyton rubrum*.
   d. **Tinea capitis:** Affects the scalp. Most common dermatophytosis in children. *Trichophyton tonsurans* is the most common cause.
   e. **Tinea unguium:** Affects the fingernails and toenails. Also known as onychomycosis. Generally caused by *Trichophyton rubrum*, although it can also be caused by *Candida*.
   f. Other forms of tinea include tinea manuum (hands), tinea barbae (hairy facial skin), and tinea faciei (glabrous facial skin).
3. **Presentation:** Dry scaly skin, rash, erythematous plaques, papules, pruritic lesions with central clearing (tinea capitis), thickened discolored nails (tinea unguium)
4. **Labs:** Fungal hyphae on skin scrapings or hair samples, positive fungal culture
5. **Treatment:** Topical terbinafine, topical clotrimazole, topical ketoconazole, topical econazole, oral itraconazole, griseofulvin (tinea capitis)

III. Dimorphic Fungi

A. *Histoplasma capsulatum* **Infection**
1. *Histoplasma capsulatum* is a dimorphic fungus that causes histoplasmosis.
2. It is endemic in the Mississippi, Missouri, and Ohio river valleys, as well as numerous other river valleys around the world. It is found in soil as well as in bat droppings.
3. It is transmitted through inhalation of airborne spores, which may remain dormant for years.
4. Most infected individuals are asymptomatic. Symptomatic individuals are generally immunocompromised, or they have been exposed to a very high inoculum load.

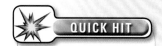

QUICK HIT

Malassezia furfur is not considered a dermatophyte. Thus, tinea versicolor is technically not classified a as dermatophytosis.

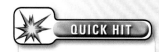

QUICK HIT

Dimorphic fungi can grow as a mold or as a yeast, depending on the growth conditions. *Histoplasma* grows as a yeast within humans.

Microbiology

5. In symptomatic patients, infection usually causes include mild pulmonary disease, which may progress to pericarditis or mediastinal fibrosis. Disseminated histoplasmosis is generally only seen in immunocompromised patients.

6. **Presentation:** Fever, headache, malaise, myalgias, abdominal pain, rales and wheezing

7. **Diagnostics:** Positive skin antigen test, pulmonary infiltrates on CXR, mild anemia, pancytopenia, elevated alkaline phosphatase (ALP), positive blood and sputum cultures

8. **Treatment:** Fluconazole, itraconazole, amphotericin B, corticosteroids

B. *Blastomyces dermatitidis* Infection

1. *Blastomyces dermatitidis* is a dimorphic fungus that cause blastomycosis.

2. Transmitted by inhalation of spores from soil. Incubation period is 20–40 days. Fifty percent of patients will never develop symptoms.

3. Extrapulmonary dissemination is rare in immunocompetent individuals.

4. Blastomycosis is not normally fatal, unless a patient is immunocompromised or the untreated infection has progressed to acute respiratory distress syndrome.

5. **Presentation:** Fever, chills, myalgias, dyspnea, cough, skin lesions, arthralgias

6. **Diagnostics:** Leukocytosis, hypoxemia, positive sputum KOH test, positive stain and culture. CXR findings are nonspecific.

7. **Treatment:** Itraconazole, amphotericin B

C. *Coccidioides immitis* Infection

1. *Coccidioides immitis* is a dimorphic fungus that causes coccidioidomycosis (also known as San Joaquin valley fever).

2. Transmission by inhalation of spores from soil. Normally seen in the southwestern United States.

3. *Coccidioides* actually forms spherules *in vivo*. Spherules are double-walled structures that are filled with many daughter endospores (*Figure 12-19*). These eventually burst, releasing the endospores into the surrounding tissue.

4. Most infected patients are asymptomatic or only mildly symptomatic.

5. Primary infection usually presents as pneumonia, with fatigue, cough, fever, and arthralgias (sometimes called desert rheumatism).

6. Immunocompromised individuals are more susceptible to disseminated infections, although it does occur in otherwise healthy individuals. Disseminated infection can involve the skin, CNS, bones, and joints.

7. **Presentation:** Fever, cough, chest pain, fatigue, dyspnea, erythema nodosum, arthralgias, rales, rhonchi. Headache, blurred vision, and altered mental status are associated with meningitis.

FIGURE
12-19 Coccidioides immitis spherules

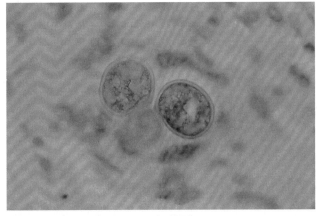

Lung granuloma with *Coccidioides* spherule. (Reprinted with permission from McClatchey KD. *Clinical Laboratory Medicine*. 2nd ed. Philadelphia, PA: Lippincott Williams & Wilkins; 2002.)

8. **Diagnostics:** Elevated sed rate, positive IgM or IgG serum titer, positive fungal culture, positive antigen skin test, elevated CSF protein (meningitis), spherules on biopsy.
9. **Treatment:** Amphotericin B, fluconazole, ketoconazole, itraconazole

D. *Paracoccidioides brasiliensis* Infection
1. *Paracoccidioides brasiliensis* is a dimorphic fungus that causes paracoccidioidomycosis when it is inhaled from the environment.
2. Endemic to Central and South America. Most cases of paracoccidioidomycosis in the United States are believed to be due to activation of latent infections that originated in Central or South America.
3. Paracoccidioidomycosis is usually asymptomatic, although it can progress to severe pulmonary infection. It may also cause fibrosis of mucous membranes, which can result in long-term sequelae.
4. Immunocompromised individuals do not have a significantly higher rate of infection, although they are at higher risk for disseminated disease once infected.
5. **Presentation:** Cough (dry or productive), dyspnea, malaise, fever, laryngeal and pharyngeal lesions, oral lesions, skin lesions, cervical lymphadenopathy.
6. **Diagnostics:** "Captain's wheel" spores in tissue or fluid samples (*Figure 12-20*), interstitial infiltrates on CXR
7. **Treatment:** Amphotericin B, itraconazole, ketoconazole, supportive care, reconstructive surgery for fibrotic sequelae

E. *Sporothrix schenckii* Infection
1. *Sporothrix schenckii* is a dimorphic fungus that causes sporotrichosis. It is found in soil and on vegetation. It is commonly transmitted through skin wounds and is informally known as rose gardener's disease.
2. Generally begins as a skin lesion or subcutaneous nodule at the wound site. It then spreads, with more lesions and nodules appearing along the draining lymphatics.
3. Disseminated sporotrichosis is very rare and usually only occurs in immunocompromised patients.

FIGURE
12-20 *Paracoccidioides* spores

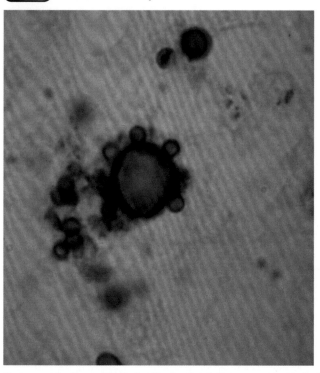

The lung contains *Paracoccidioides brasiliensis,* which displays many external buds arising circumferentially from the mother organism ("captain's wheel" spores).

4. **Presentation:** Painless skin lesions or nodules, ulcerating lesions
5. **Diagnostics:** Positive fungal cultures, positive antibody titer, granulomatous inflammation in skin biopsy
6. **Treatment:** Itraconazole, fluconazole, amphotericin B lipid formulation, saturated solution of potassium iodide (SSKI)

IV. Antifungal Drugs (Table 12-3)

TABLE 12-3 Antifungal Drugs				
Therapeutic Agent	Class—Pharmacology and Pharmacokinetics	Indications	Side or Adverse Effects	Contraindications or Precautions to Consider; Notes
Amphotericin B	**Polyene—binds ergosterol in fungal cell membrane, altering cell permeability**	Used for severe systemic fungal infections or infections where first-line antifungals are failing	**Nephrotoxicity**, fever, chills, anemia, phlebitis, arrhythmias, hypotension, hypokalemia	Administered intravenously; liposomal formulation has fewer side effects but it expensive
Nystatin	**Polyene—binds ergosterol in fungal cell membrane, altering cell permeability**	Topically for cutaneous or vulvovaginal candidiasis. "Swish and swallow" for oral thrush	**Too toxic for systemic use;** diarrhea, nausea, vomiting, and stomach pain from swallowing nystatin suspension	Topical nystatin is safe for use in pregnancy, but oral nystatin suspension is not recommended
Fluconazole	**Triazole—interferes with synthesis of the fungal membrane** by inhibiting lanosterol 14 α-demethylase, which normally converts lanosterol to ergosterol	Oropharyngeal and esophageal candidiasis, cryptococcal meningitis, vulvovaginitis	Increased LFTs, headache, nausea, abdominal pain, diarrhea	Contraindicated in pregnancy
Itraconazole	**Triazole**—(same as fluconazole)	**Life-threatening mycoses** (blastomycosis, aspergillosis, histoplasmosis), oral candidiasis, **onychomycosis**	Increased LFTs, nausea, vomiting, rash, headache	Not recommended during pregnancy
Voriconazole	**Triazole**—(same as fluconazole)	Invasive aspergillosis, candidemia, candidiasis	Visual changes, hallucinations, increased LFTs	Contraindicated in pregnancy
Posaconazole	**Triazole**—(same as fluconazole)	*Aspergillus* prophylaxis in neutropenia, refractory candidiasis	Hypokalemia, hypomagnesemia, anemia, thrombocytopenia, vaginal hemorrhage, nausea, vomiting, diarrhea	May be used in pregnancy, although it is not recommended
Ketoconazole	**Imidazole**—(same mechanism as fluconazole)	Seborrheic dermatitis, tinea versicolor, dermatophytoses, endemic mycoses. Largely replaced by newer antifungals.	Nausea, vomiting, skin irritation, hepatotoxicity, **gynecomastia**	May be used in pregnancy if necessary
Clotrimazole (Lotrimin, Mycelex)	**Imidazole**—(same mechanism as fluconazole)	Topical use for dermatophytoses and *Candida* vulvovaginitis	Abnormal LFTs as well as mild irritation at the application site	Safe for use in pregnancy
Miconazole (Desenex, Monistat)	**Imidazole**—(same mechanism as fluconazole)	Topical use for dermatophytoses and *Candida* vulvovaginitis. Oral use for oropharyngeal candidiasis.	Skin irritation at the topical application site; GI symptoms when taken orally	May be used in pregnancy, although it is not recommended

TABLE 12-3 Antifungal Drugs (Continued)

Therapeutic Agent	Class—Pharmacology and Pharmacokinetics	Indications	Side or Adverse Effects	Contraindications or Precautions to Consider; Notes
Terbinafine (Lamisil)	Allylamine—inhibits squalene epoxidase, which normally converts squalene to lanosterol → **interferes with fungal membrane synthesis**	Topically for dermatophytoses, orally for onychomycosis and tinea capitis	Skin irritation at the topical application site; GI symptoms and increased LFTs when taken orally	Safe for use in pregnancy
Caspofungin	Echinocandin—inhibits β-1,3-D-glucan synthase → **interferes with cell wall synthesis**	Candidemia, candidiasis, invasive aspergillosis	Phlebitis, fever, rash, increased LFTs	May be used in pregnancy but is not recommended
Flucytosine	Pyrimidine analog that **inhibits DNA and protein synthesis**	Candidiasis, *Cryptococcus* infections; combined with amphotericin B to treat systemic fungal infections, particularly cryptococcal meningitis	**Bone marrow suppression**, increased LFTs, some GI symptoms	May be used in pregnancy, although it is not recommended
Griseofulvin	**Inhibits microtubule function**, interfering with mitosis	Used orally to treat dermatophytoses	**GI symptoms, headache**, confusion	**Induces cytochrome P450;** contraindicated in pregnancy (teratogenic)

GI, gastrointestinal; LFTs, liver function tests.

PROTOZOA (Table 12-4)

TABLE 12-4 Protozoa

Organism	Clinical Features	Transmission	Labs	Treatment
Cryptosporidium	Chronic diarrhea in HIV-positive patients, possible respiratory or biliary tract infections. (Immunocompetent patients have only mild, self-limited diarrhea)	Contaminated water or person-to-person contact	*Cryptosporidium* in stool, elevated ALP (biliary involvement), dilated biliary ducts and/or enlarged gall bladder (biliary involvement). CXR for respiratory involvement is nonspecific.	Nitazoxanide, paromomycin, antidiarrheals, supportive therapy
Giardia lamblia	Diarrhea, greasy stool flatulence, abdominal distention	Water contaminated with animal feces, commonly affects campers and hikers	Trophozoites (pear-shaped cysts with double nuclei) in stool (*Figure 12-21*), increased fecal fat.	Metronidazole, tinidazole, paromomycin
Entamoeba histolytica	Invasion of the colon causes bloody diarrhea. May also cause liver abscesses (RUQ abdominal pain)	Contaminated water or food	Leukocytosis, elevated ALP, RBCs in trophozoites, anti-*Entamoeba* Ab in serum	Metronidazole, nitazoxanide, tinidazole, paromomycin, surgical intervention if liver abscesses are refractory to medication
Trichomonas vaginalis	Vaginal irritation, malodorous green vaginal discharge, dyspareunia, dysuria. (Men may also be infected, but are generally asymptomatic.)	Sexual contact	Low vaginal pH, flagellated protozoa in vaginal discharge	Metronidazole, tinidazole

Microbiology

(continued)

TABLE **12-4** **Protozoa** *(Continued)*

Organism	Clinical Features	Transmission	Labs	Treatment
Toxoplasma gondii	Brain abscesses in HIV-positive patients. Crosses the placenta to cause fetal chorioretinitis, hydrocephalus, and intracranial calcifications.	Normally contracted from cat feces	Ring-enhancing brain lesions on MRI, anti-*Toxoplasma* Ab in serum, tachyzoites or cysts in tissues or fluids.	Sulfadiazine, pyrimethamine, folinic acid
Plasmodium species (*P. vivax*, *P. malariae*, *P. ovale*, *P. falciparum*)	Malaria: cyclical fever, sweats, chills, headache, cough, hemoglobinuria, arthralgias, myalgias, altered mental status (*P. falciparum*)	*Anopheles* mosquito	Hemolytic anemia, merozoites on blood smear, banana-shaped gametocyte (*P. falciparum*) (*Figure 12-22*)	Primaquine, chloroquine, quinine, mefloquine, atovaquone/proguanil, artemether/lumefantrine
Naegleria fowleri	Flagellated protozoan that causes primary amebic meningoencephalitis: fever, ageusia, headache, stiff neck, mental status changes, seizures, cranial nerve palsies	Contracted from freshwater lakes.	Trophozoites in CSF or brain biopsy, positive CSF culture, elevated CSF protein	Intravenous and intrathecal amphotericin B. (Almost universally fatal. Death occurs within 5–10 days)
Trypanosoma brucei	African sleeping sickness; chancre at bite site; early stage has mild symptoms like fever, malaise, rash appear; late stage CNS involvement, leading to headaches, somnolence, and seizures	Transmitted by the tsetse fly. Endemic to sub-Saharan Africa.	*T. brucei* on smear, hypoalbuminemia, hypergammaglobulinemia, elevated ESR, anemia, thrombocytopenia, elevated CSF protein	Suramin, or melarsoprol or eflornithine for CNS involvement
Trypanosoma cruzi	Chagas disease: fever, lymphadenopathy, dilated cardiomyopathy, megaesophagus, megacolon	Transmitted by reduviid bug ("kissing bug"). Endemic to North and South America.	*T. cruzi* on blood smear	Nifurtimox, benznidazole
Leishmania donovani	Intracellular protozoa that cause cutaneous leishmaniasis (ulcerating papules, hyperpigmentation) and visceral leishmaniasis (spiking fever, night sweats, splenomegaly)	Transmitted by the female sandfly	Pancytopenia, anemia, macrophages containing amastigotes, positive tissue culture, positive PCR test	Amphotericin B lipid formulation for visceral leishmaniasis. Sodium stibogluconate for cutaneous leishmaniasis.
Babesia microti	Babesiosis, which is clinically similar to malaria, without cyclical fevers	Transmitted by *Ixodes* ticks	Anemia, hemoglobinuria, ring forms in red blood cells, crossshaped tetrad merozoites in RBCs (*Figure 12-23*)	Atovaquone plus azithromycin, or quinine plus clindamycin

Ab, antibodies; ALP, alkaline phosphatase; CXR, chest x-ray; CNS, central nervous system; CSF, cerebrospinal fluid; ESR, erythrocyte sedimentation rate; PCR, polymerase chain reaction; RBCs, red blood cells; RUQ, right upper quadrant.

FIGURE
12-21 *Giardia* trophozoites

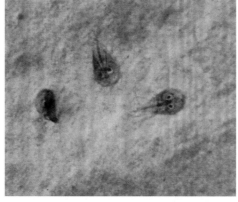

(Reprinted with permission from Sun T. *Parasitic Disorders*. 2nd ed. Baltimore, MD: Williams & Wilkins; 1998.)

FIGURE 12-22 *Plasmodium* stages

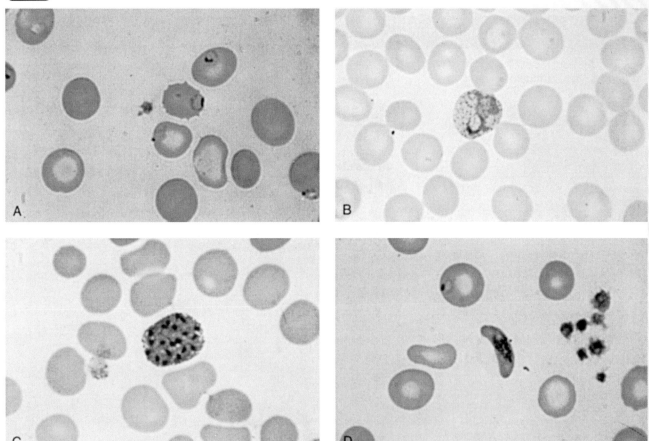

Stages in the life cycle of plasmodia that infect humans. **A.** Merozoite (ring stage) of *P. falciparum*. **B.** Trophozoite of *P. vivax*. **C.** Schizont of *P. vivax,* containing merozoites. **D.** Pathognomonic banana-shaped gametocyte of *P. falciparum*. (Reprinted with permission from Gorbach SL, Bartlett JG, et al. *Infectious Diseases*. Philadelphia, PA: Lippincott Williams & Wilkins; 2004.)

FIGURE 12-23 Babesiosis

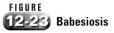
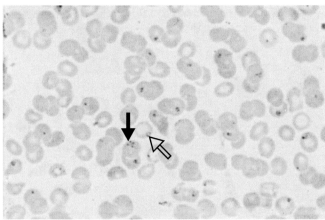

Babesia microti–infected erythrocytes from a case of transfusion-transmitted babesiosis. Note the ring form (*open arrow*) and the characteristic tetrad or "Maltese cross" (*closed arrow*). (Reprinted with permission from Gorbach SL, Bartlett JG, et al. *Infectious Diseases*. Philadelphia, PA: Lippincott Williams & Wilkins; 2004.)

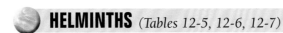

HELMINTHS (Tables 12-5, 12-6, 12-7)

TABLE 12-5 Nematodes (Roundworms)

Organism	Clinical Features	Transmission/ Life Cycle	Labs	Treatment
Enterobius vermicularis (pinworm)	Anal pruritus	**Fecal–oral transmission**; worms reside in the colon and migrate to the rectum at night to lay eggs, which hatch in 6 hours	Worms in stool, **positive "tape test"** (place transparent tape over the anus at night, then examine for eggs)	Albendazole, mebendazole
Ascaris lumbricoides (giant round-worm)	Abdominal pain and distention, nausea, diarrhea; Löeffler syndrome (wheezing, cough, dyspnea, chest pain)	**Fecal–oral transmission**; eggs hatch in the small intestine, enter bloodstream, go to the lungs, move up into the oropharynx, then down into the GI tract and begin to lay eggs	Eggs in stool, larvae in sputum, peripheral eosinophilia, intraluminal worms on abdominal x-ray	Albendazole, mebendazole, pyrantel pamoate
Trichinella spiralis	Diarrhea (initially), fever, headache, fatigue, weakness, periorbital edema, myalgias, myositis	Contracted from **consumption of undercooked pork** or wild game; larvae migrate from the GI tract into the muscles	Eosinophilia, elevated CK and LDH, myoglobinuria, anti-*Trichinella* Ab in serum, larvae on muscle biopsy	Albendazole, mebendazole, corticosteroids
Strongyloides stercoralis	**Pruritic rash at the entry site ("ground itch")**, nonspecific GI symptoms, wheezing and mild cough; altered mental status and seizures only appear in patients with the disseminated form	**Reside in soil, enter humans by penetrating the skin**; enters bloodstream, travels to lungs, then migrates through oropharynx to the intestine to lay eggs; eggs hatch in the intestine, and larvae are excreted in the feces	Eosinophilia, *Strongyloides* larvae in stool, antibodies in serum	Ivermectin, albendazole, mebendazole
Ancylostoma duodenale and *Necator americanus* (hookworms)	**Pruritic rash at the entry site ("ground itch")**, diarrhea, abdominal pain, and **symptoms of anemia**	**Reside in soil, enter humans by penetrating the skin**; life cycle similar to *Strongyloides*	**Anemia**, hookworm eggs in stool, eosinophilia (acute phase)	Albendazole, mebendazole
Wuchereria bancrofti	Lymphatic filariasis and elephantiasis: fever, lymphadenopathy, testicular pain, edema, hydrocele, elephantiasis of limbs or genitals	Transmitted by mosquitoes; larvae migrate to the lymphatics, where they cause inflammation and lymphatic obstruction	*Worms*, blood or hydrocele fluid, antigen in peripheral blood, eosinophilia	Diethylcarbamazine, doxycycline, ivermectin, albendazole; surgical excision for large hydroceles and scrotal elephantiasis

Ab, antibodies; CK, creatine kinase; GI, gastrointestinal; LDH, lactate dehydrogenase.

Microbiology

TABLE 12-6 Cestodes (Tapeworms)

Organism	Clinical Features	Transmission/Life Cycle	Labs	Treatment
Taenia solium	GI tract infection with the tapeworm causes abdominal pain, anorexia, weight loss; **larval cyst formation in host organs or tissues (cysticercosis); CNS involvement (neurocysticercosis)** can cause seizures and altered mental status	GI infection with the tapeworm results from eating undercooked pork containing larval cysts. Cysticercosis results from ingesting food/water containing tapeworm eggs.	Eosinophilia, *Taenia* eggs in stool; cysts on CT or MRI, abnormal CSF findings (neurocysticercosis)	Albendazole, praziquantel, dexamethasone. Surgical removal of cysts as needed.
Diphyllobothrium latum	Usually asymptomatic; may cause abdominal pain or indigestion may be seen; worms may absorb nutrients in the intestine (may lead to B_{12} deficiency)	Contracted by **eating undercooked fish**, mature in the small intestine	Megaloblastic anemia, eosinophilia, decreased vitamin B_{12}, eggs or worm segments in stool	Praziquantel
Echinococcus granulosus	Pulmonary cystic echinococcosis (cough, chest pain, dyspnea); hepatic echinococcosis (RUQ abdominal pain, jaundice, hepatomegaly)	Contracted from ingestion of food or water contaminated with dog feces; eggs hatch in the GI tract and larvae form hydatid cysts throughout the body	Lymphopenia, thrombocytopenia, elevated LFTs, hydatid cysts on imaging	Albendazole, surgical removal of cysts, aspiration of cyst fluid and injection of a scolicidal agent

CNS, central nervous system; CSF, cerebrospinal fluid; CT, computed tomography; GI, gastrointestinal; LFTs, liver function tests; MRI, magnetic resonance imaging; RUQ, right upper quadrant.

TABLE 12-7 Trematodes (Flatworms)

Organism	Clinical Features	Transmission/Life Cycle	Labs	Treatment
Schistosoma mansoni, Schistosoma haematobium (blood flukes)	Acute infection can present with fever, lethargy, myalgias, dysuria, abdominal pain, diarrhea, lymphadenopathy, hepatosplenomegaly; **squamous cell CA of the bladder (S. haematobium)**	Eggs hatch in water; larvae are ingested by **freshwater snails** and mature into the infectious form (cercariae); cercariae penetrate the skin of a new human host; they mature in the lungs or the liver; mature flukes migrate to the mesenteric vessels (*S. mansoni*) or the urinary tract (*S. haematobium*).	Hematuria (*S. haematobium*), peripheral eosinophilia, elevated LFTs, *Schistosoma* eggs in urine or stool, serum antibodies, positive urine PCR test	Praziquantel
Paragonimus westermani (lung fluke)	Resides in the lungs of the host, causing **chronic bronchitis and hemoptysis**; fever, cough, dyspnea, chest pain	Contracted from ingestion of **undercooked crab meat**; eggs expelled through coughing, or are swallowed and expelled in the stool	Eosinophilia, eggs in sputum and stool, ring shadows and nodules on CXR, pleural thickening	Praziquantel
Clonorchis sinensis (liver fluke)	*Clonorchis* lives in the biliary tract and is associated with **pigmented gallstones and cholangiocarcinoma**; fever, RUQ abdominal pain, diarrhea	Contracted from ingestion of undercooked fish; endemic in Far East and Southeast Asia.	Eosinophilia, eggs in stool, anti-*Clonorchis* Ab in serum	Praziquantel, albendazole

Ab, antibodies; CA, carcinoma; CXR, chest x-ray; LFT, liver function test; PCR, polymerase chain reaction; RUQ, right upper quadrant.

Microbiology

Crunch Time Review

The following pages contain high-yield information designed for review in the days just preceding the Step 1 examination.

MOST COMMON

Often on the USMLE exam, the student finds two responses that could potentially answer a question. The National Board of Medical Examiners (NBME) is testing the student to identify the more common of the two responses; for example, the more common cause, site, or type. The following is a high-yield summary of the most common characteristics of the various disorders listed in this text.

Nervous System

Most Common . . .

Aneurysm of circle of Willis	**Anterior communicating artery, bitemporal hemianopsia**
Blindness	**Diabetic retinopathy**
Blindness—preventable	***Chlamydia trachomatis***
Bacterial meningitis—elderly	***Streptococcus pneumoniae***
Bacterial meningitis—newborns	***Escherichia coli***
Bacterial meningitis—toddlers	***Haemophilus influenzae* type b**
Bacterial meningitis—young adults	***Neisseria meningitidis***
Primary cancer of the brain—child	**Medulloblastoma (cerebellum)**
Primary cancer of the brain—adult	**Astrocytoma (specifically glioblastoma)**, meningioma, schwannoma
Dementia	1. **Alzheimer** 2. Multi-infarct dementia
Demyelinating disease	**Multiple sclerosis**
Location of adult brain tumors	**Above tentorium**
Location of childhood brain tumors	**Below tentorium** (Mnemonic: Children are short, they cannot reach above the tentorium.)
Mental retardation	1. **Fetal alcohol syndrome** (most common overall cause) 2. Down syndrome (females) or fragile X (in males) (most common genetic causes)
Motor neuron disease	**Amyotrophic lateral sclerosis (ALS)**
Viral encephalitis	**Herpes simplex virus (HSV)**

Cardiovascular System

Most Common . . .

Acute mitral insufficiency—children	**Kawasaki disease**
Aneurysm	**Abdominal aorta**
AV fistula	**Penetrating knife wound**
Cancer of the heart—adults	**Metastases**
Cancer of the heart—primary—adults	**Myxoma "ball valve"**
Cancer of the heart—primary—kids	**Rhabdomyoma**
Cardiomyopathy	**Dilated (congestive) cardiomyopathy**
Cause of acute endocarditis	***Staphylococcus aureus***
Cause of subacute endocarditis	**Viridans streptococci**
Congenital cardiac anomaly	**Ventricular septal defect** (membranous > muscular)
Congenital early cyanosis	**Tetralogy of Fallot**
Coronary artery thrombosis	**Left anterior descending**
Death in hypertension	1. **Acute mitral insufficiency** 2. Lenticulostriate stroke 3. Renal failure (benign nephrosclerosis)
Death in the United States	**Ischemic heart disease**
Heart murmur	**Mitral valve prolapse**
Heart valve in bacterial endocarditis	**Mitral**
Heart valve in bacterial endocarditis in IV drug users	**Tricuspid**
Heart valve involved in rheumatic fever	**Mitral** > aortic
Hypertension	1. **Essential (95%)** 2. Renal disease
Hypertension—children	**Renal disease**, cystic disease, Wilms tumor
Hypertension—young women	**Oral contraceptives**
Myocarditis	**Coxsackie B virus**
Right heart failure	**Left heart failure**
Secondary hypertension	**Renal disease**
Sites of atherosclerosis	**Abdominal aorta** > coronary > popliteal > carotid
Vasculitis (of medium and small arteries)	**Temporal arteritis**

AV, atrioventricular; IV, intravenous.

Respiratory System

Most Common . . .

Cause of pneumonia in debilitated, hospitalized patient	***Klebsiella***
Cause of epiglottitis	***Haemophilus influenzae* type b**
Cause of IV drug user bacteremia/pneumonia	***Staphylococcus aureus***
Cause of opportunistic infection of AIDS	***Pneumocystis jirovecii* is most common overall.**
Death in patients with Alzheimer disease	**Pneumonia**
Fatal genetic defect in Caucasians	**Cystic fibrosis**
Pneumonia—community—atypical	1. ***Mycoplasma*** 2. *Legionella*
Pneumonia—community—typical	1. ***Streptococcus pneumoniae*** 2. *H. influenzae* 3. *Klebsiella*
Pneumonia—hospital acquired	1. ***Klebsiella*** 2. ***Pseudomonas*** 3. ***Escherichia coli***
Pulmonary hypertension	**Chronic obstructive pulmonary disease (COPD)**
Cancer associated with syndrome of inappropriate secretion of antidiuretic hormone (SIADH)	**Small cell carcinoma of the lung**
Tracheoesophageal fistula	**Lower esophagus communicates with trachea; upper esophagus ends in blind pouch.**

Gastrointestinal System

Most Common . . .

Bug in food poisoning	***Staphylococcus aureus***
Bug in gastrointestinal (GI) tract	1. ***Bacteroides*** 2. *Escherichia coli*
Cancer of the appendix	**Carcinoid—rarely metastasizes**
Cancer of the esophagus—malignant	**Adenocarcinoma** > squamous cell carcinoma (in United States)
Cancer of the liver	**Metastasis**; lung > GI
Tumor of the liver—primary, benign	**Cavernous hemangioma**
Cancer of the liver—primary	**Hepatocellular carcinoma**
Cancer of the mouth	**Squamous cell carcinoma or mucoepidermoid carcinoma**
Cancer of the mouth—upper lip	**Basal cell carcinoma**
Cancer of the nasal cavities	**Squamous cell carcinoma**
Cancer of the pancreas	**Adenocarcinoma** (usually in the head of pancreas)
Cancer of the salivary glands	**Pleomorphic adenoma**
Cancer of the small bowel	**Carcinoid**—frequent metastasis from ileum
Cancer of the spleen—benign	**Cavernous hemangioma**
Cancer of the stomach	**Gastric adenocarcinoma** (intestinal type or diffuse type)
Cirrhosis	**Alcohol**
Congenital GI anomaly	**Meckel diverticulum**
Diarrhea—children	**Rotavirus**
Dietary deficiency	**Iron**
GI obstruction	1. **Adhesions** 2. Indirect inguinal hernia
Intussusception	**Terminal ileum into cecum**
Liver disease	**Alcoholic liver disease**
Liver infection	**Viral hepatitis (HAV and HBV)**
Lysosomal storage disease	**Gaucher disease**
Portal hypertension	**Cirrhosis**
Protozoal diarrhea	***Giardia***
Site of diverticula	**Sigmoid colon**
Surgical emergency	**Acute appendicitis**
Worm infection in the United States	1. **Pinworm** 2. *Ascaris*

HAV, hepatitis A virus; HBV, hepatitis B virus.

Renal System

Most Common . . .

Amyloidosis	**Immunologic** (Bence Jones protein in multiple myeloma is also called the amyloid light chain.)
Death in patients with systemic lupus erythematosus (SLE)	Lupus nephropathy type IV (diffuse proliferative)
End-stage renal disease	**Diabetes**
Glomerulonephritis	**IgA nephropathy (also known as Berger disease)**
Nephrotic syndrome—adults	**Focal segmental glomerulosclerosis**
Nephrotic syndrome—kids	**Minimal change disease**
Renal failure	**Acute tubular necrosis**

Ig, immunoglobulin.

Endocrine System

Most Common . . .

Addison disease	1. **Autoimmune** 2. Infection
Cancer of the adrenal medulla—adults	**Pheochromocytoma**
Cancer of the adrenal medulla—kids	**Neuroblastoma**
Cancer of the pituitary	1. **Prolactinoma** 2. Somatotropic "acidophilic" adenoma
Cancer of the thyroid	**Papillary carcinoma**
Congenital adrenal hyperplasia	1. **21-Hydroxylase deficiency** 2. 11-Hydroxylase deficiency
Cushing	1. **Exogenous steroid therapy** 2. Primary adrenocorticotropic hormone (ACTH) tumor 3. Adrenal adenoma 4. Ectopic ACTH tumor
Enzyme deficiency	**21-Hydroxylase—95% of congenital adrenal hyperplasia**
Hypercalcemia	**Hyperparathyroidism**
Hyperparathyroidism—primary	1. **Solitary adenomas** 2. Parathyroid hyperplasia 3. Parathyroid carcinoma
Hyperparathyroidism—secondary	**Hypocalcemia due to chronic renal failure**
Hyperthyroidism	**Graves disease**
Hypopituitarism—adults	**Nonfunctioning pituitary adenoma**
Hypopituitarism—kids	**Craniopharyngioma**
Hypothyroidism	**Hashimoto thyroiditis**
Peripheral neuropathy	**Diabetes mellitus**
Thyroid disease	**Goiter**

Reproductive System

Most Common . . .

Breast mass (premenopausal)	**Fibrocystic change (premenopausal)**
Breast mass (postmenopausal)	**Breast carcinoma**
Cancer in gynecologic—malignancy	**Endometrial carcinoma**
Cancer in men	**Prostate carcinoma**
Cancer in women	**Uterine leiomyoma (fibroids)**
Cancer in women—malignant	**Breast carcinoma**
Cancer of the breast	**Infiltrating ductal adenocarcinoma**
Cancer of the ovary—benign	**Serous cystadenoma**
Cancer of the ovary—malignant	**Serous cystadenocarcinoma**
Cancer of the placenta—benign	**Cavernous hemangioma**
Cancer of the testicles	**Seminoma**
Cancer that invades the female genitourinary (GU) tract	**Endometrial adenocarcinoma**
Cause of pelvic inflammatory disease (PID)	***Neisseria gonorrhoeae* or *Chlamydia trachomatis***
Chromosomal disorder	**Down syndrome**
Hernia	**Indirect**
Opportunistic infection in AIDS	***Pneumocystis jirovecii***
Sexually transmitted disease	***C. trachomatis***

Musculoskeletal System

Most Common . . .

Bacterial arthritis in young adults	***Neisseria gonorrhoeae***
Cancer of the bone	**Metastases from breast and prostate**
Cancer of the bone—primary—adults	**Multiple myeloma**
Cancer of the connective tissue—benign	**Lipoma**
Cancer of the skin	**Basal cell carcinoma**
Carpal bone dislocation	**Lunate**
Carpal bone fracture	**Scaphoid**
Disk herniation	**L4–L5**

The Hematopoietic and Lymphoreticular System

Most Common . . .

Cancer—leukemia—14-year-old	**Acute lymphoblastic leukemia (ALL)**
Cancer—leukemia—15–39-year-old	**Acute myeloid leukemia (AML)**
Cancer—leukemia—40–60-year-old	**Chronic myelogenous leukemia (CML)**
Cancer—leukemia—>60-year-old	**Chronic lymphocytic leukemia (CLL)**
Cancer in infancy	**Hemangioma**
Cancer in children	1. **Leukemia** 2. Medulloblastoma of cerebellum
Cancer; genetic alteration	**p53**
Cancer; malignant lymphoma in children	**Burkitt lymphoma**
Cancer; site of metastasis	**Regional lymph nodes**
Cancer; site of metastasis (second most common)	**Liver**
Hereditary bleeding disorder	**von Willebrand disease**
Single-gene disorder	**Thalassemia**
Type of Hodgkin lymphoma	**Nodular sclerosis Hodgkin lymphoma**
Type of non-Hodgkin lymphoma	**Diffuse large B-cell lymphoma**

QUICK LISTS

The following Quick Lists contain high-yield information organized by basic science subject.

Physiology

Quick List: Important Formulas

	Formula	Notes
Cardiac output	$CO = $ Rate of O_2 consumption / (arterial O_2 content − venous O_2 content) $CO = SV \times HR$	$SV = $ Stroke volume $HR = $ Heart rate
Mean arterial pressure	$MAP = CO \times TPR$ $MAP = 1/3\ SBP + 2/3\ DBP$	$CO = $ Cardiac output $TPR = $ Total peripheral resistance $SBP = $ Systolic blood pressure $DBP = $ Diastolic blood pressure
Stroke volume	$EDV - ESV$	$EDV = $ End diastolic volume $ESV = $ End systolic volume
Ejection fraction	$SV\ /\ EDV \times 100$	$SV = $ Stroke volume $EDV = $ End diastolic volume
Resistance	$8\eta L\ /\ \pi r^4$	$\eta = $ Viscosity $L = $ Length $r = $ Radius
Net filtration pressure	$(P_C - P_I) - (\pi_C - \pi_I)$	$P_C = $ Hydrostatic capillary pressure $P_I = $ Hydrostatic interstitial pressure $\pi_C = $ Osmotic capillary pressure $\pi_I = $ Osmotic interstitial pressure
Glomerular filtration rate	$GFR = K_f(P_{GC} - P_{BS}) - (\pi_{GC} - \pi_{BS})$ $GFR = C_{inulin} = U_{inulin} \times V\ /\ P_{inulin}$	$K_f = $ Filtration constant $P_{GC} = $ Hydrostatic pressure in glomerular capillaries $P_{BS} = $ Hydrostatic pressure in Bowman space $\pi_{GC} = $ Osmotic pressure in glomerular capillaries $\pi_{BS} = $ Osmotic pressure in Bowman space $C_{inulin} = $ Clearance of para-aminohippuric acid (PAH) $U_{inulin} = $ Urine concentration of PAH $V = $ Urine flow rate $P_{inulin} = $ Plasma concentration of PAH
Effective renal plasma flow	$C_{PAH} = U_{PAH} \times V\ /\ P_{PAH}$	$C_{PAH} = $ Clearance of PAH $U_{PAH} = $ Urine concentration of PAH $V = $ Urine flow rate $P_{PAH} = $ Plasma concentration of PAH
Renal blood flow	$RPF\ /\ (1 - Hct)$	$RPF = $ Renal plasma flow $Hct = $ Hematocrit
Filtration fraction	$GFR\ /\ RPF$	$GFR = $ Glomerular filtration rate $RPF = $ Renal plasma flow
Free water clearance	$CH_2O = V - C_{osm}$, where $C_{osm} = U_{osm}\ V\ /\ P_{osm}$	$CH_2O = $ Clearance of water $U_{osm} = $ Urine osmolarity $P_{osm} = $ Plasma osmolarity $V = $ Urine flow rate

Biostatistics

Quick List: Important Formulas

	Formula
Sensitivity	TP / (TP + FN)
Specificity	TN / (TN + FP)
Positive predictive value	TP / (TP + FP)
Negative predictive value	TN / (TN + FN)
Prevalence	TP + FN / (TP + FP + TN + FN) Generally calculated by incidence × duration of disease
Incidence	Generally calculated by number of new cases / susceptible population
Relative risk (RR)	RR = [TP / (TP + FP)] / [FN / (FN + TN)]
Attributable risk (AR)	AR = [TP / (TP + FP)] − [FN / (FN + TN)]

FN, false negative; FP, false positive; TN, true negative; TP, true positive.

Genetics

Quick List: Inherited Diseases

Mode of Inheritance	Diseases
Autosomal dominant diseases	Adult polycystic kidney disease, familial hypercholesterolemia, Marfan syndrome, neurofibromatosis type 1, neurofibromatosis type 2, tuberous sclerosis, von Hippel–Lindau disease, Huntington disease, familial adenomatous polyposis, hereditary spherocytosis, achondroplasia
Autosomal recessive diseases	Cystic fibrosis, albinism, α_1-antitrypsin deficiency, phenylketonuria, thalassemias, sickle cell anemia, glycogen storage disease, mucopolysaccharidoses (except Hunter syndrome), sphingolipidoses (except Fabry disease), infant polycystic kidney disease, hemochromatosis
X-linked dominant diseases	Hypophosphatemic rickets
X-linked recessive diseases	Bruton agammaglobulinemia, Wiskott–Aldrich syndrome, fragile X syndrome, G6PD deficiency, ocular albinism, Lesch–Nyhan syndrome, Duchenne muscular dystrophy, hemophilia A and B, Fabry disease, Hunter syndrome
Mitochondrial diseases	Leber hereditary optic neuropathy, mitochondrial myopathies
Trisomies	Down syndrome (chromosome 21), Edward syndrome (chromosome 18), Patau syndrome (chromosome 13)
Trinucleotide repeat diseases	Huntington disease, myotonic dystrophy, Friedreich ataxia, fragile X syndrome

G6PD, glucose-6-phosphate dehydrogenase.

Pharmacology

Quick List: Important Formulas

	Formula	Notes
Volume of distribution	Total drug in body / plasma concentration	
Clearance	Rate of elimination of drug / plasma concentration	
Half-life	0.7 × volume of distribution / clearance	
Loading dose	Target plasma concentration × volume of distribution / bioavailability	Bioavailability = 1, when medication given IV
Maintenance dose	Target plasma concentration × clearance / bioavailability	Bioavailability = 1, when medication given IV

IV, intravenous.

Quick List: Important Drug Side Effects Based on Organ System *(Figure 1)*

FIGURE
1 **Important drug side effects based on organ system**

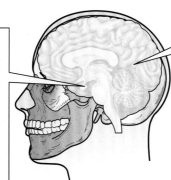

SKIN
1. Photosensitivity—sulfonamides, amiodarone, tetracycline
2. Lupus-like syndrome—hydralazine, isoniazid, procainamide, phenytoin

VASCULAR
1. Facial flushing—niacin, verapamil, nifedipine, diltiazem, adenosine, vancomycin

CARDIAC
1. Coronary vasospasm—cocaine, sumatriptan
2. Dilated cardiomyopathy—doxorubicin, daunorubicin
3. Torsades de pointes—antiarrhythmics (sotalol, quinidine), cisapride

PULMONARY
1. Cough—ACE inhibitors
2. Pulmonary fibrosis—bleomycin, busulfan, amiodarone

HEPATOBILIARY
1. Hepatitis—isoniazid
2. Hepatic necrosis—halothane, valproic acid, acetaminophen
3. Acute cholestatic hepatitis—erythromycin, azithromycin, clarithromycin

HEMATOPOIETIC
1. Agranulocytosis—clozapine, carbamazepine, colchicine, propylthiouracil, methimazole
2. Aplastic anemia—chloramphenicol, benzene, NSAIDs, propylthiouracil, methimazole
3. Hemolytic anemia (direct Coombs-positive)—methyldopa
4. Hemolytic anemia in patients with G6PD deficiency—isoniazid, sulfonamide, Primaquine, aspirin, ibuprofen, nitrofurantoin
5. Gray baby syndrome—chloramphenicol
6. Thrombosis—oral contraceptives

GENITOURINARY
1. Interstitial nephritis—methicillin, NSAIDs
2. Hemorrhagic cystitis—cyclophosphamide, ifosfamide
3. Fanconi syndrome—expired tetracycline

INTESTINAL
1. Pseudomembrane colitis—clindamycin, ampicillin

MUSCULOSKELETAL
1. Osteoporosis—corticosteroids, heparin
2. Gout—furosemide, thiazide diuretic
3. Tendonitis, tendon rupture, cartilage damage—fluoroquinolones
4. Gingival hyperplasia—phenytoin

NERVOUS SYSTEM
1. Seizures—bupropion, imipenem/cilastatin
2. Tardive dyskinesia—antipsychotics
3. Reaction with alcohol intake (headache, nausea, vomiting, flushing)—metronidazole, specific cephalosporins, procarbazine, sulfonylureas (first generation)
4. Neurotoxicity/nephrotoxicity—polymyxins
5. Ototoxicity/nephrotoxicity—cisplatin, furosemide, bumetanide, ethacrynic acid, gentamicin, neomycin, tobramycin, amikacin

ENDOCRINE
1. Adrenocortical insufficiency—glucocorticoid withdrawal
2. Gynecomastia—spironolactone, digitalis, cimetidine, alcohol (chronic use), estrogens, ketoconazole
3. Hot flashes—tamoxifen, clomiphene
4. Diabetes insipidus—lithium, demeclocycline

ACE, angiotensin-converting enzyme; G6PD, glucose-6-phosphate dehydrogenase; NSAIDs, nonsteroidal anti-inflammatory drugs.

Quick List: Drugs to Avoid in Pregnancy

Drug	Reason
ACE inhibitors	Fetal renal malformations
Aminoglycosides	Ototoxicity
Atorvastatin	Congenital defects, termination of pregnancy
Fluoroquinolones	Cartilage damage
Griseofulvin	Teratogenic
Methysergide	Oxytocic effects
Metronidazole	Mutagenesis
Ribavirin	Teratogenic
Sulfonamides	Kernicterus
Tetracyclines	Discolored teeth, inhibition of bone growth
Warfarin	Teratogenic

ACE, angiotensin-converting enzyme.

Quick List: Cytochrome P450 Interactions

Effect	Agent
Inhibitors	Cimetidine, ritonavir (protease inhibitors), amiodarone, ciprofloxacin, ketoconazole, acute alcohol use, macrolides, isoniazid, grapefruit juice, omeprazole, sulfonamides
Inducers	Phenytoin, rifampin, St. John's wort, barbiturates, griseofulvin, carbamazepine

Quick List: Antidotes

Toxic agent	Treatment
Acetaminophen	*N*-acetylcysteine
Amphetamine	Ammonium chloride (acidify urine)
Arsenic	Dimercaprol (BAL), succimer, penicillamine
Aspirin	Activated charcoal, sodium bicarbonate (alkalinize urine), dialysis
Atropine	Physostigmine
Benzodiazepines	Flumazenil
β-Blockers	Atropine, activated charcoal, glucagon, $CaCl_2$
Carbon monoxide	100% oxygen, hyperbaric oxygen
Cocaine	Supportive care, benzodiazepines, calcium channel blockers
Copper	Penicillamine
Cyanide	Sodium thiosulfate; amyl nitrate plus sodium nitrite
Digitalis	Activated charcoal, digoxin immune Fab, potassium (if serum K^+ level is low), possibly atropine
Ethylene glycol (antifreeze)	Fomepizole, ethanol, dialysis
Heparin	Protamine sulfate
Iron	Deferoxamine
Isoniazid	Vitamin B_6
Isopropyl alcohol	Supportive care
Lead	Succimer, EDTA, dimercaprol
Mercury	Dimercaprol
Methanol	Fomepizole, ethanol, dialysis
Methemoglobin	Methylene blue
Opioids	Naloxone, naltrexone
Organophosphates	Atropine, pralidoxime
Streptokinase	Aminocaproic acid
Sulfonylureas	Dextrose, octreotide
tPA	Aminocaproic acid
Tricyclic antidepressants	Gastric lavage, sodium bicarbonate (serum alkalinization), diazepam for seizures
Warfarin	Vitamin K, fresh frozen plasma

BAL, British anti-Lewisite; $CaCl_2$, calcium chloride; EDTA, ethylenediaminetetraacetic acid; tPA, tissue plasminogen activator.

Crunch Time Review

Microbiology

Quick List: Buzzwords for Microbiologic Infections

Clinical Characteristics	Organism
Branching rods in oral infections	*Actinomyces israelii*
Burn infections	*Pseudomonas aeruginosa*
Cat bite	*Pasteurella multocida*
Chancroid	*Haemophilus ducreyi*
Clue cells	*Gardnerella vaginalis*
Cold agglutinins	*Mycoplasma pneumoniae*
Currant jelly sputum	*Klebsiella*
Erythema chronicum migrans	Lyme disease
Ghon focus	Primary tuberculosis
Jarisch–Herxheimer reaction	Syphilis—treatment of an asymptomatic patient results in rapid lysis leading to symptoms
Negri bodies	Rabies
Owl's eye	CMV
Pediatric infection (in an unvaccinated patient)	*Haemophilus influenzae*
Pneumonia in cystic fibrosis	*P. aeruginosa*
Rash on palms or soles	Rocky Mountain spotted fever, secondary syphilis
Reactive arthritis (Reiter syndrome)	Urethritis, conjunctivitis, arthritis
Roth spots in retina	Endocarditis
Slapped cheeks	Parvovirus B19 (erythema infectiosum)
Splinter hemorrhages in fingernails	Endocarditis
Strawberry tongue	Scarlet fever
Suboccipital lymphadenopathy	Rubella
Sulfur granules	*A. israelii*
Tabes dorsalis	Tertiary syphilis
Thumb sign on lateral x-ray	Epiglottis (usually with *H. influenzae*)
Traumatic open wound	*Clostridium perfringens*

CMV, cytomegalovirus.

Quick List: Gram Stain Characteristics of Various Bacteria

Gram Stain Characteristics	Organisms
Gram-positive cocci	*Staphylococcus* (catalase +), *Streptococcus* (catalase −), *Enterococcus* (catalase −)
Gram-positive rods	*Clostridium* (anaerobe), *Corynebacterium, Listeria, Bacillus*
Gram-negative cocci	*Neisseria*
Gram-negative coccoid rods	*Haemophilus influenzae, Pasteurella, Brucella, Bordetella pertussis*
Gram-negative rods	**Lactose fermenters**: *Klebsiella* (fast[a]), *Escherichia coli* (fast), *Enterobacter* (fast), *Citrobacter* (slow), *Serratia* (slow) **Lactose nonfermenters**: *Shigella* (oxidase −), *Salmonella* (oxidase −), *Proteus* (oxidase −), *Pseudomonas* (oxidase +)

[a]Fast fermenter, slow fermenter.

APPENDIX I: Drug Index

The therapeutic agents shown in boldface type are those that are often emphasized in the classroom and the clinic. Particular attention should be paid to the information about these agents.

Therapeutic Agent (common name, if relevant) [trade name, where appropriate]	Class—Pharmacology and Pharmacokinetics	Indications	Side Effects or Adverse Effects	Contraindications or Precautions to Consider; Notes
Abacavir (ABC)	**Antiviral, nucleoside reverse transcriptase inhibitor—guanosine analog** → inhibits viral reverse transcriptase → prevents integration of DNA copy of viral genome into host DNA	**AIDS (used in HAART)**	**Neutropenia, anemia, peripheral neuropathy, pancreatitis, lactic acidosis, and hypersensitivity reaction (can be fatal)**	Check HLA-B*5701 test prior to starting ABC to avoid giving to patients at risk for hypersensitivity reactions
Acarbose [Precose]	Hypoglycemic agent; α-glucosidase inhibitor—inhibits intestinal brush border enzyme α-glucosidase → delays sugar hydrolysis and glucose absorption from gut → decreases postprandial hyperglycemia	Oral treatment for type 2 diabetes postprandially	Flatulence, cramps, diarrhea; may reduce absorption of iron	Does not cause reactive hypoglycemia; decreases HbA_{1c}
Acebutolol [Sectral]	Antiarrhythmic (class II)—antihypertensive; β-blocker	Hypertension, PVCs		Cardioselective; intrinsic sympathomimetic activity (useful in treating patients with hypertension who also have bradycardia)
Acetaminophen [Tylenol]	Analgesic, antipyretic—reversibly inhibits COX centrally (inactivated peripherally); prostaglandin inhibitor, **not anti-inflammatory**	Pain, fever	Liver toxicity in high doses (high levels deplete glutathione)	**Overdose treated with *N*-acetylcysteine** (regenerates glutathione); **unlike aspirin, can be used in children and patients with gout, peptic ulcer, and platelet dysfunction**
Acetazolamide [Diamox]	**Carbonic anhydrase inhibitor, diuretic—inhibits carbonic anhydrase on PCT and DCT,** which prevents HCO_3^- reabsorption; lose Na^+, HCO_3^-, and K^+ in urine	**Glaucoma, high altitude, metabolic alkalosis, alkalinization of urine, epilepsy**	**Hyperchloremic metabolic acidosis, sulfa drug allergy,** neuropathy, and ammonium toxicity	**Weak diuretic because other sites further downstream along the nephron can compensate for sodium loss;** causes decreased secretion of HCO_3^- in aqueous humor

Drug	Mechanism	Use	Side effects	Notes
Acetylcholine	**Muscarinic and nicotinic agonist**	Eye surgery (miotic)	**Increased cholinergic stimulation (MNEMONIC: DUMBBELSS**—Diarrhea, Urination, Miosis, Bronchoconstriction, Bradycardia, Excitation of skeletal muscle, Lacrimation, **S**alivation, **S**weating)	Contraindicated for patients with **peptic ulcer, asthma, hyperthyroidism, or parkinsonism**
Acetylsalicylic acid (aspirin)	**Anti-inflammatory, antipyretic, analgesic**—acetylates COX irreversibly	Articular, musculoskeletal pain; chronic pain; **maintenance therapy for preventing clot formation**	GI distress, **GI ulcers; inhibits platelet aggregation;** causes **hypersensitivity reactions (rash)**; reversible hepatic dysfunction	**Contraindicated** for **children** with flu or chicken pox (leads to **Reye syndrome**) and **patients with gout**
ACTH (corticotropin)	Increases production of steroids by the adrenal cortex	Test adrenal function in adrenocortical insufficiency		**Increased cortisol** indicates pituitary defect; **unchanged cortisol** indicates adrenal defect
Acyclovir [Zovirax]	**Antiviral**—guanosine analog; monophosphorylated by viral **thymidine kinase**; triphosphorylated form **inhibits viral DNA polymerase**	HSV, VZV, EBV, CMV (at high doses); HSV-induced mucocutaneous genital lesions and encephalitis	**Side effects depend on the route of administration: IV**—**neurotoxicity, renal problems, tremor;** oral—**diarrhea,** headache; topical—**local skin irritation**	**Resistant forms lack thymidine kinase**
Adenosine [Adenocard]	**Antiarrhythmic**—**increases potassium efflux → hyperpolarizes cell**	**Diagnosis and treatment of AV nodal arrhythmias**	**Flushing, hypotension, and chest pain**	Very short acting
Albendazole [Albenza]	**Anthelmintic**—blocks glucose uptake, resulting in eventual depletion of the parasite's energy stores	*Ascaris* (roundworm), *Ancylostoma* (hookworm), *Trichuris* (whipworm), *Strongyloides*; **cysticercosis, hydatid disease**	**Teratogenic; embryotoxic;** mild nausea, vomiting, and dizziness	Contraindicated in pregnant patients
Albuterol [Proventil, Ventolin]	**Bronchodilation**—β_2-agonist, **leads to relaxation of smooth muscle**	Asthma, COPD, bronchitis	**Tremor, tachycardia, arrhythmia,** headache, nausea, and vomiting	

(continued)

395

APPENDIX I: Drug Index

Therapeutic Agent (common name, if relevant) [trade name, where appropriate]	Class—Pharmacology and Pharmacokinetics	Indications	Side Effects or Adverse Effects	Contraindications or Precautions to Consider; Notes
Alcohol (EtOH)	Acts at GABA$_A$ receptor	Sedative; hypnotic; depressive action on brain; **indicated for methanol and ethylene glycol overdose**	**Intoxication (in order of increasing BAL)**: fine motor, coordination, ataxia, lethargy, coma, and respiratory depression **Withdrawal**: nausea, diaphoresis, delirium tremens, and seizures **Fetal alcohol syndrome**: mental retardation, growth deficiencies, microcephaly, and smooth philtrum **Chronic effects of alcoholism:** decreased liver function; Wernicke–Korsakoff syndrome, dilated cardiomyopathy, gynecomastia, and testicular atrophy	Benzodiazepines used for withdrawal symptoms; intoxication treated by thiamine, glucose, folic acid, and multivitamins
Aldesleukin [Proleukin]	Recombinant cytokine—human recombinant IL-2	**Metastatic renal cell carcinoma, metastatic melanoma, AML**		
Alendronate [Fosamax]	Bone stabilizer—bisphosphonate; **pyrophosphate analog**: reduces hydroxyapatite crystal formation, growth, and dissolution, which reduces bone turnover	**Hypercalcemia of malignancy, Paget disease, osteoporosis, hyperparathyroidism**	**Pill-induced esophagitis**	
Allopurinol [Zyloprim]	**Antigout—competitive inhibitor of xanthine oxidase**: converted to oxypurinol by xanthine oxidase, which also produces uric acid → allopurinol and oxypurinol inhibit xanthine oxidase → decreased uric acid production	**Chronic gout therapy**: lymphoma, leukemia (prevents tumor lysis–associated urate nephropathy), and uric acid stones; rheumatic arthritis	Rash; fever; GI problems, hepatotoxicity; inhibition of the metabolism of other drugs; enhances the effect of azathioprine	Should not be used to treat acute gout; inhibition of the metabolism of other drugs; enhances the effect of azathioprine
Alprazolam [Xanax]	Antianxiety—intermediate-acting benzodiazepine	**Panic attack; phobia; MNEMONIC:** AL PRAYS when he's in fear	Sedation	Respiratory depression if taken with alcohol
Alprostadil [Vasoprost]	Impotency therapy; **PGE$_1$ agonist**	**Impotency; maintains PDA**	Penile pain; prolonged erection; flushing, bradycardia, tachycardia, hypotension, and apnea	

Drug	Mechanism	Indications	Side effects	Notes
Aluminum hydroxide	**Antacid**—buffers gastric acid by raising the pH; **antidiarrheal—delays gastric emptying**	Peptic ulcer, gastritis, esophageal reflux, and diarrhea	**Constipation**, hypophosphatemia, muscle weakness, **osteodystrophy**, seizures, and **hypokalemia**	Can affect the **absorption, bioavailability**, or **urinary excretion** of drugs by changing **gastric pH, urinary pH**, or **gastric emptying**
Amantadine [Symmetrel]	**Antiviral—antiparkinsonian; inhibits** fusion of lysosomes; inhibits viral penetration and uncoating; increases release of endogenous dopamine	**Influenza A** (prophylaxis and treatment), **Parkinson disease**	**CNS effects** (ataxia, dizziness, slurred speech, nervousness, and seizure), **anticholinergic**, orthostatic hypotension, **livedo reticularis**	Mechanism of viral resistance is mutated M2 protein
Amikacin [Amikin]	**Antibiotic—aminoglycoside**, protein synthesis inhibitor; **irreversibly binds 30S ribosome** subunits; **bacteriostatic** at low concentration; **bactericidal** at high concentration	**Broad spectrum**: gram-negative rods; good for **bone** and **eye** infections; Proteus, Pseudomonas, Enterobacter, Klebsiella, Escherichia coli	**Ototoxicity, renal toxicity, neuromuscular blockade**, nausea, vomiting, vertigo, allergic rash	Does not cover anaerobes
Amiloride [Midamor]	Potassium-sparing diuretic—binds to intracellular aldosterone steroid receptors in **collecting tubules**; blocks induction of Na^+ channels and Na^+/ATPase synthesis and blocks Na^+ channels directly; lose Na^+ and Cl^- in urine	Hyperaldosteronism, potassium depletion, CHF	**Hyperkalemic metabolic acidosis, gynecomastia** (spironolactone), and antiandrogen effects	Results in decreased secretion of K^+ and H^+, which can lead to **hyperkalemic metabolic acidosis**; often given in combination with a thiazide
Aminocaproic acid [Amicar]	Competitive inhibition of plasminogen activation	Inhibits fibrinolysis; promotes thrombosis		Oral administration
Aminoglutethimide [Cytadren]	Antineoplastic—aromatase inhibitor; cytochrome P450 inhibitor that catalyzes the rate-limiting step of adrenal steroid synthesis	Breast cancer, Cushing syndrome	GI and neurological side effects; transient maculopapular rash	
Aminoglycosides	Antibiotic—**irreversibly binds 30S ribosome** subunits; **bacteriostatic** at low concentration; **bactericidal** at high concentration	**Broad spectrum**: gram-negative rods; good for **bone** and **eye** infections; Proteus, Pseudomonas, Enterobacter, Klebsiella, and Escherichia coli; also used for tuberculosis	**Ototoxicity, renal toxicity, neuromuscular blockade**, nausea, vomiting, vertigo, allergic rash	Do not cover anaerobes because oxidative metabolism is required for uptake of these drugs
Amiodarone [Cordarone]	**Antiarrhythmic (class III)—** K^+ **channel blocker**	**Ventricular/supraventricular arrhythmias**	**Hepatotoxicity, thyroid toxicity, pulmonary fibrosis, photodermatitis**	Examples include gentamycin, neomycin, and streptomycin

(continued)

Therapeutic Agent (common name, if relevant) [trade name, where appropriate]	Class—Pharmacology and Pharmacokinetics	Indications	Side Effects or Adverse Effects	Contraindications or Precautions to Consider; Notes
Amitriptyline [Elavil]	TCAs—inhibit **reuptake** of NE and 5-HT at neuronal synapses	Major depression, panic disorder; sedative; prophylaxis for migraines	Sedation, **α-blocking effects** (orthostatic hypotension), **anticholinergic** (tachycardia, dry mouth, and urinary retention), hallucinations (in elderly), and confusion (in elderly); overdose toxicity results in **convulsions, coma, cardiotoxicity** (arrhythmias), respiratory depression, and hyperpyrexia	
Amlodipine [Norvasc]	**Dihydropyridine Ca²⁺ channel blocker**—block voltage-gated Ca²⁺ channels of **vascular** smooth muscle	**Hypertension, angina pectoris, Prinzmetal angina, Raynaud phenomenon**	Peripheral edema, **flushing, dizziness,** and constipation	
Amobarbital [Amytal sodium]	Sedative-hypnotic; barbiturate; prolongs IPSP duration for GABA receptor	Antiepileptic, cerebral edema, anesthetic	Sedation, respiratory depression	
Amodiaquine	Antimalarial—uncertain mechanism	Suppression and treatment of acute attacks	Headache; GI and visual disturbances; pruritus; prolonged therapy may lead to retinopathy	
Amoxapine	TCAs—inhibit **reuptake** of NE and 5-HT at neuronal synapses	Major depression, panic disorder	Sedation, **α-blocking effects** (orthostatic hypotension), **anticholinergic** (tachycardia, dry mouth, and urinary retention), hallucinations (in elderly), and confusion (in elderly); overdose toxicity results in **convulsions, coma, cardiotoxicity** (arrhythmias), respiratory depression, and hyperpyrexia	
Amoxicillin	**Antibiotic–β-lactam, penicillin derivative,** cell wall inhibitor; same mechanism as penicillin; distinguished by activity against **gram-negative rods:** bactericidal	Gram-positive cocci, gram-positive rods, gram-negative cocci, and **gram-negative rods— extended spectrum:** *E. coli, Proteus, Salmonella, Shigella,* and *Haemophilus influenzae*	**Hypersensitivity reaction; rash when given to mononucleosis patients**	Orally administered; not effective against penicillin-resistant *Staphylococcus;* **can be combined with clavulanic acid** (β-lactamase inhibitor) to enhance spectrum
Amoxicillin/clavulanic acid [Augmentin]	Antibiotic—clavulanic acid inhibits β-lactamase			

Drug	Mechanism	Clinical use	Side effects	Notes
Amphetamine	**Stimulant—releases NE, dopamine**, and 5-HT	Narcolepsy, attention deficit disorder, weight reduction	Dilated pupils, psychosis, hallucinations, increased BP	Contraindicated with MAOI; metabolized by liver
Amphotericin B [Fungizone]	**Antifungal—binds to cell membrane sterols** (especially ergosterol); forms pores in membrane; fungicidal	Wide spectrum fungal coverage: *Candida, Histoplasma, Cryptococcus, Blastomyces, Aspergillus, Coccidioides, Sporothrix,* and *Mucor*	Impairment of renal function, hypersensitivity, flushing, fever, shaking chills, hypotension, thrombophlebitis, anemia, arrhythmias, hypokalemia	**Penetrates CNS poorly**: poor GI absorption, so given IV
Ampicillin	**Antibiotic—β-lactam, penicillin derivative,** cell wall inhibitor; same mechanism as penicillin; distinguished by activity against **gram-negative rods**: bactericidal	Gram-positive cocci, gram-positive rods, gram-negative cocci, and **gram-negatives rods—extended spectrum:** *E. coli, Proteus, Salmonella, Shigella,* and *H. influenzae*	Hypersensitivity reaction: rash, when given to mononucleosis patients	IV administration; not effective against penicillin-resistant *Staphylococcus*; **can be combined with clavulanic acid** (β-lactamase inhibitor) to enhance spectrum
Amprenavir	**Antiviral, protease inhibitor—**protease responsible for final step of viral proliferation; inhibits protease in progeny virions → assembly of nonfunctional viruses	AIDS (used in HAART)	GI irritation (nausea, diarrhea), hyperglycemia, hyperlipidemia, and lipodystrophy	**All protease inhibitors end in -navir; metabolism occurs by cytochrome P450**
Amrinone [Inocor]	Inotropic agent—**phosphodiesterase inhibitor;** increases contractility via increase in intracellular Ca^{2+}	Acute CHF	**Thrombocytopenia,** arrhythmias, hepatotoxicity, and GI disturbances	Rarely used today because of the side effects
Anastrozole [Arimidex]	Aromatase inhibitor	**Breast cancer** in postmenopausal women, endometriosis	Hot flashes, nausea, and vomiting	Can be used in estrogen receptor–positive or hormone receptor–unknown breast cancer
Anistreplase (APSAC) [Eminase]	**Thrombolytic—plasminogen activator**	Lysis of clots	Hemorrhage	Active compound via deacylation by esterase
Anthraquinone	**Simulant laxative—**reduces absorption of electrolytes and water from gut	Constipation		
α$_2$-Antiplasmin	Inhibits fibrinolysis			
Aprotinin [Trasylol]	Hemostatic agent—antiplasmin activator	Inhibits fibrinolysis; promotes thrombosis		
Asparaginase [Elspar]	Antineoplastic—deprives cells of asparagines	Cancer	Fever, mental depression, coma, hepatotoxicity	
Aspart [NovoLog]	**Rapid-acting insulin—***see mechanism for regular insulin*	**Diabetes mellitus** (typically type 1), hyperkalemia, and stress-induced hyperglycemia	**Hypoglycemia** (diaphoresis, vertigo, and tachycardia), insulin allergy, insulin antibodies, lipodystrophy	

(continued)

Therapeutic Agent (common name, if relevant) [trade name, where appropriate]	Class—Pharmacology and Pharmacokinetics	Indications	Side Effects or Adverse Effects	Contraindications or Precautions to Consider; Notes
Atenolol [Tenormin]	Antihypertensive—**β₁-blocker**	Hypertension, angina	Bradycardia, heart block, fatigue, impotence; **masks signs of hypoglycemia in diabetics**	**Cardioselective**
Atorvastatin [Lipitor]	Lipid-lowering agent—**HMG-CoA reductase inhibitor**, inhibits synthesis of cholesterol precursor mevalonate; **decreases LDL, increases HDL, and decreases TG**	**High LDL, preventative after thrombotic event (e.g., MI or stroke)**	Reversible increase in LFTs; myositis	**Contraindicated in pregnant** or lactating women and children; **increased incidence of rhabdomyolysis when taken with fibric acid, niacin, cyclosporine, and erythromycin**
Atracurium [Tracrium injection]	**Nondepolarizing** neuromuscular blocker			Minimal histamine release
Atropine	Reversible cholinergic muscarinic blocker	Dries salivary secretions; Parkinson disease; peptic ulcer; diarrhea; GI spasm; bladder spasm; COPD; asthma; cholinomimetic poisoning; antidiarrheal; antiemetic; high dose: vasodilation as a result of histamine release; mydriasis and cycloplegia (thorough fundus exam, accurate refraction)	Dry mouth, hyperthermia, mydriasis, tachycardia, hot and flushed skin, agitation, delirium; **MNEMONIC: Dry as a bone (dry mouth), hot as a hare (inhibition of sweating), red as a beet (tachycardia, cutaneous vasodilation), blind as a bat (blurring vision), mad as a hatter (hallucinations and delirium)**	Contraindicated in patients with glaucoma and elderly men with BPH
Aurothioglucose [Solganal]	Antirheumatic—gold salt	Rheumatic arthritis	Skin eruption, itching, toxic nephritis, bone marrow suppression	
Aurothiomalate	Antirheumatic—gold salt	Rheumatic arthritis	Skin eruption, itching, toxic nephritis, bone marrow suppression	
Azathioprine [Imuran]	Immunosuppressant—purine **antagonist**; inhibits nucleic acid metabolism; blocks both CMI and humoral response	**Transplant** (especially kidney), **acute glomerulonephritis, renal component of lupus, rheumatoid arthritis**	Bone marrow depression, rash, fever, nausea, vomiting, hepatotoxicity, malignancy, GI intolerance	**Metabolized by xanthine oxidase**
Azithromycin [Zithromax]	**Antibiotic—macrolide**, protein synthesis inhibitor; binds to the 23S RNA of the 50S ribosome subunits → blocks translocation → prevents protein synthesis; bacteriostatic	**First choice for cell wall–deficient bugs: *Mycoplasma, Rickettsia, Chlamydia, Legionella; Corynebacterium diphtheriae;* gram-positive cocci (*Streptococcus*)**	GI discomfort, **acute cholestatic hepatitis, rashes;** increases the concentration of **oral anticoagulants** and theophyllines	Can be used in patients with **streptococcal infections** and **penicillin allergies**

Drug	Class/Mechanism	Clinical Use	Side Effects	Notes
Aztreonam [Azactam]	**Antibiotic—monocyclic β-lactam,** cell wall inhibitor; same mechanism as penicillin (binds to PBP3); bactericidal	**Gram-negative bacteria, especially *Pseudomonas, Klebsiella, Serratia,* and Enterobacteriaceae; no activity against gram-positives or anaerobes**	Rash, GI distress (nausea, vomiting, etc.)	**Does not cross-react with penicillin; synergistic with aminoglycosides;** can be used in patients with **penicillin allergies and renal insufficiency who cannot take aminoglycosides**
Bacitracin	Antibiotic—**inhibits cell wall formation; bactericidal**	Gram-positive bacteria	**Nephrotoxic**	Topical only
Baclofen [Lioresal]	Skeletal muscle relaxant—**GABA mimetic;** works at the GABA$_B$ receptor	**Muscle spasms,** tetanus contractions, orthopedic manipulation		
BCNU (carmustine)	Antineoplastic—**DNA alkylation**	Cancer	Delayed bone marrow suppression, lung and kidney damage	
Beclomethasone	Corticosteroids—inhibit leukotriene synthesis → reduces inflammation and leads to bronchodilation	Asthma, COPD	**Osteoporosis, cushingoid reaction, psychosis, glucose intolerance, infection, hypertension, cataracts**	
Benserazide	Antiparkinsonian—inhibits decarboxylase (L-dopa to dopamine) in periphery	Parkinson disease		
Benztropine [Cogentin]	**Antiparkinsonian—muscarinic blocker; H$_1$ blocker**	Parkinson disease	Sedation, urinary retention, dry mouth, constipation, and mental confusion	Less effective than levodopa in Parkinson disease
Bephenium hydroxynaphthoate	Anthelmintic—cholinergic agonist causing contraction, then relaxation in worm	*Necator* and *Ancylostoma* (hookworms)	Vomiting	
Betamethasone	Glucocorticoid	**Induction of surfactant synthesis in premature infants**		One of two steroids to cross placenta
Bethanechol [Urecholine, Duvoid]	**Muscarinic agonist**	**Atony of bladder; paralytic ileus; MNEMONIC: Bethanechol** stimulates the **b**ladder and **b**owel	Diarrhea/**D**ecreased BP, **U**rination, **M**iosis, **B**ronchoconstriction, **E**xcitation of skeletal muscle, **L**acrimation, **S**alivation/**S**weating—**MNEMONIC: DUMBELS**	**Contraindicated in patients with peptic ulcer, asthma, hyperthyroidism, and Parkinson disease**
Bisacodyl [Dulcolax]	**Stimulant laxative,** increases peristalsis	Constipation	Electrolyte imbalances (chronic use), gastric irritation	
Bischloroethylamines (nitrogen mustards) [Mustargen]	Antineoplastic—**DNA alkylation and cross-linking**	Cancer	Nausea, vomiting, bone marrow suppression, alopecia, teratogenicity, carcinogenicity	

(continued)

APPENDIX I: Drug Index

Therapeutic Agent (common name, if relevant) [trade name, where appropriate]	Class—Pharmacology and Pharmacokinetics	Indications	Side Effects or Adverse Effects	Contraindications or Precautions to Consider; Notes
Bismuth [Pepto-Bismol]	**Cytoprotectant—binds to ulcer base → protection; allows bicarbonate ion secretion to reestablish pH gradient in the mucous layer**	**Traveler's diarrhea**, peptic ulcer disease		
Black widow spider venom	Presynaptic neuromuscular junction blocker—overstimulates acetylcholine release			
Bleomycin [Blenoxane]	**Antineoplastic—generates free radicals that bind, intercalate, and cut DNA**	**Testicular cancer and Hodgkin lymphoma**	**Pulmonary fibrosis**, fever, blistering, stomatitis, hypersensitivity reactions (anaphylaxis)	
Botulinum [Botox, Dysport]	**Neuromuscular blocker— presynaptic neuromuscular junction blocker; prevents acetylcholine release**	Wrinkles, muscle spasm	Paralysis	
Bretylium [Bretylol]	Antiarrhythmic (class III)—K+ channel blocker; prolongs ventricular action potential, effective refractory period, and blocks NE release	Arrhythmias; refractory ventricular fibrillation and ventricular tachycardia during cardiac arrest	Orthostatic hypotension, nausea, vomiting	
Bromocriptine [Parlodel]	**Antiparkinsonian—agonist at D_2; partial antagonist at D_1**	**Parkinson disease, hyperprolactinemia, acromegaly** (paradoxical effect—releases growth hormone from normal pituitary)	**Inhibits prolactin release**; hallucination, delirium, nausea, vomiting, cardiac arrhythmia, postural hypotension, and erythromelalgia	
Buclizine	Antiemetic	Sedation, parkinsonism		
Budesonide [Rhinocort]	Intranasal glucocorticoids—decrease cytokine synthesis; downregulate inflammatory response in the nasal mucosa	Nasal congestion, allergic rhinitis	Local irritation of nasal mucosa, epistaxis	
Bumetanide [Bumex]	Loop diuretic—inhibits $Na^+/K^+/2Cl^-$ reabsorption in the loop of Henle	CHF, diuresis, pulmonary edema, acute hypercalcemia, acute hyperkalemia, acute renal failure	Ototoxicity, interstitial nephritis, hyperuricemia, acute hypovolemia, hypokalemia, metabolic alkalosis, hyperglycemia, hypocalcemia, hypomagnesemia	
α-Bungarotoxin	Postsynaptic neuromuscular junction blocker; irreversibly binds nicotinic receptor		Paralysis	Component of snake venom

Drug	Mechanism/Class	Clinical Use	Side Effects/Toxicity	Notes
Bupivacaine	Anesthetic—blocks Na$^+$ channel intracellularly	Local anesthetic	Sleepiness, light-headedness, myocardial depression, hypotension, visual/audio disturbances, restlessness, nystagmus, shivering, tonic-clonic convulsions, death	
Buprenorphine [Buprenex]	Opioid analog—mixed agonist/antagonist action	Treatment of opioid/cocaine dependence	Respiratory depression, sedation, and nausea/vomiting	
Bupropion [Wellbutrin, Zyban]	**Antidepressant—unknown mechanism; thought to be an agonist at D$_2$, 5-HT**	Major depression, **smoking cessation**	Tachycardia, insomnia, headache, and seizure (especially patients with bulimia)	Does not have sexual side effects such as those occurring with SSRIs
Buspirone [Buspar]	Antidepressant partial agonist at serotonin receptors	Generalized anxiety		**2 weeks for effects to become apparent**
Caffeine [NoDoz]	Stimulant—**adenosine receptor blocker**: stimulates CNS and cardiac muscle; relaxes smooth muscle; produces diuresis; increases cerebrovascular resistance	**Acute migraine attack**	Crosses placenta and into breast milk	**Avoid in patients with peptic ulcer** because it stimulates gastric mucosal secretions
Calcitonin [Calcimar, Miacalcin]	Hypocalcemic agent—anti-osteoporotic agent; **lowers plasma Ca^{2+} and phosphate**; inhibits bone and kidney reabsorption	**Hypercalcemia, Paget disease, osteoporosis**		
Calcium carbonate [TUMS, Caltrate]	**Antacid**—buffers gastric acid by raising pH	Peptic ulcer, gastritis, esophageal reflux, and calcium deficiency	**Hypercalcemia, rebound acid increase, and hypokalemia**	**Can affect the absorption, bioavailability, or urinary excretion of drugs by changing gastric pH, urinary pH, or gastric emptying**
Calcium citrate	Dietary Ca^{2+} supplement	Ca^{2+} deficiency		
Calcium gluconate	Dietary Ca^{2+} supplement	Ca^{2+} deficiency		
Calcium lactate	Dietary Ca^{2+} supplement	Ca^{2+} deficiency		
Captopril [Capoten]	**Antihypertensive—ACE inhibitor** → inhibits conversion of angiotensin I to II → decreases angiotensin II (Ang II) levels → prevents vasoconstriction from Ang II	Hypertension, CHF, post-MI; prevention/treatment of diabetic nephropathy	**Cough, angioedema, hyperkalemia**, renal insufficiency (especially in bilateral renal artery stenosis)	Contraindicated in pregnancy (fetal renal malformation)
Carbachol [Isopto Carbachol]	Antiglaucoma agent—muscarinic cholinergic agonist, works on both muscarinic and nicotinic receptors	Miotic, glaucoma	**DUMBBELSS** (see Acetylcholine)	Contraindicated in patients with peptic ulcer, asthma, hyperthyroidism, and Parkinson disease

(continued)

APPENDIX I: **Drug Index**

Therapeutic Agent (common name, if relevant) [trade name, where appropriate]	Class—Pharmacology and Pharmacokinetics	Indications	Side Effects or Adverse Effects	Contraindications or Precautions to Consider; Notes
Carbamazepine [Tegretol]	Antiepileptic—prolongs inactivated state of Na^+ channels; decreases release of glutamate (and other excitatory neurotransmitters)	Epilepsy (partial and **tonic–clonic** [drug of choice]), **trigeminal neuralgia** (drug of choice)	**Agranulocytosis, liver toxicity (check LFTs), and aplastic anemia**	**Induces cytochrome P450**
Carbenicillin	**Antibiotic—β-lactam, penicillin derivative,** cell wall inhibitor; same mechanism as penicillin; distinguished by activity against **Pseudomonas;** bactericidal	**Extended spectrum—** *Pseudomonas, Proteus,* and *Enterobacter* species	**Hypersensitivity reactions,** decreased platelet function	Not effective against penicillin-resistant *Staphylococcus;* **can be combined with clavulanic acid** (β-lactamase inhibitor) to enhance spectrum; administered IV
Carbidopa-levodopa [Sinemet]	Antiparkinsonian—inhibits decarboxylase (L-dopa to dopamine) **in periphery; does not cross BBB**	**Parkinson disease; used with levodopa,** which reduces metabolism of dopamine in periphery and increases its availability in CNS; especially effective for bradykinesia	**Treatment efficacy declines with progression of disease** due to a decrease in healthy dopaminergic neurons required for levodopa's MOA	
Carboplatin [Paraplatin]	Antineoplastic—**cross-links DNA**	Ovarian cancer	Bone marrow suppression and anemia	Contains platinum
Carboprost [Prostin]	Abortive agent—PGF_{2a}	Therapeutic abortion	Nausea, vomiting, diarrhea	
Carvedilol	**Antihypertensive,** antiarrhythmic (class II)—α- and β-blocker	**Hypertension, angina, MI, and antiarrhythmic**	**Impotence, asthma, bradycardia,** AV block, heart failure, sedation, and sleep alterations	
Caspofungin	**Antifungal—**inhibits cell wall synthesis	Invasive aspergillosis or *Candida*	GI irritation, flushing	Administered IV
Castor oil	**Stimulant laxative—**reduces absorption of electrolytes and water from gut; active component is ricinoleic acid	Constipation, labor induction		
Celecoxib [Celebrex]	**NSAID—selectively inhibits COX-2**	Rheumatoid arthritis, osteoarthritis; pain, inflammation	**Increased risk of thrombosis, sulfa allergy, and less toxic to GI mucosa**	COX-2 selectivity reduces inflammation while minimizing GI adverse effects (ulcers)

Drug	Class/Mechanism	Clinical use	Side effects	Notes
Cephalosporins	**Antibiotic—β-lactam**, cell wall inhibitor; same mechanism as penicillin, bactericidal; **from first generation to third generation: a. Gram-positive** coverage **decreases b. Gram-negative** coverage **increases c. CNS penetration increases d. β-Lactamase resistance increases**	**First generation: Gram-positive cocci and PEcK** (*Proteus mirabilis*, *Escherichia coli*, and *Klebsiella*; **second generation**: same as first generation + **HENPEcK** (*H. influenzae*, *Enterobacter*, and *Neisseria*); **third generation: cephalosporins are used for meningitis**; *Klebsiella*, **Lyme disease, and gram-negative bacteria**	**Hypersensitivity reaction, pain at injection site, intolerance to alcohol** (cefamandole, cefotetan, moxalactam, and cefoperazone), **hypothrombinemia** (cefamandole, cefoperazone, and moxalactam, due to vitamin K inhibition), **thrombophlebitis, positive Coombs test**	**First generation**: cefazolin, cephalexin; **second generation**: cefaclor, cefoxitin, and cefuroxime; **third generation**: ceftriaxone, cefotaxime, and ceftazidime; **fourth generation**: cefepime; ***Pseudomonas* coverage**: cefepime; ceftazidime and cefepime; **cross-hypersensitivity with penicillins occurs in 5%–10% of patients**
Chloral hydrate	Anesthetic agent	Sedative (in children), hypnotic	Bitter taste, GI distress	Inexpensive
Chlorambucil [Leukeran]	Antineoplastic—DNA alkylation and **cross-linking**	Cancer	Nausea, vomiting, bone marrow suppression (mild), alopecia, teratogenicity, carcinogenicity, and **pulmonary fibrosis**	
Chloramphenicol [Chloromycetin]	**Antibiotic—protein synthesis inhibitor; inhibits 50S peptidyl transferase activity; bacteriostatic** but bactericidal versus *H. influenzae* and *Neisseria meningitidis*	Meningitis (*H. influenzae*, *N. meningitidis*, and *Streptococcus pneumoniae*), typhoid fever, *Salmonella*, *Rickettsia* (Rocky Mountain spotted fever in children), *Bacteroides*	**Fatal aplastic anemia, bone marrow suppression, gray baby syndrome** (cyanosis, vomiting, green stools, and vasomotor collapse due to insufficient glucuronidase in neonatal liver)	
Chlordiazepoxide [Librium]	Long-acting benzodiazepine; antianxiety; enhances GABA; increases IPSP amplitude	Sedative, hypnotic, antianxiety, antiepileptic; alcohol withdrawal		
Chlorguanide	Antimalarial—inhibits dihydrofolate reductase	**Prophylaxis for falciparum** malaria; **suppression of vivax** malaria	Minor GI upset	
Chloroquine phosphate [Aralen]	Antimalarial—uncertain mechanism	**Suppression of malaria** and treatment of **acute** attack; **amebiasis; clonorchis; rheumatoid arthritis; SLE**	Headache, GI disturbances, visual disturbances, **pruritus**; prolonged therapy may lead to **retinopathy**	
Chloroprocaine	Anesthetic—block Na⁺ channel intracellularly	Local anesthetic	Sleepiness, light-headedness, visual/audio disturbances, restlessness, nystagmus, shivering, tonic–clonic convulsions, death	
Chlorpheniramine [Chlor-Trimeton]	Antihistamine—H₁ blocker	Allergies, **motion sickness**	Sedation, CNS depression, atropine-like effects, allergic dermatitis, blood dyscrasias, teratogenicity, acute antihistamine poisoning	

(continued)

Therapeutic Agent (common name, if relevant) [trade name, where appropriate]	Class—Pharmacology and Pharmacokinetics	Indications	Side Effects or Adverse Effects	Contraindications or Precautions to Consider; Notes
Chlorpromazine [Thorazine]	Antiemetic, antipsychotic—phenothiazines; blocks D_2, α_1, and H_1 receptors	Antipsychotic, antiemetic, hiccups	**Extrapyramidal** (dystonia, akinesia, akathisia, and tardive dyskinesia), **anticholinergic** (dry mouth, constipation), **alpha blockade** (hypotension), **histamine** (sedation); toxicity results in neuroleptic malignant syndrome (rigidity, myoglobinuria, autonomic instability, and hyperpyrexia)	Atropine-like effects fairly common
Chlorpropamide	**Hypoglycemic agent, first-generation sulfonylurea**—closes potassium channel in β-cell membrane → reduces K^+ efflux, increases Ca^{2+} influx → increases secretion of insulin	Oral treatment for type 2 diabetes	**Hypoglycemia**, GI disturbances, muscle weakness, mental confusion	Rarely used due to toxicity
Cholestyramine [Questran]	Lipid-lowering agent—**bile acid resins** act by binding bile acids in the small intestine, forming insoluble complexes that are excreted; decreased bile acids stimulate the liver to increase conversion of cholesterol to bile acids, increasing hepatic LDL receptors, decreasing serum LDL	Reduction of cholesterol	Steatorrhea, constipation, impairment of absorption of drugs/vitamins	**Inhibits warfarin absorption**
Chorionic gonadotropin [Pregnyl]	Infertility therapy—LH-like in action	Treats infertility, induces ovulation, induces masculinization in infertile men, diagnostic for cryptorchidism in young boys		
Cimetidine [Tagamet]	**H_2 blocker**—blocks histamine H_2 receptors reversibly → decreases proton secretion by parietal cells	Peptic ulcer disease, gastritis, esophageal reflux	**Gynecomastia, impotence**, decreased libido in males, **confusion, dizziness, and headaches**	**Crosses placenta, decreases renal excretion of creatinine, CYP450 inhibitor**
Ciprofloxacin [Cipro]	**Antibiotic—quinolone, DNA synthesis inhibitor; inhibits DNA gyrase** (topoisomerase II) and **topoisomerase IV** → blocks DNA synthesis; bactericidal	**Gram-negative infections** (especially UTI and bone): *Pseudomonas*, Enterobacteriaceae, and *Neisseria*; **gram-positive infections** (staphylococci); **intracellular:** *Legionella*	**GI disturbances, headache, dizziness, phototoxicity, cartilage damage (children, fetus), tendonitis** and **tendon rupture (adults), myalgias (children)**	May elevate theophylline to toxic levels, causing seizure; divalent cations inhibit gut absorption; therefore, quinolones cannot be taken with milk, iron-containing preparations, or antacids.

Drug	Class/Mechanism	Clinical Use	Notes/Side Effects
Cisapride [Propulsid]	**GI stimulant—prokinetic; increases acetylcholine release at myenteric plexus →** increases esophageal tone, gastric/duodenal contractility (improves colon transit time)	Constipation	Rarely used; interacts with **erythromycin, ketoconazole, nefazodone, and fluconazole** to produce **torsades de pointes**
Cisplatin [Platinol]	Antineoplastic—cross-links DNA	Cancer	Bone marrow and renal toxicity, **cystitis, peripheral neuropathy, ototoxicity**; alopecia (severe)
Citalopram	SSRIs—inhibit **reuptake** of 5-HT at neuronal synapses	Major depression, OCD, anorexia, and bulimia	Inhibits liver enzymes, nausea, agitation, **sexual dysfunction** (anorgasmia), and dystonic reactions	Contraindicated with **MAOIs** secondary to **serotonin syndrome** (hyperthermia, muscle rigidity, and cardiovascular collapse); allows time for antidepressant effect, usually takes 2–3 weeks
Clarithromycin [Biaxin]	**Antibiotic—macrolide**, protein synthesis inhibitor; binds to the 23S RNA of the 50S ribosome subunits → blocks translocation → prevents protein synthesis; bacteriostatic	**First choice for cell wall–deficient bugs: *Mycoplasma, Rickettsia, Chlamydia,* and *Legionella; Corynebacterium diphtheriae;* gram-positive cocci (*Streptococcus*)**	GI discomfort, **acute cholestatic hepatitis,** and **rashes**; increases concentration of **oral anticoagulants** and theophyllines	Can be used in patients with **streptococcal infections** and **penicillin allergies**
Clavulanic acid	β-Lactamase inhibitor; synergistic with penicillins		
Clindamycin [Cleocin]	**Antibiotic—protein synthesis inhibitor; binds to 50S subunits →** blocks peptide bond formation; bacteriostatic or bactericidal depending on concentration, site, and organism	**Gram-positive bacteria (*Streptococcus* and *Staphylococcus*); treats anaerobic** infections	Severe diarrhea; **potentially fatal pseudomembranous colitis caused by *Clostridium difficile***
Clofazimine [Lamprene]	Antibiotic—antileprosy; unknown mechanism	*Mycobacterium leprae*	Turns skin red-brown or black
Clofibrate [Atromid-S]	Lipid-lowering agent—**upregulates lipoprotein lipase (periphery) → increases TG clearance; decreases LDL, increases HDL, and decreases TG**	Increased TG, increased LDL	Myositis, increased LFTs; increased risk of GI and liver cancer; potentiates anticoagulant drugs; gallstones; mild GI disturbances
Clomiphene [Clomid]	**Selective estrogen receptor modulator—binds** estrogen receptors in pituitary → prevents normal feedback inhibition, increases LH and FSH release from pituitary → stimulates ovulation	Stimulates ovulation in infertility, **PCOS**	**Hot flashes, ovarian enlargement, multiple gestation pregnancy,** and **visual disturbances**

(continued)

Therapeutic Agent (common name, if relevant) [trade name, where appropriate]	Class—Pharmacology and Pharmacokinetics	Indications	Side Effects or Adverse Effects	Contraindications or Precautions to Consider; Notes
Clomipramine	TCAs—inhibit **reuptake** of NE and 5-HT at neuronal synapses	Major depression, OCD, and panic disorder	Sedation, **α-blocking effects** (orthostatic hypotension), **anticholinergic** (tachycardia, dry mouth, and urinary retention), hallucinations (in elderly), and confusion (in elderly); overdose toxicity results in **convulsions, coma, cardiotoxicity** (arrhythmias), respiratory depression, and hyperpyrexia	
Clonazepam [Klonopin]	**Antiepileptic—benzodiazepine**	**Epilepsy (absence of seizures)**		
Clonidine [Catapres]	**Antihypertensive**—centrally acting sympathetic agent (α_2-agonist) → decreases sympathetic outflow from CNS → decreases peripheral resistance	Hypertension, smoking withdrawal, heroin and cocaine withdrawal	Drowsiness, **dry mouth; rebound hypertension after abrupt withdrawal**	
Clotrimazole [Lotrimin, Mycelex]	Antifungal—inhibits ergosterol synthesis, preventing cell membrane formation	**Topical use against yeasts, dermatophytes, ringworm, fungi, mold, and oral candidiasis in AIDS**	Burning, itching, and redness when used topically	
Clozapine [Clozaril]	Atypical antipsychotic—blocks D_4, α_1, 5-HT, muscarinic receptors	Schizophrenia, useful for positive and negative symptoms	Agranulocytosis, **extrapyramidal** (occurs at a lower rate than typicals), **anticholinergic** (dry mouth, constipation), **alpha blockade** (hypotension), **histamine** (sedation); toxicity results in neuroleptic malignant syndrome (occurs at a lower rate than typicals)	Second-line agent used for refractory schizophrenia; weekly blood counts for patients on this agent due to agranulocytosis
Cocaine	**CNS stimulant—blocks NE, 5-HT, and dopamine reuptake**	**Local anesthetic**	**Vasoconstriction, hypertension, nasal mucus ischemia**	
Codeine	**Opioid agonist**	**Pain,** antitussive	**Constipation**	Converted to morphine 10%
Colchicine	Anti-inflammatory—interrupts **microtubule formation,** thereby interfering with normal mitosis and inhibiting WBC migration and phagocytosis	Acute gout therapy	Diarrhea (common)	Contraindicated in elderly and feeble patients and in patients with GI disturbances, cardiac anomalies, or renal problems

Drug	Mechanism	Use	Side Effects / Notes
Colestipol [Colestid]	Lipid-lowering agent—**bile acid resin**, impedes fat absorption; **lowers LDL**, binds cholesterol metabolites	Reduction of cholesterol	Steatorrhea, constipation, impaired absorption of drugs and vitamins
Corticotropin-releasing hormone (CRH)	Increases ACTH production by anterior pituitary	Used in diagnosis of Cushing syndrome	
Cortisol (hydrocortisone) [Hydrocortone, Nutracort]	**Glucocorticoid—induces new protein synthesis; increases gluconeogenesis and lipolysis; reduces peripheral glucose use; catabolic effect on muscle, bone, skin, fat, and lymph tissue; anti-inflammatory; immunosuppressant**	**Adrenal insufficiency, congenital adrenal hyperplasia, diagnosis of pituitary–adrenal disorder, reduces inflammation (especially chronic), leukemia, decreases hypercalcemia**	**Iatrogenic Cushing syndrome, redistribution of fat, acne, insomnia, weight gain, hypokalemia, decrease in skeletal muscle, osteoporosis, hyperglycemia, ulcers, psychosis, cataracts, increased susceptibility to infections, growth suppression in children**
Cosyntropin [Cortrosyn]	ACTH analog—increases production of steroids by adrenal	Used in diagnosis of adrenocortical insufficiency	
Cromolyn [Nasalcrom, Gastrocrom]	**Antiasthmatic—prevents release** of mediators from mast cells → prevents bronchoconstriction and inflammation	Asthma prophylaxis	**Laryngeal edema (rare)** Not used during acute exacerbation
Cyanocobalamin (Anacobin)	Supplies vitamin B_{12}	B_{12} deficiency	
Cyclobenzaprine [Flexeril]	Centrally acting muscle relaxant	Muscle spasms, tetanus contractions, orthopedic manipulation	Antimuscarinic effects
Cyclophosphamide [Cytoxan]	**Immunosuppressant—alkylating agent; destroys proliferating lymphoid cells; alkylates resting cells**	**Transplant rejection, rheumatic arthritis**	GI and bone marrow toxicity, **hemorrhagic cystitis** Coadministration of mesna will prevent hemorrhagic cystitis
Cycloserine [Seromycin]	Antibiotic—analog of o-alanine; interferes with cell wall synthesis	*Mycobacterium*	Psychotic reactions
Cyclosporine [Sandimmune]	**Immunosuppressant—inhibits T-helper cell activity; inhibits IL-2, IL-3, and IFN-γ formation by T-helper cells**	**Transplant rejection**	**Nephrotoxic, hepatotoxic; hypertension; increased incidence of viral infection and lymphoma**
Cyproheptadine [Periactin]	Antihistamine—antipruritic; 5-HT$_3$ agonist; histamine blocker	Decreases diarrhea in carcinoid tumors, decreases dumping syndrome	Weight gain
Cytosine arabinoside [Cytosar-U]	Antineoplastic—inhibits DNA replication and RNA polymerization; competitive inhibitor of dCTP; inhibits chain elongation	Cancer, AML	Severe myelosuppression, stomatitis, alopecia

(continued)

APPENDIX I: **Drug Index**

Therapeutic Agent (common name, if relevant) [trade name, where appropriate]	Class—Pharmacology and Pharmacokinetics	Indications	Side Effects or Adverse Effects	Contraindications or Precautions to Consider; Notes
Dacarbazine (DTIC-Dome)	Antineoplastic—DNA alkylation; strand breakage; inhibits nucleic acid and protein synthesis	Cancer		
Dactinomycin [Cosmegen]	Antineoplastic—intercalates into DNA	Cancer	Skin eruptions, hyperkeratosis	
Danazol [Danocrine]	**Testosterone derivative—weak agonist for androgen, progesterone, and glucocorticoid receptors**	**Endometriosis and fibrocystic disease**	**Masculinization in women, gynecomastia** in men	
Dantrolene [Dantrium]	**Non-centrally acting muscle relaxant—decreases Ca²⁺ from sarcoplasmic reticulum**	**Malignant hyperthermia**	**Hepatotoxic**	
Dapsone [Dapsone]	Antibiotic—related to sulfonamides	*Mycobacterium leprae*	GI disturbances, hemolysis, methemoglobinemia	
Daunorubicin [DaunoXome, Cerubidine]	Antineoplastic—**oxidizes free radicals; intercalates into DNA; breaks DNA;** affects plasma membrane	Cancer	Cardiac changes resulting in cumulative **cardiotoxicity**	
Deferoxamine [Desferal]	**Metal chelator**	**Acute toxicity of iron**	**Hypotensive shock; neurotoxic if long-term use**	
Delavirdine	**Antiviral, nonnucleoside reverse transcriptase inhibitor**—binds viral reverse transcriptase and inhibits movement of protein domains → terminates viral DNA synthesis → prevents integration of viral genome into host DNA	**AIDS (used in HAART)**	**Neutropenia, anemia, peripheral neuropathy, and rash**	
Desflurane [Suprane]	Anesthetic	General anesthetic	Irritating to airway	
Desipramine [Norpramin]	TCAs—inhibit **reuptake** of NE and 5-HT at neuronal synapses	Major depression, panic disorder, and anxiety	Sedation, **α-blocking effects** (orthostatic hypotension), **anticholinergic** (tachycardia, dry mouth, and urinary retention), hallucinations (in elderly), and confusion (in elderly); overdose toxicity results in **convulsions, coma, cardiotoxicity** (arrhythmias), respiratory depression, and hyperpyrexia	Desipramine is the least sedating of the TCA

Drug	Mechanism	Clinical use	Side effects	Notes
Desmopressin [DDAVP]	Antidiuretic—synthetic analog of antidiuretic hormone; recruits water channels to luminal membrane in collecting duct	Antidiuresis, central (pituitary) diabetes insipidus	Overhydration; allergic reaction; larger doses result in pallor, diarrhea, and hypertension; coronary constriction; chronic rhinopharyngitis	Synthetic analog to vasopressin, intranasal administration
Desogestrel	Progesterone—binds progesterone receptors	Endometrial cancer, amenorrhea, abnormal uterine bleeding, and prevention of pregnancy		Also used to prevent endometrial hyperplasia in postmenopausal women taking estrogen
Detemir [Levemir]	Long-acting insulin—see mechanism for regular insulin	Diabetes mellitus (typically type 1)	Hypoglycemia (diaphoresis, vertigo, tachycardia), insulin allergy, insulin antibodies, lipodystrophy	
Dexamethasone [Decadron, Maxidex]	Corticosteroid—reduces lymph node and spleen size; inhibits cell cycle activity of lymphoid cells; lyses T cells; suppresses antibody, prostaglandin, and leukotriene synthesis; blocks monocyte production of IL-1	Antiemetic, autoimmune disorders, allergic reactions, asthma, organ transplantation (especially during rejection crisis), test for etiology of hypercortisolism	Insomnia, epigastric disturbances, cushingoid reaction, psychosis, glucose intolerance, infection, hypertension, cataracts	
DHEA	Androgen and estrogen precursor		Acne, hair loss, hirsutism, deepening of voice	
Diazepam [Valium]	Antianxiety, benzodiazepine—enhances GABA; increases IPSP amplitude	Sedative, hypnotic, antianxiety, antiepileptic (status epilepticus, grand mal)	Sedation	
Diazepam-binding inhibitor (DBI)	Benzodiazepine receptor antagonist			
Diazoxide	K^+ channel opener—hyperpolarizes and relaxes vascular smooth muscle	Hypertension	Hypoglycemia (reduces insulin release), hypotension	
Diclofenac [Cataflam, Voltaren]	NSAID—enteric coated			
Dicloxacillin [Dynapen, Pathocil]	Antibiotic—β-lactam, penicillin derivative, cell wall inhibitor; same mechanism as penicillin; distinguished by activity against penicillinase-producing Staphylococcus; bactericidal	Staphylococcal infections (except MRSA)	Hypersensitivity reactions; interstitial nephritis (methicillin)	Penicillinase resistant; MRSA is resistant to methicillin because of altered penicillin-binding protein target site
Dicyclomine [Bentyl]	Antimuscarinic	Bladder/GI spasm; decreases acid in ulcer		
Didanosine (ddI) [Videx]	Nucleoside reverse transcriptase inhibitor—guanosine analog → inhibits viral reverse transcriptase → prevents integration of DNA copy of viral genome into host DNA	AIDS (used in HAART)	Neutropenia, anemia, peripheral neuropathy, pancreatitis, and lactic acidosis	

(continued)

Therapeutic Agent (common name, if relevant) [trade name, where appropriate]	Class—Pharmacology and Pharmacokinetics	Indications	Side Effects or Adverse Effects	Contraindications or Precautions to Consider; Notes
Diethylcarbamazine [Hetrazan]	Anthelmintic—sensitizes helminths	Filariasis to phagocytosis by macrophages	Headache, malaise, joint pain, anorexia; death of filaria causes swelling and edema of skin, enlarged lymph nodes, hyperpyrexia, and tachycardia	
Digitoxin [Crystodigin]	Inotropic agent—cardiac glycoside; increases cardiac contractility	Severe left ventricular systolic dysfunction, antiarrhythmic	Progressive dysrhythmia, anorexia, nausea, vomiting, headache, fatigue, confusion, blurred vision, altered color perception, halos around dark objects	Contraindicated in patients with right-sided heart failure, diastolic failure; Wolff–Parkinson–White syndrome; ECG changes: increases PR, decreases QT, depresses ST, and inverts T
Digoxin [Lanoxin]	**Inotropic agent—cardiac glycoside; inhibits Na/K/ATPase → indirect inhibition of Na⁺/Ca²⁺ exchanger → increases Ca²⁺ → increases cardiac contractility**	**Severe left ventricular systolic dysfunction** (increases contractility), **atrial fibrillation** (decreases conduction at AV node and depresses SA node)	**Progressive dysrhythmia**, anorexia, nausea, vomiting, headache, fatigue, **confusion, blurred vision, altered color perception, halos around dark objects**	Contraindicated in patients with right-sided heart failure, diastolic failure; **ECG changes: increases PR, decreases QT, depresses ST, and inverts T; toxicities of digoxin are increased by renal failure** (decreases excretion), **hypokalemia** (potentiates drug's effects), and **quinidine** (decreases clearance, displaces digoxin)
Diiodohydroxyquin [Yodoxin]	Antiprotozoal—direct action	Amebiasis	Subacute myelo-optic neuropathy	
Diltiazem [Cardizem, Dilacor]	**Non-dihydropyridine Ca²⁺ channel blocker**—block voltage-gated Ca²⁺ channels of **cardiac** smooth muscle	**Hypertension, angina pectoris, arrhythmia**	Cardiac depression, peripheral edema, **flushing, dizziness,** and constipation	
Dimenhydrinate [Dramamine]	Antivertigo—antiemetic; H₁ blocker	Emesis, dizziness		
Dimercaprol [British anti-lewisite]	Metal chelator	Arsenic, mercury, or cadmium poisoning	Hypertension, tachycardia, headaches, nausea, vomiting, pain at injection site	
Dinoprostone [Cervidil, Prepidil]	Prostaglandin—PGE₂ analog → cervical dilation, uterine contraction	Induction of labor, termination of pregnancy		
Diphenhydramine [Benadryl]	**Antihistamine—antiemetic; muscarinic blocker; H₁ blocker (first generation)**	**Allergic reactions, asthma, motion sickness, antiemetic, insomnia**	Sedation, CNS depression, **atropine-like effects, allergic dermatitis, blood dyscrasias, teratogenicity,** acute antihistamine poisoning	Rarely used as antiparkinsonian agent

Drug [Brand]	Mechanism/Class	Clinical use	Adverse effects	Notes
Disopyramide [Norpace]	Antiarrhythmic (class IA)—Na$^+$ channel blocker	Wolff–Parkinson–White syndrome	Heart failure	Contraindicated in patients with sick sinus syndrome
Disulfiram [Antabuse]	**Antialcoholic agent—inhibits aldehyde dehydrogenase**	**Alcoholism**	**Tachycardia, hyperventilation, nausea**	
Dobutamine [Dobutrex]	**Inotropic agent—β-agonist; positive inotropic effects on the heart and vasodilation**	**Acute heart failure; increases cardiac output**		
Docusate	**Stool softener** by emulsifying stool, makes passage of stool easier	Constipation	Rash	
Doxazosin [Cardura]	Antihypertensive—α_1-blocker	Hypertension, BPH	**Orthostatic hypotension**, dizziness, and headache	First-dose orthostatic hypotension
Doxepin [Sinequan]	TCAs—inhibit **reuptake** of NE and 5-HT at neuronal synapses	Major depression, panic disorder, and potent antihistamine	Sedation, **α-blocking effects** (orthostatic hypotension), **anticholinergic** (tachycardia, dry mouth, and urinary retention), hallucinations (in elderly), and confusion (in elderly); overdose toxicity results in **convulsions, coma, cardiotoxicity** (arrhythmias), respiratory depression, and hyperpyrexia	
Doxorubicin [Adriamycin]	Antineoplastic—oxidizes free radicals; intercalates into DNA; breaks DNA; affects plasma membrane	Cancer	Cardiac changes resulting in cumulative cardiotoxicity	
Doxycycline	**Tetracycline antibiotic—protein synthesis inhibitor; binds 30S ribosome subunits → prevents attachment of tRNA; bacteriostatic**	**Broad spectrum including atypical pathogens: *Chlamydia, Rickettsia, Mycoplasma pneumoniae, Vibrio cholerae, Ureaplasma urealyticum, Francisella tularensis, Helicobacter pylori,* and *Borrelia burgdorferi*** (Lyme disease)	**Liver toxicity, GI distress, depression of bone/teeth development** (less than with tetracycline), **photosensitivity** (less than with tetracycline), **Fanconi syndrome**	**Contraindicated in pregnancy and children; divalent cations inhibit gut absorption, therefore cannot take with milk, antacids, or iron-containing preparations; fecally eliminated**
Dronabinol [Marinol]	Antiemetic—unknown mechanism; binds cannabinoid receptors and inhibits vomiting center in medulla	Antiemetic, appetite stimulant in patients with AIDS	Dry mouth, dizziness, inability to concentrate, disorientation, anxiety, tachycardia, depression, paranoia, psychosis	THC derivative
Echothiophate [Phospholine Iodide]	Antiglaucoma—inhibits cholinesterase; nicotinic receptor stimulator; irreversible	Closed-angle glaucoma	Open-angle glaucoma	
Edetate calcium disodium (calcium EDTA) [Calcium Disodium Versenate]	Metal chelator	Lead toxicity	Nephrotoxic	

(continued)

APPENDIX I: **Drug Index**

Therapeutic Agent (common name, if relevant) [trade name, where appropriate]	Class—Pharmacology and Pharmacokinetics	Indications	Side Effects or Adverse Effects	Contraindications or Precautions to Consider; Notes
Edrophonium [Enlon, Tensilon]	Cholinesterase inhibitor	Diagnosis of myasthenia gravis, emergency anesthetic		
Efavirenz	Antiviral, nonnucleoside reverse transcriptase inhibitor—**binds viral reverse transcriptase and inhibits movement of protein domains → terminates viral DNA synthesis → prevents integration of viral genome into host DNA**	AIDS (used in HAART)	Depression, dizziness, vivid dreams; **teratogenic**	
Emetine	Antiprotozoal—causes degeneration of nucleus and reticulation of cytoplasm; directly lethal	Severe amebic infection	Diarrhea, nausea, vomiting, abdominal pain; cardiac effects: hypotension, precordial pain, ECG changes	
Emtricitabine (FTC)	Antiviral, nucleoside reverse transcriptase inhibitor—**cytidine analog** → inhibits viral reverse transcriptase → prevents integration of DNA copy of the viral genome into the host DNA	AIDS (used in HAART)	**Neutropenia, anemia, peripheral neuropathy, pancreatitis, and lactic acidosis**	
Enalapril [Vasotec]	**Antihypertensive—ACE inhibitor** → inhibits conversion of angiotensin I to II → decreases Ang II levels → prevents vasoconstriction from Ang II	Hypertension, CHF, post-MI; prevention/treatment of diabetic nephropathy	**Cough, angioedema, hyperkalemia,** renal insufficiency (especially in bilateral renal artery stenosis)	Contraindicated in pregnancy (fetal renal malformation)
Encainide	Antiarrhythmia (class IC)—Na⁺ channel blocker	Wolff–Parkinson–White syndrome		No antimuscarinic action; no effect on action potential
Enflurane [Ethrane]	Anesthetic agent	General anesthetic	Seizure	Abnormal ECG or seizures
Enfuvirtide	Antiviral, fusion inhibitor—**binds viral gp41 subunit → inhibits conformation change (required for fusion with CD4 cell) → blocks viral entry and replication**	AIDS (used in patients on antiretroviral therapy with persistent viral replication)	**Hypersensitivity reactions, reaction at injection site, and bacterial pneumonia**	**Used in combination with other antiretroviral drugs**

Drug	Description	Clinical use	Adverse effects	Notes
Enoxaparin [Lovenox]	Low-molecular-weight heparin; enhances **inhibition of factor Xa and thrombin by increasing antithrombin activity** (preferentially increases the inhibition of factor Xa)	Prophylaxis of thrombosis	**Elevated AST/ALT (reversible), heparin-associated thrombocytopenia**	Caution in recent surgery or active bleeding ulcers or internal hemorrhages; fewer bleeding complications, more bioavailable, and longer half-life than unfractionated heparin; no requirement for monitoring
Ephedrine	Bronchodilation—mixed adrenergic agonist	Stimulates NE release, antitussive, myasthenia gravis	Increases BP	
Epinephrine	Adrenergic agonist	Acute asthma, anaphylactic shock		Activates both α- and β-receptors, but is preferential for β
Eplerenone	**Potassium-sparing diuretic**—binds to intracellular aldosterone steroid receptors in **collecting tubules;** blocks induction of Na$^+$ channels and Na$^+$/ATPase synthesis; loss of Na$^+$, Cl$^-$ in urine	Hyperaldosteronism, potassium depletion, and CHF	**Hyperkalemic metabolic acidosis, gynecomastia** (spironolactone), and antiandrogen effects	Like spironolactone but more selective for mineralocorticoid receptors; results in decreased secretion of K$^+$ and H$^+$, which can lead to **hyperkalemic metabolic acidosis;** often given in combination with a thiazide
Epoetin alfa [Procrit, Epogen]	**Colony-stimulating factor**—erythropoietin produced via recombinant DNA technology	Anemia (especially in renal failure), AIDS	**Hypertension**	
Epoprostenol [Flolan]	**Prostacyclin**—increases cardiac index and stroke volume; **decreases pulmonary vascular resistance and mean systemic pressure**	Pulmonary hypertension		
Ergotamine [Ergomar]	**Antimigraine**—vasoconstriction	**Acute attack of migraine**	**Gangrene** as a result of vasoconstriction	**Contraindicated in pregnant patients or patients with cardiovascular disease or coronary artery disease**
Erythromycin	**Antibiotic**—**macrolide,** protein synthesis inhibitor; binds to the 23S RNA of the 50S ribosome subunits → blocks translocation → prevents protein synthesis; bacteriostatic	**First choice for cell wall–deficient bugs: *Mycoplasma, Rickettsia, Chlamydia,* and *Legionella; Corynebacterium diphtheriae;*** gram-positive cocci (*Streptococcus*)	GI discomfort, **acute cholestatic hepatitis,** and **rashes;** increases concentration of oral anticoagulants and theophyllines	Can be used in patients with **streptococcal infections** and **penicillin allergies**
Esmolol [Brevibloc]	**Antiarrhythmic (class II)**—β$_1$-selective blocker	**Blocks the effect of catecholamines on heart, decreases the activity of nodal tissue, slows sinus rate, depresses AV conduction**	**Asthma, negative inotropic agent**	Short duration

APPENDIX I: **Drug Index**

(continued)

Therapeutic Agent (common name, if relevant) [trade name, where appropriate]	Class—Pharmacology and Pharmacokinetics	Indications	Side Effects or Adverse Effects	Contraindications or Precautions to Consider; Notes
Estrogen [Estratab, Premarin]	Growth and development of female organs; linear bone growth; epiphyseal closure; endometrial growth; maintains responsiveness of breasts, uterus, and vagina; inhibits bone resorption; increases hepatic production of α_2-globulins, coagulation factors II, VII, IX, and X, and HDL; decreases antithrombin and cholesterol	Osteoporosis; contraception; can be used in combination with progesterone	**Small increased incidence of breast and endometrial cancers; blood clots; may lead to sodium and water retention; nausea; breast tenderness; hyperpigmentation; increased risk of bleeding, gallbladder disease, migraines, hypertension**	
Etanercept	Recombinant form of human TNF receptor → binds TNF → decreases inflammatory response	Rheumatoid arthritis, psoriasis, and ankylosing spondylitis	Infections	
Ethacrynic acid [Edecrin]	Phenoxyacetic acid derivative diuretic—prevents cotransport of Na$^+$, K$^+$, and Cl$^-$ in **thick ascending limb**; loss of Na$^+$, Cl$^-$, Ca^{2+}, and K$^+$ in urine	**Diuresis in patients with sulfa drug allergy**	**Ototoxicity, hypokalemic metabolic alkalosis,** and dehydration	**Can be given to patients with sulfa drug allergy,** hyperuricemia, and acute gout
Ethambutol [Myambutol]	Antibiotic—unknown mechanism	*Mycobacterium*		
Ether	**Anesthetic agent**	**General anesthetic**	Fire/explosion	No longer used
Ethinyl estradiol	Estrogen—binds estrogen receptor	In women: **hypogonadism, ovarian failure, contraception,** and menstrual abnormalities; in men: **androgen-dependent prostate cancer**	**Endometrial cancer, bleeding, and thrombosis**	Used in combination with progestin in patients with intact uterus; increased risk of endometrial cancer with unopposed estrogen therapy; females exposed to diethylstilbestrol in utero have an increased risk of **vaginal clear cell adenocarcinoma**
Ethosuximide	Antiepileptic—**decreases Ca^{2+} conduction**	Epilepsy **(absence seizures)**		
Etidocaine [Duranest]	Anesthetic agent—blocks Na$^+$ intracellularly	Local anesthetic	Sleepiness, light-headedness, visual/audio disturbances, restlessness, nystagmus, shivering, tonic–clonic convulsions, death, greater toxicity than other local anesthetics	

Drug	Mechanism	Clinical use	Side effects	Notes
Etidronate [Didronel]	Bone stabilizer—pyrophosphate analog; reduces hydroxyapatite crystal formation, growth, and dissolution, which reduces bone turnover	Hypercalcemia of malignancy, Paget disease, osteoporosis, hyperparathyroidism		
Etomidate [Amidate]	Anesthetic agent	Induces stage 3 anesthesia	Painful injection, myoclonic movements	
Etoposide	**Antineoplastic—G2 phase specific—inhibits topoisomerase II → increases DNA degradation**	**Small cell lung cancer**, prostate and testicular carcinoma	**Myelosuppression**, nausea, vomiting, **alopecia**	
Etretinate	Vitamin A analog	Severe acne, psoriasis		
Exenatide [Byetta]	Hypoglycemic agent, **incretin mimetic**—agonizes GLP-1 receptors → decreases glucagon, increases insulin, delays gastric emptying	Injectable treatment for **type 2 diabetes**	Mild weight loss, nausea, **hypoglycemia**, constipation, slight risk of pancreatitis	Derived from exendin, a hormone found in Gila monster saliva
Ezetimibe [Zetia]	Antihyperlipidemia; **cholesterol absorption blocker**—prevents cholesterol reabsorption at brush border in small intestine; **decreases LDL; no effect on HDL or TG**	**Increased LDL, hypertriglyceridemia**, cardiac event risk reduction	**Increases LFT (rarely): myopathy,** hepatotoxicity, pancreatitis; abdominal symptoms	No proven clinical benefit; may increase plaque thickness
Famotidine [Pepcid]	**H$_2$ blocker—reversibly blocks histamine H$_2$ receptors → reduces gastric acid secretion**	**Peptic ulcer disease, gastritis, and esophageal reflux**	**Gynecomastia**: rare: confusion, dizziness, and headaches	**Crosses placenta; milder side effect profile** than cimetidine and ranitidine
Felodipine [Plendil]	**Dihydropyridine Ca^{2+} channel blocker**—block voltage-gated Ca^{2+} channels of **vascular** smooth muscle	**Hypertension, angina pectoris, Prinzmetal angina, Raynaud phenomenon**	Peripheral edema, **flushing, dizziness,** and constipation	
Fenofibrate	**Lipid-lowering agent—upregulates lipoprotein lipase (periphery) → increases TG clearance; decreases LDL, increases HDL, and decreases TG**	**Increased TG, increased LDL**	Myositis, increased LFTs	Reduces TG more than other agents
Fentanyl	**Opioid agonist**	**Pain**, general anesthetic	Prolonged recovery, nausea	
Fexofenadine hydrochloride [Allegra]	Antihistamine			
Filgrastim [Neupogen]	**Granulocyte-macrophage colony–stimulating factor**	**Recovery of bone marrow (e.g., chemotherapy-induced neutropenia)**		

(continued)

APPENDIX I: Drug Index

Therapeutic Agent (common name, if relevant) [trade name, where appropriate]	Class—Pharmacology and Pharmacokinetics	Indications	Side Effects or Adverse Effects	Contraindications or Precautions to Consider; Notes
Finasteride [Proscar]	**Antiandrogen—5α-reductase inhibitor** → decreases the conversion of testosterone to dihydrotestosterone	**BPH**, male pattern baldness	Decreased libido, decreased ejaculate volume	
Flecainide [Tambocor]	**Antiarrhythmic (class IC)—Na⁺ channel blocker**			
Fluconazole [Diflucan]	**Antifungal—inhibits ergosterol synthesis**, preventing cell membrane formation	**Cryptococcal meningitis, mucosal candidiasis, coccidioidomycosis**	**Abdominal pain, nausea, hepatotoxicity**	
Flucytosine [Ancobon]	Antifungal—competitive inhibitor of thymidylate synthetase; impairs DNA synthesis	*Candida, Cryptococcus*	Nausea, vomiting, diarrhea, rash, bone marrow and liver toxicity, enterocolitis	Imported in the fungus via permease
Fludrocortisone [Florinef]	Mineralocorticoid—aldosterone analog	Used with cortisol in adrenal insufficiency		
Flumazenil [Romazicon]	Benzodiazepine receptor antagonist	Alcohol abuse, anxiety		IV only
Flunarizine [Sibelium]	Weak Ca²⁺ channel blocker	Prophylaxis for migraine		
Fluoride	Stabilizes hydroxyapatite crystal structure; stimulates new growth of bone (unknown mechanism)		Nausea, vomiting, neurologic symptoms, arthralgias, arthritis	Stains teeth in toxic amounts
5-Fluorouracil (5-FU)	Antineoplastic—**inhibits thymidylate synthetase; inhibits RNA synthesis**	**Colon and breast cancer**	**Delayed toxicity: nausea, oral and GI ulcers, and bone marrow depression**	
Fluoxetine [Prozac]	SSRIs—inhibit **reuptake** of 5-HT at neuronal synapses	Major depression, OCD, anorexia, bulimia, anxiety	Inhibits liver enzymes, nausea, agitation, **sexual dysfunction** (anorgasmia), and dystonic reactions	Contraindicated with **MAOIs** secondary to **serotonin syndrome** (hyperthermia, muscle rigidity, and cardiovascular collapse); allows time for antidepressant effect, usually takes 2–3 weeks
Fluphenazine [Prolixin]	Antipsychotic—phenothiazine; blocks D₂, α₁, and H₁ receptors	Psychosis	**Extrapyramidal** (dystonia, akinesia, akathisia, and tardive dyskinesia), **anticholinergic** (dry mouth, constipation), **alpha blockade** (hypotension), and **histamine** (sedation); toxicity results in neuroleptic malignant syndrome (rigidity, myoglobinuria, autonomic instability, and hyperpyrexia)	**Extrapyramidal** side effects are more common

Drug [Brand]	Class / Mechanism	Clinical Use	Side Effects / Notes
Flurazepam [Dalmane]	Benzodiazepine—enhances GABA; increases IPSP amplitude	Sedative, hypnotic, antianxiety, antiepileptic	
Flutamide [Eulexin]	**Antiandrogen**—nonsteroidal, competitive androgen receptor blocker	**Metastatic prostate cancer**	
Fluticasone [Flonase]	Intranasal glucocorticoids—decrease cytokine synthesis, downregulate inflammatory response in the nasal mucosa	Nasal congestion, allergic rhinitis	Local irritation of nasal mucosa, epistaxis
Fluvastatin [Lescol]	Lipid-lowering agent—inhibits HMG-CoA reductase; lowers LDL	Hyperlipidemia (especially type II)	Liver toxicity, myopathy, mild GI disturbances
Fluvoxamine [Luvox]	Antidepressant—SSRI	Anxiety, OCD	Contraindicated in pregnant or lactating women and children
Folic acid [Folvite]	**Vitamin—one carbon carrier; nucleic acid synthesis**	**Given to pregnant women to prevent neural tube defects in utero**	**Decreased in pregnancy or with the use of phenytoin and isoniazid**
Foscarnet [Foscavir]	**Antiviral**—nonnucleoside inhibitor of DNA polymerase	**CMV retinitis (resistant to ganciclovir), HSV (resistant to acyclovir)**	Hypocalcemia; CNS, cardiac, and **renal toxicity**; anemia / **Does not require activation by viral kinase**
Fosinopril [Monopril]	**Antihypertensive—ACE inhibitor** → inhibits conversion of angiotensin I to II → decreases Ang II levels → prevents vasoconstriction from Ang II	Hypertension, CHF, post-MI; prevention/treatment of diabetic nephropathy	**Cough, angioedema, hyperkalemia**, renal insufficiency (especially in bilateral renal artery stenosis) / Contraindicated in pregnancy (fetal renal malformation)
Furosemide [Lasix]	Loop diuretic—prevents cotransport of Na^+, K^+, and Cl^- in **thick ascending limb**; loss of Na^+, Cl^-, Ca^{2+}, and K^+ in urine	**Hypertension, CHF**, cirrhosis, nephrotic syndrome, **pulmonary edema**, hypercalcemia	**Potassium wasting, metabolic alkalosis**, hypotension, dehydration, ototoxicity, nephritis, and gout / Do not give in patients with **sulfa drug allergy**; rapid onset and short duration of action, which is ideal for relieving acute edema
Gabapentin [Neurontin]	Antiepileptic—blocks Na^+ channels	Add-on drug for epilepsy	
Ganciclovir [Cytovene]	**Antiviral—guanosine analog**; inhibits viral DNA polymerase	**CMV (especially CMV retinitis in AIDS)**	**Bone marrow suppression** (leukopenia, neutropenia, and thrombocytopenia), **renal impairment, seizures** / **Resistance from lack of thymidine kinase or mutation of viral DNA polymerase; more toxic than acyclovir**
Gemfibrozil	**Lipid-lowering agent—upregulates lipoprotein lipase (periphery)** → **increases TG clearance; decreases LDL, increases HDL, and decreases TG**	**Increased TG, increased LDL**	Myositis, increased LFTs; potentiates **anticoagulant drugs**; gallstones; mild GI disturbances / Reduces TG more than other agents; contraindicated in patients with impaired renal or hepatic function and pregnant or lactating women
Gentamicin [Garamycin]	**Antibiotic—aminoglycoside**, protein synthesis inhibitor; irreversibly binds **30S ribosome subunits**; **bacteriostatic** at low concentration; **bactericidal** at high concentration	**Broad spectrum**: gram-negative rods; good for **bone** and **eye** infections; *Proteus, Pseudomonas, Enterobacter, Klebsiella,* and *Escherichia coli*	**Ototoxicity, renal toxicity, neuromuscular blockade,** nausea, vomiting, vertigo, allergic rash

(continued)

Therapeutic Agent (common name, if relevant) [trade name, where appropriate]	Class—Pharmacology and Pharmacokinetics	Indications	Side Effects or Adverse Effects	Contraindications or Precautions to Consider; Notes
Gestodene	**Progesterone**—binds progesterone receptors	**Endometrial cancer**, amenorrhea, abnormal uterine bleeding, and **prevention of pregnancy**		Also used to prevent endometrial hyperplasia in postmenopausal women taking estrogen
Glargine [Lantus]	**Long-acting insulin**—*see mechanism for regular insulin*	**Diabetes mellitus** (typically **type 1**)	**Hypoglycemia** (diaphoresis, vertigo, and tachycardia), insulin allergy, insulin antibodies, lipodystrophy	
Glimepiride [Amaryl]	**Hypoglycemic agent, second-generation sulfonylurea**—closes potassium channel in pancreatic β-islet cell membrane → reduces K⁺ efflux, increases Ca²⁺ influx → increases secretion of insulin	Oral treatment for **type 2 diabetes**	**Hypoglycemia**, GI disturbances, muscle weakness, mental confusion, weight gain	Not useful in type 1 diabetes mellitus because it requires some β-cell function
Glipizide [Glucotrol]	**Hypoglycemic agent, second-generation sulfonylurea**—closes potassium channel in pancreatic β-islet cell membrane → reduces K⁺ efflux, increases Ca²⁺ influx → increases secretion of insulin	Oral treatment for **type 2 diabetes**	**Hypoglycemia**, GI disturbances, muscle weakness, mental confusion, weight gain	Not useful in type 1 diabetes mellitus because it requires some β-cell function
Glyburide [DiaBeta, Micronase]	**Hypoglycemic agent, second-generation sulfonylurea**—closes potassium channel in pancreatic β-islet cell membrane → reduces K⁺ efflux, increases Ca²⁺ influx → increases secretion of insulin	Oral treatment for **type 2 diabetes**	**Hypoglycemia**, GI disturbances, muscle weakness, mental confusion, weight gain	Not useful in type 1 diabetes mellitus because it requires some β-cell function
Glyceryl guaiacolate [Fenesin]	**Expectorant**—increases bronchial secretions	**Promotes cough**		
Glycopyrrolate [Robinul]	**Antimuscarinic**	**Bladder/GI spasm, decreases acid in ulcer**		Quaternary amine
GnRH	**Controls release of FSH, LH**	**Stimulates pituitary function**		
Gonadorelin [Lutrepulse]	**Analog of GnRH**—controls release of FSH, LH	**Stimulates pituitary function**		

Drug	Mechanism/Class	Clinical Use	Side Effects/Toxicity	Notes
Griseofulvin [Fulvicin, Grifulvin, Grisactin]	**Antifungal**—inhibits cell mitosis by disrupting mitotic spindles; binds to tubulin	**Dermatophytes (especially *Trichophyton rubrum*)**	**Headache, mental confusion, rash, GI irritation, hepatotoxic, photosensitivity, carcinogenic, teratogenic**	Increases **cytochrome P450** and warfarin metabolism
Growth hormone (somatotropin, somatrem)	**Synthetic analog of growth hormone—causes liver to produce insulin-like growth factors (somatomedins)**	Replacement therapy in children with **growth hormone deficiency, Turner syndrome; burn victims**		
Growth hormone—releasing hormone (GHRH)	**Synthetic analog of GHRH—stimulates the release of growth hormone**	Dwarfism	Pain at injection site	
Guaifenesin [Robitussin]	Expectorant—thins mucus and lubricates irritated respiratory tract	Cough associated with common cold and minor upper respiratory tract infections		Does not suppress cough reflex
Guanethidine [Ismelin]	**Antihypertensive**—interferes with NE release	**Severe hypertension**	Orthostatic hypotension, exercise hypotension, impotence, and diarrhea	**Contraindicated in patients taking TCAs**
Haloperidol [Haldol]	**Antipsychotic**—butyrophenone; blocks D and α_1 receptors	**Schizophrenia, psychosis, acute mania, and Tourette syndrome**	**Extrapyramidal** (dystonia, akinesia, akathisia, and tardive dyskinesia), **endocrine** (galactorrhea), **anticholinergic** (dry mouth, constipation), **alpha blockade** (hypotension), and **histamine** (sedation); prolonged QT syndrome; toxicity results in neuroleptic malignant syndrome (rigidity, myoglobinuria, autonomic instability, and hyperpyrexia)	Extrapyramidal side effects are more common; neuroleptic malignant syndrome is treated with dantrolene and dopamine agonists
Haloprogin [Halotex]	**Antifungal—unknown mechanism; fungistatic**	**Topical for tinea pedis**		
Halothane	Anesthetic agent	General anesthetic	**Hepatotoxic, malignant hyperthermia (with succinylcholine), arrhythmia**	**Contraindicated in adults**
Heparin	**Anticoagulant**—increases PTT by accelerating antithrombin	**Deep vein thrombosis, pulmonary thrombosis, MI**	Overdose reversed by IV protamine sulfate, osteoporosis	**Fast acting; does not cross placenta**
Heroin	**Metabolized to morphine**			**More lipid soluble than morphine**
Hexamethonium	Nicotinic ganglionic blocker	Hypertensive emergency	Severe orthostatic hypotension, blurred vision, constipation, and sexual dysfunction	

(continued)

Therapeutic Agent (common name, if relevant) [trade name, where appropriate]	Class—Pharmacology and Pharmacokinetics	Indications	Side Effects or Adverse Effects	Contraindications or Precautions to Consider; Notes
Hydralazine [Apresoline]	**Antihypertensive**—increases cGMP smooth muscle relaxation → vasodilates arterioles → afterload reduction	**Severe hypertension, CHF**	**Compensatory tachycardia**, fluid retention, **lupus-like syndrome**	**First-line therapy for hypertension in pregnancy**, used with methyl-dopa; contraindicated in angina/coronary artery disease because of compensatory tachycardia
Hydrochlorothiazide (HCTZ) [HydroDIURIL]	Thiazide diuretic—inhibits transport of Na$^+$ and Cl$^-$ into the cells of DCT	**Hypertension, CHF**, idiopathic hypercalciuria, and nephrogenic diabetes insipidus	**Hypokalemia, metabolic alkalosis, mild hyperlipidemia, hyperuricemia**, malaise, **hypercalcemia**, hyperglycemia, and hyponatremia	Do not give in patients with sulfa drug allergy
Hydrocodone and acetaminophen [Bancap-HC]	Opioid agonist	Antitussive, analgesic		
Hydromorphone [Dilaudid]	Opioid agonist	Antitussive, analgesic	Respiratory depression, constipation, nausea	
Hydroxychloroquine [Plaquenil]	Antiprotozoal—antirheumatic	Rheumatic arthritis, malaria	Ocular toxicity (blurred vision)	Contraindicated in patients with psoriasis
Hydroxyurea [Hydrea]	**Antineoplastic—binds ribonucleotide reductase; inhibits formation of DNA**	**Melanoma, chronic myelogenous leukemia, sickle cell disease**	Nausea, vomiting, bone marrow suppression	
Ibuprofen [Advil, Motrin]	**NSAID—reversibly inhibits COX** (both COX-1 and COX-2) → decreases prostaglandin synthesis	**Inflammation, pain**	GI distress, **GI ulcers**, coagulation disorders, aplastic anemia, metabolic abnormalities, hypersensitivity, renal damage	
Ibutilide [Corvert]	Antiarrhythmic (class III)—K$^+$ channel blocker	Terminates atrial fibrillation and flutter	Prolongs QT interval	
Idazoxan	Antihypertensive—α_2-blocker			
Idoxuridine [Herplex Liquifilm]	Antiviral—thymidine analog; inhibits DNA polymerase; inhibits DNA synthesis	Topical for HSV keratitis	Local irritation, allergic contact keratitis	
Ifosfamide [Ifex]	Antineoplastic—DNA alkylation and cross-linking	Cancer	**Hemorrhagic cystitis**, nephrotoxicity, nausea, vomiting, bone marrow suppression, alopecia, teratogenicity, carcinogenicity	Coadministration of mesna will prevent hemorrhagic cystitis

Drug	Action/Mechanism	Clinical Uses	Side Effects	Notes
Imipenem and cilastatin [Primaxin]	Antibiotic—carbapenem, cell wall inhibitor; same mechanism as penicillin; bactericidal	Broad spectrum—gram-positive cocci (MSSA and Streptococcus), gram-negative rods (Pseudomonas and Enterobacter spp.), anaerobes	Hypersensitivity reaction, seizure, confusion state, and superinfection (pseudomembranous colitis)	Significant side effects limit use to when other drugs have failed or in the case of life-threatening infections; always administered with cilastatin (inhibits renal dehydropeptidase) to reduce inactivation in renal tubules
Imipramine [Tofranil]	TCAs—inhibit reuptake of NE and 5-HT at neuronal synapses	Major depression, nocturnal enuresis, and panic disorder	Sedation, α-blocking effects (orthostatic hypotension), anticholinergic (tachycardia, dry mouth, and urinary retention), hallucinations (in elderly), and confusion (in elderly); overdose toxicity results in convulsions, coma, cardiotoxicity (arrhythmias), respiratory depression, and hyperpyrexia	
Indecainide	Antiarrhythmic (class IC) Na$^+$ channel blockers			No antimuscarinic action; no effect on action potential
Indinavir [Crixivan]	Antiviral, protease inhibitor—protease responsible for final step of viral proliferation; inhibits protease in progeny virions → assembly of nonfunctional viruses	AIDS (used in HAART)	GI irritation (nausea, diarrhea), hyperglycemia, hyperlipidemia, lipodystrophy, thrombocytopenia	All protease inhibitors ending in -navir; metabolism occurs by cytochrome P450
Indomethacin [Indocin]	Anti-inflammatory, NSAID—reversibly inhibits COX (both COX-1 and COX-2)→ decreases prostaglandin synthesis	Acute gout therapy; closes PDA	GI distress, GI ulcers, coagulation disorders, aplastic anemia, metabolic abnormalities, hypersensitivity, renal damage	
Infliximab	Anti-inflammatory—monoclonal antibody that binds TNF → inhibits proinflammatory effects of TNF	Crohn disease, rheumatoid arthritis, and ankylosing spondylitis	Infections, fever, hypotension, and reactivation of latent tuberculosis	
Insulin, regular [Humulin R, Novolin R]	Short-acting insulin—Liver: promotes glucose storage as glycogen; increases TG synthesis. Muscle: facilitates protein and glycogen synthesis. Adipose tissue: improves TG storage by activating plasma lipoprotein lipase; reduces circulating free fatty acids	Diabetes mellitus (typically type 1), hyperkalemia, and stress-induced hyperglycemia	Hypoglycemia (diaphoresis, vertigo, and tachycardia), insulin allergy, insulin antibodies, lipodystrophy	

(continued)

Therapeutic Agent (common name, if relevant) [trade name, where appropriate]	Class—Pharmacology and Pharmacokinetics	Indications	Side Effects or Adverse Effects	Contraindications or Precautions to Consider; Notes
Interferon α-2a [Roferon A], α-2b [Intron A], and α-n3 [Alferon-N]	Antiviral—glycoproteins—block viral RNA, DNA, and protein synthesis	Genital warts, chronic hepatitis B and C, AIDS-related Kaposi sarcoma, laryngeal papillomatosis, hairy cell leukemia	Flulike symptoms, neutropenia, depression	
Interferon β-1a [Avonex, Rebif]	Antiviral—glycoproteins—block viral RNA, DNA, and protein synthesis	Multiple sclerosis	Flulike symptoms, neutropenia, depression	
Interferon γ-1b [Actimmune]	Antiviral—glycoproteins—block viral RNA, DNA, and protein synthesis	Chronic granulomatous disease	Flulike symptoms, neutropenia	
Ipecac (syrup) [Quelidrine]	Expectorant—increases bronchial secretions	Promotes cough		
Ipratropium [Atrovent]	Bronchodilator—muscarinic antagonist; competitively blocks muscarinic receptors → prevents bronchoconstriction	Asthma, COPD		
Isocarboxazid [Marplan]	MAOIs—inhibit **degradation** of NE and 5-HT at neuronal synapses	**Atypical depression** (with hypersomnia, anxiety, sensitivity to rejection, and hypochondriasis)	**Hypertensive episodes** with ingestion of tyramine-containing foods or β-agonists, hyperthermia, and convulsions	Contraindicated with **SSRIs** and **meperidine** secondary to **serotonin syndrome** (hyperthermia, muscle rigidity, and cardiovascular collapse)
Isoflurane	Anesthetic	General anesthetic		Best muscle relaxant, most widely used
Isoniazid (INH)	**Antibiotic**—inhibits synthesis of mycolic acids	***Mycobacterium* treatment (*Mycobacterium tuberculosis* and *Mycobacterium kansasii*); *Mycobacterium tuberculosis* prophylaxis**	**Peripheral and CNS effects as a result of pyridoxine deficiency; liver damage; hemolytic anemia in G6PD deficiency; SLE-like syndromes**	Pyridoxine (vitamin B_6) can prevent neurotoxicity
Isoproterenol [Isuprel]	Bronchodilator—β-agonist (non-selective); relaxes bronchial smooth muscle through $β_2$-receptor activity	Asthma	Tachycardia ($β_1$-receptor activity)	
Isosorbide dinitrate [Isordil]	Antianginal—stimulates the synthesis of cGMP, leading to muscle relaxation via NO formation; vasodilator	Angina, CHF	Headache, orthostatic hypotension, syncope	Long acting
Isotretinoin [Accutane]	**Vitamin A analog**	**Severe acne, psoriasis**	**Keratinization, teratogenic**	

Drug	Mechanism	Clinical use	Adverse effects	Notes
Itraconazole [Sporanox]	**Antifungal—inhibits ergosterol synthesis, preventing cell membrane formation**	Oral for dermatophytoses and onychomycosis; **drug of choice for histoplasmosis, blastomycosis, sporotrichosis, paracoccidioidomycosis**	**GI disturbances, hepatotoxicity**	Contraindicated in pregnancy
Ivermectin	**Anthelmintic**—binds to invertebrate chloride channels → hyperpolarizes parasite nerve and muscle cells → parasite paralysis	Onchocerciasis, strongyloidiasis		Mazzotti-like reaction
Ketamine [Ketalar]	**Anesthetic agent; blocks NMDA-type glutamate receptors**	General anesthetic	**Dissociative anesthesia, catatonia, hallucinations**	
Ketoconazole [Nizoral]	**Antifungal**—inhibits ergosterol synthesis, preventing cell membrane formation; inhibits adrenal and gonadal steroid synthesis	Chronic mucocutaneous candidiasis, blastomycosis, histoplasmosis, coccidioidomycosis, hypercortisolism, prostate carcinoma	**GI irritation, gynecomastia, thrombocytopenia, hepatotoxic, rash, fever, chills**	**Inhibits cytochrome P450**
Ketorolac [Toradol]	**NSAID—reversibly inhibits COX** (both COX-1 and COX-2) → decreases prostaglandin synthesis; relieves pain and reduces swelling	**Postoperative pain**, severe pain	GI distress, **GI ulcers**, coagulation disorders, aplastic anemia, metabolic abnormalities, hypersensitivity, renal damage	
Labetalol [Normodyne, Trandate]	**Antihypertensive—nonselective β- and α₁-blocker**	Hypertension	**Bronchospasm, bradycardia**, AV block, heart failure, sedation, and sleep alterations	
Lactulose	**Osmotic laxative**	Decreases ammonia in hepatic encephalopathy; constipation	Abdominal bloating, flatulence	Lowers colon pH so that ammonia is trapped and then excreted
Lamivudine (3TC) [Epivir]	**Antiviral, nucleoside reverse transcriptase inhibitor—cytidine analog** → inhibits viral reverse transcriptase → prevents integration of DNA copy of viral genome into host DNA	**AIDS (used in HAART)**	**Neutropenia, anemia, peripheral neuropathy, pancreatitis, and lactic acidosis**	
Lamotrigine [Lamictal]	Antiepileptic—blocks Na⁺ channels	Add-on drug for epilepsy		
Lansoprazole	**Proton pump inhibitor—irreversibly inhibits H⁺/K⁺-ATPase in gastric parietal cells → decreases proton secretion by parietal cells**	Peptic ulcer disease, gastritis, esophageal reflux, **Zollinger–Ellison syndrome**		**Inhibits cytochrome P450;** given with **clarithromycin** and **amoxicillin** for *H. pylori*
Latanoprost [Xalatan]	PGF₂ₐ: increases aqueous humor outflow	Glaucoma	Blurred vision, burning, hyperemia, itching, hyperpigmentation of iris, keratitis	

(continued)

Therapeutic Agent (common name, if relevant) [trade name, where appropriate]	Class—Pharmacology and Pharmacokinetics	Indications	Side Effects or Adverse Effects	Contraindications or Precautions to Consider; Notes
Leucovorin	Allows stem cells to bypass the inhibition of dihydrofolate reductase caused by methotrexate	Treats acute toxicity of methotrexate		
Leuprolide [Lupron]	GnRH analog—agonist (when given pulsatile), antagonist (when given continuously)	Infertility (given pulsatile), prostate cancer (given continuous), uterine fibroids, endometriosis, precocious puberty	Nausea, vomiting, and antiandrogen effects (testicular atrophy); menopausal symptoms	
Levamisole [Ergamisol]	Anthelmintic—immunostimulatory to host; helps rid the host of parasite	Ascaris (roundworm), Ancylostoma (hookworm), therapy for immunodeficiency	GI disturbances, rashes, neutropenia	
Levodopa	Antiparkinsonian agent—precursor of dopamine; administered with carbidopa (most often) or benserazide to inhibit carboxylase deactivation of levodopa in periphery	Parkinson disease		Inhibited by vitamin B_6; do not give with MAOI or pyridoxine
Levofloxacin [Levaquin]	Antibiotic—quinolone; inhibits DNA gyrase (topoisomerase II) and topoisomerase IV → blocks DNA synthesis; bactericidal	Gram-negative infections (especially UTI and bone): Pseudomonas, Enterobacteriaceae, and Neisseria; gram-positive infections (Staphylococcus, Streptococcus); intracellular: Legionella	GI disturbances, headache, dizziness, phototoxicity, cartilage damage (children, fetus), tendonitis and tendon rupture (adults), myalgias (children)	May elevate theophylline to toxic levels, causing seizure; contraindicated in pregnant women; divalent cations inhibit gut absorption, therefore cannot be taken with milk, antacids, or iron-containing preparations
Levomethadyl [Orlaam]	Opioid agonist	Long-lasting maintenance therapy for heroin addiction		
Levonorgestrel [Plan B]	Progesterone—binds progesterone receptors	Endometrial cancer, amenorrhea, abnormal uterine bleeding, and prevention of pregnancy		Also used to prevent endometrial hyperplasia in postmenopausal women taking estrogen
Levothyroxine (T_4) [Levothroid, Synthroid]	Synthetic analog of thyroxine (T_4)	Hypothyroidism	Tachycardia, heat intolerance, tremors, and arrhythmia	
Lidocaine [Xylocaine]	Antiarrhythmic (class IB), anesthetic agent—blocks Na^+ channels intracellularly	Local anesthetic, ventricular tachycardia	Sleepiness, light-headedness, visual/audio disturbances, restlessness, nystagmus, shivering, tonic–clonic convulsion, death	Given with epinephrine to maintain locality and increase duration of anesthetic properties via epinephrine-mediated vasoconstriction

APPENDIX I: Drug Index

Drug	Mechanism/Class	Clinical use	Adverse effects/Notes
Linagliptin [Tradjenta]	**Hypoglycemic agent, DPP-IV inhibitor**—prevents degradation of incretin hormones → decreased glucagon, increased insulin	Oral treatment for **type 2 diabetes**	Diarrhea, constipation, edema
Liraglutide [Victoza]	Hypoglycemic agent, **incretin mimetic**—agonizes GLP-1 receptors → decreases glucagon, increases insulin, delays gastric emptying	Injectable treatment for **type 2 diabetes**	Mild weight loss, nausea, vomiting, diarrhea, slight risk of pancreatitis	Increased incidence of medullary thyroid cancer in animal models
Lisinopril [Prinivil, Zestril]	**Antihypertensive—ACE inhibitor** → inhibits conversion of angiotensin I to II → decreases Ang II levels → prevents vasoconstriction from Ang II	Hypertension, CHF, post-MI; prevention/treatment of diabetic nephropathy	**Cough, angioedema, hyperkalemia**, renal insufficiency (especially in bilateral renal artery stenosis)	Contraindicated in pregnancy (fetal renal malformation)
Lispro [Humalog]	**Rapid-acting insulin**—*see mechanism for regular insulin*	**Diabetes mellitus** (typically **type 1**), **hyperkalemia, and stress-induced hyperglycemia**	**Hypoglycemia** (diaphoresis, vertigo, and tachycardia), insulin allergy, insulin antibodies, lipodystrophy
Lithium [Eskalith, Lithobid, Lithotabs, Lithonate]	Antimanic—unclear mechanism; inhibits regeneration of IP_3 and DAG; important for many second-messenger systems	Bipolar disorder, acute manic events	Tremor, hypothyroidism, polyuria, and teratogenesis	Close monitoring of serum levels required due to narrow therapeutic window
Loperamide [Imodium]	**Antidiarrheal—similar to opioid agonist**	**Oral antidiarrheal**	
Loratadine [Claritin]	**Antihistamine**—H_1 blocker (second generation)	**Seasonal allergies**	**Sedating**; rare: headache, dizziness, fatigue, CNS, weak antiandrogenic effect, leukopenia, and reduced sperm count	**Inhibits metabolism or absorption of some drugs**; less sedating than first-generation H_1 blocker due to decreased CNS entry
Lorazepam [Ativan]	Antianxiety—benzodiazepine; enhances GABA, increases IPSP amplitude	Sedative, hypnotic, antianxiety, antiepileptic; panic attack	
Losartan [Cozaar]	**Antihypertensive**—Ang II receptor blockers → prevents vasoconstriction from Ang II	**Hypertension**	Fetal renal toxicity, **hyperkalemia**
Lovastatin [Mevacor]	**Lipid-lowering agent—HMG-CoA reductase inhibitors**—inhibits synthesis of cholesterol precursor mevalonate; **decreases LDL, increases HDL, and decreases TG**	**High LDL, preventative after thrombotic event (e.g., MI, stroke)**	Reversible increase in LFTs; myositis	**Contraindicated in pregnant or lactating women and children**
α_2-Macroglobulin	Inhibits fibrinolysis		

(continued)

Therapeutic Agent (common name, if relevant) [trade name, where appropriate]	Class—Pharmacology and Pharmacokinetics	Indications	Side Effects or Adverse Effects	Contraindications or Precautions to Consider; Notes
Magnesium hydroxide (milk of magnesia)	**Antacid, osmotic laxative**—buffers gastric acid by raising pH	Peptic ulcer, gastritis, esophageal reflux, and constipation	**Diarrhea, hyporeflexia, hypotension, cardiac arrest, and hypokalemia**	**Can affect the absorption, bioavailability, or urinary excretion of drugs by changing the gastric pH, urinary pH, or gastric emptying**
Magnesium sulfate, magnesium citrate	**Osmotic laxative**		Magnesium toxicity (in renal insufficiency)	
Malathion	Organophosphate—inhibits cholinesterase	Least toxic organophosphate		
Mannitol [Osmitrol]	Osmotic diuretic—prevents isosmotic reabsorption of filtrate in **PCT, loop of Henle,** and **collecting tubule;** loss of Na$^+$ and all other filtered solutes in urine	Shock, drug overdose, decreased intracranial or intraocular pressure; maintenance of urine flow in rhabdomyolysis	Pulmonary edema, dehydration; contraindicated in anuria and CHF	Results in increased urine volume; readily filtered and not reabsorbed
Maprotiline	Blocks NE uptake	Major depression	Sedation, orthostatic hypotension	
Maraviroc	**Antiviral, CCR5 antagonist**—inhibits viral CCR5 coreceptor → blocks viral entry to host cell	**AIDS; patients on antiretroviral therapy with persistent viral replication**	**Fever, cough, upper respiratory infections, peripheral neuropathy, dizziness**	
Mebendazole [Vermox]	Anthelmintic—irreversible; inhibits glucose uptake	Hookworm, roundworm, threadworm, some cestodes		
Mecamylamine [Inversine]	Antihypertensive—nicotinic ganglionic blocker	Hypertension emergency; smoking cessation	Decreases GI motility, cycloplegia, hypotension, xerostomia	
Mechlorethamine (nitrogen mustard) [Mustargen]	Antineoplastic—DNA alkylation and cross-linking	Cancer	Nausea, vomiting, bone marrow suppression, alopecia, teratogenicity, carcinogenicity	
Meclizine [Antivert, Bonine]	Antiemetic agent—H$_1$ blocker	Emesis, vertigo	Teratogenic	
Mefloquine [Lariam]	Antimalarial—uncertain mechanism	Treatment of acute attack of chloroquine-resistant organisms	CNS: dizziness, disorientation, hallucinations, seizure, and depression; GI disturbances; nausea; vomiting; abdominal pain	
Melatonin	Promotes sleep	Clock shifting		Pineal hormone

Drug [Brand]	Mechanism / Class	Indications	Adverse Effects	Notes
Melphalan [Alkeran]	Antineoplastic—DNA alkylation and cross-linking	Cancer	Nausea, vomiting, bone marrow suppression (serious), alopecia, teratogenicity, carcinogenicity, pulmonary fibrosis, hypersensitivity	
Menotropin [Pergonal]	Mixture of FSH and LH	Secondary hypogonadism with infertility		
Meperidine [Demerol]	**Opioid agonist**	**Pain**, acute migraine attacks	**CNS excitation at high doses:** histamine release; antimuscarinic effects	**Contraindicated in patients with MAOI** (results in hyperpyrexia)
Mephenesin	Centrally acting muscle relaxant	Muscle spasms, tetanus contractions, orthopedic manipulation	Sedation	
Mepivacaine [Isocaine]	Anesthetic agent—blocks Na^+ channels intracellularly	Local anesthetic	Sleepiness, light-headedness, visual/audio disturbances, restlessness, nystagmus, shivering, tonic–clonic convulsion, death	
6-Mercaptopurine [Purinethol]	Antineoplastic—inhibits purine synthesis; disrupts DNA and RNA synthesis	Childhood leukemias	Myelosuppression	
Meropenem [Merrem]	**Carbapenem**—cell wall inhibitor; same mechanism as penicillin; bactericidal	**Broad spectrum—gram-positive cocci** (MSSA and *Streptococcus*), **gram-negative rods** (*Pseudomonas* and *Enterobacter* spp.), **anaerobes**	Reduced risk of seizure compared to imipenem	Stable to dihydropeptidase I, unlike imipenem
Metformin [Glucophage]	**Hypoglycemic agent, biguanide**—decreases hepatic gluconeogenesis, increases glycolysis → decreases serum glucose levels	First-line oral treatment for **type 2 diabetes**	**Lactic acidosis**, GI upset (diarrhea, nausea, and abdominal pain), metallic taste; decreased vitamin B_{12} absorption	Stop drug in patients undergoing studies or procedures involving **contrast**; contraindicated in patients with renal dysfunction
Methadone [Dolophine]	**Opioid agonist—synthetic**	**Maintenance therapy for heroin addiction, pain**	Respiratory depression, histamine release, constipation, nausea, miosis	
Methicillin	**Antibiotic—β-lactam, penicillin derivative**, cell wall inhibitor; same mechanism as penicillin; distinguished by activity against **penicillinase-producing** *Staphylococcus*; bactericidal	**Staphylococcal infections** (except MRSA)	**Hypersensitivity reactions;** interstitial nephritis (methicillin)	Penicillinase resistant; MRSA is resistant to methicillin because of altered penicillin-binding protein target site
Methimazole [Tapazole]	**Antithyroid agent**—inhibits peroxidase enzyme in thyroid → decreases synthesis of thyroid hormone	Hyperthyroidism	**Agranulocytosis**	**Crosses the placenta; can cause fetal goiter, hypothyroidism, and aplasia cutis (fetal scalp defect)**

(continued)

Therapeutic Agent (common name, if relevant) [trade name, where appropriate]	Class—Pharmacology and Pharmacokinetics	Indications	Side Effects or Adverse Effects	Contraindications or Precautions to Consider; Notes
Methohexital [Brevital]	Anesthetic agent—barbiturate; prolongs IPSP duration	Antiepileptic, cerebral edema, anesthetic (stage 3 anesthetic)		Ultrashort acting
Methotrexate [Rheumatrex]	Antineoplastic—**folic acid analog (dihydrofolate reductase inhibitor); immunosuppressant**	**Rheumatoid arthritis**, bone marrow transplant, acute lymphocytic and my-elogenous leukemia, choriocarcinoma, lung cancer, ectopic pregnancy	Oral and GI ulceration, **myelo-suppression**, thrombocytopenia; leukopenia, hepatotoxicity, **fibrotic lung disease**	**Leucovorin is given as an adjuvant after treatment**
Methoxyflurane [Penthrane]	Anesthetic agent	General anesthetic	Nephrotoxic	No longer used
Methylcellulose [Citrucel]	**Bulk-forming laxative**—dietary fiber	Constipation	Impaction above strictures, fluid overload, gas, and bloating	
Methyldopa [Aldomet]	**Antihypertensive**—centrally acting sympathetic agent (α-agonist) → decreases sympathetic outflow from CNS	**Hypertension**	Sedation, hemolytic anemia	**Positive Coombs test**
Methylphenidate [Ritalin]	CNS stimulant—amphetamine; releases neurotransmitter from synapse	Stimulant; treatment of choice for **attention deficit hyperactivity disorder**		
Methyltestosterone [Android, Virilon]	**Androgen**—androgen receptor agonist	In men: hypogonadism, delayed puberty (promotes secondary sex characteristics), and impotence; in women: estrogen receptor–positive breast cancer	**Masculinization (hirsutism)**, **testicular atrophy**, prostate hyperplasia, prostate cancer, impotence, **stunt growth** (premature epiphyseal plate closure), and hyperlipidemia	Decreases testicular testosterone, leading to Leydig cell inhibition and gonadal atrophy
Methysergide [Sansert]	**Antimigraine**—5-HT antagonist and weak vasoconstrictor	Prophylaxis of migraine	GI distress; inflammatory fibrosis of kidney, lung, and cardiac valves	**Contraindicated in patients with peripheral vascular disease, coronary artery disease, and pregnancy; patient placed on a drug holiday to prevent tachyphylaxis**
Metoclopramide [Reglan]	**GI stimulant—prokinetic agent; D₂-receptor antagonist; central and peripheral D₂ antagonism at low doses**, weak 5-HT₃ antagonism at high doses; enhances acetyl-choline release, increases resting tone, contractility, lower esophageal sphincter tone, and motility (does not affect colon transit time)	**Diabetic** and **postoperative gastroparesis, nausea,** counteracts nausea of **migraine,** increases stomach motility	Sleepiness, fatigue, headache, insomnia, dizziness, nausea, akathisia, **dystonia,** and tardive dyskinesia	Interacts with digoxin and **diabetic agents; contraindicated in small bowel obstruction**

Drug	Mechanism / Class	Clinical use	Adverse effects / Notes
Metocurine [Metubine Iodide]	**Nondepolarizing neuromuscular blocker**		
Metolazone [Mykrox, Zaroxolyn]	Diuretic—decreases Na⁺ reabsorption in the distal tubule by inhibiting the Na/Cl⁻ cotransporter; reduced peripheral resistance	Hypertension, CHF	Hypokalemia, hyperuricemia, hypovolemia, hyperglycemia (especially in diabetics), hypercalcemia, hypersensitivity reaction, Na⁺ excretion in advanced renal failure
Metoprolol [Lopressor, Toprol XL]	**Antihypertensive,** antiarrhythmic (class II)—β₁-selective blocker	**Hypertension, angina, MI, and antiarrhythmic**	**Impotence, asthma, bradycardia,** AV block, heart failure, sedation, and sleep alterations
Metronidazole [Flagyl]	**Antibiotic, antiprotozoal**—penetrates cell membrane and gives off nitro moiety → forms toxic metabolites → reacts and damages DNA; bactericidal	*Bacteroides fragilis* (especially for endocarditis and CNS); **pseudomembranous colitis** (*C. difficile*); **amebiasis; giardiasis; trichomoniasis; bacterial vaginosis** (*Gardnerella vaginalis*), **peptic ulcer disease** (part of *H. pylori* triple therapy)	Nausea, vomiting, **disulfiram-like reaction to alcohol,** metallic taste, paresthesia, stomatitis, carcinogenic and mutagenic **Contraindicated in pregnancy**
Metyrapone [Metopirone]	Inhibits cortisol synthesis	Diagnosis of pituitary dysfunction	
Mevastatin	Lipid-lowering agent—inhibits **HMG-CoA reductase; lowers LDL**	Hyperlipidemia (especially type II)	**Liver toxicity, myopathy,** mild GI disturbances **Contraindicated in pregnant** or lactating women or in children
Mexiletine [Mexitil]	Antiarrhythmic (class IB)—Na⁺ channel blocker		
Midazolam [Versed]	**Benzodiazepine; short acting**	**Preanesthetic medication; produces antegrade amnesia** (loss of memory of events after administration) **calming down the patient**	Circulatory and respiratory depression **Flumazenil antagonizes CNS depression caused by benzodiazepines**
Mifepristone (RU-486)	**Antiprogesterone**—synthetic steroid, progesterone receptor blocker → blocks the effects of progesterone → myometrium contraction	**Termination of intrauterine pregnancy** (emergency postcoital contraceptive)	**Heavy bleeding, uterine cramping,** GI effects (nausea, vomiting, and anorexia) Controversial "morning after" drug
Miglitol	Hypoglycemic agent, α-glucosidase inhibitor—inhibits intestinal brush border enzyme α-glucosidase → delays sugar hydrolysis and glucose absorption → decreases postprandial hyperglycemia	Oral treatment for type 2 diabetes postprandially	Flatulence, cramps, and diarrhea; may reduce absorption of iron Does not cause reactive hypoglycemia; decreases HbA₁c
Milrinone [Primacor]	Inotropic agent—phosphodiesterase inhibitor; increases contractility via increase in intracellular Ca²⁺	CHF	

(continued)

APPENDIX I: Drug Index

Therapeutic Agent (common name, if relevant) [trade name, where appropriate]	Class—Pharmacology and Pharmacokinetics	Indications	Side Effects or Adverse Effects	Contraindications or Precautions to Consider; Notes
Mineral oil [Fleet Mineral Oil Enema]	**Laxative—hyperosmolar agent;** draws water into gut lumen → gut distension → promotes peristalsis and evacuation of bowel	**Preoperative patients,** short-term treatment of constipation		May interfere with the absorption of fat-soluble vitamins
Minoxidil [Loniten, Rogaine]	Antihypertensive—**K$^+$ channel opener** → hyperpolarizes and relaxes vascular smooth muscle	**Severe hypertension**	**Hypertrichosis,** pericardial effusion	
Mirtazapine	α_2-Antagonist → increases release of NE and 5-HT	Major depression (especially with insomnia)	**Weight gain,** dry mouth, increased appetite, and sedation	
Misoprostol [Cytotec]	**Cytoprotectant—PGE$_1$ analog →** increased production and secretion of gastric mucosa barrier; decreased acid production; cervical dilation, uterine contractions	**Prevents NSAID-induced peptic ulcers;** maintains PDA; **induction of labor,** termination of pregnancy	Diarrhea	**Abortion-inducing drug,** contraindicated in women of childbearing age
Molindone [Moban]	Antipsychotic—blocks D$_2$ receptors	Psychosis	Parkinsonism, tardive dyskinesia	
Montelukast [Singulair]	**Leukotriene inhibitor;** reduces inflammation	**Asthma**		Not for acute attacks
Moricizine [Ethmozine]	Antiarrhythmic (class IC)—Na$^+$ channel blockers	Ventricular arrhythmia	Dizziness, nausea	
Morphine [Astramorph, Duramorph, Infumorph, Kadian, MS Contin, Oramorph, MSIR, Roxanol]	Opioid agonist—chronic oral dose converted to more potent morphine-6-glucuronide	Severe pain, general anesthetic, antitussive, antidiarrheal	Respiratory depression, histamine release, constipation, nausea, miosis	
Moxifloxacin [Avelox]	**Antibiotic—quinolone; inhibits DNA gyrase** (topoisomerase II) and **topoisomerase IV** → **blocks DNA** synthesis; bactericidal	**Less activity against gram-negative infections than other fluoroquinolones; gram-positive infections** (*Staphylococcus, Streptococcus*); **intracellular:** *Legionella;* **anaerobes**	**GI disturbances, headache, dizziness, phototoxicity, cartilage damage (children, fetus), tendonitis and tendon rupture (adults), myalgias (children)**	**May elevate theophylline to toxic levels, causing seizure; contraindicated in pregnant women; divalent cations inhibit gut absorption, therefore cannot be taken with milk, antacids, or iron-containing preparations**
Muromonab (OKT3)	Immunosuppressant—monoclonal antibody against CD3 on T lymphocytes	Acute rejection of **renal transplants**		

Muscarine	Muscarinic agonist		Abdominal pain, diarrhea, bronchoconstriction	Contraindicated in patients with peptic ulcer, asthma, hyperthyroidism, and Parkinson disease
Nabilone [Cesamet]	Antiemetic—unknown mechanism; binds cannabinoid receptors and inhibits vomiting center in medulla	Emesis	Dry mouth, dizziness, inability to concentrate, disorientation, anxiety, tachycardia, depression, paranoia, psychosis	THC derivative
N-Acetylcysteine [Mucomyst]	Breaks disulfide bonds; mucolytic (loosens mucus plugs)— replenishes glutathione	Overdose of acetaminophen; liquefies sputum to assist expulsion; also used to prevent contrast nephropathy	Unpleasant odor during administration	
Nadolol [Corgard]	Antihypertensive—antianginal; blocker	Hypertension, angina, esophageal varices		
Nafcillin	Antibiotic—β-lactam, penicillin derivative, cell wall inhibitor; same mechanism as penicillin; distinguished by activity against penicillinase-producing Staphylococcus; bactericidal	Staphylococcal infections (except MRSA)	Hypersensitivity reactions	Penicillinase resistant; MRSA is resistant to methicillin and nafcillin because of altered penicillin-binding protein target site
Nalbuphine [Nubain]	Mixed agonist/antagonist of opioids	Similar to pentazocine		
Nalorphine	Mixed agonist/antagonist of opioids	Antagonizes the effects of morphine	Respiratory depression, analgesia	
Naloxone [Narcan]	Antagonist of all opioids	Drug of choice for opioid antagonism	Ineffective to use against barbiturate overdose but safe	
Naltrexone [ReVia]	Antagonist of all opioids	Longer action than naloxone; can be used orally		
Naproxen [Naprosyn, Aleve]	NSAID—reversibly inhibits COX (both COX-1 and COX-2) → decreases prostaglandin synthesis	Inflammation, pain	GI distress, GI ulcers, coagulation disorders, aplastic anemia, metabolic abnormalities, hypersensitivity, renal damage	
Natamycin [Natacyn]	Antifungal—binds to cell membrane sterols (especially ergosterol); forms pores in membrane; fungicidal	Topical for fungal keratitis (eye)		
Nedocromil [Tilade]	Antiasthmatic; stabilizes membranes of mast cells and prevents mediator release	Asthma	Unpleasant taste	Not for acute asthmatic attacks
Nefazodone [Serzone]	Antidepressant—postsynaptic 5-HT$_2$ antagonist	Depression		

(continued)

APPENDIX I: **Drug Index**

Therapeutic Agent (common name, if relevant) [trade name, where appropriate]	Class—Pharmacology and Pharmacokinetics	Indications	Side Effects or Adverse Effects	Contraindications or Precautions to Consider; Notes
Nelfinavir	**Antiviral, protease inhibitor**—protease responsible for final step of viral proliferation; inhibits protease in progeny virions → assembly of nonfunctional viruses	**AIDS (used in HAART)**	GI irritation (nausea, diarrhea), hyperglycemia, hyperlipidemia, and lipodystrophy	All protease inhibitors end in -navir; metabolism occurs by cytochrome P450
Neomycin [Mycifradin, Neosporin]	Antibiotic—aminoglycoside; binds 30S ribosome subunits; bacteriostatic at low concentration; bactericidal at high concentration	Reduction of gut flora	Renal damage, deafness	Inhibits absorption of digitalis; topical use
Neostigmine [Prostigmin]	Inhibits cholinesterase	**Paralytic ileus, neurogenic bladder, myasthenia gravis**		
Nevirapine	**Antiviral, nonnucleoside reverse transcriptase inhibitor**—binds viral reverse transcriptase and inhibits movement of protein domains → terminates viral DNA synthesis → prevents integration of viral genome into the host DNA	**AIDS (used in HAART)**	Neutropenia, anemia, peripheral neuropathy, and rash	
Niclosamide [Niclocide]	Anthelmintic—inhibits anaerobic metabolism	Tapeworms: *Taenia solium*, *Taenia saginata*, *Hymenolepis nana*		
Nicotine [Habitrol, NicoDerm, Nicotrol]	Nicotinic agonist	**Stops smoking**		
Nifedipine [Adalat, Procardia]	**Dihydropyridine Ca^{2+} channel blocker**—blocks voltage-gated Ca^{2+} channels of **vascular** smooth muscle	**Hypertension, angina pectoris, Prinzmetal angina, Raynaud phenomenon**	Peripheral edema, **flushing, dizziness,** and constipation	
Nitrofurantoin [Macrobid]	Antibiotic—urinary antiseptic; unknown mechanism of action	Gram-positive and gram-negative bacteria		Contraindicated in patients with renal insufficiency
Nitroglycerin	**Antianginal—stimulates synthesis of cGMP, leading to muscle relaxation via NO formation**	**Angina**	Headache, orthostatic hypotension, syncope	**Monday disease; short acting**
Nitrosoureas	Antineoplastic—alkylating agent; lipid soluble	CNS tumors		
Nitrous oxide	Anesthetic agent	General anesthetic	Hypoxia	

Drug	Mechanism	Clinical use	Side effects	Notes
Nizatidine [Axid]	**H₂ blocker—reversibly blocks histamine H₂ receptors → reduces gastric acid secretion**	**Peptic ulcer disease, gastritis, and esophageal reflux**	**Gynecomastia**; rare: confusion, dizziness, and headaches	**Crosses placenta; milder side effect profile** than cimetidine and ranitidine
Norethindrone	**Progesterone**—binds progesterone receptors	**Endometrial cancer**, amenorrhea, abnormal uterine bleeding, and **prevention of pregnancy**		Also used to prevent endometrial hyperplasia in postmenopausal women taking estrogen
Norfloxacin	**Antibiotic—quinolone; inhibits DNA gyrase** (topoisomerase II) and **topoisomerase IV** → blocks DNA synthesis; bactericidal	**Gram-negative infections** (especially UTI and bone): *Pseudomonas*, Enterobacteriaceae, and *Neisseria*; **gram-positive infections** (staphylococci)	**GI disturbances, headache, dizziness, phototoxicity, cartilage damage (children, fetus), tendonitis** and **tendon rupture (adults), myalgias (children)**	May elevate theophylline to toxic levels, causing seizure; divalent cations **inhibit gut absorption, therefore cannot be taken with milk, antacids, or iron-containing preparations**
Norgestimate	**Progesterone**—binds progesterone receptors	**Endometrial cancer**, amenorrhea, abnormal uterine bleeding, and **prevention of pregnancy**		Also used to prevent endometrial hyperplasia in postmenopausal women taking estrogen
Nortriptyline [Pamelor]	TCAs—inhibit **reuptake** of NE and 5-HT at neuronal synapses	Major depression, panic disorder, and anxiety	Sedation, **α-blocking effects** (orthostatic hypotension), **anticholinergic** (tachycardia, dry mouth, and urinary retention), hallucinations (in elderly), and confusion (in elderly); overdose toxicity results in **convulsions, coma, cardiotoxicity** (arrhythmias), respiratory depression, and hyperpyrexia	
NPH [Humulin N, Novolin N]	**Intermediate-acting insulin**—*see mechanism for regular insulin*	**Diabetes mellitus** (typically **type 1**)	**Hypoglycemia** (diaphoresis, vertigo, and tachycardia), insulin allergy, insulin antibodies, lipodystrophy	
Nystatin [Mycostatin]	Antifungal—binds to cell membrane sterols (especially ergosterol) → disrupting fungal membranes; fungicidal	**Mucosal candidal** infections (skin, vaginal, and GI)	Few	Used topically or as mouth rinse; too toxic for systemic use
Octreotide [Sandostatin]	**Synthetic analog of somatostatin**— decreases release of growth hormone, gastrin, secretin, VIP, CCK, glucagon, and insulin	**Acromegaly, glucagonoma, insulinoma carcinoid syndrome**	Nausea, cramps, and gallstones	
Ofloxacin [Floxin]	**Antibiotic—quinolone, DNA synthesis inhibitor; inhibits DNA gyrase** (topoisomerase II) and **topoisomerase IV** → blocks DNA synthesis; bactericidal	**Gram-negative infections** (especially UTI and bone): *Pseudomonas*, Enterobacteriaceae, and *Neisseria*; **gram-positive infections** (staphylococci); **intracellular: *Legionella***	**GI disturbances, headache, dizziness, phototoxicity, cartilage damage (children, fetus), tendonitis** and **tendon rupture (adults), myalgias (children)**	May elevate theophylline to toxic levels, causing seizure; divalent cations **inhibit gut absorption, therefore cannot be taken with milk, antacids, or iron-containing preparations**

(continued)

Therapeutic Agent (common name, if relevant) [trade name, where appropriate]	Class—Pharmacology and Pharmacokinetics	Indications	Side Effects or Adverse Effects	Contraindications or Precautions to Consider; Notes
Olanzapine [Zyprexa]	Atypical antipsychotic—blocks D_4, α_1, 5-HT, and muscarinic receptors	Schizophrenia, OCD, anxiety disorder, depression, mania, and Tourette syndrome	Agranulocytosis, **weight gain, diabetes; extrapyramidal** (occurs at a lower rate than typicals), **anticholinergic** (dry mouth, constipation), **alpha blockade** (hypotension), **histamine** (sedation); toxicity results in neuroleptic malignant syndrome (occurs at a lower rate than typicals)	
Omeprazole [Prilosec]	**Proton pump inhibitors— irreversibly inhibits H^+/K^+-ATPase in gastric parietal cells → decreases proton secretion by parietal cells**	Peptic ulcer disease, gastritis, esophageal reflux, and **Zollinger–Ellison syndrome**		**Inhibits cytochrome P450**; given with **clarithromycin** and **amoxicillin** for *H. pylori*
Ondansetron [Zofran]	**Antiemetic—serotonin antagonist, 5-HT$_3$ blocker**	**Nausea** (caused by **cancer therapy** or **postoperative state**)	Headache, constipation, dizziness	
Oprelvekin [Neumega]	IL-11 stimulates multiple stages of **thrombopoiesis**, increasing platelet production	**Thrombocytopenia**		
Orlistat [Xenical]	**Inhibits pancreatic lipases →** alters fat metabolism	**Obesity** (long term)	**Steatorrhea**, GI irritation, reduced absorption of fat-soluble vitamins, and headache	**Used in conjunction with modified diet**
Oseltamivir [Tamiflu]	**Antiviral—inhibits neuraminidase →** decreases release of progeny viruses	**Influenza A and B treatment and prophylaxis**		Begin within 2 days of onset of flu symptoms to decrease the duration and intensity of symptoms
Oxacillin [Bactocill]	Antibiotic—β-lactam; penicillinase resistant	Staphylococcal infections		
Oxaprozin [Daypro]	NSAID—mildly uricosuric	Acute gout		Contraindicated in patients with kidney stones
Oxazepam [Serax]	Antianxiety—benzodiazepine; enhances GABA; increases IPSP amplitude	Sedative, hypnotic, antiepileptic, anxiolytic		Recommended for use in elderly
Oxybutynin [Ditropan]	Antimuscarinic	Bladder/GI spasm; decreases acid in ulcer		

Drug	Mechanism	Clinical use	Side effects	Notes
Oxycodone [Roxicodone]	**Partial opioid agonist** at mu receptor	Severe pain, general anesthetic	Respiratory depression, constipation, nausea	
Oxytocin [Pitocin, Syntocinon]	**Synthetic analog of oxytocin—stimulates uterine contraction and contraction of breast myo-epithelial cells; milk letdown reflex**	**Induces labor, controls uterine hemorrhage**		
Paclitaxel [Taxol]	Antineoplastic—stabilizes polymerization of microtubules	Ovarian and breast cancer		
Pamidronate [Aredia]	Bone stabilizer—pyrophosphate analog; reduces hydroxyapatite crystal formation, growth, and dissolution, which reduces bone turnover	Hypercalcemia of malignancy, Paget disease, osteoporosis, hyperparathyroidism		
Pancuronium [Pavulon]	Nondepolarizing neuromuscular blocker		Minimal histamine release	
Paroxetine [Paxil]	SSRIs—inhibit **reuptake** of 5-HT at neuronal synapses	Major depression, OCD, anorexia, and bulimia	Inhibits liver enzymes, nausea, agitation, **sexual dysfunction** (anorgasmia), and dystonic reactions	Contraindicated with **MAOIs** secondary to **serotonin syndrome** (hyperthermia, muscle rigidity, and cardiovascular collapse); allows time for antidepressant effect, usually takes 2–3 weeks
Penicillamine [Cuprimine, Depen]	Antiarthritis—anti-gold medicine; not specific; unknown mechanism; arthritis relief	**Rheumatic arthritis, copper poisoning, metal chelator**	Decreases vitamin B_6; bone marrow suppression; proteinuria; autoimmune syndrome	
Penicillin	**Antibiotic—β-lactam, cell wall inhibitor; binds penicillin-binding protein → inhibits transpeptidase** cross-linking of cell wall **→ inhibits bacterial cell wall synthesis → activates autolytic enzymes;** bactericidal	**Gram-positive cocci, gram-positive rods, gram-negative cocci, some anaerobes, enterococci, and spirochetes**	**Hypersensitivity reactions, neutropenia, thrombocytopenia, anemia, CNS effects, superinfection** (pseudomembranous colitis)	Not penicillinase resistant
Pentazocine [Talwin]	Mixed agonist/antagonist of opioids	Analgesia		Only mixed agonist/antagonist available orally
Pentobarbital [Nembutal Sodium]	Barbiturate—prolongs IPSP duration	Cerebral edema, anesthetic		
Pergolide [Permax]	Antiparkinsonian—dopamine agonist; inhibits prolactin release	Treats breast engorgement, inhibits lactation		
Phenazocine	Opioid agonist			

(continued)

Therapeutic Agent (common name, if relevant) [trade name, where appropriate]	Class—Pharmacology and Pharmacokinetics	Indications	Side Effects or Adverse Effects	Contraindications or Precautions to Consider; Notes
Phenelzine	**Antidepressant, MAOIs**—inhibits **degradation** of NE and 5-HT at neuronal synapses	**Atypical depression** (with hypersomnia, anxiety, sensitivity to rejection, and hypochondriasis)	**Hypertensive episodes** with ingestion of tyramine-containing foods or β-agonists, hyperthermia, and convulsions	Contraindicated with **SSRIs** and **meperidine** secondary to **serotonin syndrome** (hyperthermia, muscle rigidity, and cardiovascular collapse)
Phenobarbital	**Barbiturate**—prolongs IPSP duration	**Antiepileptic (partial and tonic–clonic), cerebral edema, anesthetic**	Sedation	Many drug interactions
Phenolphthalein [Ex-Lax]	**Stimulant laxative**—reduces absorption of electrolytes and water from gut	Constipation	Tumorigenic	
Phenoxybenzamine [Dibenzyline]	Antihypertensive—α-blocker; long acting; irreversible	Pheochromocytoma	Nasal congestion, miosis, orthostatic hypotension	
Phentolamine [Regitine]	**Antihypertensive—α-blocker**	**Diagnosis of pheochromocytoma**; hypertension (especially tyrosine induced)		
Phenylbutazone [Butazolidin]	**NSAID**	**Rheumatic arthritis, acute gout**	**Agranulocytosis, aplastic anemia**	
Phenylephrine [Neo-Synephrine, Nostril]	Nasal decongestant—α_1-agonist	Nasal decongestant	Hypertension	
Phenylzin	Antidepressant—MAOI; nonselective but isoenzyme A most important; irreversible	Depression		
Phenytoin [Dilantin]	**Antiepileptic—decreases Na$^+$ flux**	**Epilepsy (partial and tonic–clonic), digitalis-induced arrhythmia**	**Decreases folic acid, gingival hyperplasia, hirsutism, nystagmus**	**Induces cytochrome P450; saturable elimination**
Physostigmine [Eserine]	**Inhibits cholinesterase**	**Intestinal or bladder atony, glaucoma**		
Pilocarpine [Ocusert]	**Antiglaucoma—muscarinic agonist**	**Xerostomia, narrow- and open-angle glaucoma**	**Focusing problems, nausea, abdominal pain, sweating; high dose: bradycardia, hypotension**	**Contraindicated in patients with peptic ulcer, asthma, hyperthyroidism, and Parkinson disease**
Pindolol [Visken]	Antihypertensive, antiarrhythmic (class II)—β-blocker	Hypertension		

Drug	Mechanism	Clinical Use	Side Effects / Notes	
Pioglitazone [Actos]	Hypoglycemic agent, thiazolidinedione—binds PPARγ receptors; improves target cell response to insulin	Oral treatment for **type 2 diabetes**	**Weight gain**, edema, hepatotoxicity; increases LDL and TGs	Contraindicated in CHF
Piperacillin [Pipracil] **piperacillin-tazobactam** [Zosyn]	**Antibiotic—β-lactam, penicillin derivative**, cell wall inhibitor; same mechanism as penicillin; distinguished by activity against ***Pseudomonas***; bactericidal	**Extended spectrum**—*Pseudomonas, Proteus,* and *Enterobacter* species	**Hypersensitivity reactions**, decreased platelet function	Not effective against penicillin-resistant *Staphylococcus*, **can be combined with clavulanic acid** (β-lactamase inhibitor) to enhance spectrum; administered IV
Pirenzepine	**Muscarinic antagonist—blocks M₁ receptors on ECL cells → decreases histamine secretion; blocks M₃ receptors on parietal cells → decreases acid secretion**	Peptic ulcer	**Tachycardia, dry mouth, and blurry vision** (difficulty accommodating)	
Piroxicam [Feldene]	NSAID			Long acting; contraindicated in the elderly
Platelet-activating factor (PAF)	Activation of platelets and PMN aggregation; increases vascular permeability			
Plicamycin [Mithracin]	Antineoplastic—inhibits DNA-directed RNA synthesis; decreases protein synthesis needed for bone reabsorption	Paget disease, hypercalcemia		
Polymyxins (colistin)	**Antibiotic—binds to cell membranes → disrupt osmotic properties; bactericidal**	**Gram-negative bacteria: *Pseudomonas* and coliforms; usually topical; can be used IV or nebulized for difficult-to-treat gram-negative infections**	**Neurotoxic, nephrotoxic** (acute renal tubular necrosis)	
Potassium	**Depresses ectopic pacemaker in hypokalemia**	**Digoxin toxicity**		
Potassium iodide [Thyro-Block]	Expectorant—increases bronchial secretions; high doses decrease release of thyroid hormone	Promotes cough; hyperthyroidism		
Pralidoxime (2-PAM) [Protopam]	Acetylcholinesterase reactivator	**Overdose of malathion/parathion organophosphates; must be used before aging occurs**		
Pramlintide [Symlin]	**Hypoglycemic agent, analog of amylin**—a pancreatic hormone secreted with insulin that decreases glucagon and delays gastric emptying	Injectable treatment for **type 2 diabetes**	Nausea, vomiting, hypoglycemia	

(continued)

Therapeutic Agent (common name, if relevant) [trade name, where appropriate]	Class—Pharmacology and Pharmacokinetics	Indications	Side Effects or Adverse Effects	Contraindications or Precautions to Consider; Notes
Pravastatin [Pravachol]	Lipid-lowering agent—**HMG-CoA reductase inhibitor**—inhibits synthesis of cholesterol precursor mevalonate; **decreases LDL, increases HDL, and decreases TG**	**High LDL, preventative after thrombotic event (e.g., MI, stroke)**	Reversible increase in LFTs; myositis	Contraindicated in pregnant or lactating women and children
Praziquantel [Biltricide]	Anthelmintic—increases membrane permeability causing loss of Ca^{2+}	Schistosomes, flukes	GI disturbances, headache, fever, urticaria	
Prazosin [Minipress]	Antihypertensive—α_1-**blocker** → vasodilation → decreases total peripheral resistance	Pheochromocytoma, hypertension, BPH	**Orthostatic hypotension**, dizziness, headache	First-dose orthostatic hypotension
Prednisone [Deltasone]	Glucocorticoid—inhibits protein synthesis; reduces lymph node and spleen size; inhibits cell cycle activity of lymphoid cells; lyses T cells; suppresses antibody, prostaglandin, and leukotriene synthesis; **blocks monocyte production of IL-1**	Rheumatic arthritis, autoimmune disorders, allergic reaction, asthma, COPD, organ transplantation (especially during rejection crisis)	Osteoporosis, cushingoid reaction, psychosis, glucose intolerance, infection, hypertension, cataracts	
Prilocaine [Citanest]	Anesthetic agent—blocks Na^+ channels intracellularly	Local anesthetic	Sleepiness, light-headedness, visual/audio disturbances, restlessness, nystagmus, shivering, tonic–clonic convulsions, death	
Primaquine phosphate	Antimalarial—unknown mechanism	Prevents relapse of *Plasmodium ovale* and *Plasmodium vivax* malaria; prophylaxis for *Plasmodium falciparum* malaria	GI disturbances, mild anemia; **marked hemolysis in G6PD-deficient individuals; prolongs QT interval**	
Probenecid [Benemid]	Antigout—increased secretion of uric acid (uricosuric)—competes with uric acid for **reabsorption in the kidney**	Chronic gout therapy	**Caution: should not be used in patients with sulfa allergies;** rash; GI disturbances; drowsiness	Should not be used to treat acute gout or patients with uric acid stones
Probucol [Bifenabid, Lesterol]	Lipid-lowering agent—lowers HDL and LDL; mechanism unknown	Hyperlipidemia	Prolongs QT interval; GI disturbances	Contraindicated in patients with heart disease
Procainamide [Pronestyl, Procanbid]	Antiarrhythmic (class IA)—Na^+ **channel blocker**	Ventricular arrhythmia	Lupus-like syndrome	

Drug	Mechanism/Class	Use	Side effects	Notes
Procaine [Novocain]	Anesthetic agent—blocks Na$^+$ intracellularly	Local anesthetic	Sleepiness, light-headedness, visual/audio disturbances, restlessness, nystagmus, shivering, tonic–clonic convulsions, death	
Procarbazine [Matulane]	Antineoplastic—DNA alkylation and strand breakage; inhibits nucleic acid and protein synthesis	Cancer		
Prochlorperazine [Compazine]	**Antiemetic—dopamine (D$_2$-receptor) antagonist**	**Nausea**; counteracts nausea of **migraine**	Teratogenic	
Progesterone [Progestasert]	**Hormone—causes secretory changes in endometrium and breast; necessary to maintain pregnancy**	**Endometrial cancer**, amenorrhea, abnormal uterine bleeding, and **prevention of pregnancy**	**Long-lasting suppression of menses, endometriosis, hirsutism, bleeding disorders, nausea, breast tenderness, hyperpigmentation, gallbladder disease, migraines, hypertension**	Also used to prevent endometrial hyperplasia in postmenopausal women taking estrogen
Prolactin	**Hormone—stimulates lactation**			
Promethazine [Phenergan]	**Antihistamine, antiemetic**—D$_2$-receptor antagonist; H$_1$ blocker	Counteracts nausea of **migraine**; allergies; **motion sickness**	Sedation, CNS depression, atropine-like effects, allergic dermatitis, blood dyscrasias, **teratogenicity**, acute antihistamine poisoning	
Propafenone [Rythmol]	Antiarrhythmic (class IC)—Na$^+$ channel blocker			
Propantheline	**Muscarinic antagonist—blocks M$_1$ receptors on ECL cells → decreases histamine secretion; blocks M$_3$ receptors on parietal cells → decreases acid secretion**	Peptic ulcer	**Tachycardia, dry mouth, and blurry vision** (difficulty accommodating)	
Propofol [Diprivan]	Anesthetic agent	General anesthetic; fast acting for ambulatory or outpatients	Seizure	
Propranolol [Inderal]	β-Blocker, antimigraine—decreases cAMP and calcium currents → increases PR interval, suppresses abnormal pacemakers, especially in AV node	**Ventricular tachycardia, supraventricular tachycardia, and slowing ventricular rate during atrial fibrillation and atrial flutter**	**Impotence, exacerbation of asthma, bradycardia,** AV block, CHF, sedation, and sleep alteration	

(continued)

Therapeutic Agent (common name, if relevant) [trade name, where appropriate]	Class—Pharmacology and Pharmacokinetics	Indications	Side Effects or Adverse Effects	Contraindications or Precautions to Consider; Notes
Propylthiouracil [Propyl-Thyracil]	Antithyroid agent—inhibits peroxidase enzyme in thyroid → decreases synthesis of thyroid hormone	**Hyperthyroidism**	**Agranulocytosis**	**Crosses the placenta and can cause fetal goiter and hypothyroidism;** preferred to methimazole in treating pregnant women with moderate to severe hyperthyroidism
Protriptyline [Vivactil]	Antidepressant—TCA; blocks NE, 5-HT, muscarinic, α_1, and histamine receptors	Depression, anxiety	Tremors (NE block), anorexia (5-HT block), anticholinergic (muscarinic block), hypotension (α_1-block), drowsiness (histamine block)	
Pseudoephedrine [Sudafed]	α- and β-Adrenergic agonist; stimulates bronchial relaxation (β), increases heart rate (β), and vasoconstriction (α)	Nasal decongestant; sinusitis, upper respiratory tract infection	Tachycardia, increased BP, hypersensitivity	Sales limited; precursor for illicit methamphetamine synthesis
Psyllium [Perdiem Fiber]	**Bulk-forming laxative**—dietary fiber	Constipation	Impaction above strictures, fluid overload, gas, and bloating	
PTH	Increases plasma Ca^{2+} levels by increasing reabsorption in kidney; activates vitamin D, which aids in Ca^{2+} absorption from gut; resorbs Ca^{2+} from bone; decreases phosphate reabsorption by kidney	Used to distinguish between hypoparathyroidism and pseudohypoparathyroidism		
Pyrantel [Antiminth, Reese's Pinworm Medicine]	Anthelmintic—depolarizing neuromuscular blocker causing spastic paralysis in worms	*Ascaris* (roundworm), *Ancylostoma* (hookworm), threadworm		
Pyrazinamide	Antibiotic—postulated mechanism involves inhibition of enzyme pyrazinamidase → inhibition of fatty acid synthesis	*Mycobacterium*	Impairs liver function	
Pyridostigmine [Mestinon]	**Inhibits cholinesterase**	**Myasthenia gravis**		
Pyrimethamine [Daraprim]	Antimalarial—inhibits dihydrofolate reductase	Malaria	Large doses causes megaloblastic anemia	

Drug	Mechanism	Clinical Use	Side Effects/Notes
Quetiapine [Seroquel]	Atypical antipsychotic—blocks D_2, 5-HT, α_1, and H_1 receptors	Schizophrenia, acute mania	Suicide attempt in major depression, arrhythmia, **extrapyramidal** (occurs at a lower rate than typicals), **anticholinergic** (occurs at lower rate than other agents), **alpha blockade** (hypotension), and **histamine** (sedation); toxicity results in neuroleptic malignant syndrome (occurs at a lower rate than typicals)
Quinapril [Accupril]	**Antihypertensive—ACE inhibitor** → inhibits conversion of angiotensin I to II → decreases Ang II levels → prevents vasoconstriction from Ang II	Hypertension, CHF, post-MI; prevention/treatment of diabetic nephropathy	**Cough, angioedema, hyperkalemia**, renal insufficiency (especially in bilateral renal artery stenosis) Contraindicated in pregnancy (fetal renal malformation)
Quinidine [Quinaglute]	**Antiarrhythmic (class IA)—Na^+ channel blocker**	Arrhythmias, acute malarial infection	**May precipitate arrhythmias at high doses; nausea; vomiting; diarrhea; cinchonism: tinnitus, headache, nausea, disturbed vision; renal damage; hemolytic anemia; purpura; agranulocytosis** Torsades de pointes, inhibits cytochrome P450
Quinine	**Antimalarial—unknown mechanism**	**Suppression and treatment of acute attack of chloroquine-resistant organism; leg cramps**	**Cinchonism: tinnitus, headache, nausea, disturbed vision; renal damage; hemolytic anemia; purpura; agranulocytosis**
Quinolones	**Antibiotic—blocks DNA synthesis by inhibiting DNA gyrase**	Gram-negative infections (especially UTI and bone): *Pseudomonas*, Enterobacteriaceae, and *Neisseria*; gram-positive infections; intracellular: *Legionella*	GI disturbances, headache, dizziness, phototoxicity, cartilage damage **May elevate theophylline to toxic levels, causing seizure; divalent cations inhibit gut absorption, therefore cannot be taken with milk antacids, or iron-containing preparations**
Radioiodide (I-131)	**Destroys thyroid gland**	Hyperthyroidism	Hypothyroidism
Raloxifene [Evista]	**Selective estrogen receptor modulator—breast (estrogen antagonist); endometrium (estrogen antagonist)**: prevents proliferation of endometrium; **bone (estrogen agonist)**: decreases bone turnover, increases bone density; **cardiovascular (estrogen agonist)**: decreases LDL	Osteoporosis, breast cancer	Hot flashes, sinusitis, weight gain, muscle pain, leg cramps, **increased risk of blood clots** Unlike estrogen, raloxifene does **not decrease HDL**

(continued)

443

Therapeutic Agent (common name, if relevant) [trade name, where appropriate]	Class—Pharmacology and Pharmacokinetics	Indications	Side Effects or Adverse Effects	Contraindications or Precautions to Consider; Notes
Raltegravir	**Antiviral, integrase inhibitor**—inhibits the final step in integration of viral DNA into host DNA	**HAART**	**Neutropenia, pancreatitis, hepatotoxicity, hyperglycemia**	
Ranitidine [Zantac]	**H₂ blocker—blocks histamine H₂ receptors reversibly → decreases proton secretion by parietal cells**	**Peptic ulcer disease, gastritis, and esophageal reflux**	**Gynecomastia, impotence,** decreased libido in males, **confusion, dizziness, and headaches**	**Crosses placenta, decreases renal excretion of creatinine, cytochrome P450 inhibitor**
Repaglinide [Prandin]	Hypoglycemic agent—**meglitinide; acts at pancreatic islet cell** to reduce K⁺ efflux, increases Ca²⁺ influx, **increases secretion of insulin**	Oral treatment for **type 2 diabetes**	Hypoglycemia	
Reserpine [Rauserfia]	Antihypertensive—prevents storage of monoamines in synaptic vesicle	Hypertension	**Mental depression**, sedation, nasal stuffiness, and diarrhea	
RhoGAM	**Rh immunoglobulin**	**Prevents hemolytic disease of the newborn**		
Ribavirin	Antiviral—**guanosine analog;** inhibits IMP dehydrogenase → decreases synthesis of guanine nucleotides	**Hepatitis C when given with interferon**	Hemolytic anemia, elevated bilirubin; teratogen	
Rifampin [Rifadin]	**Antibiotic—inhibits DNA-dependent RNA polymerase**	*Mycobacterium;* reduces resistance to dapsone when used in treatment of leprosy; prophylaxis in close contacts of people with *N. meningitidis* meningitis	Turns body fluid orange in color; liver damage	**Interferes with birth control pills by increasing estrogen metabolism; induces cytochrome P450**
Risedronate [Actonel]	**Bone stabilizer—bisphosphonate; pyrophosphate analog;** reduces hydroxyapatite crystal formation, growth, and dissolution, which reduces bone turnover	**Hypercalcemia of malignancy, Paget disease, osteoporosis, hyperparathyroidism**	**Pill-induced esophagitis**	

Drug	Mechanism	Clinical use	Side effects/toxicity	Notes
Risperidone	Atypical antipsychotic—blocks D_2, 5-HT, α_1, and H_2 receptors	Schizophrenia, useful for positive and negative symptoms	Agranulocytosis, **extrapyramidal** (occurs at a lower rate than typicals), **anticholinergic** (occurs at lower rate than other agents), **alpha blockade** (hypotension), and **histamine** (sedation); toxicity results in neuroleptic malignant syndrome (occurs at a lower rate than typicals)	Second-line agent used for refractory schizophrenia
Ritodrine [Yutopar]	B_2-Agonist → uterine relaxation	Inhibits preterm labor		
Ritonavir [Norvir]	**Antiviral, protease inhibitor**—protease responsible for final step of viral proliferation; inhibits protease in progeny virions → assembly of nonfunctional viruses	**AIDS (used in HAART)**	**GI irritation (nausea, diarrhea), hyperglycemia, hyperlipidemia, and lipodystrophy**	**All protease inhibitors end in -navir; metabolism occurs by cytochrome P450**
Rituximab	Monoclonal antibodies; binds to CD20 receptor on tumor cells, resulting in lysis	Non-Hodgkin lymphoma	Fever, rigor, chills; nausea, hypersensitivity; tumor lysis syndrome; irregular heart rhythms; infection; pancytopenia	
Ropivacaine	Anesthetic agent—blocks Na^+ intracellularly	Local anesthetic	Sleepiness, light-headedness, visual/audio disturbances, restlessness, nystagmus, shivering, tonic–clonic convulsion, death	
Rosiglitazone [Avandia]	Hypoglycemic agent, thiazolidinedione—binds PPARγ receptors, improves target cell response to insulin	Oral treatment for **type 2 diabetes**	**Weight gain**, edema, hepatotoxicity; increases LDL and TGs; **may increase risk of MI**	Contraindicated in CHF
Salmeterol [Serevent]	**Antiasthmatic—long-acting β_2-agonist, leads to relaxation of smooth muscle**	Asthma prophylaxis	**Hand tremor**, headache, nervousness, dizziness, cough, stuffed nose, runny nose, ear pain, muscle pain/cramps, sore throat	Not in acute asthmatic attack
Saquinavir [Invirase]	**Antiviral, protease inhibitor**—protease responsible for final step of viral proliferation; inhibits protease in progeny virions → assembly of nonfunctional viruses	**AIDS (used in HAART)**	**GI irritation (nausea, diarrhea), hyperglycemia, hyperlipidemia, and lipodystrophy**	**All protease inhibitors end in -navir; metabolism occurs by cytochrome P450**
Sargramostim [Leukine]	Granulocyte-macrophage colony-stimulating factor	**Recovery of bone marrow (e.g., bone marrow transplant failure)**	Hypertension	
Sarin/soman	Irreversibly inhibits cholinesterase	Rapidly fatal	"Nerve gas"	

(continued)

APPENDIX I: Drug Index

Therapeutic Agent (common name, if relevant) [trade name, where appropriate]	Class—Pharmacology and Pharmacokinetics	Indications	Side Effects or Adverse Effects	Contraindications or Precautions to Consider; Notes
Saxagliptin [Onglyza]	**Hypoglycemic agent, DPP-IV inhibitor**—prevents degradation of incretin hormones → decreased glucagon, increased insulin	Oral treatment for **type 2 diabetes**	Diarrhea, constipation, edema	
Scopolamine	**Anticholinergic**—M_1-muscarinic receptor antagonist	**Motion sickness** prophylaxis	**Dry mouth**, drowsiness, and **vision disturbances**	**Delivered transdermally**
Scorpion toxin	Presynaptic neuromuscular junction blocker; overstimulates acetylcholine release			
Secobarbital [Seconal Sodium]	Antiepileptic—anesthetic agent; barbiturate; prolongs IPSP duration	Epilepsy, cerebral edema		
Selegiline [Eldepryl]	Antiparkinsonian—increases dopamine by inhibiting MAO, irreversibly	Parkinson disease		
Senna [Senokot]	**Stimulant laxative**; increases peristalsis	Constipation	Electrolyte imbalances (chronic use), melanosis coli	
Sertraline [Zoloft]	SSRIs—inhibit **reuptake** of 5-HT at neuronal synapses	Major depression, OCD, anorexia, bulimia, and anxiety	Inhibits liver enzymes, nausea, agitation, **sexual dysfunction** (anorgasmia), and dystonic reactions	Contraindicated with **MAOIs** secondary to **serotonin syndrome** (hyperthermia, muscle rigidity, and cardiovascular collapse); allows time for antidepressant effect, usually takes 2–3 weeks
Sevoflurane [Sevorane, Ultane]	Anesthetic agent	General anesthetic		
Sibutramine [Meridia]	**Sympathomimetic serotonin and NE reuptake inhibitor**	**Obesity** (short term and long term)	Hypertension, tachycardia	
Sildenafil [Viagra]	**Phosphodiesterase type 5 inhibitor (cGMP-specific)—increased cGMP** → smooth muscle relaxation → increased blood flow in the corpus cavernosum → penile erection	**Erectile dysfunction**	**Abnormal vision** (impaired bluegreen color vision), **UTIs, cardiovascular events, priapism, dyspepsia,** headache, and flushing	Risk of hypotension (fatal) in patient taking nitrates
Simvastatin [Zocor]	Lipid-lowering agent—HMG-CoA **reductase inhibitors**—inhibit synthesis of cholesterol precursor mevalonate; **decreases LDL, increases HDL, and decreases TG**	**High LDL, preventative after thrombotic event (e.g., MI, stroke)**	Reversible increase in LFTs; myositis	Contraindicated in pregnant and lactating women and children

Drug	Mechanism	Clinical use	Adverse effects	Notes
Sitagliptin [Januvia]	**Hypoglycemic agent, DPP-IV inhibitor**—prevents degradation of incretin hormones → decreased glucagon, increased insulin	Oral treatment for **type 2 diabetes**	Diarrhea, constipation, edema	
Sodium nitroprusside	Antianginal—direct release of NO → increases cGMP → vasodilator (arterial dilation)	**Hypertensive emergency, CHF, and angina**	Cyanide toxicity, hypotension	Short acting, given IV
Somatostatin [Zecnil]	Hormone—**decreases release of growth hormone, gastrin, secretin, VIP, CCK, glucagon, and insulin**	Acromegaly, glucagonoma, insulinoma	**Nausea, cramps, gallstones**	
Sotalol [Betapace]	Antiarrhythmic (class III)—K^+ channel blocker	Torsades de pointes		
Spectinomycin [Trobicin]	Aminoglycoside antibiotic—protein synthesis inhibitor; **irreversibly binds 30S ribosome** subunits; **bacteriostatic** at low concentration; **bactericidal** at high concentration	**Broad spectrum**: gram-negative rods; good for **bone and eye** infections; *Proteus, Pseudomonas, Enterobacter, Klebsiella,* and *Escherichia coli*	**Ototoxicity, renal toxicity, neuromuscular blockade,** nausea, vomiting, vertigo, allergic rash, superinfections	Used to treat gonorrhea in those allergic to penicillin
Spironolactone [Aldactone]	Potassium-sparing diuretic—binds to intracellular aldosterone steroid receptors in **collecting tubules;** blocks induction of Na^+ channels and Na^+/ATPase synthesis or blocks Na^+ channels directly (amiloride, triamterene); loss of Na^+, Cl^- in urine	Hyperaldosteronism, potassium depletion, and CHF	**Hyperkalemic metabolic acidosis, gynecomastia** (spironolactone), and antiandrogen effects	Results in decreased secretion of K^+ and H^+, which can lead to **hyperkalemic metabolic acidosis;** often given in combination with a thiazide
Streptokinase [Streptase]	**Thrombolytic—plasminogen activator**	**Lysis of clots**	**Hemorrhage**	
Streptomycin	Aminoglycoside antibiotic—protein synthesis inhibitor; **irreversibly binds 30S ribosome** subunits; **bacteriostatic** at low concentration; **bactericidal** at high concentration	**Broad spectrum**: gram-negative rods; good for **bone and eye** infections; *Proteus, Pseudomonas, Enterobacter, Klebsiella,* and *Escherichia coli;* **tuberculosis and other mycobacteria**	**Ototoxicity, renal toxicity, neuromuscular blockade, nausea,** vomiting, vertigo, allergic rash, superinfections	
Strychnine	Acts on the postsynaptic Renshaw cell; binds to glycine receptor (mimics effect of tetanus)	Depression	Fatal seizures	Rat poison
Succinylcholine [Anectine]	**Depolarizing neuromuscular blocker**	**Rapid-sequence intubation**	Increases intraocular pressure; succinylcholine apnea in genetically defective pseudocholinesterase; malignant hyperthermia if given with halothane	**Contraindicated in patients with glaucoma and patients taking antibiotics**

(continued)

Therapeutic Agent (common name, if relevant) [trade name, where appropriate]	Class—Pharmacology and Pharmacokinetics	Indications	Side Effects or Adverse Effects	Contraindications or Precautions to Consider; Notes
Sucralfate [Carafate]	Antiulcer—protective coating of GI lining	Reduces the effect of gastric acid on mucosa	Constipation	
Sulfamethoxazole, sulfisoxazole, sulfadiazine	**Antibiotic—sulfonamide, DNA synthesis inhibitor; competitive inhibitor of dihydropteroate synthetase (blocks folic acid synthesis);** bacteriostatic	**Broad spectrum: gram-positive UTI; chlamydial infection of genital tract and eye; treatment of nocardiosis**	**Forms crystals in kidney and bladder, causing damage; hypersensitivity reaction; pho-tosensitivity; kernicterus (in infants); hemolysis (in G6PD deficiency)**	Displaces other drugs such as warfarin from albumin
Sulfasalazine	**Anti-inflammatory—sulfapyridine (antibacterial) and mesalamine (anti-inflammatory)**	Ulcerative colitis, Crohn disease	Malaise, nausea, **sulfonamide toxicity,** and reversible **oligospermia**	**Activated by colonic bacteria**
Sulfinpyrazone [Anturane]	Antigout—increased secretion of uric acid (uricosuric)—competes with uric acid for **reabsorption in the kidney**	Chronic gout therapy	**Caution: should not be used in patients with sulfa allergies;** GI irritation; hypersensitivity reaction; agranulocytosis	Should not be used to treat acute gout or patients with uric acid stones
Sulindac [Clinoril]	Anti-inflammatory—prodrug sulfide	Chronic inflammation (arthritis)		
Sumatriptan [Imitrex]	**Antimigraine—agonist at 5-HT$_{1d}$ receptors**	**Acute attack of migraine**		
Tacrolimus (FK506) [Prograf]	**Immunosuppressant—blocks activation of T-cell transcription factors; involved in IL synthesis**	**Transplant rejection**	**Nephrotoxic; neurotoxic; hyper-glycemia; GI disturbances**	
Tamoxifen [Nolvadex]	**Selective estrogen receptor modulator—competitively binds estrogen receptors; breast (estrogen antagonist):** prevents proliferation of estrogen receptor positive tumor cells; **endometrium (partial agonist); bone (agonist):** decreases bone turnover, increases bone density	**Treats estrogen-dependent breast cancer in postmenopausal women;** reduces contralateral breast cancer; osteoporosis prevention	**May increase risk of endometrial cancer;** increased risk of blood clots; **hot flashes;** flushing	
Temazepam [Restoril]	Benzodiazepine—enhances GABA, increases IPSP amplitude	Sedative, hypnotic, antianxiety, antiepileptic		

Drug	Mechanism/Class	Clinical Use	Side Effects/Notes
Tenofovir disoproxil fumarate (TDF)	**Antiviral, nucleoside reverse transcriptase inhibitor—adenosine analog** → inhibits viral reverse transcriptase	**HAART**	**Nausea, vomiting, headache, renal dysfunction**
Terazosin [Hytrin]	Antihypertensive—α_1-blocker	Pheochromocytoma, hypertension, BPH	Postural hypotension
Terbinafine [Lamisil]	Antifungal—inhibits squalene-2,3-epoxidase	Orally for onychomycosis, topically for dermatophytes	Hepatotoxicity
Terbutaline [Brethine, Bricanyl, Brethaire]	**β_2-Agonist**—bronchodilator; relaxes uterus	**Bronchodilates to treat asthma; inhibits preterm labor;** treatment of uterine hyperstimulation	
Tetanus toxin	**Acts at the presynaptic Renshaw cell; prevents glycine release**		Seizures
Tetracaine [Pontocaine]	Anesthetic agent—blocks Na$^+$ channels intracellularly	Local anesthetic	Sleepiness, light-headedness, visual/audio disturbances, restlessness, nystagmus, shivering, tonic–clonic convulsions, death
Tetracycline [Achromycin, Sumycin, Topicycline]	**Tetracycline antibiotic—protein synthesis inhibitor; binds 30S ribosome subunits** → prevents attachment of tRNA; bacteriostatic	**Broad-spectrum including atypical pathogens: *Chlamydia, Rickettsia, M. pneumoniae, V. cholerae, U. urealyticum, Francisella tularensis, H. pylori,* and *B. burgdorferi*** (Lyme disease)	**Liver toxicity, GI distress, depression of bone/teeth development, photosensitivity, Fanconi syndrome**	**Contraindicated in pregnancy and children; divalent cations inhibit gut absorption, therefore cannot take with milk, antacids, or iron-containing preparations; renally eliminated**
THC (active ingredient in marijuana)	Unknown mechanism; binds cannabinoid receptors and inhibits vomiting center in medulla	Antiemetic	Dry mouth, dizziness, inability to concentrate, disorientation, anxiety, tachycardia, depression, paranoia, psychosis
Theophylline [Aerolate, Elixophyllin, Respbid, Slo-bid, Slo-Phyllin, Theo-24, Theo-Dur, Theolair, Uniphyl]	Methylxanthines—unknown mechanism; postulated to inhibit phosphodiesterase → decreases cAMP hydrolysis → promotes bronchodilation; stimulates CNS, cardiac muscle; relaxes smooth muscle; produces diuresis; increases cerebral vascular resistance	Asthma	Cardiotoxicity, neurotoxicity	Metabolized by cytochrome P450; narrow therapeutic window; tolerance develops
Thiabendazole [Mintezol]	**Anthelmintic**	***Strongyloides, Ancylostoma*** (hookworm), ***Enterobius*** (pinworm), ***Trichuris*** (whipworm)	Vomiting, diarrhea, dizziness, bradycardia, hypotension, paresthesia, yellow vision, angioneurotic edema, perianal rashes

(continued)

APPENDIX I: Drug Index

Therapeutic Agent (common name, if relevant) [trade name, where appropriate]	Class—Pharmacology and Pharmacokinetics	Indications	Side Effects or Adverse Effects	Contraindications or Precautions to Consider; Notes
6-Thioguanine	Antineoplastic—inhibits purine synthesis; disrupts DNA and RNA synthesis	Adult leukemias	Bone marrow suppression	
Thiopental [Pentothal]	Anesthetic agent—barbiturate; prolongs IPSP duration	Antiepileptic, cerebral edema, anesthetic (stage 3 anesthetic)	Laryngospasm during stage 3 induction	
Thioridazine [Mellaril]	Antipsychotic—phenothiazines; muscarinic, blocks D_2 and α_1 receptors	Psychosis	**Extrapyramidal** (dystonia, akinesia, akathisia, and tardive dyskinesia), **anticholinergic** (dry mouth, constipation), **alpha blockade** (hypotension), and **histamine** (sedation); toxicity results in neuroleptic malignant syndrome (rigidity, myoglobinuria, autonomic instability, and hyperpyrexia)	**Cardiac toxicity (prolongs QT interval); atropine-like effects** are very common; antimuscarinic effects exacerbate tardive dyskinesia; visual impairment has been reported
Thiotepa [Thioplex]	Antineoplastic—unknown mechanism	Cancer		
Thiothixene [Navane]	Antipsychotic—thioxanthene; blocks D_2, α_1, and H_1 receptors	Psychosis	Anticholinergic effects	
Thrombopoietin	Recombinant human thrombopoietin	**Thrombocytopenia**		
Ticarcillin [Ticar], **ticarcillin-clavulanate** [Timentin]	**Antibiotic—β-lactam, penicillin derivative,** cell wall inhibitor; same mechanism as penicillin; distinguished by activity against *Pseudomonas*, bactericidal	**Extended spectrum—***Pseudomonas*, *Proteus*, and *Enterobacter* spp.	**Hypersensitivity reactions,** decreased platelet function	Not effective against penicillin-resistant *Staphylococcus*, can be **combined with clavulanic acid** (β-lactamase inhibitor) to enhance spectrum; administered IV
Ticlopidine [Ticlid]	**Inhibits ADP-induced platelet aggregation;** acts on ADP receptor	**Transient ischemic attack, stroke**		
Timolol [Betimol, Blocadren, Timoptic]	Antiglaucoma—antihypertensive; β-blocker	Hypertension, MI, glaucoma	Asthma, bradycardia	
Tizanidine [Zanaflex]	Centrally acting muscle relaxant—presynaptic inhibition of motor neurons; acts like clonidine on α_2 receptor	Muscle spasms from spinal cord injury; multiple sclerosis		
Tocainide [Tonocard]	Antiarrhythmic (class IB)—Na^+ channel blocker			

Drug	Mechanism	Indication	Side Effects / Notes
Tolbutamide [Orinase]	**Hypoglycemic agent, first-generation sulfonylurea**—closes potassium channels located in β-cell membrane → reduces K⁺ efflux, increases Ca²⁺ influx → increases secretion of insulin	Oral treatment for **type 2 diabetes**	Rarely used due to toxicity
Tolnaftate [Tinactin, Desenex]	Antifungal—unknown mechanism; bactericidal	Topical against *Trichophyton rubrum*, *Trichophyton tonsurans*, and *Trichophyton mentagrophytes*	
Topiramate [Topamax]	Antiepileptic—blocks Na⁺ channels	Add-on drug for epilepsy	
Torsemide [Demadex]	Loop diuretic; inhibits Na⁺/K⁺/Cl⁻ channels	Diuresis	Ototoxicity, metabolic alkalosis, hypokalemia, hyperglycemia, hyperuricemia
tPA (alteplase) [Activase]	**Thrombolytic—plasminogen activator**	**Lysis of clots**	**Hemorrhage**
Tramadol [Ultram]	Analgesic—similar to opioid agonist	Chronic pain of osteoarthritis	Nausea, vomiting, constipation, and drowsiness
Tranexamic acid (AMCHA) [Cyklokapron]	Thrombotic agent—competitive inhibitor of plasminogen activation	Inhibits fibrinolysis; promotes thrombosis	
Tranylcypromine [Parnate]	Antidepressant—MAOI; inhibits degradation of NE and 5-HT at neuronal synapses; nonselective, but isoenzyme A most important; reversible	**Atypical depression** (with hypersomnia, anxiety, sensitivity to rejection, and hypochondriasis)	**Hypertensive episodes** with ingestion of tyramine-containing foods or β-agonists, hyperthermia, and convulsions Contraindicated with **SSRIs** and **meperidine** secondary to **serotonin syndrome** (hyperthermia, muscle rigidity, and cardiovascular collapse); only reversible MAOI
Trazodone [Desyrel]	Atypical antidepressant—inhibits reuptake of serotonin	Major depression (especially with insomnia), insomnia	Sedation, nausea, **priapism**, and postural hypotension
Tretinoin [Retin-A]	Retinoids—inhibits microcomedo formation and existing lesions; makes keratinocytes in sebaceous follicles less adherent and easier to remove	Acne, skin cancer	Photosensitivity
TRH (protirelin) [Relefact TRH]	Stimulates TSH and prolactin release	Diagnosis of thyroid disease	
Triamcinolone	**Glucocorticoid**—inhibits protein synthesis; reduces lymph node and spleen size; inhibits cell cycle activity of lymphoid cells; lyses T cells; suppresses antibody, prostaglandin, and leukotriene synthesis; blocks monocyte production of IL-1	Addison disease, rheumatic arthritis, autoimmune disorders, allergic reaction, asthma, organ transplantation (especially during rejection crisis)	**Osteoporosis, cushingoid reaction, psychosis, glucose intolerance, infection, hypertension, cataracts, peptic ulcers**

(continued)

Therapeutic Agent (common name, if relevant) [trade name, where appropriate]	Class—Pharmacology and Pharmacokinetics	Indications	Side Effects or Adverse Effects	Contraindications or Precautions to Consider; Notes
Triamterene [Dyrenium]	Potassium-sparing diuretic—binds to intracellular aldosterone steroid receptors in **collecting tubules**; blocks induction of Na^+ channels and Na^+/ATPase synthesis and blocks Na channels directly; loss of Na^+, Cl^- in urine	Hyperaldosteronism, potassium depletion, and CHF	**Hyperkalemic metabolic acidosis, gynecomastia** (spironolactone), and antiandrogen effects	Results in decreased secretion of K^+ and H^+, which can lead to **hyperkalemic metabolic acidosis**; often given in combination with a thiazide
Triazolam [Halcion]	Benzodiazepine—enhances GABA; increases IPSP amplitude	Sedative, hypnotic, antianxiety	Paranoia, violent behavior, antiepileptic	
Trientine	Metal chelator	Copper poisoning, Wilson disease		
Trifluridine ophthalmic [Viroptic]	Antiviral—thymidine derivative; inhibits DNA polymerase; inhibits DNA synthesis	DNA viruses		
Trihexphenidyl [Artane]	Antiparkinsonian—muscarinic blocker	Parkinson disease		
Triiodothyronine (T_3) [Triostat]	Synthetic analog of thyroid hormone T_3	**Hypothyroidism**	Tachycardia, heat intolerance, tremors, and arrhythmia	
Trimethaphan [Arfonad]	Antihypertensive—nondepolarizing nicotinic blocker	Hypertension (short term)		
Trimethoprim [Proloprim, Trimpex]	**Antibiotic—DNA synthesis inhibitor; competitive inhibition of dihydrofolate reductase** (blocks folic acid synthesis); bacteriostatic	**Gram-negative UTI; combined with sulfonamides to treat UTI, otitis media, chronic bronchitis, shigellosis, *Salmonella*, and PCP**	Megaloblastic anemia, leukopenia, and granulocytopenia	Supplementation with folic acid may help pancytopenia
TSH (thyrotropin) [Thyrogen]	**Increases output of thyroid hormone**	**Assesses thyroid function; increases uptake of I-131 in thyroid carcinoma**		
d-Tubocurarine [Tubarine]	**Nondepolarizing neuromuscular blocker**	Topical for dermatophytes (especially tinea pedis)	Paralysis	
Undecylenic acid [Desenex]	Antifungal—unknown mechanism; fungistatic			
Urofollitropin [Metrodin]	FSH analog	Infertility		
Urokinase [Abbokinase]	**Thrombolytic agent—plasminogen activator**	**Lysis of clots**	**Hemorrhage**	

Drug	Mechanism/Class	Clinical Use	Side Effects	Notes
Valacyclovir [Valtrex]	**Antiviral—guanosine analog;** inhibits DNA polymerase	**HSV, VZV, EBV, and CMV at high doses**	**GI disturbances, CNS and renal problems, headache, tremor, rash**	**Longer lasting than acyclovir**
Valproic acid [Depakene]	**Antiepileptic—blocks Na⁺ channels and increases GABA**	**Epilepsy: partial, absence, and tonic–clonic**	Liver toxicity, pancreatitis; potentially fatal	
Valsartan [Diovan]	**Antihypertensive**—Ang II receptor blockers → prevents vasoconstriction from Ang II	**Hypertension**	Fetal renal toxicity, **hyperkalemia**	
Vancomycin [Vancocin]	**Antibiotic—cell wall inhibitor,** binds to D-alanyl-D-alanine portion of cell wall → inhibits cell wall glycopeptide polymerization → stops bacterial cell wall synthesis; usually bactericidal	**Serious infections by gram-positive bacteria:** _**Streptococcus, Staphylococcus,**_ **and some anaerobes (especially** _**C. difficile**_**)**	**Ototoxicity, nephrotoxicity, thrombophlebitis, and diffuse flushing—"red man syndrome" caused by histamine release**	Can prevent red man syndrome by pretreatment with antihistamines and slow infusion; resistance occurs when bacteria change amino acid in cell wall to D-alanyl-D-lactate
Vardenafil	**Phosphodiesterase type 5 inhibitor (cGMP-specific)**—increased cGMP → smooth muscle relaxation → increased blood flow in the corpus cavernosum → penile erection	**Erectile dysfunction**	**Abnormal vision** (impaired blue-green color vision), **UTIs, cardiovascular events, priapism, dyspepsia,** headache, and flushing	Risk of hypotension (fatal) in patient taking nitrates
Vasopressin [Pitressin]	**Antidiuretic—recruits water channels to luminal membrane in collecting duct**	**Antidiuresis; treats central diabetes insipidus**	**Overhydration; allergic reaction; larger doses: pallor, diarrhea, and hypertension; coronary constriction; chronic rhinopharyngitis**	**Also known as antidiuretic hormone**
Vecuronium [Norcuron]	Nondepolarizing neuromuscular blocker			
Venlafaxine [Effexor]	**Antidepressant, anti-anxiolytic—serotonin and NE reuptake inhibitor**	**Depression, generalized anxiety disorder, social phobia**	Sweating, **nausea, constipation,** anorexia, somnolence, dry mouth, dizziness, **insomnia, and hypertension;** nervousness, abnormal dreams, tremor, abnormal vision, impotence, and anorgasmia	
Verapamil [Calan, Isoptin]	**Non-dihydropyridine Ca²⁺ channel blockers**—block voltage-gated Ca²⁺ channels of **cardiac** smooth muscle	**Hypertension, angina pectoris, arrhythmia**	Cardiac depression, peripheral edema, **flushing, dizziness,** and constipation	
Vidarabine [Vira-A]	Antiviral—adenosine analog; inhibits DNA polymerase	Herpes (also topical for HSV keratitis); varicella	GI disturbances; CNS, bone marrow suppression; liver and kidney dysfunction	
Vinblastine [Velban]	**Antineoplastic—blocks polymerization of microtubules**	**Hodgkin disease**	Peripheral neuritis	

(continued)

Therapeutic Agent (common name, if relevant) [trade name, where appropriate]	Class—Pharmacology and Pharmacokinetics	Indications	Side Effects or Adverse Effects	Contraindications or Precautions to Consider; Notes
Vincristine [Oncovin]	**Antineoplastic—blocks polymerization of microtubules**	**Acute leukemia**	**Peripheral neuritis**	
Vitamin A (retinol) [Aquasol A]	Vitamin	Night blindness, xerophthalmia	Hyperkeratosis	
Vitamin B$_1$ (thiamine)	**Vitamin**	**Alcoholics (prophylaxis for Wernicke–Korsakoff syndrome)**		**Decrease results in beriberi**
Vitamin B$_2$ (riboflavin)	Vitamin—component of flavin compounds: FMN, FAD			Inhibits chlorpromazine; decreased results in skin, oral, and ocular lesions
Vitamin B$_3$ (nicotinic acid, niacin)	Vitamin—component of nicotinic compounds: NAD, NADH	Maintains integrity of skin, decreases VLDL and LDL, increases HDL	Flushing, pruritus, myopathy, hepatotoxicity	Decrease results in dermatitis, diarrhea, dementia, and death
Vitamin B$_5$ (pantothenic acid)	Vitamin—component of CoA			
Vitamin B$_6$ (pyridoxine)	Vitamin	Protein metabolism, neurotransmitter synthesis	Neuritis, convulsions	Isoniazid decreases amount
Vitamin B$_{12}$ [Cyanocobalamin]	**Vitamin**	**Megaloblastic anemia**		
Vitamin C (ascorbic acid)	Vitamin	Maintains collagen; oxidation-reduction reactions		Decrease results in scurvy
Vitamin D (calcitriol) [Rocaltrol]	**Vitamin—binds to receptors in cytoplasm; alters gene expression and protein synthesis; increases bone resorption of Ca^{2+}; increases renal and intestinal absorption of Ca^{2+} and phosphate**	**Rickets, osteomalacia, hypocalcemia, hypoparathyroidism, osteoporosis**		
Vitamin E	**Vitamin—antioxidant**	**Possible prophylaxis for heart disease**		**Decrease results in abortion, creatinuria, and ceroid pigment**
Vitamin K (phytonadione) [Mephyton]	**Vitamin—enhances clotting factors**	**Bleeding disorders**		**Decreased in children of mothers taking phenytoin or phenobarbital**
Voriconazole [Vfend]	**Antifungal—inhibits ergosterol synthesis,** preventing cell membrane formation	Serious invasive fungal infections (**invasive aspergillosis,** invasive candidiasis)	**Vision disturbances (blurred vision, light sensitivity),** GI disturbances, hepatotoxicity	

Drug	Mechanism	Clinical use	Toxicity	Notes
Warfarin [Coumadin]	Anticoagulant—inhibits potassium epoxide regeneration	Thrombosis	Bleeding	Contraindicated in pregnancy, patients with liver, CNS, and hemostatic disease; 99% exists protein bound; extremely sensitive to cytochrome P450 system
Yohimbine	Impotence therapy—α_2 antagonist			
Zafirlukast [Accolate], montelukast [Singulair]	Antiasthma agent—antileukotriene; blocks leukotriene receptors (leukotriene D_4 [LTD_4]) → prevents bronchoconstriction and inflammatory cell infiltrate	Asthma (especially aspirin-induced asthma)		
Zanamivir [Relenza]	Antiviral—inhibits neuraminidase → decreases release of progeny viruses	Influenza A and B treatment and prophylaxis		Begin within 2 days of onset of flu symptoms to decrease the duration and intensity of symptoms
Zidovudine (ZDV; formerly azidothymidine [AZT]) [Retrovir]	Antiviral, nucleoside reverse transcriptase inhibitor—inhibits viral reverse transcriptase → prevents integration of DNA copy of viral genome into the host DNA	AIDS (used in HAART); pregnant women with HIV to reduce fetal transmission	Neutropenia, anemia (megaloblastic anemia), peripheral neuropathy, pancreatitis, and lactic acidosis	
Zileuton	Antiasthma agent-5-lipoxygenase inhibitor → inhibits conversion of arachidonic acid to leukotriene → prevents bronchoconstriction and inflammatory cell infiltrate	Improves asthma		
Zolpidem [Ambien]	Binds to benzodiazepine receptor but is not a benzodiazepine	Insomnia		

APPENDIX I: Drug Index

5-HT, 5-hydroxytryptamine (serotonin); ACE, angiotensin-converting enzyme; ACTH, adrenocorticotropic hormone; ADP, adenosine diphosphate; AMCHA, 4-(aminomethyl) cyclohexane carboxylic acid; AML, acute myelocytic leukemia; APSAC, anisoylated plasminogen streptokinase activator complex; AST/ALT, aspartate aminotransferase/alanine aminotransferase; ATPase, adenosine triphosphatase; AV, atrioventricular; BAL, blood alcohol level; BBB, blood–brain barrier; BCNU, bischloroethylnitrosourea; BP, blood pressure; BPH, benign prostatic hypertrophy; cAMP, cyclic adenosine monophosphate; CCK, cholecystokinin; CCR5, C-C chemokine receptor 5; cGMP, cyclic guanosine monophosphate; CHF, congestive heart failure; CMI, cell-mediated immunity; CMV, cytomegalovirus; CNS, central nervous system; CoA, coenzyme A; COPD, chronic obstructive pulmonary disease; COX, cyclooxygenase; DAG, diacylglycerol; DCT, distal convoluted tubule; dCTP, deoxycytidine triphosphate; DHEA, dehydroepiandrosterone; DPP-IV, dipeptidyl peptidase-IV; EBV, Epstein–Barr virus; ECG, electrocardiogram; electrocardiography; ECL, enterochromaffin-like; EtOH, ethanol; FAD, flavin adenine dinucleotide; FMN, flavin mononucleotide; FSH, follicle-stimulating hormone; G6PD, glucose-6-phosphate dehydrogenase; GABA, γ-aminobutyric acid; GI, gastrointestinal; GLP-1, glucagon-like peptide-1; GnRH, gonadotropin-releasing hormone; HAART, highly active antiretroviral therapy; HDL, high-density lipoprotein; HLA, human leukocyte antigen; HMG-CoA, 3-hydroxy-3-methylglutaryl coenzyme A; HSV, herpes simplex virus; IFN, interferon; IL, interleukin; IMP, inosine 5′ monophosphate; IP_3, inositol triphosphate; IPSP, inhibitory postsynaptic potential; IV, intravenous; LDL, low-density lipoprotein; L-dopa, levodopa (levo-3, 4-dihydroxyphenylalanine); LFT, liver function test; LH, luteinizing hormone; MAO, monoamine oxidase; MAOI, monoamine oxidase inhibitor; MI, myocardial infarction; MOA, mechanism of action; MRSA, methicillin-resistant *Staphylococcus aureus*; MSIR, morphine sulfate instant release; MSSA, methicillin-sensitive *Staphylococcus aureus*; NAD, nicotinamide adenine dinucleotide; NADH, reduced nicotinamide adenine dinucleotide; NE, norepinephrine; NMDA, *N*-methyl-D-aspartate; NO, nitric oxide; NPH, neutral protamine Hagedorn; NSAID, nonsteroidal anti-inflammatory drug; OCD, obsessive-compulsive disorder; PCOS, polycystic ovary syndrome; PCP, *Pneumocystis carinii* pneumonia; PCT, proximal convoluted tubule; PDA, patent ductus arteriosus; PGE_1, prostaglandin E_1; PGE_2, prostaglandin E_2; $PGF_{2\alpha}$, prostaglandin $F_{2\alpha}$; PMN, polymorphonuclear; PPAR-γ, peroxisome proliferator-activated receptor-γ; PTH, parathyroid hormone; PTT, partial thromboplastin time; PVC, premature ventricular contraction; Rh, rhesus [factor]; SA, sinoatrial; SLE, systemic lupus erythematosus; SSRI, selective serotonin reuptake inhibitor; TCA, tricyclic antidepressant; TG, triglycerides; THC, tetrahydrocannabinol; TNF, tumor necrosis factor; tPA, tissue plasminogen activator; TRH, thyrotropin-releasing hormone; TSH, thyrotropin-stimulating hormone; tRNA, transfer RNA; TSH, thyroid-stimulating hormone; UTI, urinary tract infection; VIP, vasoactive intestinal peptide; VLDL, very low-density lipoprotein; VZV, varicella-zoster virus; WBC, white blood cell.

APPENDIX II: **Bug Index**

BACTERIA

Name	Morphology	Pathogenesis	Description of Disease	Laboratory Findings, Notes	Transmission	Prevention and Therapy
Actinomyces israelii	Gram-positive; filamentous; anaerobic	Unknown	Actinomycosis—oral, thoracic, pelvic, or peritoneal abscesses with draining sinus tracts	Forms filaments; sulfur granules	Dental disease or trauma	Penicillin and drainage
Bacillus anthracis	Gram-positive; rod with square ends; capsule of D-glutamate (only protein capsule); non-motile; spore former; aerobic	Anthrax toxin—edema factor (exotoxin); protective antigen for cell entry; lethal factor (zinc MP increases TNF)	Anthrax—three clinical syndromes: cutaneous (black eschar), inhalational (respiratory symptoms and widened mediastinum), and GI (abdominal pain)	Medusa head colonies; catalase positive	Spores from animals (usually cattle)	Attenuated strain human vaccine; penicillin; ciprofloxacin; doxycycline
Bacillus cereus	Gram-positive; rod; spore former; aerobic	Spores germinate when rice is reheated; enterotoxins—emetic toxin (heat stable), diarrhea toxin (heat labile)	Food poisoning—early vomiting and late diarrhea		Enters through the GI tract via reheated rice	Avoid reheated rice and beans; treatment is symptomatic; cephalosporin
Bacteroides fragilis	Gram-negative; bacilli; anaerobic; capsulated; no exotoxin	Capsule; weak endotoxin	Infections below diaphragm; peritonitis; bacteremia; pelvic inflammatory disease; foul-smelling abscess; sepsis	Mixed infections; pleomorphic	Deep penetrating wounds; wound debridement	Metronidazole, clindamycin
Bordetella pertussis	Gram-negative; coccobacilli; capsule	Noninvasive infection of bronchial epithelium; pertussis toxin (two subunits)—A sub-unit ADP ribosylates adenylate cyclase, increasing cAMP, whereas B subunit causes attachment; tracheal cytotoxin destroys ciliated epithelial cells, resulting in cough	Whooping cough; three stages of disease: catarrhal, paroxysmal coughing, and convalescent	Culture nasopharynx onto 10%–15% blood agar (Bordet-Gengou agar); slide agglutination test	Droplet nuclei	Acellular pertussis vaccine (at 2, 4, and 6 months) or whole inactive cells; erythromycin (use in catarrhal stage or prophylaxis for sick contacts); treatment in paroxysmal coughing stage is supportive
Borrelia burgdorferi	Spirochete; microaero-philic; flagella	Invasion and replication in the bloodstream; immune response to organism results in pathology	Lyme disease—erythema chronicum migrans with involvement of the heart, joints, and CNS	Common in the northeastern, midwestern, and western United States	Deer ticks; serology	Avoid ticks; wear long pants in wooded areas; doxycycline and penicillin

Organism	Characteristics	Mechanism	Presentation	Diagnosis	Transmission	Treatment
Brucella spp.	Gram-negative; coccobacillus; facultative; intracellular	Catalase; LPS; inhibits release of peroxidase in macrophages	Undulant fever—macrophages engulf and then rerelease into the bloodstream; granulomas; drenching night sweats	Serology	Contaminated milk and cheese; droplets; contact with infected animals	Pasteurization of dairy products; tetracycline plus streptomycin
Campylobacter jejuni	Gram-negative; comma-shaped bacilli; motile	Enterotoxin with antigenic diversity stimulates cAMP; incubation 2–6 days	Gastroenteritis—greenish, watery, foul-smelling diarrhea followed by bloody stools with fever	Microaerophilic; Campy plate; diarrhea in college students; oxidase positive	Milk, water, poultry	Symptomatic; self-limiting
Chlamydia trachomatis	Obligate intracellular	Replicates within host lysosomes, using host's cellular machinery	Strains A–C: blindness; strains D–K: nongonococcal urethritis, cervicitis; strains L1–L3: lymphogranuloma venereum	Leading cause of preventable blindness in the world; inactive form extracellular (elementary body) and metabolically active form intracellular (reticulate body)	Sexual contact or via birth canal	Tetracycline, azithromycin
Chlamydophila pneumoniae	Obligate intracellular	Replicates within host lysosomes, using host's cellular machinery	Pneumonia, bronchitis, and pharyngitis; rarely, Guillain–Barré syndrome, arthritis, and meningoencephalitis	Cell culture or other advanced lab testing required to make a definitive diagnosis; treatment is usually empiric	Person-to-person	Macrolides (azithromycin, clarithromycin), doxycycline
Chlamydophila psittaci	Obligate intracellular	Replicates within host lysosomes, using host's cellular machinery	Psittacosis—dry cough with CNS symptoms (photophobia and headache)	Giemsa stain; inactive form extracellular (elementary body) and metabolically active form intracellular (reticulate body)	Aerosol of dried bird feces	Tetracycline, quinolones, azithromycin
Clostridium botulinum	Gram-positive; rod; spore former; anaerobic	Botulinum toxin inhibits release of acetylcholine at neuromuscular junction resulting in flaccid paralysis; exotoxins A, B, and E	Botulism (weakness and respiratory paralysis); food, wound, and infant types; floppy baby syndrome; dysphagia; constipation	Toxin in blood	Spores from contaminated food/canned foods	Trivalent antitoxin; sterilization of canned foods; cook to inactivate toxin; respiratory support
Clostridium difficile	Gram-positive; rod; spore former; anaerobic	Exotoxins A and B—A (cholera-like) causes fluid release and hemorrhagic necrosis; B (diphtheria-like) damages mucosa and causes pseudomembrane formation	Antibiotic-associated pseudomembranous colitis; bloody diarrhea	ELISA detects toxin B in the stool sample	Hospital workers	Withdraw causative antibiotics (classically clindamycin); oral metronidazole, oral vancomycin

(continued)

BACTERIA *(Continued)*

Name	Morphology	Pathogenesis	Description of Disease	Laboratory Findings, Notes	Transmission	Prevention and Therapy
Clostridium perfringens	Gram-positive; rod; spore former, anaerobic	α-Toxin (damages cell membranes); γ-toxin (tissue necrosis and hemolysis); cholera-like heat-labile enterotoxin (food poisoning—watery diarrhea); spores establish in GI and produce enterotoxins	Gas gangrene; food poisoning; anaerobic cellulites	Large rods found in food; double zone of hemolysis	Grows in traumatized tissue (muscle); spores in food and soil germinate in reheated foods (stews, soups)	Clean and debride wounds; cook food well
Clostridium tetani	Gram-positive; rod; spore former (tennis racquet shaped); anaerobic	Tetanus toxin (exotoxin)—blocks release of inhibitory neurotransmitters	Tetanus: lockjaw (trismus), spastic paralysis (opisthotonos), and sardonic grin (risus sardonicus)	Usually not recovered by culture	Spore entry via wound (e.g., a rusty nail)	Toxoid vaccine (2, 4, 6, and 18 months); booster every 10 years; tetanus Ig (passive immunity); penicillin
Corynebacterium diphtheriae	Gram-positive; rod; club shaped; arranged in V or L form; not spore former	Exotoxin—A subunit ADP ribosylates EF-2, and B subunit binds toxin to the cell; phage conversion	Diphtheria—pseudomembrane forms in the throat; bull neck; systemic toxemia	Tellurite plate (Loffler's medium) grows black colonies	Airborne droplets	Inactivated toxoid vaccine; antitoxin (neutralizes unbound toxin); penicillin; erythromycin
Coxiella burnetii	Obligate intracellular	Unknown	Q fever	Only rickettsia not transmitted to humans by an arthropod vector; occupational hazard for tanners, sheep shearers, and dairy farmers	Inhalation of aerosols of urine and feces; transplacental	Tetracycline
Enterococcus faecalis	Gram-positive; cocci	Lipoteichoic acid	Urinary, biliary, and cardiovascular infections; endocarditis	Catalase negative; bacitracin resistant; variable hemolysis; grows in 6.5% NaCl/Lancefield group D	Normal flora of gut gaining access to blood	Penicillin or ampicillin and an aminoglycoside
Escherichia coli	Gram-negative; bacilli	Endotoxin—septic shock; heat-labile enterotoxin (LT): increased cAMP leads to diarrhea; heat-stable enterotoxin (ST) stimulates guanylate cyclase to cause diarrhea; pili: adhere to epithelium especially in UTIs; verotoxin (O157:H7): Shigella-like toxin in enterohemorrhagic *E. coli* (EHEC) that inhibits 28S rRNA to cause bloody diarrhea	UTI; sepsis; neonatal meningitis; enteropathogenic *E. coli* (EPEC): traveler's diarrhea; enterotoxigenic *E. coli* (ETEC): watery diarrhea; enteroinvasive *E. coli* (EIEC): dysentery; EHEC: bloody diarrhea, hemolytic uremic syndrome	Oxidase—cysteine agar	Transplacental; fecal–oral route; foodborne	UTIs: trimethoprim-sulfamethoxazole, ciprofloxacin; sepsis: cephalosporins; traveler's diarrhea: rehydration

Organism	Morphology	Pathogenesis	Disease	Diagnosis	Transmission	Treatment
Francisella tularensis	Gram-negative; rod; intracellular	Capsule; intracellular within macrophages; granuloma formation	Painful lymph nodes; glandular and ocular ulcers	Serology	Zoonotic via rabbits and ticks	Live attenuated vaccine; streptomycin; thorough cooking of meat
Gardnerella vaginalis	Gram variable; bacillus; anaerobic	Unknown	Vaginosis—watery discharge, fishy odor	Clue cells (epithelial cells coated with bacteria; whiff test		Metronidazole
Haemophilus ducreyi	Gram-negative; bacilli	Virulence via pili	Chancroid with pain and purulent exudate	Lesions similar to those of syphilis; lymphadenopathy	Sexually transmitted	Azithromycin, ceftriaxone
Haemophilus influenzae	Gram-negative; coccobacilli; polysaccharide capsule (polyribitol phosphate)	IgA protease degrades antibody and attaches to respiratory tract; capsule (type B) prevents phagocytosis	Infantile meningitis; epiglottitis; number 2 cause of otitis media and sinusitis	Needs heme (factor X) and NAD (factor V) to grow; chocolate agar; check CSF	Respiratory droplets	Hib vaccine (β-type capsule conjugated to diphtheria toxoid as a carrier protein); ceftriaxone
Helicobacter pylori	Gram-negative; bacilli; motile; flagella	Urease results in ammonia production and subsequent gastric damage	Peptic ulcers (type B gastritis)	Microaerophilic; Campy plate; urea breath test; urease positive; serology ELISA; biopsy	Ingestion	Triple therapy: amoxicillin, omeprazole, and clarithromycin; quadruple therapy: bismuth, tetracycline, metronidazole, and omeprazole
Klebsiella pneumoniae	Gram-negative; bacilli; capsule; positive quellung reaction	Large capsule hinders phagocytosis	Pneumonia, particularly in malnourished alcoholics; UTI; bacteremia	Currant jelly sputum (thick bloody sputum)	Aspiration of respiratory droplets	Cephalosporins
Legionella pneumophila	Gram-negative; bacilli	Endotoxin affects smokers, alcoholics, and those older than 55 years of age	Legionnaire disease (atypical pneumonia)	Dieterle silver stain; cysteine required for culture; urine test for Legionella antigen	Aerosol from environmental water sources and contaminated air conditioning system	Erythromycin, quinolones
Listeria monocytogenes	Gram-positive; rod; arranged in V or L form; tumbling motility; not spore former	Grows intracellularly in macrophages; listeriolysin-O cytotoxic	Meningitis and sepsis in newborns and immunocompromised individuals	Small, gray colonies; β-hemolysis; motility; serology	Transferred to humans by animals or their feces; unpasteurized milk; contaminated vegetables, cheese, and cabbage	Ampicillin and gentamicin; trimethoprim-sulfamethoxazole
Moraxella catarrhalis	Gram-negative; diplococcus		Upper respiratory tract infection; number 3 cause of otitis media and sinusitis		Transmitted by respiratory secretions	Azithromycin; penicillin resistant (100% strains make β-lactamase)

(continued)

BACTERIA *(Continued)*

Name	Morphology	Pathogenesis	Description of Disease	Laboratory Findings, Notes	Transmission	Prevention and Therapy
Mycobacterium avium-intracellulare (MAC)	Acid-fast bacilli	Unknown	TB-like disease in immunocompromised individuals		From the soil and water to immunocompromised individuals	Azithromycin plus ethambutol plus rifampin
Mycobacterium leprae	Acid-fast bacilli; obligate intracellular	Tuberculoid: cell-mediated response causes damage; lepromatous: anergy of CD8 cells leads to uncontrolled replication	Leprosy—tuberculoid and lepromatous; lesions in cool parts of body	Cannot be grown in culture but is harvested in the footpads of armadillos; acid-fast stain of infected areas; lepra cells (modified mononuclear epithelioid cells containing acid-fast bacilli)	Prolonged contact, especially with the lepromatous form	Dapsone and rifampin for tuberculoid form (6-month treatment); clofazimine, dapsone, and rifampin for lepromatous form (2-year treatment)
Mycobacterium tuberculosis	Acid-fast bacilli; aerobic; high lipid cell walls (mycotic acids and wax D)	Cord factor; granulomas and caseation	Primary TB (chronic pneumonia), secondary TB (reactivation, hemoptysis), miliary TB (disseminated), latent TB	Ziehl-Neelsen stain; slow-growing (3–8 weeks) on Lowenstein-Jensen medium; niacin positive; PPD positive if >10 cm after 48 h	Droplets from coughing	BCG vaccine with live attenuated organisms (rarely used in the United States); isoniazid, rifampin, ethambutol, pyrazinamide initially, then isoniazid plus rifampin to complete 6–9 months of therapy
Mycoplasma pneumoniae	Obligate intracellular; not seen on a Gram stain; smallest free-living organism; only bacteria with cholesterol in membrane (no cell wall)	Hydrogen peroxide and lytic enzymes resulting in damage to the respiratory tract	Walking pneumonia; bullous myringitis (inflamed tympanic membrane); common in young adults (college)	Positive cold agglutinin; highest incidence in 5- to 15-year-olds	Respiratory droplets	Erythromycin
Neisseria gonorrhoeae (gonococcus)	Gram-negative; cocci; coffee bean–shaped pairs; no polysaccharide capsule	Endotoxin (lipid A); pili with variation; proteins I, II, III (porin, adhesin, autoagglutination); IgA protease penicillinase plasmid	Urethral and vaginal infections; discharge; salpingitis and PID; neonatal conjunctivitis; septic arthritis	Thayer-Martin agar; only glucose fermentation; oxidase positive; also check for chlamydia caused by common coinfection	Sexual contact; newborns; symptomatic in men but not usually in women	Condoms; erythromycin or silver nitrate in neonates; ceftriaxone; spectinomycin and tetracycline
Neisseria meningitidis (meningococcus)	Gram-negative; diplococci; coffee bean–shaped pairs; polysaccharide capsule (antiphagocytic)	Endotoxin (LPS) contains lipid A; capsule; IgA protease; pili variation; deficiencies in late-acting complement components; asplenic patients	Meningitis; petechial rash; pharyngitis; Waterhouse–Friderichsen syndrome	Glucose and maltose fermentation; oxidase positive; lumbar puncture with high protein and low glucose; grows on Thayer-Martin agar	Respiratory droplets	Vaccine, rifampin, or ciprofloxacin (prophylaxis for close contacts); penicillin G or ceftriaxone

APPENDIX II: **Bug Index**

Organism	Morphology	Pathogenesis	Disease	Identification	Transmission	Treatment
Nocardia asteroides	Acid-fast; gram-positive branching bacillus; aerobic	Lysosome-phagosome fusion inhibited; immunocompromised individuals at risk	Nocardiosis—lung, heart, kidney, and brain abscesses	Forms filaments	Airborne particles from soil; noncommunicable	Sulfonamides
Pasteurella multocida	Gram-negative; coccobacillus;		Diffuse cellulitis, chronic abscess	Nonhemolytic mucoid colonies on blood agar	Bite/scratch of a dog or cat	
Proteus vulgaris and *mirabilis*	Gram-negative; bacillus	Pili (adherence to renal pelvis); urease (alkalinization urine, increased precipitation, resulting in increased stone formation)	UTI	Urease positive; swarming motility colonies	GU flora	Ciprofloxacin, trimethoprim-sulfamethoxazole (TMP–SMX)
Pseudomonas aeruginosa	Gram-negative; coccobacilli	Pili; A/B toxin similar to diphtheria; flagella; hemolysin	UTI; septicemia; burn infections	Fruity smell; blue-green pigment	Water; environment; opportunistic: patients with catheters, leukemia, burns, cystic fibrosis, ventilatory assistance, neutropenia, chronic lung disease	May express broad resistance to antibiotics
Rickettsia prowazekii	Obligate intracellular	Invasion of the endothelial lining; possible endotoxin	Epidemic typhus		Louse	Tetracycline
Rickettsia rickettsii	Obligate intracellular	Invasion of endothelial lining	Rocky Mountain spotted fever: vasculitis, rash spreads from periphery inward	Weil-Felix reaction (agglutination when patient's serum mixed with OX strain of *Proteus vulgaris*)	*Dermacentor* ticks	Tetracycline
Rickettsia typhi	Obligate intracellular	Invasion of endothelial lining; possible endotoxin	Endemic typhus—rash spreads from the trunk outward		Spread by fleas	Tetracycline
Salmonella spp.	Gram-negative; rod; multiple flagella	Invades mucosa of GI tract; penetration of layers and systemic infection (typhoid fever); flagellar proteins; endotoxin	Typhoid fever, gastroenteritis, sepsis	Lactose-negative; polysaccharide, somatic O antigens and protein flagellar H antigens; (usually poultry) encapsulated; Widal test	Fecal–oral; contaminated food	Fluoroquinolone, ceftriaxone, azithromycin
Shigella spp.	Gram-negative; rod; nonmotile; not spore former	Invades mucosal M cells; presented to macrophage, which increase TNF and IL-1; produces microabscesses and ulcers; begins in small intestine and invades lower colon; Shiga toxin (A/B toxin); works on 28S ribosome and removes the base; low infective dose; invasion into blood is rare	Bacterial dysentery (shigellosis): ulcerative colitis of large intestine, fever, chills, cramps, tenesmus, bloody stool	Rectal swab; three types: *dysenteriae* (rare, most severe), *sonnei* (most common, day care), *flexneri* (gay men)	Fecal–oral route	Public health measures; significant resistance; fluoroquinolone, ceftriaxone, azithromycin

(continued)

BACTERIA (Continued)

Name	Morphology	Pathogenesis	Description of Disease	Laboratory Findings, Notes	Transmission	Prevention and Therapy
Staphylococcus aureus	Gram-positive; cocci; capsule; protein A in the cell wall; yellow, creamy, grapelike clusters on culture	Rapid growth; protein A (antiphagocytic); enterotoxin (watery diarrhea); toxic shock syndrome toxin; exfoliation; α-toxin; coagulase	Abscesses; pyogenic infections (endocarditis, osteomyelitis); food poisoning; toxic shock syndrome; scalded skin syndrome	Coagulase positive; catalase positive; β-hemolytic; novobiocin sensitive; ferment mannitol	Via the hands from the skin, nasal mucosa; enterotoxin: ham, chicken salad, cottage cheese, processed food	Hand washing; 80% penicillin resistant (make β-lactamase); vancomycin; first-generation cephalosporin; nafcillin, oxacillin
Staphylococcus epidermidis	Gram-positive; cocci; white, creamy, grapelike clusters on culture	Surface glycocalyx	Endocarditis; infection on catheters and implant sites; sepsis in neonates	Coagulase negative; catalase positive; no hemolysis; novobiocin sensitive	On skin; IV drug users	Vancomycin
Staphylococcus saprophyticus	Gram-positive; cocci; creamy, grapelike clusters	Selectively adheres to transitional epithelium	UTI in young women	Coagulase negative; catalase positive; no hemolysis; novobiocin resistant	Many sexual partners	Quinolones, oral cephalosporin
Streptococcus agalactiae	Gram-positive; cocci; diploid; group B *Streptococcus*	Capsular antigen (contains sialic acid blocks opsonization)	Number 1 cause of neonatal sepsis and meningitis	Catalase negative; bacitracin resistant; β-hemolysis; Lancefield group B; hippurate hydrolysis positive	Genital tract of some women	Ampicillin before delivery; penicillin G
Streptococcus pneumoniae	Gram-positive; cocci; lancet shaped; in pairs; polysaccharide capsule (85 different types)	Capsule prevents phagocytosis; IgA protease; adheres to mucosa	Pneumonia; meningitis; bacteremia; upper respiratory infection; otitis media	Catalase negative; α-hemolysis bile soluble; inhibited by optochin; quellung reaction (capsular swelling)	Inhalation of aerosols, which leads to colonization of oropharynx	Polysaccharide capsular vaccine available for high-risk groups; penicillin and erythromycin
Streptococcus pyogenes	Gram-positive; cocci; chains or pairs; rough or smooth hyaluronic acid capsule	M protein (pili); streptokinase (dissolves fibrin); DNase; hyaluronidase; hemolysins: erythrogenic toxin (scarlet fever rash); streptolysin-O and streptolysin-S; exotoxin A (superantigen causing TSS-like syndrome)	Pharyngitis; cellulitis; rheumatic fever; acute glomerulonephritis; TSS-like syndrome	Catalase negative; bacitracin (A disk) sensitive; (β-hemolytic; antistreptolysin-O for serotyping; Lancefield group A; rapid antigen detection test	May colonize skin, throat	Penicillin G (increasing resistance to erythromycin)

Organism						
Treponema pallidum	Spirochete	Multiplication followed by blood vessel involvement	Syphilis—primary with painless sores, purulent exudate, and induration; secondary with a rash; tertiary (rare) includes CNS involvement and aortitis	Dark field microscopy; screen with RPR or VDRL test for cardiolipin (nontreponemal tests); confirm with FTA-abs or MHA-tp (treponemal specific test); systemic illness can occur with treatment (Jarisch–Herxheimer reaction)	Sexually transmitted; transplacental	Penicillin
Tropheryma whipplei	Gram-positive; rod actinomycete	Foamy macrophages found in the lamina propria of the jejunum	Whipple disease—steatorrhea, lymphadenopathy, fever, and cough	Visualization of the organism in a biopsy of the small bowel	Unknown	Trimethoprim-sulfamethoxazole
Vibrio cholerae	Gram-negative; comma-shaped rod; polar flagella ADP ribosylates G protein	Pili adhere to gut mucosa; phage-coded cholera toxin: two A active subunits and five B-binding units (A subunit increasing cAMP and causing movement of ions and water out of the cell)	Rice water stools	Fecal specimens culture; agglutination assays	Fecal–oral route via water and food	Vaccine not available in the United States; rehydration; tetracycline, fluoroquinolones, trimethoprim-sulfamethoxazole
Vibrio parahaemolyticus	Gram-negative; comma-shaped rod	Toxin	Explosive diarrhea, cramps, nausea	High-infective dose required	Shellfish; raw or undercooked seafood	Self-limited
Yersinia pestis	Gram-negative; bacillus; intracellular	V and W antigens (active within macrophages); fibrinolysin; F1 protein inhibits phagocytosis	Bubonic plague (with lymph node swelling and bubol); fever; conjunctivitis	Cultures are hazardous and precautions must be taken	Zoonotic via rat fleas	Vaccine; gentamicin, doxycycline

ADP, adenosine diphosphate; BCG, bacille Calmette–Guérin; cAMP, cyclic adenosine monophosphate; CNS, central nervous system; CSF, cerebrospinal fluid; DNase, deoxyribonuclease; ELISA, enzyme-linked immunosorbent assay; FTA-abs, fluorescent treponemal antibody absorption test; GI, gastrointestinal; GU, genitourinary; Hib, *Haemophilus influenzae* type b; Ig, immunoglobulin; IL, interleukin; IV, intravenous; LPS, lipopolysaccharide; MHA-tp, microhemagglutination assay test; MP, metalloproteinase; NaCl, sodium chloride; NAD, nicotinamide adenine dinucleotide; PPD, purified protein derivative; RPR, rapid plasma reagin; TB, tuberculosis; TNF, tumor necrosis factor; TSS, toxic shock syndrome; UTI, urinary tract infection; VDRL, Venereal Disease Research Laboratory.

VIRUSES

Name	Morphology	Description of Disease	Pathogenesis	Laboratory Findings, Notes	Transmission	Prevention and Therapy
Adenovirus	Nonenveloped DNA virus; double stranded	Pharyngitis or pneumonia; acute gastroenteritis; conjunctivitis	Infects the epithelium of the eyes, respiratory tract, and GI tract	Complement fixation	Respiratory droplets; hand-to-eye; also fecal–oral	Live vaccine for military populations; no treatments
Coronavirus	Enveloped single-stranded positive RNA virus	Common cold	Infects upper respiratory tract	None	Respiratory secretions	None
Coxsackie B virus	Nonenveloped RNA virus; single stranded; linear; positive polarity	Myocarditis, pericarditis, spastic paralysis	Replicates in the pharynx and GI tract and spreads to other tissues	Isolating virus in cell culture; rise in convalescent antibody	Fecal–oral and respiratory	No therapy or prevention
Cytomegalovirus	Enveloped DNA virus; linear; double stranded	Pneumonia, retinitis, and hepatitis in immuno-compromised patients; mononucleosis-like syndrome in immunocompromised patients; cytomegalic inclusion disease of fetus	Infects the oropharynx initially; involves lymphocytes	"Owl's eye" nuclear inclusions	Human body fluids; transplacental, organ transplantation	Ganciclovir
Ebola virus	Enveloped RNA virus; single stranded; linear; negative polarity	African hemorrhagic fever—often rapidly fatal	Viral replication in all organs leads to necrosis	Virus isolation; rise in antibody titer	Contact with blood and body secretions	None
Epstein–Barr virus	Enveloped DNA virus; linear; double stranded	Infectious mononucleosis; causes Burkitt lymphoma	Spreads via the lymph nodes and bloodstream to the liver and spleen from the pharyngeal epithelium	Atypical lymphocytes; positive heterophil antibody (Monospot test); common infection of college students	Saliva	None
Hantavirus	Enveloped RNA virus; single stranded; circular, segmented; negative polarity	Hanta pulmonary syndrome—influenza-like followed by acute respiratory failure	Invasion of the respiratory epithelium	PCR assay of viral RNA from lung tissue	Airborne (inhalation of rodent urine and feces); found in southwestern United States	None
Hepatitis A virus	Nonenveloped RNA virus; single stranded; positive polarity	Hepatitis A; causes acute hepatitis; no chronic infection	Replicates in the GI tract; spreads to the liver; hepatocellular injury via cytotoxic T-cell response	Detect IgM antibody	Fecal–oral route	Killed viral vaccine; immune globulin during the incubation period may hinder disease

Virus	Characteristics	Disease	Pathogenesis	Diagnosis	Transmission	Treatment/Prevention
Hepatitis B virus (HBV)	Enveloped DNA virus; incomplete circular double stranded; polymerase in virion (virion called the Dane particle); surface antigen (HBsAg); core antigen (HBcAg)	Hepatitis B; arthritis; rash; glomerulonephritis; may result in hepatocellular carcinoma	Immune response (CD8 cells) to the virus results in hepatocellular injury; Ag–Ab complexes form	Serologic tests for HBsAg, HBsAb, HBcAb, and HBeAb	Blood, perinatal, sexual	Vaccine; interferon-α; tenofovir, lamivudine inhibit HBV DNA synthesis
Hepatitis C virus (HCV)	Enveloped RNA virus; single stranded; positive polarity	Hepatitis C; possible predisposition to hepatocellular carcinoma	Cytotoxic T cells result in hepatocellular injury	HCV RNA or anti-HCV Ab; currently the most common cause of transfusion-related hepatitis	Blood, perinatal, sexual	Interferon-α; ribavirin
Hepatitis D virus (delta virus)	Enveloped defective RNA virus; single stranded; negative polarity; no polymerase	Hepatitis D	Cytotoxic T cells result in hepatocellular injury; uses HBsAg as a protein coat and can only replicate in hosts already infected with HBV	Serologic testing for delta antigen	Blood, perinatal, sexual	Interferon-α; prevention of hepatitis B
Hepatitis E virus (HEV)	Enveloped; single-stranded RNA virus; positive polarity	Hepatitis E; acute hepatitis no chronic disease		Anti-HEV IgM antibody by ELISA	Fecal–oral route	
Herpes simplex virus type 1	Enveloped DNA virus; linear; double stranded	Herpes labialis (fever blisters and cold sores); keratitis; encephalitis	Lesions on the mouth and face initially; travels retrograde and becomes latent in the trigeminal ganglion; recurrences induced by sunlight, stress, and fever	Multinucleated giant cells on Tzanck smear; immunofluorescence of infected cells; in situ hybridization defects; viral DNA	Saliva; direct contact with the lesion	Acyclovir, trifluorothymidine for keratitis
Herpes simplex virus type 2	Enveloped DNA virus; linear; double stranded	Herpes genitalis; meningitis	Vesicular lesions on the genitalia; retrograde passage through the axon and latency in the sacral ganglion; stress-induced recurrences	Multinucleated giant cells on Tzanck smear; immunofluorescence of infected cells; in situ hybridization defects; viral DNA	Sexual, transplacental	Acyclovir
Human herpes virus 6	Enveloped DNA virus; linear; double stranded	Roseola infantum (exanthem subitum)—common disease of children characterized by high fever and rash	Infects T and B cells	PCR or acute and convalescent antibody titers	Saliva	Symptomatic

(continued)

APPENDIX II: Bug Index

Name	Morphology	Description of Disease	Pathogenesis	Laboratory Findings, Notes	Transmission	Prevention and Therapy
HIV	Enveloped RNA virus; diploid; single stranded; positive polarity; reverse transcriptase, retrovirus	AIDS	Infects and kills helper T cells via the CD4 receptors and gp120 protein	Screen with ELISA; Western blot test confirms	Sexual, body fluids, perinatal; blood products	AZT to HIV-infected mothers and newborns; HAART; treat opportunistic infections such as pneumonia or Kaposi sarcoma
Influenza virus	Enveloped RNA virus; segmented; single stranded; negative polarity; polymerase in virion	Influenza	Infects the epithelium of the respiratory tract via hemagglutinin and neuraminidase on surface spikes; antigenic shift and drift of surface spikes lead to epidemics	Cell culture; hemagglutination inhibition; complement fixation; H and N protein spikes	Respiratory droplets; vaccine composed of inactivated strains of current virus, which causes disease	Zanamivir and oseltamivir for both prevention and treatment; vaccine composed of inactivated strains of current virus, which causes disease
Measles virus	Enveloped RNA virus; single stranded; negative polarity; polymerase in virion	Measles, subacute sclerosing panencephalitis (SSPE)	Infection spreads via the bloodstream from the upper respiratory tract to the organs; maculopapular rash caused by an immune response (Koplik spots)	Usually not done	Respiratory droplets	Attenuated vaccine; no treatment
Mumps virus	Enveloped RNA virus; single stranded; negative polarity; polymerase in virion	Mumps; sterility owing to bilateral orchitis	Spreads from the upper respiratory tract to the organs (parotid glands, testes, ovaries, and CNS) via the bloodstream	Cell culture and hemadsorption; rise in antiviral antibody	Respiratory droplets	Attenuated vaccine; no treatment
Norwalk virus	Nonenveloped; RNA virus; single stranded; linear; positive polarity	Gastroenteritis	Binds to cells of intestinal brush border; prevents absorption of water and nutrients; blunted villi in jejunum; infiltration with mononuclear cells	Not performed; serology; ELISA for Ag; stool EM	Fecal–oral	Symptomatic treatment
Papillomavirus	Nonenveloped DNA virus; circular; double stranded	Papillomas (warts); condylomata acuminata; cervical and penile carcinoma	dsDNA incorporates into host DNA; E1 and E2 promote DNA replication; E6 and E7 early viral genes inhibit activity of p53 and Rb tumor suppressor genes, respectively	Koilocytes (squamous cell with perinuclear clearing) in lesions; to define type use in situ DNA hybridization	Sexual via direct contact with genital lesions	Interferon-α; liquid nitrogen for warts; vaccine; annual Pap smear for cervical cancer screening

	Characteristics	Disease	Mechanism	Diagnosis	Transmission	Treatment
Parainfluenza	Enveloped; single stranded–RNA virus	Upper respiratory tract infection, croup (laryngotracheobronchitis), bronchiolitis, pneumonia	Two major surface glycoproteins fusion and HN; replication limited to respiratory epithelial cells		Direct person-to-person contact and large droplet aerosols	Supportive
Parvovirus B19	Nonenveloped; DNA virus; single stranded; linear	Erythema infectiosum (fifth disease)—characterized by "slapped cheek" appearance; may cause aplastic crisis in sickle cell disease	Erythema infectiosum—virus causes immune complex deposition; aplastic anemia: virus infects immature RBCs and kills them	Parvovirus-specific IgG/IgM antibody levels; laboratory analysis for viral DNA	Unknown—may be respiratory or direct contact	Self-limited
Poliovirus	Nonenveloped RNA virus; single stranded; positive polarity	Abortive poliomyelitis, aseptic meningitis (more common), paralytic poliomyelitis, progressive postpoliomyelitis muscle atrophy (very rare)	Replicates in the pharynx and GI tract and spreads to the CNS; death of the anterior horn cells in the spinal cord; neurotropic for motor cortex	Isolation from CSF	Fecal–oral	Salk vaccine: inactivated injection; Sabin vaccine: attenuated oral vaccine, given in childhood immunizations; no treatment; **MNEMONIC:** Saber tooth tiger is alive and eats (Sabin vaccine is live oral vaccine)
Rabies virus	Enveloped RNA virus; bullet shape; single stranded; negative polarity RNA; polymerase in virion	Rabies	ACh receptor of neuron binds virus; the virus follows the retrograde direction to invade the CNS and brain, resulting in encephalitis	Negri bodies (eosinophilic inclusion in nerve cell)	Animal (skunks, bats) bites; domestic dogs in developing countries	Before exposure: vaccine; after exposure: antirabies Ig plus inactivated vaccine from human cell culture; no treatment
Reovirus (*Rotavirus*)	Nonenveloped RNA virus; 11 segments; double stranded; RNA polymerase in virion	Gastroenteritis in children	Resistant to stomach acid, thus infects the small intestine	ELISA detects the virus in stool	Respiratory droplets; fecal–oral route	Rehydration with fluids and electrolytes
Respiratory syncytial virus	Enveloped RNA virus; single stranded; negative polarity; polymerase in virion	Pneumonia or bronchiolitis in children	Immune response to lower respiratory tract infection	Multinucleated giant cells	Direct person-to-person contact	Supportive; ribavirin no longer recommended for children
Rhinovirus	Nonenveloped RNA virus; single stranded; positive polarity; numerous serotypes	Common cold	Upper respiratory tract mucosa and conjunctiva infected; replicates at temperatures <37°C; killed by stomach acid	None	Aerosol droplets with hand-to-nose transmission	None

(continued)

VIRUSES *(Continued)*

Name	Morphology	Description of Disease	Pathogenesis	Laboratory Findings, Notes	Transmission	Prevention and Therapy
Rubella virus	Enveloped RNA virus; single stranded; positive polarity	Rubella; congenital: cardiovascular and neurologic malformations, especially if infection occurs during the first trimester	Spreads from the nasopharynx to the skin via the bloodstream; rash caused by replication and immune injury; German measles	Growth in cell culture via interference of Coxsackie virus; recent infection in the mother is detected by IgM, IgA	Respiratory droplets	Attenuated vaccine; no treatment
Varicella-zoster virus	Enveloped DNA virus; linear; double stranded	Chicken pox (varicella) in children; shingles (zoster) in adults	Infects respiratory tract and spreads to the liver and skin via the blood; an acute episode followed by latency in the sensory ganglia; numerous crop of vesicles in different stages at different times	Intranuclear inclusions; shingles is usually unilateral and generally follows the distribution of the dermatomes	Chicken pox: respiratory droplets; shingles: reactivation of the latent virus	Attenuated vaccine; famciclovir, valacyclovir
Variola virus	Double stranded; DNA	Smallpox (rare)	Respiratory infection; initially replicates in URT; systemic dissemination by lymphatics; replication in multiple organs; extensive rash to hemorrhage of small blood vessels; single crop of vesicles in one stage all at once			Vaccinia variola

ACh, acetylcholine; Ag–Ab, antigen–antibody; AZT, azidothymidine; CD, cluster of differentiation; CNS, central nervous system; CSF, cerebrospinal fluid; dsDNA, double-stranded DNA; ELISA, enzyme-linked immunosorbent assay; EM, electron microscopy; GI, gastrointestinal; HAART, highly active antiretroviral therapy; HBcAb, hepatitis B core antibody; HBeAb, hepatitis B e antibody; HBsAb, hepatitis B surface antibody; HN, hemagglutinin-neuraminidase; Ig, immunoglobulin; PCR, polymerase chain reaction; Rb, retinoblastoma; RBC, red blood cell; URT, upper respiratory tract.

FUNGI

Name	Morphology	Pathogenesis	Description of Disease	Laboratory Findings, Notes	Transmission	Prevention and Therapy
Aspergillus fumigatus	Filamentous; septate hyphae and dichotomous branching; mold only	Opportunistic; growth of *Aspergillus* in a pre-existing cavitary lesion in the lung	Aspergilloma—hemoptysis; invasive aspergillosis in neutropenic individuals	Septate, branching hyphae; "fungus ball" seen on a radiograph	Airborne spores	Amphotericin B, voriconazole; surgery to remove a "fungus ball"
Blastomyces dermatitidis	Dimorphic fungus—mold in the soil but a yeast in tissue	Invades the respiratory tract and may invade the skin or bone	Blastomycosis—granulomatous and suppurative infection of the respiratory tract	Tissue biopsy showing circular yeast with a broad-based bud	Airborne; endemic to North America	Itraconazole; amphotericin B for serious infections
Candida albicans	Pseudohyphae and hyphae on invasion; yeast in normal flora; germ tubes at 37° C; yeast only	Opportunistic in immunosuppressed patients and those with foreign bodies (e.g., catheters); mucocutaneous lesions in children with a T-cell defect	Thrush, chronic mucocutaneous candidiasis, vaginal candidiasis	Colonies on Sabouraud agar; germ tube formation	Part of the normal flora	Oral form can be prevented by nystatin "swish and swallow"; treatment with nystatin; miconazole; amphotericin B; IV amphotericin B, fluconazole, or caspofungin for bloodborne infection
Coccidioides immitis	Dimorphic—mold in the soil, spherule in tissue; barrel-shaped hyphae	Inhalation, spherules, releasing endospores within the respiratory tract	Coccidioidomycosis—an influenza-like illness with fever and cough	Tissue specimen showing spherules	Airborne; endemic to southwestern United States and Latin America	Amphotericin B, itraconazole, ketoconazole
Cryptococcus neoformans	Encapsulated; not dimorphic; yeast only	Usually immunocompromised patients; spreads via the bloodstream	Cryptococcosis, cryptococcal meningitis	Organism with a capsule seen on an India ink preparation; latex agglutination test	Inhalation of airborne yeast cells	Oral fluconazole as preventative in patients with AIDS; amphotericin B with flucytosine as initial therapy for cryptococcal meningitis
Histoplasma capsulatum	Dimorphic—a mold in the soil, a yeast in tissue; septate hyphae	Inhaled spores are engulfed by macrophages and develop into yeast forms intracellularly	Histoplasmosis—granulomas in the lung tissue	Tissue biopsy showing yeast cells visible in macrophages; radioimmunoassay for *Histoplasma* RNA and DNA	Airborne; endemic to Ohio and Mississippi River valleys; found in bird droppings	Amphotericin B, itraconazole
Mucor spp.	Nonseptate hyphae that branch at near right angles; mold only	Invades the nasal sinuses, lungs, and GI tract	Tissue necrosis	Nonseptate hyphae seen microscopically	Airborne	Amphotericin B; debridement of necrotic tissue
Pneumocystis jirovecii	Respiratory pathogen	Alveolar inflammation	Pneumonia	Silver stain	Inhalation by immunocompromised individual	Trimethoprim-sulfamethoxazole; pentamidine
Sporothrix schenckii	Thermally dimorphic fungus	Inflammation and swelling of the lymph nodes and vessels	Sporotrichosis ("rose gardener's disease")	Cigar-shaped budding cells	Thorn prick	Protection during gardening; potassium iodide; itraconazole

GI, gastrointestinal; IV, intravenous.

APPENDIX II: Bug Index

PARASITES AND PROTOZOA

Name	Morphology	Pathogenesis	Description of Disease	Laboratory Findings, Notes	Transmission	Prevention and Therapy
Ascaris lumbricoides	Intestinal parasite	Larvae in the lung and a heavy worm burden in gastrointestinal tract	Ascariasis—intestinal obstruction, abdominal pain, coughing, nausea	Eosinophilia; eggs in feces	Contaminated food or soil	Maintain sanitary conditions; ivermectin or mebendazole
Entamoeba histolytica	Intestinal protozoan; cigar-shaped cysts; four nuclei	Trophozoite form invades the colon	Amebic dysentery, liver abscess, flask-shaped ulcers	Trophozoites or cysts seen in stool	Fecal–oral	Maintain sanitary conditions; metronidazole with iodoquinol or paromomycin; steroids exacerbate
Enterobius vermicularis	Intestinal parasite	Worms migrate to anus at night to lay eggs; results in perianal pruritus	Pinworm infection—anal pruritus, vaginal irritation, and cystitis	Eggs on "Scotch tape" test (tape applied to the anus and then viewed under a microscope)	Reinfection by self; fecal–oral contact; egg ingestion	Mebendazole
Giardia lamblia	Intestinal protozoan; pear shaped; flagella; tumbling motility; two nuclei; four flagella	Interfere with fat and protein absorption	Giardiasis—acute diarrhea, flatulence, bloating	Trophozoites or cysts in stool	Fecal–oral	Do not drink untreated water from streams or rivers; metronidazole
Leishmania donovani	Protozoan	Organs of the reticuloendothelial system are destroyed by macrophages infected with the protozoan	Cutaneous leishmaniasis—ulcerating papules that heal slowly; visceral leishmaniasis ("kala-azar")—hyperpigmentation of the skin, massive splenomegaly, fever, anemia, and malaise	Biopsy of reticuloendothelial tissue shows the infected macrophages	Female *Phlebotomus* sandfly transmits the disease from the infected host to a human	Protection from sandfly bites; sodium stibogluconate (antimony compound) for cutaneous form; liposomal amphotericin B for visceral form
Plasmodium spp.	Blood and tissue protozoan; signet ring trophozoites in RBCs; banana-shaped gametocytes (*Plasmodium falciparum*)	Sporozoites from bite enter the bloodstream and invade hepatocytes (exoerythrocytic phase); merozoites invade the RBCs (erythrocytic phase)	Malaria—fever, chills, hepatomegaly, splenomegaly; symptoms in cyclical pattern (3 days for *P. malariae*; 2 days for *P. ovale*, *P. falciparum*, *P. vivax*); tissue anoxia	Blood smear shows organisms; *P. falciparum* is acute and needs immediate treatment	Female *Anopheles* mosquito	Insecticides or protection from bites; chloroquine, quinine, atovaquone-proguanil, mefloquine, artemether/lumefantrine

470

Organism	Characteristics	Mechanism	Disease	Diagnosis	Transmission	Treatment/Prevention
Schistosoma spp.	Blood fluke; eggs have spine (*S. mansoni* has large lateral spine, *S. haematobium* has a terminal spine, *S. japonicum* has a small lateral spine); two sexes	Eggs lead to inflammation, fibrosis, and granuloma formation	Schistosomiasis—pipestem fibrosis of liver; *S. haematobium* affects the bladder; *S. mansoni* affects the mesenteric vessels	Eggs in the stool or urine	Penetration of the skin by cercariae	Maintain sanitary conditions; praziquantel
Taenia sp.	Cestode: *T. solium*—pork tapeworm; *T. saginata*—beef; *Diphyllobothrium latum*—fish; four suckers and circle of hooks; 5–10 uterine branches	Encyst in tissue (eyes, brain, muscle) resulting in mass lesions	Taeniasis and cysticercosis	Gravid proglottids in stool	Eating raw or undercooked meat (taeniasis), or fecal–oral (cysticercosis)	Cook meat and maintain sanitary conditions; albendazole or praziquantel
Toxoplasma gondii	Tissue protozoan	Infects macrophages; infects the brain, liver, eyes	Toxoplasmosis	Serologic; high morbidity and mortality	Ingestion of cysts; cat feces; transplacental	Cook meat and avoid cat feces; sulfadiazine positive, pyrimethamine
Trichinella spiralis	Intestinal parasite	Muscle inflammation	Trichinosis—periorbital edema, myositis, fever, and diarrhea	Larvae on muscle biopsy; eosinophilia by 14th day; double-barreled egg	Eating raw or undercooked meat	Cook meat; thiabendazole
Trichomonas vaginalis	Urogenital protozoan; pear shaped; flagella; trophozoites	Attaches to the wall of the vagina	Trichomoniasis—itching and burning with greenish discharge from the vagina (strawberry cervix)	Visible in secretions	Sexual transmission	Treat both partners; metronidazole
Trypanosoma brucei (African)	Blood and tissue protozoan	Infects the brain and leads to encephalitis	Sleeping sickness—fever, enlarged lymph nodes, somnolence, coma, death	Visible in the blood	Tsetse fly (in Africa)	Protection from bites; insecticide; suramin
Trypanosoma cruzi (American)	Blood and tissue protozoan	Amastigotes attack cells, especially cardiac muscle cells	Chagas disease—dilated cardiomyopathy, megaesophagus, megacolon	Visible in the blood	Reduviid bugs (in Latin America) (also known as "kissing bugs")	Protect from bites; insecticide; nifurtimox

RBC, red blood cell.

471

Index

NOTE: Page numbers followed by *f* indicate figures; *t* indicates tables.